SIXTH EDITION

Beauty Therapy

THE FOUNDATIONS

The official guide to beauty therapy at level 2 VRQ

LORRAINE NORDMANN & MARIAN NEWMAN

CENGAGE
Learning®

Australia • Brazil • Japan • Korea • Mexico • Singapore • Spain • United Kingdom • United States

HABIA SERIES LIST

Hairdressing

Student textbooks

Begin Hairdressing: The Official Guide to Level 1 REVISED 2e *Martin Green*

Hairdressing – The Foundations: The Official Guide to Level 2 7e *Leo Palladino and Martin Green*

Professional Hairdressing: The Official Guide to Level 3 REVISED 6e *Martin Green and Leo Palladino*

The Pocket Guide to Key Terms for Hairdressing *Martin Green*

The Official Guide to the City & Guilds Certificate in Salon Service 1e *John Armstrong with Anita Crosland, Martin Green and Lorraine Nordmann*

The Colour Book: The Official Guide to Colour for NVQ Levels 2 & 3 1e *Tracey Lloyd with Christine McMillan-Bodell*

eXtensions: The Official Guide to Hair Extensions 1e *Theresa Bullock*

Salon Management *Martin Green*

Men's Hairdressing: Traditional and Modern Barbering 2e *Maurice Lister*

African-Caribbean Hairdressing 2e *Sandra Gittens*

The World of Hair Colour 1e *John Gray*

The Cutting Book: The Official Guide to Cutting at S/NVQ Levels 2 and 3 *Jane Goldsbro and Elaine White*

Professional Hairdressing titles

Trevor Sorbie: The Bridal Hair Book 1e *Trevor Sorbie and Jacki Wadeson*

The Art of Dressing Long Hair 1e *Guy Kremer and Jacki Wadeson*

Patrick Cameron: Dressing Long Hair 1e *Patrick Cameron and Jacki Wadeson*

Patrick Cameron: Dressing Long Hair 2 1e *Patrick Cameron and Jacki Wadeson*

Bridal Hair 1e *Pat Dixon and Jacki Wadeson*

Balmain Hair, *Hair Extensions: Additions and Integrations 1/e*

Professional Men's Hairdressing: The Art of Cutting and Styling 1e *Guy Kremer and Jacki Wadeson*

Essensuals, the Next Generation Toni and Guy: Step by Step 1e *Sacha Mascolo, Christian Mascolo and Stuart Wesson*

Mahogany Hairdressing: Step to Cutting, Colouring and Finishing Hair 1e *Martin Gannon and Richard Thompson*

Mahogany Hairdressing: Advanced Looks 1e *Martin Gannon and Richard Thompson*

The Total Look: The Style Guide for Hair and Make-up Professional 1e *Ian Mistlin*

Trevor Sorbie: Visions in Hair 1e *Trevor Sorbie, Kris Sorbie and Jacki Wadeson*

The Art of Hair Colouring 1e *David Adams and Jacki Wadeson*

Beauty therapy

Beauty Basics: The Official Guide to Level 1 3e *Lorraine Nordmann*

Beauty Therapy – The Foundations: The Official Guide to Level 2 VRQ 5e *Lorraine Nordmann*

Beauty Therapy – The Foundations: The Official Guide to Level 2 5e *Lorraine Nordmann*

Professional Beauty Therapy – The Official Guide to Level 3 4e *Lorraine Nordmann*

The Pocket Guide to Key Terms for Beauty Therapy *Lorraine Nordmann and Marian Newman*

The Official Guide to the City & Guilds Certificate in Salon Services 1e *John Armstrong with Anita Crosland, Martin Green and Lorraine Nordmann*

The Complete Guide to Make-Up 1e *Suzanne Le Quesne*

The Encyclopedia of Nails 1e *Jacqui Jefford and Anne Swain*

The Art of Nails: A Comprehensive Style Guide to Nail Treatments and Nail Art 1e *Jacqui Jefford*

Nail Artistry 1e *Jacqui Jefford*

The Complete Nail Technician 3e *Marian Newman*

Manicure, Pedicure and Advanced Nail Techniques 1e *Elaine Almond*

The Official Guide to Body Massage 2e *Adele O'Keefe*

An Holistic Guide to Massage 1e *Tina Parsons*

Indian Head Massage 2e *Muriel Burnham-Airey and Adele O'Keefe*

Aromatherapy for the Beauty Therapist 1e *Valerie Worwood*

An Holistic Guide to Reflexology 1e *Tina Parsons*

An Holistic Guide to Anatomy and Physiology 1e *Tina Parsons*

The Essential Guide to Holistic and Complementary Therapy 1e *Helen Beckmann and Suzanne Le Quesne*

The Spa Book 1e *Jane Crebbin-Bailey, Dr John Harcup, and John Harrington*

SPA: The Official Guide to Spa Therapy at Levels 2 and 3, *Joan Scott and Andrea Harrison*

Nutrition: A Practical Approach 1e *Suzanne Le Quesne*

Hands on Sports Therapy 1e *Keith Ward*

Encyclopedia of Hair Removal: A Complete Reference to Methods, Techniques and Career Opportunities, *Gill Morris and Janice Brown*

The Anatomy and Physiology Workbook: For Beauty and Holistic Therapies Levels 1–3. *Tina Parsons*

The Anatomy and Physiology CD-Rom

Beautiful Selling: The Complete Guide to Sales Success in the Salon *Rath Langley*

The Official Guide to the Diploma in Hair and Beauty Studies at Foundation Level 1e *Jane Goldsbro and Elaine White*

The Official Guide to the Diploma in Hair and Beauty Studies at Higher Level 1e *Jane Goldsbro and Elaine White*

The Official Guide to Foundation Learning in Hair and Beauty 1e *Jane Goldsbro and Elaine White*

**Beauty Therapy The Foundations –
The Official Guide to Level 2 VRQ, 6th Edition**
Lorraine Nordmann and Marian Newman

Development Editor: Lauren Darby

Senior Production Editor: Alison Burt

Senior Manufacturing Buyer: Eyvett Davis

Typesetter: MPS Limited

Cover design: HCT Creative

Text design: Design Deluxe

For product information and technology assistance,
contact **emea.info@cengage.com.**
For permission to use material from this text or product,
and for permission queries,
email **emea.permissions@cengage.com.**

British Library Cataloguing-in-Publication Data
A catalogue record for this book is available from the British Library.

ISBN: 978-1-4080-7113-7

Cengage Learning EMEA
Cheriton House, North Way, Andover, Hampshire SP10 5BE,
United Kingdom

Cengage Learning products are represented in Canada by Nelson Education Ltd.

For your lifelong learning solutions, visit **www.cengage.co.uk**

Purchase your next print book, e-book or e-chapter at
www.Cengagebrain.com

Printed in Malta by Melita Press
1 2 3 4 5 6 7 8 9 10 – 16 15 14

Contents

Foreword

Beauty Therapy, The Foundations, The Official Guide to Level 2 VRQ, Sixth Edition

N othing stands still; time has the effect of showing your age, not necessarily in a positive way. One beneficial aspect of the beauty industry is that advances in products and techniques with well trained beauty therapists mean that, as an industry, we can offer clients a service that not only provides them with positive results but has a cascading effect on their family, friends and ultimately the general public.

So it's no surprise that the number one beauty author, Lorraine Nordmann, takes all of this in her stride and produces a superb book that reflects industry expectations, best practice and a strong focus on client care and professional attitudes.

Lorraine is never one for holding back, and her sense of understanding the complexity of the industry shows by the way she has the ability to write in an engaging style; keeping the content simple yet making you feel that her considerable knowledge and experience are at your fingertips and you're fired up ready to go. Lorraine has excelled herself again, making sure that this edition will be well read and will leave a lasting impression on what the industry requirements are.

As Director of Standards and Qualifications for Habia, I'm delighted that Lorraine reflects the standards and ethos of Habia.

Jane Goldsbro
Director of Standards & Qualifications
Habia

About our partners

Habia, the Hair and Beauty Industry Authority is appointed by government to represent employers in the Hair and Beauty Sector. Habia's main role is to manage the development of the National Occupational Standards (NOS) for hairdressing, barbering, beauty therapy, nails and spa. They are developed by industry for industry and represent best practice to achieving skills and knowledge for a particular job role. The NOS are used as the building blocks for the development of all qualifications that are developed by Awarding Organizations and by Cengage to develop textbooks and support products for learners.

Habia is also responsible for the development and implementation of Apprenticeship Frameworks and issuing the apprenticeship certificates. Alongside providing information to employers on government initiatives that may affect the hair and beauty industry be it educational, environmental or financial. A central point of contact for information, Habia provides guidance on careers, business development, legislation, salon health and safety.

Habia is part of SkillsActive, the Sector Skills Council that covers Hair & Beauty, Sports and the Active Leisure Sector.

VTCT is a government approved specialist awarding organisation responsible for qualifications in the beauty therapy, complementary therapy, hairdressing, sports, fitness, hospitality and catering sectors.

VTCT has been in existence for over 50 years, and in fact it was VTCT who originally coined the phrase *Beauty Therapy*. VTCT has remained at the forefront of developing the vocational system of qualifications in the UK and internationally.

VTCT invests in many charitable projects which support education and training in the beauty therapy industry. VTCT is the main sponsor and organiser of Worldskills UK (Beauty Therapy competitions) and VTCT also fund the development of the European and British Standard for Beauty Salon Services. In addition, VTCT donates charitable funds to disfigurement charities, prison education and other worthwhile causes linked to the beauty therapy sector.

VTCT has the widest and most diverse range of qualifications in the beauty industry and are leading on many new initiatives in education, including online assessment and registration, e-portfolio and e-resources.

VTCT develops innovative, fit for purpose qualifications via beauty therapy technical expert panels made up of employers, industry experts and educationalists from all over the UK.

About the book

Throughout this textbook you will find many colourful text boxes designed to aid your learning and understanding as well as highlight key points. Here are examples and descriptions of each:

HEALTH & SAFETY

Draws your attention to related health and safety information essential for each technical skill.

ACTIVITY

Feature within all chapters and provide additional tasks for you to further your understanding.

Directional arrows point you to other parts of the book that explore similar topics, in order for you to expand your learning.

CourseMate video boxes highlight some techniques which are available to view online.

TOP TIP

These share the author's experience and provide positive suggestions to improve knowledge and skills for each unit.

ANATOMY & PHYSIOLOGY BOX
Highlight essential anatomy and physiology knowledge needed for the unit.

Knowledge Check

These boxes are designed to check your knowledge of the subject being discussed on the page. These will often include information about the current laws surrounding a topic.

ALWAYS REMEMBER

Suggests good working practice and help you develop your skills and awareness during your training.

ASSESSMENT OF KNOWLEDGE AND UNDERSTANDING

Are provided at the end of all core chapters. You can use the questions to prepare for oral and written assessments and help test your own knowledge throughout. Seek guidance from your supervisor/assessor if there are areas you are unsure of.

INDUSTRY ROLE MODEL

LORRAINE NORDMANN, Author of Beauty Therapy Textbooks

" Feature throughout the book and are your insight into the exciting beauty industry. This profile is included at the start of the chapter and they provide subject specific tips that are both practical and inspiring.

" Role model quotes are included throughout a number of core chapters. Each quote provides valuable insight into the world of work, providing helpful and practical advice about work in such a varied and innovative industry.

Role Model Quotes

Products, tools and equipment

◆ Help you prepare for each practical treatment and show you the tools, materials and products required.

About the website

se Beauty Therapy Level 2 VRQ CourseMate alongside *Beauty Therapy The Foundations: The Official Guide to Level 2 VRQ 6th Edition* textbook for a complete blended learning solution!

This highly interactive resource brings course concepts to life and is designed to support lecturers and students through the range of online resources which can be perfectly integrated into the classroom to cover the guided learning hours for each unit.

For Students:

- Searchable eBook
- Step-by-step videos
- Interactive multiple choice quizzes
- Interactive activities and games

For Lecturers:

- Lessons plans
- PowerPoint slides
- Activity handouts
- 'Engagement Tracker' tools so students' progression and comprehension can be fully monitored

For more information please email emea.fesales@cengage.com

About the authors

I am proud to have worked in beauty therapy for the past 30 years and am amazed at the technological advances that have been made. The beauty therapy industry is never boring, offers immense job satisfaction, clear progression opportunities and is increasingly diverse allowing you to specialize in what have effectively become micro-industries within what was traditionally termed beauty therapy, i.e. nails, make-up, massage and spa. This allows you to excel in the area of the industry that you feel passionate about, which ultimately raises the profile of our industry. Industry role models feature in each chapter to share their experiences, offering practical advice throughout.

This VRQ Level 2 book aims to support you as you develop the capability and knowledge required when preparing to gain employment and work in the beauty therapy industry.

Enjoy your training and I wish you great success in the industry.

Lorraine Nordmann

I was delighted to be invited to contribute to the VRQ edition of Lorraine's book, *Beauty Therapy – The Foundations*. I feel very strongly about the standards of education and skills of nail technicians working in the professional industry.

Hopefully these nail chapters provide many answers but also encourage further research. For those interested in a career as a nail technician I recommend the third edition of my book *The Complete Nail Technician* as the next step.

Marian Newman

About the contributor

I joined the Beauty Industry in 1995 with excitement and enthusiasm. My aim was to become an educator so I set my plan into place and after 9 years as a therapist I began to teach the ITEC Diploma courses at a local college.

During this time, I was already providing an eyebrow threading service to my private clients and so in 2006, with an ever-growing demand for quality education and training in threading, I set up The National School of Threading and formulated the first BABTAC accredited threading course in UK.

Since then I have had the opportunity to work with many high profile companies, colleges, spas and beauty academies around the UK, Ireland and Europe. I have been providing not only training but advice, guidance and assistance with brand development, business start-ups and consultancy.

I was particularly proud to be asked to collaborate with The Guild, Boots No7 Brand, Nails Inc. and then Habia in the development of the standards for the NVQ in Threading which is now being taught in many colleges around the country.

I have been a role model for threading for many years and intend to remain so as I have great passion for education and strive to provide exceptional training to this wonderfully diverse industry.

I will continue to provide this service throughout UK and Europe whilst introducing my own branded product line and a new and exciting workshop... BrowRehab.

Lorraine Onorato

Acknowledgements

The author and publishers would like to thank the following:

For their help with the photoshoot and videoshoot:

Nathan Allan Photography, **nathanallanphotography.com**

Ken Franklin, Video4 Ltd. **www.video4.co.uk**

For their contribution as industry role models:

Samantha Sweet

Gill Morris

Tina Rooks

Danielle Norman

Shavata Singh

Charlotte Savoury

Marian Newman

Margaret Dabbs

Liza Smith

Nataliya

Janice Brown

Kathryn Darwin

Eleanor Wright

Nichola Joss

The author would personally like to thank:

Elizabeth and Norman Whiteside

Kathryn Leach

Shane Noden – personal trainer, The Personal Training People, Kenyons Lane South, Haydock, St Helens, Merseyside

Clare Kirkman

Christine Berry

Mike Turner – Photographer

Helen Eastwood

Chloe Eastwood

Gemma Hanlon

Vicky Kennedy – salon owner and beauty therapist, New Woman, New Man and Evolve, Westhoughton

Jacqueline Davi

xx

Credit list

© Beauty Express – 464 tl; © Marian Newman Nails – 502 br, 516 tm1, 516 tr1, 516 tm2, 516 tr2, 517 bl, 517 bm, 517 br; © Mundo Professional (www.mundoproducts.co.uk) – 466 tl, 468 tl, 470 ml1; © Nevit Dilman – 67 mr; Aqua Sana, Center Parcs – 172 tl; Australian Bodycare – 522 bl; Beauty Express – 213 tr, 213 mr, 213 br, 213 mr, 488 tl; Beauty Express Ltd – 414 ml1, 438 ml, 527 mr, 527 br, 536 ml1, 613 mr; Beauty Guild – 9tr4; Caflon – 561 bm1, 561 br; Cengage Learning EMEA – 581 tr; Claire Napoli for Cengage Learning – 67 mr; Collin UK – 8tr1; Courtesy Collin UK © Collin Paris – 145 bl; Courtesy of Aircare Europe – 463 br1, 463 br2; Courtesy of Grafton – 485 tr; Courtesy of Salon Iris www.saloniris.co.uk – 187 tl; Courtesy of Simon Jersey www .simonjersey.com – 113 tr; Dale Sauna Ltd, www.dalessauna.co.uk – 8r3, 13 mr; Depilex – 14 tr; Dermalogica – 137 bl, 159 mr, 167 tl, 223 mr, 224 ml, 231 tr, 237 mr, 252 tl; Dr A L Wright – 49 tr, 50 bl, 52 tl, 52 ml, 53 mr, 60 bl, 61 mr, 62 bl, 396 tl2, 397 tl2, 397 tl4, 397 tl5, 398 tl1, 398 tl3, 398 tl4, 399 tl1, 399 tl2, 440 tl2, 440 tl3, 441 tl1, 441 tl3; Dr John Gray, The World of Skincare – 41 tr, 60 tl, 60 ml, 61 ml, 61 mr, 138 bl, 208 tl, 217 mr, 399 mr; Dr M H Beck – 48 tl, 50 br, 51 mr, 54 ml, 54 ml, 55 br, 57 tr, 57 mr, 58 tl, 59 tr, 59 br, 61 mr, 62 ml, 63 tr, 395 tl2, 396 tl1, 396 tl4, 535 bl2; Ellisons – 9tr1, 18 mr, 118 tl, 118 tr, 119 br, 122 ml, 124 ml, 142 br, 143 tm, 148 bl, 213 bm, 225 mr, 236 br, 267 br, 268 tl, 272 bl, 276 tr, 318 bm, 390 ml, 412 tl, 412 ml, 415 mr, 432 bl, 433 br, 530 tl, 530 bl, 546 ml, 548 tl, 549 tr, 555 tr, 555 bl1, 555 bm1, 555 br1, 555 bl2, 555 bm2, 555 br2, 556 tl, 556 tr, 561 tr, 575 br, 586 tl; Gill Morris and Janice Brown/Cengage Learning – 524 tl2, 553 ml, 553 mc, 553 mr, 554 bl1, 554 br1, 554 bl2, 554 br2; Habia – 9 tr2, 9tr2, 391 tr, 524 tl1, 624 bl, 624 bm, 624 br, 625 tl, 625 tr; HSE – 62 tr, 111 bl, 473 tr; Hugh Rushton – 42 br; ISA – 9tr3; iStock – 15 tr (Lise Gagne), 17 br (James Tutor), 18 tr (Helene Vallee), 38 tl (Stephane Bidouze), 55 tr (Wolfgang Lienbacker), 98 bl (Jacob Wackerhausen), 179 br ((©Rich Legg), 208 bl (Milan M Jurkovic), 328 bl (©SZE FEI WONG), 423 tl; Jane Iredale/Iredale Mineral Make-up – 357 mr, 361 br; Jefford and Swain, The Encyclopedia of Nails – 119 tr; Jessica – 390 tl; Ken Franklin/Media Select International for Cengage Learning' – 266 mr, 268 mr, 309 br, 306 tl2, 312 tl, 312 tr, 426 tl1, 426 tl2, 426 tr2, 442 bl, 548 tm, 548 tr; Korres Natural Products, www.korres.com – 347 tl, 356 ml, 357 br, 361 br; Make-up and photo by Diana Estrada – 380 bm2; Make-up by Andrea Perry-Bevan, photo by Steve Collinson – 380 br2; Make-up by Angela Dicarlo – 380 bl1; Make-up by Bridget Taylor, photo by Rob Mcgrory – 380 bl2, 380 bm1; Make-up by Roque Cozzette – 380 br1; Marian Newman – 409 ml, 409 mb, 409 mr; Mavala – 384 tr, 423 mr, 423 bl; Mediscan – 50 ml, 53 mr, 55 mr, 56 ml, 93 mr, 394 bl1, 440 bl2, 441 tl2; Milady, a part of Cengage Learning, photography by Visual Recollection – 6 tm1, 150 bl, 156 tl, 157 tl, 157 br, 276 br, 275 mr, 283 tl, 308 tl1, 308 tm2, 308 tr3, 308 ml4, 308 m5, 308 mr6, 308 bl7, 308 bm8, 308 br9, 332 tl1, 332 tl2, 332 tl3, 332 tl4, 332 tl5, 332 tl6, 332 tl7, 332 tl8, 332 tl9, 332 tl10, 332 tl12, 333 ml, 333 bl, 333 br, 334 ml2, 344 ml2, 345 mr, 351 tl1, 351 tm1, 351 tm2, 351 tr1, 351 tl2, 351 tm3, 355 mr, 432 ml; Moom www .moom-uk.com – 525 tr, 528 tl; Mystic Tan – 608 bl; Nail Creations – 504 tm1, 512 tl1, 512 tl2, 512 tl3; Nail Delights – 504 tl3, 504 tm3, 513 tr1, 513 tr2; Nathan Portlock Allan Photography/Media Select International for Cengage Learning' – 12 br, 13 br, 14 mr,

1 Introduction

LEARNING OBJECTIVES

There are two learning outcomes to achieve for this unit:

1 Be able to describe the key characteristics of the beauty related industries

2 Be able to describe working practices in the beauty related industries.

Your assessment range applied requires you to:

◆ Understand different organizations, main treatments and occupational roles in the beauty industry.

◆ Be familiar with legislation, employment characteristics and **employment rights and responsibilities**.

◆ Be familiar with how to source information relating to educational developments, and employment progression opportunities and continual professional development related to the beauty industry

◆ Understand the importance of personal presentation and good working practices related to the range of treatments to be carried out

◆ Identify the different marketing and publicity methods which may be used to promote the products and treatments available in the workplace.

◆ Be familiar with the different financial procedures that may be used to purchase treatments and products and the workplace.

◆ Identify retail opportunities to promote products and treatments to a client which benefit both the client and organization.

KEY TERMS

camouflage

Habia

employment rights and responsibilities

equal opportunities

grievance

massage

nail polish

pedicure

Unit Topic

Working in beauty related industries

INTRODUCTION

A career in beauty therapy provides you with the opportunity to work across a range of diverse skill areas offering treatments to enhance the appearance of the facial skin, the nails, the eye area in fact every treatment offered should make the client feel more confident in their appearance with the final result of the treatment meeting their overall treatment requirements. To be successful there are practical skills to master and knowledge to learn which will be applied when carrying out any treatment or workplace service.

This chapter informs you about the requirements for working in the beauty related industries, helping you to learn about key features and working practices required.

You will learn about:

◆ different qualifications and training routes within the beauty therapy sector

◆ where to find out more information about working in the beauty related industry

◆ the different types of organisations offering employment in the industry

◆ the main beauty treatments offered in the beauty workplace

◆ the different legislation and workplace policies and your responsibilities in observing it in your day to day work role

◆ the marketing, publicity necessary to inform your clients about the products and treatments available

◆ how to handle different types of payments.

Introduction

This book covers the essential practical skills and knowledge necessary to become a beauty therapist qualified at Diploma Level 2, VRQ (Vocationally Related Qualification).

What is a VRQ?

The VRQ is a nationally recognized Vocationally Related Qualification. Where relevant units relate to the Beauty Therapy National Occupational Standards (NOS) this is identified throughout the book. The VRQ assesses the skills and abilities required for the beauty therapy workplace, in particular the knowledge and understanding requirements, preparing you for your career in beauty therapy. VRQs may take place in an imitation, although realistic, beauty therapy learning environment, complying with all relevant health and safety legislation requirements. This may include schools, colleges and the workplace. Practical assessment is recommended to be performed on a client but some awarding organizations allow the practical assessment to be carried out on colleagues, friends and family.

Habia (Hair and Beauty Therapy Industry Authority) is the industry lead body. The Habia website provides a list of the awarding organization qualifications that can be studied. See www.habia.org. A list of approved training centres can also be found on the website.

The VRQ helps you to develop the skills and knowledge required when preparing to gain employment and work in the beauty therapy industry. Assessment judgement is made upon your level of practical skills and knowledge. Commercial competence requirements are less important initially, as it is recognized that these will be achieved with experience in the workplace.

Units and learning outcomes

Your qualification is made up of a number of units. Each unit describes a specific activity or skill.

Each unit is divided into learning outcomes, which list the practical skills and knowledge which underpin it, and are required to carry out the activity or skill.

Each awarding organization will specify a structure (rules of combination) for their own Level 2 Beauty Therapy VRQ Diploma(s). There will be mandatory (compulsory) units which must be studied and achieved and there may be further optional units to select from. Refer to your awarding organization qualification handbook which will detail the units which are mandatory and optional for your qualification.

Beauty Therapy – The Foundations VRQ covers the following list of units which includes all the mandatory units across all the awarding organizations and the most popular optional units. Where anatomy and physiology knowledge is required in a unit, this is identified and signposted with the key to where it is covered in Chapter 2.

ANATOMY & PHYSIOLOGY

TOP TIP

Units carry a credit weighting and the optional units you can select from must achieve the required total credit figure for the qualification.

Qualification unit	Chapter
Working in beauty related industries	Chapter 1
Follow health and safety practice in the salon	Chapter 3
Promote products and services to clients in the salon	Chapter 4

Qualification unit	Chapter
Client care and communication in beauty related industries	Chapter 5
Salon reception duties	Chapter 6
Provide facial skincare	Chapter 7
Remove hair using waxing techniques	Chapter 15
Provide eyelash and brow treatments	Chapter 8
Provide manicure treatments	Chapter 11
Provide pedicure treatments	Chapter 12
Shaping and colouring eyebrows	Chapter 8
Provide eyelash perming	Chapter 8
Provide threading services for hair removal	Chapter 9
Apply make-up	Chapter 10
Create an image based on a theme	Chapter 10
Provide and maintain nail enhancements	Chapter 13
Provide nail art	Chapter 14
Provide ear piercing	Chapter 16
Provide head massage	Chapter 17
Apply skin tanning techniques	Chapter 18
Facial skin care for men	Online

Practical skills – what you can do

Practical skills are listed as practical activities or tasks to be carried out which will show your practical skills and capabilities to the assessor.

Range – what you must cover

Range statements are identified for each outcome. The range relates to what you must cover and the different conditions under which a skill or knowledge requirement of the unit must be demonstrated.

Where evidence has been achieved, this is cross-referenced (directed) in the portfolio (a place where you store your evidence) to where the evidence can be found.

To achieve each unit, all practical skills and knowledge requirements must have been met and evidence presented as necessary. Evidence is provided by completion of practical and written tasks or knowledge tests which are often completed electronically with an online test. Evidence is usually provided in your assessment book and portfolio and may be paper-based or electronic.

This edition of *Beauty Therapy – The Foundations* follows the Beauty Therapy VRQ Level 2 Diploma practical skills and knowledge requirements, for both the mandatory and optional units.

Professional beauty therapist/
make-up artist

When you qualify and receive your VRQ Level 2 Diploma certificate you may gain employment in the beauty therapy workplace and study further towards an NVQ, although this is not an essential requirement.

Each chapter introduction lists the unit learning objectives, outcomes, range and knowledge requirements.

Sources of information

You can access the following to supply you with further information about working in the beauty therapy related industries:

◆ the Internet

◆ professional beauty therapy journals

◆ Habia: **www.habia.org.uk**

◆ beauty training providers

◆ further education colleges

◆ qualification awarding bodies, i.e. City and Guilds (C&G); Vocational Training Charitable Trust (VTCT); International Therapy Examination Council (ITEC); Edexcel

◆ career guidance providers, e.g. Connexions

◆ professional beauty membership organizations.

Employment opportunities

Employment opportunities in the beauty therapy industry include:

◆ business owner

◆ freelance working for yourself

- manager or senior beauty therapist in a salon
- junior beauty therapist in a salon
- retailing (selling) cosmetics and skincare, referred to as a cosmetic consultant
- specializing in a particular beauty therapy skill such as facial skincare or waxing hair removal
- employment in a spa or leisure centre providing beauty therapy treatments.

The treatments you deliver and responsibilities you have when working in the beauty industry will be dependent upon your industry qualification and level of attainment.

> **TOP TIP**
>
> While training for your VRQ, completing work placements, either voluntary or paid, is vital to improve your confidence and help you gain a greater understanding of the requirements for working in the beauty related industries 'on the job'. This will enhance your CV, helping you to build an impressive work experience-related portfolio.

Level	Qualification description	Related practical skills and knowledge
Level 1	Introduction to beauty therapy industry developing understanding and preparation for employment in the beauty therapy industry	Health and safety and legal responsibilities. Different career and progression opportunities available. Theory and practical application of basic: - make-up - face painting techniques - nail art
Level 2	Develops a varied range of beauty therapy knowledge and skills applied requiring the use of initiative, decision-making skills and individual responsibility	Health and safety and legal responsibilities. Anatomy and physiology. Retail and promotional activities. Reception duties. Facial and make-up treatments. Eye treatment treatments. Hair removal techniques including waxing and threading. Nail treatments to both the hands and feet, including artificial nail application. Skin tanning techniques. Ear piercing
Level 3	Develops a broad knowledge of complex beauty therapy treatments and combines practical and theoretical study	Health and safety and legal responsibilities. Anatomy and physiology. Retail and promotional activities. Financial management. Application of facial and body electrotherapy treatments. **Massage** treatment to the different parts of the body using various techniques and massage mediums to achieve different effects. Hair removal using epilation technique. Specialist make-up techniques including **camouflage** make-up

The beauty related industries

Different types of organizations offering employment within the beauty related industries are listed on the following page.

Beauty organization	Description	
Manufacturer	These are different companies who make or supply the different tools, products and equipment that you work with	
Salon	Salons employ staff to deliver beauty therapy treatments to meet the needs of their clients. Some salons choose to specialize in particular areas of beauty therapy, for example, hair removal treatment. It is popular for hairdressing salons to offer a variety of beauty therapy treatments too, for example, make-up and nail treatments to provide a complete 'make-over' treatment package	
Health spa	Health spas provide facial and body health and well-being treatments in a relaxing environment. Specialist products and treatments achieve different therapeutic effects	
Hotel	Some hotels offer a range of beauty/spa based treatments onsite which may include facials, massages and body treatments	
Cruise liners	Cruise liners employ beauty therapists to provide many different types of beauty treatment and promotional activities to cruise liner passengers. Retail of both products and treatments is a key work target for the beauty therapist, so good selling skills are essential	

(Continued)

Beauty organization	Description	
Fitness and leisure providers	Some fitness and leisure centres offer a range of beauty treatments onsite to support the total achievement of health and well-being	
Professional membership organizations	As a professional beauty therapist, it is important that you adhere to a code of ethical (correct) practice and keep up-to-date in your skills and knowledge. You may wish to become a member of a professional organization or body, which will issue you with a copy of its agreed standards and provide industry updates through training opportunities and journals. Some membership organizations offer insurance benefits also	
Suppliers	Suppliers provide you with all the resources you need to carry out your treatments. These range from general consumables, such as cotton wool etc., to specialist suppliers of products, tools and equipment	

(Continued)

Beauty organization	Description	
Industry leading bodies	Habia is the government-appointed standards-setting body for hair, beauty, nails, spa therapy, barbering and African-type hair, and creates the standards that form the basis of all qualifications including NVQs, SVQs, apprenticeships, diplomas and foundation degrees, as well as industry codes of practice. Habia provides guidance on industry related organization qualifications such as VRQs, careers, business development, legislation, salon safety and **equal opportunities,** and is responsible to government on industry issues such as education and skills. Habia raises the profile of its industries through the press and media, and is the first port of call for news organizations and broadcasters on news items and background information. **www.habia.org**	**habia.** hair and beauty industry authority

ACTIVITY

Research and list different treatments that are offered in a health spa.

TOP TIP

Hotel beauty/spa breaks

Special offer day and weekend treatment packages are popular. They also attract clients to stay at the hotel in quieter months of the year such as September and January.

TOP TIP

Professional membership organizations include:

◆ Habia (Hair and Beauty Industry Authority) **www.habia.com**

◆ International Spa Association (ISA) **www.experienceispa.com**

◆ The Beauty Guild **www.beautyguild.com**

◆ BABTAC (British Association of Beauty Therapists and Cosmetologists) **www.babtac.com**

◆ FHT (The Federation of Holistic Therapists) **www.fht.org.uk**

Beauty treatments

Some of the main treatments and services offered by the beauty related industries are listed below.

Beauty treatment	Description	
Manicure	A treatment to care for, maintain and improve the condition and appearance of the hands, nails and surrounding skin	

(Continued)

Beauty treatment	Description	
Pedicure	A treatment to care for, maintain and improve the condition and appearance of the feet, nails and surrounding skin	
Waxing	The temporary removal of excess or unwanted hair from a body area using a choice of wax suited to the body area, skin sensitivity and hair type	
Nail enhancement	Artificial nail structures applied to enhance the natural nail by: increasing its length; improving overall appearance and to strengthen and repair	
Make-up	Cosmetics applied to the skin of the face to enhance and accentuate, or to minimize facial features. Make-up products create balance in the face. Application technique and choice of product will depend upon the result to be achieved	
Basic facial	A treatment used to improve the appearance, condition and functioning of the skin and underlying structures	

(Continued)

Beauty treatment	Description	
Electrical facial	Also referred to as electrotherapy. Specialist mechanical or electrical equipment is applied to improve the condition and appearance of the face and neck area. Each piece of equipment creates different effects and results	
Electrolysis	Total destruction of the hair follicle using an electric current to permanently stop unwanted hair growth	
Eyelash and eyebrow treatments	Treatments applied to enhance the eye area including eyebrow shaping, permanent eyelash and eyebrow tinting, and artificial eyelash application	
Body massage	Manipulation of the soft tissues of the body, producing heat in the area of application. It also benefits by stimulating the body's muscular, circulatory and nervous systems	

(Continued)

Beauty treatment	Description	
Aromatherapy	The use of essential oils – aromatic substances that have a vast range of aromas extracted from flowers, seeds, roots, fruits and bark. Usually combined with massage to influence the client's mood and create a feeling of well-being	
Reflexology	A treatment using finger point pressure applied to different parts of the feet and hands called zones, to improve energy flow through the body and health and well-being. Derived from Ancient Chinese, Egyptian and Indian techniques	
Heat and water therapy	*Heat therapy* – skin warming treatments including the use of moist and dry heat; includes sauna and steam treatments. *Water therapy* – also known as hydrotherapy (derived from the Greek *hydor* 'water' and *therapia* 'therapy' meaning 'the therapeutic use of water'). Treatments include hydrotherapy baths; water jet tunnel and wet flotation treatments; spa pools; pools and showers	
Hot stone therapy	Massage using a variety of volcanic stones, which may be cold or heated to stimulate or relax; used in conjunction with massage they help to restore the flow of energy in the body by using a variety of application techniques	
Indian head massage	A massage treatment traditionally practised in India. It is applied to the upper body using the hands. The massage helps to relieve stress and tension, creating a feeling of well-being. Oils may be applied to the scalp and hair to improve their condition	

(Continued)

Beauty treatment	Description	
Electrical body treatments	Also referred to as electrotherapy. Mechanical or electrical equipment Is used to improve the condition and appearance of the limbs and trunk areas or overall appearance of the body. Each piece of equipment creates specific effects and results	
Body wrapping	A body treatment where the body is wrapped in bandages, plastic sheets or thermal blankets to achieve different therapeutic effects	
Tanning	A treatment which makes the skin become darker in colour. Achieved through UV tanning or self tanning. In UV tanning the skin is exposed to artificially produced ultraviolet light and the skin darkens creating a tan. Self tanning uses cosmetic products containing an ingredient which creates a healthy, tanned appearance of the skin. Different methods can be used to apply self-tan products including automated spray, manual and airbrush application	

Beauty related work roles

There are a wide range of different job opportunities available in the beauty related industries. A brief explanation of these various occupational beauty related work roles are described below.

Occupational work role	Description of activities	
Beauty therapist	Beauty therapists provide beauty treatments and treatments which, if qualified to Level 3 (VRQ or NVQ), may include those listed in the chart on pages 10–14. They also give advice to clients and promote retail beauty products to support the treatments they offer. Beauty therapists may be salon based, work from their own home or travel to a location such as the client's home	

(Continued)

Occupational work role	Description of activities	
Make-up artist	Make-up artists apply make-up and often also style the hair of performers and presenters for TV, film, theatre, fashion shows, live performances and photo shoots	
Electrologist	A specialist in hair removal who uses electrolysis to permanently destroy the hair follicle to stop hair growth. A sterile needle is used to apply an electric current with galvanic or short wave diathermy electrical equipment	
Nail technician	A specialist in nail treatments including care of the natural nail with manicures and pedicures, nail art application and artificial nail enhancement techniques	
Manicurist/pedicurist	A manicurist/pedicurist specializes in applying treatments for the hands (manicure) and feet (pedicure) with the aim of improving or maintaining their health and appearance through the provision of specialized treatments	
Massage therapist	The massage therapist provides massage treatments to the face, head and body. This may be performed *manually*, where the beauty therapist's hands manipulate the client's skin, tissue and underlying muscles, or *mechanically* using a machine. Massage techniques can achieve a relaxing or stimulating effect and create a feeling of well-being	

(Continued)

Occupational work role	Description of activities	
Aromatherapist	Aromatherapists treat a variety of physical conditions and psychological disorders using essential aromatic oils that are extracted from flowers, trees, fruit and herbs, selected for their therapeutic properties	
Reflexologist	In reflexology every part of the body is reflected in a precise area, or reflex point, on the feet and hands. The reflexologist works on the foot or the hand as appropriate, using a precise technique based upon the application of finger point pressure on the reflex zones of the feet and hands to restore the flow of energy through the body	
Complementary therapist	A practitioner providing treatment alongside or in addition to conventional medicine. This is referred to as 'complementary medicine' as the two practices *complement* each other. The practitioner treats the client's body and mind as a whole and this is often referred to as an 'holistic approach'	

(Continued)

Occupational work role	Description of activities	
Cosmetic consultant	Usually employed by a cosmetic company in a retail environment or freelance, cosmetic consultants sell cosmetics and advise customers on the right products to meet their requirements	
Sales representative	Promotes a particular product, treatment or company 'brand'. They are often experts in their field and can offer technical support and training within the beauty related industries through continuing professional development (CPD). CPD maintains an individual's expertise and awareness of current beauty related industry practice	
Receptionist	The receptionist receives clients entering the beauty work area, handles enquiries, makes appointments, deals with client payments and maintains the appearance of the reception area. The receptionist should always take care of clients in a polite, efficient manner, particularly while questioning them to find out what they require	
Salon manager	The salon manager supervises and supports other colleagues with additional responsibilities for the day-to-day running of the business, complying with all workplace legislation, maintaining resource levels and monitoring staff performance and attainment towards any specific targets	

(Continued)

Occupational work role	Description of activities	
Teacher	Teachers are qualified and trained to teach their occupational skills and assess their learners' competence or capability across a variety of courses and levels	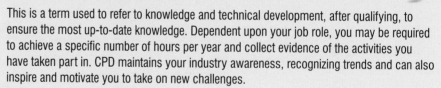
Trainer	Trainers are qualified to train learners in a variety of courses, often in specific CPD courses	

TOP TIP

Continuing Professional Development (CPD)

This is a term used to refer to knowledge and technical development, after qualifying, to ensure the most up-to-date knowledge. Dependent upon your job role, you may be required to achieve a specific number of hours per year and collect evidence of the activities you have taken part in. CPD maintains your industry awareness, recognizing trends and can also inspire and motivate you to take on new challenges.

TOP TIP

Visiting trade shows and subscribing to professional trade magazines provide an excellent opportunity to keep up-to-date with new products, equipment and treatments. The Internet also allows you to follow current and future trends.

Legislation

There is a great deal of legislation affecting the beauty related industries. Legislation legally must be provided, so it is important to understand what affects you and the treatments you provide.

Legislation related to this unit includes:

◆ Equal Opportunity and Discrimination Acts (2010)

◆ Working Time Regulations (2003)

◆ National Minimum Wage Act (1998)

◆ Employment Rights Act (1996)

◆ Employment Act (2008)

◆ Health and Safety at Work Act (1974)

◆ Performing Rights Regulations

◆ Data Protection Act (1998)

◆ Trade Description Act (1968 and 1972)

◆ Consumer Protection Act (1987).

Refer to CHAPTER 3 Health and Safety and CHAPTER 4 Selling Skills to find out more about what this legislation enforces.

You are required to be able to describe the basic principles of finance and selling. This includes knowing how to inform your clients about different products and treatments and the importance of having excellent product knowledge; knowing when and how to promote a product or treatment using effective communication skills which engage your client; following through the stages of the selling process identifying the client's need for the product; the most appropriate product to meet their need and demonstrating the product's features and benefits; overcoming any obstacles presented by the client; and finally closing the sale.

To learn more about selling techniques refer to CHAPTER 4 Selling Skills.

When you have achieved a sale, you need to know how to handle the different types of payments. The pricing of products and treatments is covered by different consumer protection legislation that you need to comply with. Remember, for a business to be successful it is essential that clients are aware of your business and the different treatments and products you provide.

Find out more about this in CHAPTER 6 Salon Reception.

Find out more about consumer protection legislation in CHAPTER 4 Selling Skills.

Business marketing and publicity

Marketing and publicity is necessary to make clients aware of your products or treatments and helps create or maintain interest in what you offer. These activities target existing and potential clients. A budget should be allocated for marketing and the choice of advertising will depend upon how much money is available to spend and which will be most cost-effective. Marketing activities such as promotional activities can occur internally at the business premises or off site at an external venue. Promotions are essential to the success of the business. An annual business plan should identify what promotions are intended to be implemented – an event list. This will be based upon a promotion strategy (which will involve all staff) to reach target markets in order to achieve a specific objective(s) or goal.

There may be a contribution from sponsors, such as skincare companies, who will play a part in supporting the success of a promotional event or sponsor advertising. Ideas from staff are important and appraisals provide a good opportunity for you to offer ideas such as how a new client target group can be reached or how the profile of the treatments that are on offer can be raised.

Methods of marketing and publicity include using signage in the business, fliers, direct mailings, email, text phone messaging, social media sites' website advertisement, and media such as advertisements in papers, commercial journals, radio and television. The advertising campaign needs a specific goal. This could be a short-term goal, e.g., the launch of a new product, discounted treatments, etc. or a long-term goal such as establishing the business name and familiarity with its product and treatments, 'the brand'. This would be achieved through repeat advertising. The best advert is your clients who if happy advertise through positive word-of-mouth.

TOP TIP

Keeping in contact with clients

Social media sites are popular ways of publicizing your work, i.e. make-up images and communicating any marketing information, i.e. promotions.

Texting clients is an increasingly popular way of keeping in touch with your clients; reminding them of their appointments or 'last minute' special offers. Always gain their consent for this communication method first!

Where possible, videos and photographic images of marketing activities may be shown on the business website or as an information medium in the reception area to maintain interest and awareness.

Never miss any marketing opportunities for the business when holding a promotion. The local press can be informed, if invited advise them of the best time to be there and who to contact. A journalist could be invited to receive a treatment for free and then feedback on their experience!

The beauty *trade press* can also be used which will feature new developmental areas within the sector and commentary on items such as charity-based events. If there is something new and innovative this could be reviewed by the *consumer press* who will then put it into the public domain, so the potential to raise the business profile from this opportunity is much higher.

A successful career in beauty therapy

As well as having received the necessary training and qualifications, you must also have good employability skills to gain employment within the beauty related industries. An employer regards these as being just as important as your qualification.

An employer will expect you to use good working practices at all times which require you to be:

Professional – presenting a consistent, positive image of yourself and the workplace.

Courteous – clients should be treated with respect in all communication and contact, both verbal and non-verbal, and during each stage of treatment delivery.

TOP TIP

Good working practices

These include completing treatments to the best of your ability and following all relevant legislation, codes of practice and work-related policies and procedures.

ACTIVITY

List some examples of what being courteous means to you when dealing with a client. Consider the scenarios below and state how you would deal with each in a courteous manner:

◆ a client arriving at reception when you are already busy with another client
◆ a client arriving late for a treatment
◆ a client receiving a treatment for the first time.

ACTIVITY

Write a list of the personal strengths you feel you have that would make you successful as a beauty therapist.

Write a list of any weaknesses or areas for development you have, e.g. poor punctuality, which need improvement to improve your personal employability skills.

Knowledge Check

What do you understand by the requirements of the legislation and codes of practice listed below and how do you comply with them in your everyday work?

Personal Protective Equipment (PPE) (2002)

Control of Substances Hazardous to Health (COSHH) (2002)

Manual Handling Operations Regulations (1992)

Electricity at Work Regulations (1989)

Habia Code of Practice for Waxing

Need more help? Refer to Chapter 3 Health and Safety, to find out more about the legislation and how it applies to you.

Refer to Chapter 3 Health and Safety

TOP TIP

Only ever work within your job role in any activity carried out in the workplace.

ACTIVITY

If a client could not receive a treatment because they had a skin disorder that could not be treated, how would you deal with this discreetly?

Discreet – you must be careful and tactful in how you communicate and express yourself at all times in the working environment. Certain conversation topics may not be suitable and cause embarrassment. Always 'think before you speak'. Avoid passing on personal opinions which may cause offence. In compliance with the legislation of the Data Protection Act (1998), never pass on client or staff information unless agreement has been given.

Personable – a successful business requires employees who are personable or pleasant and have people skills. This means having a positive attitude, being able to work well, co-operate and communicate with others – a team player.

Enthusiastic – employers want employees to have high aspirations and are willing to work hard to achieve them.

Responsible – your employer will expect you to think carefully when performing any tasks to avoid unnecessary error. Self-discipline is a good attribute to ensure all tasks are completed competently and meet the required deadline.

When you have successfully completed your VRQ in Beauty Therapy at Level 2 you can gain employment or progress your training, gaining further technical awards or certificates of higher qualification.

Personal health, hygiene and professional presentation

Your appearance allows the client to make their first judgement about both you and the workplace, so make sure that you create the correct impression! Employees in the workplace should always reflect the most desirable image of the profession that they work in.

ACTIVITY

List further employability skills you think are important and explain why.

HEALTH & SAFETY

Personal Protective Equipment (PPE) at Work Regulations (1992) For certain treatments, such as waxing treatments, it is necessary to wear a protective apron over the overall to protect the overall and avoid contamination. For certain treatments it also necessary to wear gloves.

HEALTH & SAFETY

Workplace policy Employers will advise you on personal presentation requirements in relation to accessories and adornment including facial piercings, tattoos, nail length and if nail polish may be worn.

HEALTH & SAFETY

Control of Substances Hazardous to Health (COSHH) (2002) Essential information for beauty therapists is available on the HSE website in a section called 'COSHH and your industry'. You will be able to find out more about how COSHH affects you. See **www.hse.gov.uk**

Due to the nature of many of the treatments offered and close working proximity to the client, the beauty therapist must wear protective, hygienic workwear. An overall is ideal and also presents a smart uniform. An overall might comprise of a dress, in a length suited to a work role a tunic top, with co-ordinating trousers or skirt. A fresh, clean overall should be worn each day. Tights may be worn to protect the leg area if exposed.

Make-up If worn, make-up should be well applied and appropriate for the type of beauty treatment being offered, correct skincare cosmetics should be selected to suit your skin type. A healthy facial appearance will be a positive advertisement for your work.

Jewellery Keep jewellery to a minimum, such as a wedding ring, a fob watch and small stud earrings. This prevents scratching the client accidentally during the treatment and for reasons of hygiene.

Nails Nails, both natural and artificial if worn, should be short, neatly manicured and free of nail polish unless the employee's main duties involve nail treatments or reception duties. **Nail polish** contains ingredients which can cause an allergic response in some people.

Hair Hair should be secured and worn away from the face if long, for reasons of both safety when performing treatments and hygiene.

Shoes Wear low heeled, well-fitting, comfortable shoes that enclose the feet fully. This will provide protection if you accidentally drop anything on your feet, e.g. hot paraffin wax. Remember that you will be on your feet for most of the day: they need to support your feet properly!

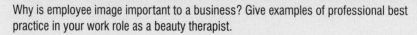

ACTIVITY

Why is employee image important to a business? Give examples of professional best practice in your work role as a beauty therapist.

An example is provided:

◆ wear a clean, neatly pressed overall uniform every day.

Employment rights and responsibilities

It is important to have a basic understanding of employment law that protects you and which employers must abide by. These laws and regulations are designed to ensure that you are not exploited or treated unfairly.

Contract of employment

Because there are so many ways that a person may be employed each person should have a contract of employment which states the 'terms and conditions' of their employment.

Your employment status may be full time (typically 37–40 hours per week), part time, freelance (self-employed) or contractual (employed for a fixed-term period).

Employment is regulated by the Employment Rights Act (1996). It may be referred to in the case of a dispute as evidence of an employee's 'terms and conditions'.

A contract of employment should be issued by the employer to the employee within 8 weeks of start of work. It will include important information such as the date your employment began; your hours of work; when and how you will be paid and your hours of work, including your holiday entitlement. Also, it will include your job title and job description; whether it is permanent or contractual, and details of sickness, pension and redundancy entitlements. It will also state how much notice you must work if you wish to leave the employment. The disciplinary and **grievance** procedures should always be included in your contract of employment. Finally, it must include the address of the place of work as you need to be informed if you are working in more than one place.

National Minimum Wage Act (1998)

Since 1998 it has been illegal to pay less than the national minimum hourly rate of pay. Every year the government amends the national minimum hourly rate to allow for inflation and average increases in wages.

Working safely

There is a good deal of legislation relating to health and safety in the workplace. It is there to provide safe working environment for all. You will need to know the laws relating to beauty therapy – your responsibilities and your rights. If you cause harm to your client or put them at risk you will be liable for prosecution. The same applies to an employer who does not provide a safe working environment for their employees.

The Health and Safety at Work Act (1974) (HASAWA) states the minimum standards of health, safety and welfare required in each area of the workplace. Refer to Chapter 3 Health and Safety, to find out more about health, safety and welfare in the workplace.

> **TOP TIP**
> To find out more about aspects of employment law visit **www.direct.gov.uk/en/ Employment/index.htm**

Education and employment progression opportunities

When qualified at VRQ Level 2 you can continue to develop your skills and knowledge as follows:

◆ VRQ or NVQ Level 3 Beauty Therapy or Make-up

◆ other associated industry qualifications in hairdressing, nails, massage or spa treatments

◆ further training to gain advanced practical techniques to maintain continuous professional development (CPD). CPD is important to keep yourself up-to-date and meet the emerging trends of the industry. This may include further VRQ awards or certificates

◆ on achievement of Level 3 qualifications you may find employment, dependent upon your training route, as a:

- ◆ business owner
- ◆ college lecturer and assessor
- ◆ salon trainer and assessor
- ◆ technician for a manufacturer providing training on products, equipment and treatments
- ◆ salon manager
- ◆ senior beauty therapist or make-up artist
- ◆ sales and marketing manager
- ◆ cruise ship or airline beauty therapist.

◆ other routes include:

- ◆ working in the media – magazines, advertisements and television
- ◆ specializing in a particular area such as electrolysis or photographic make-up
- ◆ employment as a make-up artist working on film sets, in television studio, theatre, music videos and fashion providing fashion runway make-up.

When you achieve your Level 3 qualification in beauty therapy or make-up you can continue to update and advance your skills as relevant to your career path/goals.

ACTIVITY

What would you consider your 'dream job'? Using professional journals/magazines or online job advertisements search for a vacancy and obtain a job description so you can see the qualifications, experience and personal attributes that you will need to have. Alternatively, you may already have a role model: ask their advice on what it took to get there! You can then draw up a plan of what you will need to achieve, and when and how to gain the necessary evidence and experience. This is your career path, the journey required to achieve your career goal.

TOP TIP

Industry role models have contributed 'tips of the trade' in this book, sharing their expertise and valued knowledge. On successful completion of your Level 2 qualification you will be able to work in a rewarding job full of variety with career possibilities that are endless!

TOP TIP

Beauty therapy is one of the UK's 20 happiest sectors to work in, according to City & Guilds, scoring 8 out of 10.

Industry role models

In the beauty therapy and make-up industry there are many role models who have extensive experience which has helped raise the industry profile. Their passion for their work is inspirational to our beauty therapists and make-up artists of the future.

STUDENT CASE STUDY

Name: Verity Eden

Title of Qualification:

VRQ Level 2 Beauty Therapy (nearly completed VRQ Level 3 Beauty Therapy)

What did you enjoy most about studying, and what did you find most challenging?

I have really enjoyed carrying out treatments in the college salon as this has enabled me to perfect my practical skills without the pressure of a real work environment. The anatomy and physiology knowledge is definitely the most challenging part of the course but I know how important it is so I don't mind studying hard to get it right.

What are your next steps in your career development, and where would you like to see yourself in the future?

I am due to finish my VRQ Level 3 Beauty Therapy Diploma in a couple of months. Once this has been completed, I look forward to working in a salon and building up my skills further. In the future I would like have my own salon, specializing in dermatology and facial treatments.

What inspires and motivates you?

My college tutors are inspirational; they have such a passion for the subjects they teach, you can't help but feel passionate too. I am also inspired by some of the leading professionals in the beauty therapy world such as the role models in this book.

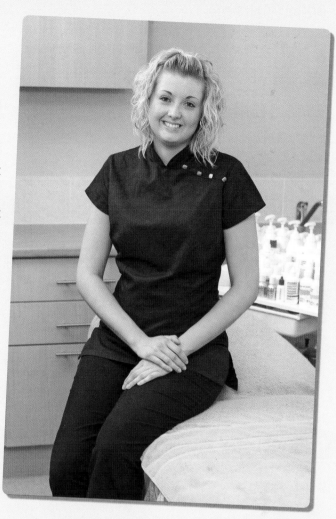

I feel motivated when I receive good feedback from a client, whether it's a family member, friend or someone who has come into the college salon. It is a really nice feeling when a client tells you that you have made them feel better and that they will come back to see you again.

What is the most important thing you have learnt from your beauty therapy qualifications?

The consultation process is the most important part of any treatment so one of the most important things I have learnt is how to communicate effectively and professionally with clients. If you can get the consultation right, the treatment should be successful, so good communication skills are the key.

What would you say to a new student starting their Level 2 qualification?

Go for it! The theory side of the course, especially the anatomy and physiology, is a lot harder than Level 1 but it all seems worth it when you're practising your treatments and getting it right. If you have any choices, make sure you choose your optional units carefully and don't just do what your friends are doing.

What do you think makes a good beauty therapist?

I think to be good beauty therapist you need to be polite and professional with your clients, and also be able to show empathy where necessary. The hygiene and appearance of the beauty therapist is also extremely important.

ROLE MODEL

WENDY NIXON

" Wendy is an Environmental Health Practitioner, specializing in health and safety enforcement. She works as Health and Safety Consultant to the hair and beauty industry.

Wendy shares her expertise in Chapter 3 Health and Safety.

ROLE MODEL

SAMANTHA SWEET

 Samantha has represented CND (Creative Nail Design) for 22 years and in 2006 founded Sweet Squared, the largest most respected nail distributor

in the UK. Samantha shares her expertise in Chapter 4 Selling Skills.

ROLE MODEL

GILL MORRIS

" Gill is a Chartered Marketer, Fellow of the RSA and a Member of the Professional Speaking Association. Since 1999 Gill has run her own highly successful training, coaching and mentoring business assisting salon

owners, managers and therapists to reach their full potential. Gill shares her expertise in Chapter 5 Client Care and Communication.

ROLE MODEL

TINA ROOKS

" Tina Rook heads up Saks Education. Tina joined Saks in 1999 with the task of creating NVQ training programmes in hairdressing and beauty therapy, so apprentices could learn their trade while working in Saks salons.

Tina shares her expertise in Chapter 6 Salon Reception.

ROLE MODEL

DANIELLE NORMAN

" As the Education Operations Manager at Dermalogica, Danielle is responsible for the overall operations of training centres located across the UK and Ireland. Danielle shares her expertise in Chapter 7 Skincare.

ROLE MODEL

SHAVATA SINGH

" Shavata Singh is Brand Director of Shavata UK (encompassing Shavata Brow Studio and LASH LOUNGE by Shavata). Shavata shares her expertise in Chapter 8 Eyelash and Brow Treatments and Chapter 9 Threading.

ROLE MODEL

CHARLOTTE SAVOURY

" As Key Artist for Illamasqua, Charlotte's role varies from designing looks inspired by specific briefs, working with and training the teams across the UK and supporting research in the development of new products and collections. Charlotte shares her expertise in Chapter 10 Make-Up.

ROLE MODEL

MARIAN NEWMAN

" Contributing author to this book, Marian is one of the leading professionals in the beauty therapy industry. Marian has worked in the professional nail industry since 1986 and comes from a scientific background. After working with several product companies, she now works independently within the media and fashion sector. Marian has a close association with Habia in the development of educational standards and skills and is the Chairperson of the Nail Services Forum. Marian shares her expertise in Chapter 11 Manicure Treatments.

ROLE MODEL

MARGARET DABBS

Margaret Dabbs is a fully trained Podiatrist. She is company founder and Chief Executive of Margaret Dabbs London, foot clinics based in London and now Dubai. Margaret shares her expertise in Chapter 12 Pedicure Treatments.

ROLE MODEL

LIZA SMITH

Liza Smith is one of the country's most respected Nail Artists. She is owner of Bodylines salon and Head educator at CND (Creative Nail Designs). Liza shares her expertise in Chapter 13 Provide and Maintain Nail Enhancements.

ROLE MODEL

NATALIYA

Nataliya works full time in her own salon N-Style in Edinburgh. She regularly contributes to the industry with her Nail Trail article in Scratch Magazine. Nataliya shares her expertise in Chapter 14 Nail Art.

ROLE MODEL

JANICE BROWN

Janice is director of Beauty (Hof Beauty Ltd), one of the leading suppliers to the Beauty industry. Janice is co-author of *Encyclopedia of Hair Removal* and *Practical Electrolysis* with Gill Morris. Janice shares her expertise in Chapter 15 Waxing Treatments.

ROLE MODEL

KATHRYN DARWIN

" Kathryn is Sales and Training Manager at Studex UK Ltd where she works on marketing material for national customers, reviewing new products and presenting our Ear Piercing Systems to local councils. Kathryn shares her expertise in Chapter 16 Ear Piercing.

ROLE MODEL

ELEANOR MONKS

" Eleanor is Training Manager at the prestigious Sanctuary Spa, Covent Garden, where she is responsible for the training and ongoing development of all team members within the business. Eleanor shares her expertise in Chapter 17 Head Massage.

ROLE MODEL

NICHOLA JOSS

" Nichola is Celebrity Beauty Therapist/Facialist and St Tropez Global Brand Ambassador. Nicola works with the film, television, beauty and fashion industries to create a natural looking, golden glow that is essential for a healthy, youthful appearance. Nichola shares her expertise in Chapter 18 Skin Tanning.

2 Anatomy and Physiology

LEARNING OBJECTIVES

◆ Understand the structure of the skin and its function.

◆ Understand the structure of the hair and types of hair growth.

◆ Understand the structure of nails and nail growth.

◆ Be familiar with the external ear structure.

◆ Be familiar with muscle groups and bones of the body.

◆ Be familiar with the composition and function of blood and the lymphatic system.

KEY TERMS

acid mantle	bones of the arm	circulatory system
anagen	bones of the foot	collagen
apocrine glands	bones of the hand	concealer
arrector pili muscle	bones of the lower leg	cortex
bacteria	camouflage products	cure
blepharitis	catagen	cuticle (hair)
blood	cells	cuticle (nail)
blood vessels	chemical reaction	cyclical pattern of growth
bone	chilblains	dermal papilla

dermis
dihydroxyacetone (DHA)
ear
eccrine glands
eczema
elastin
epidermis
external ear
facial bones
free edge
hair
hair follicle
histamine
hyperpigmentation
hypopigmentation
infestation
keloids
keratin
lymph
lymph vessels
lymphatic system

masks
melanin
melanocytes
muscle tone
muscles
muscles in the lower leg
muscles of facial expression
muscles of the foot
muscles of the hand and arm
muscles of the upper body
nail bed
nail growth
nail plate
nail structure
nails
nerve
nervous system
neurones
pigment
pilo-sebaceous unit
sebaceous gland

sebaceous glands
sebum
sensory nerve endings
shoulder girdle
skin allergy
skin appendages
skin condition
skull
styes
subcutaneous layer
superfluous hair
sweat glands
telogen
terminal hairs
tissues
tinea pedis or athlete's foot
tinea corporis or body ringworm
vellus hairs
viruses
vitamin D

INTRODUCTION

As a beauty therapist it is necessary that you have a good understanding of anatomy and physiology, as many of your treatments aim to improve the particular functioning of the different systems of the body. For example, a facial massage will improve blood and lymph circulation in the area as you massage the skin's surface, and increase cellular renewal as you improve nutrition to the living cells, while removing dead skin cells. The result is healthier, looking skin.

It is necessary for you to know and understand anatomy and physiology and apply this knowledge relevant to each beauty therapy treatment carried out.

For example when you are carrying out a waxing service observing the hairs removed will indicate if your skill technique is correct, as you will recognise what a hair will look like on removal in its different stages of hair growth.

Knowledge and understanding requirements

You are required to have knowledge and understanding of the anatomy and physiology where identified for the different units you are studying as part of your VRQ qualification. You may be assessed through written questions or assignments. To guide and support you in your study and revision, the anatomy and physiology you need to know and understand for each unit has been identified with an A&P symbol in each chapter. Simply look for the A&P symbol and check back here for your knowledge and understanding requirements.

Anatomy and physiology knowledge requirements

The beauty therapy units with anatomy and physiology knowledge requirements are:

Knowledge requirements	Chapter
Provide facial skincare	Chapter 7
Provide eyelash and brow treatments	Chapter 8
Provide eyelash perming	Chapter 8
Provide threading services for hair removal	Chapter 9
Apply make-up	Chapter 10
Provide manicure treatments	Chapter 11
Provide pedicure treatments	Chapter 12
Provide and maintain nail enhancements	Chapter 13
Provide nail art	Chapter 14
Remove hair using waxing techniques	Chapter 15
Provide ear piercing	Chapter 16
Provide head massage	Chapter 17
Apply skin tanning techniques	Chapter 18

You can find out more about hair, nails, skin, the muscular system, the **circulatory system**, cardio-vascular and lymphatic system, and the blood and lymph supply to the **ear**, in the relevant sections throughout this chapter.

Anatomical terminology

Anatomical terminology is used to describe the location and description of a body part. It is useful to know these terms, as it will assist your anatomy understanding. As you read through this chapter you will notice the terms listed in the table on page 34.

Anatomy and physiology knowledge and understanding requirements for each VRQ unit

	Provide facial skincare	Remove hair using waxing techniques	Provide manicure treatments	Provide pedicure treatments	Provide eyelash and brow treatments	Apply make-up	Provide and maintain nail enhancement	Provide nail art	Provide ear piercing	Provide eyelash perming	Provide threading treatments for hair removal	Provide head massage	Apply skin tanning techniques
Skin													
Skin structure and function	✓	✓	✓	✓	✓	✓	✓	✓	✓	✓	✓	✓	✓
Growth cycle and repair	✓	✓											
Diseases and disorders	✓	✓	✓	✓	✓	✓	✓	✓	✓	✓	✓	✓	✓
Hair													
Hair structure and function		✓			✓					✓	✓	✓	
Types of hair growth		✓									✓		
Hair growth cycle		✓			✓					✓	✓	✓	
Nails													
Nail structure and function			✓	✓			✓	✓					
Nail growth			✓	✓			✓	✓					
Diseases and disorders			✓	✓			✓	✓					
Muscular system													
Muscle groups in the treatment area of the body, position and action	✓		✓	✓		✓			✓			✓	
Skeletal system													
Bones in the treatment area of the body, position, structure and function	✓		✓	✓		✓			✓			✓	
Cardio-vascular and lymphatic system													
Composition and function of blood and lymph	✓	✓	✓	✓		✓	✓		✓			✓	
Cardio-vascular and lymphatic system structure	✓	✓	✓	✓		✓	✓		✓			✓	
External ear structure									✓				

Examples of anatomical terminology

Term	Definition	Term	Definition
Anterior	Front (usually refers to front of the body)	Superficial	Near the surface
Posterior	Back (usually refers to the back of the body)	Superior	Above
Proximal	Nearest to	Inferior	Below
Medial	Middle	Plantar	Front surface
Distal	Furthest away	Dorsal	Back surface
Lateral	Side		

Knowledge Check

What are the effects of ageing on the skin?

Refer to page 209 to help you.

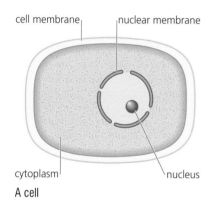

cell membrane | nuclear membrane

cytoplasm | nucleus

A cell

Cells

The human body consists of many trillions of microscopic **cells**. Each cell contains a chemical substance called protoplasm, which contains various specialized structures whose activities are essential to our health. If cells are unable to function properly, a disorder results.

Surrounding the cell is the cell membrane. This forms a border between the cell contents and their surrounding environment. The membrane has a porous surface that allows food to enter and waste materials to leave.

In the centre of the cell is the nucleus, which contains thread-like structures called chromosomes. On these are the genes we have inherited from our parents and this genetic information makes us who we are. The genes are ultimately responsible for cell reproduction and cell functioning.

The liquid within the cell membrane and surrounding the nucleus is called cytoplasm. Scattered throughout this are other small bodies, the organelles or 'little organs'; each has a specific function within the cell.

Cells in the body tend to specialize in carrying out particular functions. Groups of cells which share function, shape, size or structure are called **tissues**.

Tissues

If the tissues are damaged, for example, if the skin is accidentally broken, the tissue cells divide to repair the damage – called regeneration. The body is composed of four basic tissues. These are described in the table on the following page.

Tissues may be grouped to form the larger functional and structural units we know as organs, such as the heart.

The skin

The skin varies in appearance according to our race, gender and age. It also alters from season to season and from year to year, and reflects our general health, lifestyle and diet.

Skin functions

More information on how race, gender and age affects the skin's appearance can be found in **CHAPTER 7** Facial Skincare.

The human skin is an organ – the largest of the body. It provides a tough, flexible covering, with many different important functions. The main functions are listed on the following page.

Types of tissue and general functions

Name of tissue	Examples	General functions
Epithelial	Epidermis outer layer of skin	Forms surface and linings for protection
Connective	Dermis layer of skin Collagen fibres Bone Ligaments Tendons	A structural tissue that supports, surrounds and connects different parts of the body
Muscular nucleus muscle fibres	Voluntary or skeletal, muscle tissue Involuntary or smooth muscle tissue	Contracts and shortens producing movement. Skeletal muscle tissue moves the body and maintains posture. Smooth muscle tissue moves substances through the body
Nervous nucleus spindle-shaped cell cells separated from each other	Neurones (nerve cells)	Forms a communication system between different parts of the body, controlling and co-ordinating most body processes

By remembering the word *SHAPES* this will help you remember the functions of the skin: Sensation, Heat regulation, Absorption, Protection, Excretion, Secretion.

Sensation

The skin is a sensory organ and the sensations of touch, pressure, pain, heat and cold are identified by sensory nerves and receptors in the skin. This information is then sent to the brain for decoding and initiating the appropriate bodily response. The skin also allows us to recognize objects by their feel and shape.

Heat regulation

Humans maintain a normal body temperature of 36.8–37°C. Body temperature is controlled in part by heat loss through the skin and by sweating. If the temperature of the body is increased by 0.25–0.5°C, the sweat glands excrete sweat on to the skin's surface. The body is cooled by the loss of heat used to evaporate the sweat from the skin's surface. If the body becomes too warm there is an increase in blood flow into the blood capillaries in the skin. The blood capillaries widen (dilate), this is referred to as vasodilation and heat is lost from the skin. Hair limits heat loss from the scalp. If the external temperature becomes low and the body needs to conserve heat there is a reduction in blood flow into the blood capillaries in the skin. The blood capillaries become narrower (constrict) so less blood is brought to the skin's surface, this is called vasoconstriction.

Absorption

Although structured to protect itself from penetration by harmful substances, absorption may take place through the sweat glands, hair follicles and epidermal cells for a beneficial effect. Water and fat-soluble substances such as essential oils are examples of products used to be absorbed by the skin.

Protection

The skin protects the body from potentially harmful substances and conditions.

◆ The outer surface is bactericidal, helping to prevent the multiplication of harmful microorganisms. It also prevents the absorption of many substances (unless the surface is broken), because of the structure of the cells on its outer surface, which form a chemical and physical barrier.

◆ The skin cushions the underlying structures from physical injury.

◆ The skin provides a waterproof coating. Its natural oil, **sebum**, prevents the skin from losing vital water, and therefore helps to prevent skin dehydration (tissues lacking in water).

◆ The skin contains a pigment or colour called **melanin**. This absorbs harmful rays of ultraviolet (UV) light.

◆ The skin has a warning system against outside invasion. Redness and irritation of the skin indicate that the skin is intolerant or allergic to something, this may be either external or internal.

Excretion

Small amounts of certain waste products, such as urea, water and salt, are removed from the body in sweat by excretion from sweat glands through the surface of the skin from the skin's pores.

Secretion

The skin secretes its natural oil, sebum, which is a mixture of fats and waxes and covers the skin's entire surface except the palms of the hands and the soles of the feet, and helps to protect the skin.

TOP TIP

Skin water loss

Although the skin has a waterproof property it allows approximately 500ml of water to be lost from the tissues through evaporation every day. Application of a moisturizer reduces this loss and provides vital hydration.

HEALTH & SAFETY

Skin absorption Although the skin is structured to avoid penetration of harmful substances by absorption, certain chemicals can be absorbed through the skin. Always protect the skin when using potentially harmful substances, and wear protective gloves when using harsh chemical cleaning agents.

TOP TIP

Skin thickness

The skin accounts for one-eighth of the body's total weight. It measures approximately 1.5 m² in total, depending on body size. It is thinnest on the eyelids (0.05mm), and thickest on the soles of the feet (approximately 5mm). The thinnest areas will have less tolerance and react more quickly in order to protect the body when in contact with harmful substances. That is why skin sensitivity tests are applied to areas of the skin where it is thinnest.

Nutrition

The skin provides storage for fat, which provides an energy reserve. The skin is also responsible for producing a significant proportion of our **vitamin D**, which is created by a **chemical reaction** when sunlight is in contact with the skin.

Activity in the skin

Puberty is when the body matures sexually and the reproductive organs become functional. Age of puberty differs from child to child. The average age for most girls is 11, reaching full sexual maturity within 4 years of starting puberty.

The average age for most boys is 12, reaching full sexual maturity within 6 years of starting puberty.

Chemical substances (hormones) control these changes in our bodies at puberty and become very active at this stage.

Among other effects, this activity causes the skin to become more oily, and often blemishes appear on the skin's surface. Seven out of ten teenagers find that their skin becomes blemished with blackheads (comedones), inflamed angry spots (pustules and papules) and even scars at this time: a skin disorder called acne vulgaris.

During our twenties the skin should look its best; any hormonal imbalance that occurred at puberty should by now have stabilized.

As we grow older, the skin ages too. In our late twenties and early thirties we will see fine lines appearing on the skin's surface, especially around the eyes where the skin is thinner.

At around the age of 40, hormone activity in the body becomes slower and the skin begins to lose its strength and elasticity. The skin becomes increasingly drier, and lines and wrinkles appear on the surface. In our late fifties brown patches of discoloured skin (lentigines) may appear: these are commonly seen at the temple region of the face and on the backs of the hands and are caused by UV light damage.

Fortunately, help is at hand to care for the skin: there are an ever-increasing number of skincare products from a vast and highly profitable cosmetics industry, and there is the skill and expertise of the qualified beauty therapist.

If it is your intention to become a qualified beauty professional, you need to learn about the skin's construction, its function, the different types of skin and how and why skin is changed by both internal and external influences.

ALWAYS REMEMBER

Ultraviolet exposure and the production of vitamin D

The skin's correct functioning is essential to life. It becomes darker to protect against excessive UV exposure but can also produce vitamin D. A fatty substance in the skin is converted to vitamin D with UV light from the sun. This circulates in the blood and with the mineral salts calcium and phosphorus helps the formation and maintenance of the health of the body's bones. Lack of vitamin D can lead to a bone-softening disease called rickets.

Skin structure

If we looked within the skin using a microscope, we would be able to see two distinct layers: the **epidermis** and the **dermis**. Between these layers is a specialized membrane which acts like a 'glue', sticking the two layers together: this is the basement membrane. If the epidermis and dermis become separated, body fluids fill the space, creating a blister, a small pocket of fluid in the top layers of the skin.

Situated below the epidermis and dermis is a further layer, the **subcutaneous layer** or fat layer. The fat layer consists of cells called adipose cells, containing fatty deposits. The thickness of the subcutaneous layer varies according to the body area, and is, for example, very thin around the eyes.

Skin structure

Outer skin surface (epidermis)

The layers and zones of the epidermis

The epidermis

The epidermis is located directly above the dermis. It is composed of five layers or strata, with the surface layer forming the outer skin – what we can see and touch. The main function of the epidermis is to protect the deeper living structures from invasion and harm from the external environment.

There is no blood supply in the epidermis. Nourishment of the epidermis, essential for growth is received from a liquid called the interstitial fluid formed from blood plasma. This acts as a link between the blood and cells.

Each layer of the epidermis can be recognized by its shape and by the function of its cells. The main type of cell found in the epidermis is the keratinocyte, which produces the protein **keratin**. It is keratin that makes the skin tough and that reduces the entry of substances into or out of the body.

Over a period of about four weeks, cells move from the bottom layer of the epidermis to the top layer, the skin's surface, changing in shape and structure as they progress. The process of cellular change takes place in stages:

◆ *the cell is formed at the bottom layer* – by division of an earlier cell. This type of cell division is called mitosis.

◆ *the cell matures* – it changes structure and moves upwards and outwards.

◆ *the cell dies* – it moves upwards and becomes an empty shell, which is eventually shed from the top layer.

The process of cellular change is illustrated below.

The layers and zones of the epidermis
The thickness of the five epidermal layers varies over the body's surface. Each layer is located either in the germinative zone or keratinization zone. This is illustrated and described later:

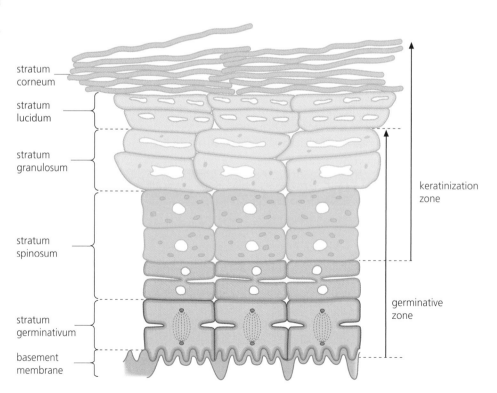

stratum corneum

stratum lucidum

stratum granulosum

keratinization zone

stratum spinosum

germinative zone

stratum germinativum

basement membrane

The germinative zone In the germinative zone the cells of the epidermis layers are living cells. The germinative zone layers of the epidermis are the stratum germinativum, stratum spinosum and stratum granulosum.

Stratum germinativum The stratum germinativum, or basal layer, is the deepest layer of the epidermis. It is formed from a single layer of column-shaped cells joined to the basement membrane. These cells divide continuously and produce new epidermal cells (keratinocytes), a process known as mitosis.

Stratum spinosum The stratum spinosum, or prickle-cell layer, is formed from two to six rows of cells which appear long in relation to their width, termed elongated; these have a surface of spiky spines which connect to surrounding cells. Each cell has a large nucleus and is filled with fluid.

Two other important cells are found in the germinative zone of the epidermis: Langerhan cells and melanocyte cells.

Langerhan cells

Special defence cells which absorb and remove foreign bodies that enter the skin. They then move from the epidermis to the dermis below, and finally enter the lymph system (the body's waste-transport system) where the foreign bodies are made safe by neutralizing them.

Melanocyte cells

Produce the skin pigment melanin, which contributes to our skin colour. About one in every ten stratum germinative cells is a melanocyte. **Melanocytes** are stimulated to produce melanin by UV rays, and their main function is to protect the other epidermal cells in this way from the harmful effects of UV light.

The quantity and distribution of melanocytes differs according to race. In a white skin the melanin tends to be destroyed when it reaches the granular layer. With stimulation from artificial or natural UV light, however, melanin will also be present in the upper epidermis.

In contrast a black skin has melanin present in larger quantities throughout *all* the epidermal layers, a level of protection that has evolved to deal with bright UV light. This increased protection allows less UV to penetrate the dermis below, reducing the possibility of premature ageing from exposure to UV light. The more even quality and distribution of melanin also means that people with dark skins are less at risk of developing skin cancer.

Another pigment, carotene, which is yellowish, also occurs in epidermal cells. Its contribution to skin colour lessens in importance as the amount of melanin in the skin increases.

Skin colour also increases when the skin becomes warm. This is because the blood capillaries at the surface dilate, bringing blood nearer to the surface so that heat can be lost – this is called vasodilation. If the temperature is cold the blood capillaries become

TOP TIP

Artificial skin tanning

Self-tanning products contain an ingredient called **dihydroxyacetone (DHA)**. This provides an artificial tanned appearance to the skin. DHA reacts with the skin's amino acids, chemical protein chains in the stratum corneum. Through desquamation the colour is lost as the skin's surface cells are removed.

ALWAYS REMEMBER

Psoriasis

A skin disorder affecting cell division. Cell division occurs much more quickly, resulting in clusters of dead skin cells appearing on the skin's surface. See page 59 for more information on psoriasis.

Knowledge Check

Name six functions of the skin. Refer to pages 35–37 to help you.

ALWAYS REMEMBER

Desquamation

When the epidermis cell dies and is eventually shed from the skin's surface this is termed desquamation.

ALWAYS REMEMBER

Stratum

Stratum is the Latin word for layer.

ALWAYS REMEMBER

Allergic reactions

Sometimes, the skin's surface intolerance to a substance is immediate. It shows as an allergic reaction, in which the skin becomes red, itchy and swollen.

Melanocyte and Langerhan cells in the stratum germinative layer of the skin

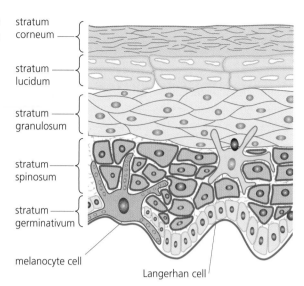

stratum corneum

stratum lucidum

stratum granulosum

stratum spinosum

stratum germinativum

melanocyte cell

Langerhan cell

Knowledge Check

What are the three main layers of the skin? Refer to page 37 to help you.

TOP TIP

Cosmetic sunscreens

Many hair and skincare products and cosmetics, including lipsticks and mascaras, now contain sunscreens. This is because research has shown that UV exposure is the principal cause of skin ageing and can also cause the hair to become dry.

HEALTH & SAFETY

Vitiligo Lack of skin pigment is called *vitiligo* or *leucoderma*. It can occur with any skin colour, but is more obvious on dark skin. Avoid exposing such skin to UV light as it does not have melanin protection. See page 55 for more information on vitiligo.

narrower so less blood is brought to the skin's surface to conserve heat – this is called vasoconstriction and the skin will lose colour.

Stratum granulosum

The stratum granulosum, or granular layer, is composed of one, two or three layers of cells that have become much flatter. The nucleus of the cell has begun to break up, creating what appear to be granules within the cell cytoplasm. These are known as keratohyaline granules and later form keratin. At this stage the cells form a new, combined layer.

The keratinization zone   The keratinization zone, or cornified zone, is where the cells begin to die and where finally they will be shed from the skin. The cells at this stage become progressively flatter, and the cell cytoplasm is replaced with the hard protein keratin.

Stratum lucidum

The stratum lucidum, clear layer or lucid layer, is only seen in non-hairy areas of the skin such as the palms of the hands and the soles of the feet. The cells here lack a nucleus and are filled with a clear substance called eledin produced at a further stage of the keratinization process.

Stratum corneum

The stratum corneum, cornified or horny layer, is formed from several layers of flattened, scale-like overlapping cells, composed mainly of keratin. These help to reflect UV light from the skin's surface; black skin, which evolved to withstand strong UV, has a thicker stratum corneum than does Caucasian skin.

It takes about three weeks for the epidermal cells to reach the stratum corneum from the stratum germinativum. The cells are then shed, a process called desquamation.

The outer layer of the epidermis, the stratum corneum, is up to 20 per cent thicker in men than women.

Every time the stratum corneum cells are removed through desquamation, the basal cell makes new cells to replace those removed. The dermis also makes more collagen and elastin. This is good news for your client! Beauty therapy treatments such as exfoliation remove dead skin cells and have a skin desquamating effect.

ALWAYS REMEMBER

Scars

When the surface has been broken, the skin at the site of the injury is replaced but may leave a scar. This initially appears red, due to the increased blood supply to the area, required while the skin heals. When healed, the redness will fade. If the skin's healing process continues for longer than necessary, too much scar tissue will be formed, resulting in a raised scar called a 'keloid' scar.

HEALTH & SAFETY

Sunburn If the skin becomes red on exposure to sunlight, this indicates that the skin has been overexposed to UV light. It will often blister and shed itself.

The dermis

The dermis is the inner portion of the skin, situated underneath the epidermis and composed of dense connective tissue containing other structures such as the lymphatic vessels which carry lymph which has a defensive action removing bacteria and waste products preventing infection; **blood vessels** which carry blood, a nutritive liquid, oxygen and hormones; and nerves which receive and respond to different stimuli.

Other appendages – structures associated with the dermis of the skin – include hair follicles, the arrector pili muscle, sweat glands, sebaceous glands and nails are all located in the dermis. It is much thicker than the epidermis and has two distinct layers: the papillary layer and the reticular layer.

The papillary layer The part of the dermis known as the papillary layer supplies the epidermis above with its nutrition. Tiny projections called dermal papillae contain both blood and lymph capillaries and nerve endings. It is these which nourish the epidermis above with blood and remove waste away through the associated lymphatic circulation.

The reticular layer The reticular layer, below the papillary layer, contains a dense network of protein fibres. These fibres allow the skin to expand, to contract, and to perform

For more information on keloid scarring see page 60

The skin

TOP TIP

Calluses

The skin will become much thicker in response to friction. A client with a manual occupation, such as a construction worker, may therefore develop hard skin (calluses) on their hands. The **skin condition** can be treated with an emollient preparation, which will moisturize and soften the dry skin. Calluses can occur on the feet also and will benefit from an emollient preparation designed for the feet.

TOP TIP

Papillae ridges – our unique fingerprint

The formation of the papillae ridges in the dermis are unique to each individual, and this provides our fingerprint.

TOP TIP

Massage – benefits the skin beneath

Appropriate external massage movements can be used to increase the blood supply within the dermis, bringing extra nutrients and oxygen to the skin and to the underlying muscle. At the same time, the lymphatic circulation is increased, improving the removal of waste products that may have accumulated.

intricate, supple movements. The reticular layer contains sweat glands, blood vessels, hair follicles, lymph vessels, the arrector pili muscles and sebaceous glands.

This network is composed of two sorts of protein fibre: yellow **elastin** fibres and white **collagen** fibres. Elastin fibres give the skin its elasticity, and collagen fibres give it its strength. The fibres are produced by specialized cells called fibroblasts, and are held in a gel called the ground substance.

While this network is strong, the skin will appear youthful and firm. As the fibres harden and fragment, however, the network begins to collapse, losing its elasticity. The skin then begins to show visible signs of ageing.

Male skin contains more collagen, a skin protein providing strength. Collagen production in females slows at the menopause which can result in sudden skin ageing. As such, skin ageing appears faster in females than males.

A major cause of damage to this network is unprotected exposure of the skin to UV light and to weather. Sometimes, too, the skin loses its elasticity because of a sudden increase in body weight, for example at puberty or pregnancy. This results in the appearance of stretch marks, streaks of thin skin that are a different colour from the surrounding skin: on white skin they appear as thin reddish streaks; on black skin they appear slightly lighter than the surrounding skin. The lost elasticity cannot be restored. Cosmetic treatments can be applied to improve their appearance.

Collagen and elastin fibres in the dermis

Sensory nerves

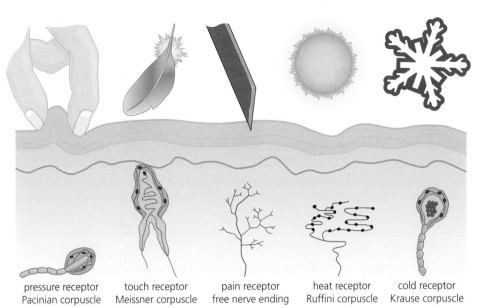

| pressure receptor Pacinian corpuscle | touch receptor Meissner corpuscle | pain receptor free nerve ending | heat receptor Ruffini corpuscle | cold receptor Krause corpuscle |

Nerve endings The dermis contains different types of sensory nerve endings, which interpret the sensations of touch, pressure, pain and temperature. These send messages to the central nervous system and the brain, informing us about the outside world and what is happening on the skin's surface. The appearance of each of these nerve endings is quite varied, as illustrated. The sensory nerve endings in the skin cause us to have a reflex, involuntary action to unpleasant stimuli protecting the skin from injury.

Growth and repair The body's blood system of arteries and veins continually brings blood to the capillary networks in the skin and takes it away again. The blood carries the nutrients and oxygen essential for the skin's health, maintenance and growth, and takes away waste products.

If the skin is damaged, it repairs itself. Blood transports repair cells to the site of the injury. These blood cells then form a clot, which dries and prevents infection from germs entering the skin. Collagen fibres are secreted by fibroblast cells in the dermis, which bind the surface of the wound together. Epithelial cells of the dermis cover the wound underneath the clot. The clot or scab is lost. The cells of the dermis grow upwards until the skin's thickness is restored.

Defence Within the dermis are the structures responsible for protecting the skin from harmful foreign bodies and irritants.

One set of cells, the mast cells, burst when stimulated during inflammation or allergic reactions, and release a chemical substance called histamine. This causes the blood vessels nearby to enlarge, thereby bringing more blood to the site of the irritation to limit skin damage and begin repair.

Knowledge Check

How many layers form the epidermis of the skin? Name these layers in order, starting with the outermost layer. Refer to page 38 to help you.

HEALTH & SAFETY

Sunbathing When sunbathing, always protect the skin with an appropriate protective sunscreen product according to skin type and natural hair/skin colouring. After UV exposure, always use an emollient aftersun preparation to minimize the cumulative effects of premature ageing, by rehydrating and soothing the skin.

ALWAYS REMEMBER

Sensory nerve endings

Sensory nerve endings are most numerous in sensitive parts of the skin, such as the fingertips and the lips.

Knowledge Check

What is the function of fibroblast cells?

Name two protein fibres found in the skin.

What does each protein provide the skin with?

In the dermis, what is this dense network of protein fibres called?

Refer to pages 41–42 to help you.

TOP TIP

Moisturizers

Cosmetic moisturizers mimic sebum in providing a protective, oily covering for the skin's surface to reduce moisture loss.

Knowledge Check

What happens at the keratinization zone of the epidermis? Which three layers of the skin make up this zone? Refer to page 38 to help you.

In the blood, and also in the lymph and the connective tissue, are another group of cells: the macrophages or 'big eaters'. These destroy microorganisms and engulf dead cells and other unwanted particles. When necessary, they travel to an area where they are needed, for example, the site of an infection. They form a role in the immune system that protects the body from disease-causing microorganisms.

Collecting waste Lymph vessels in the skin carry a fluid called lymph, a straw-coloured fluid similar in composition to blood plasma. Plasma is the liquid part of the blood that disperses from the blood capillaries into the tissue spaces. Lymph is composed of water, lymphocytes (a type of white blood cell that plays a key role in the immune system), oxygen, nutrients, hormones, salts and waste products. The waste products are removed and usable protein is recycled for further use by the body. Lymph acts as a link between the blood and the cells.

Control of skin functioning Hormones are chemical messengers transported in the blood. They control the activity of many organs in the body, including the cells and glands in the skin. These include melanosomes, cells which produce skin pigment (melanin), and the sweat glands and sebaceous glands.

Hormone imbalance at different times of our life may disturb the normal functioning of these cells and structures, causing various skin disorders.

Skin appendages Within the dermis are structures called skin appendages. These include:

◆ sweat glands

◆ sebaceous glands

◆ hair follicles, which produce hair

◆ nails.

Sweat glands Sweat glands or sudoriferous glands are composed of epithelial tissue, a specialized lining tissue which extends from the epidermis into the dermis. These glands are found all over the body, but are particularly plentiful on the palms of the hands and the soles of the feet. Their function is to regulate body temperature through the evaporation of sweat from the surface of the skin. Fluid loss and control of body temperature are important to prevent the body overheating, especially in hot, humid climates. For this reason, perhaps, sweat glands are larger and more abundant in black skins than white skins as a result of evolution.

TOP TIP

Pores

Pores allow the absorption of some facial cosmetics into the skin. Many facial treatments are therefore aimed at cleansing the pores, some with a particularly deep cleansing action, as with *cosmetic cleansers* and *facial masks*.

The pores may become enlarged due to congestion caused by dirt, poor skincare routine, dead skin cells, cosmetics and ageing. The application of an *exfoliating* and *astringent* skincare preparation creates deep cleansing and a tightening effect upon the skin's surface, slightly reducing the size of the pores.

An eccrine sweat gland

Apocrine gland

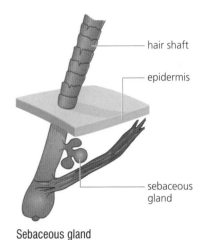

Sebaceous gland

There are two types of sweat glands: *eccrine glands* and *apocrine glands*. **Eccrine glands** are simple sweat-producing glands, found over most of the body, appearing as tiny tubes (ducts). The eccrine glands are responsive to heat. They are straight in the epidermis, and coiled in the dermis. The duct opens directly onto the surface of the skin through an opening called a pore.

Eccrine glands continuously secrete small amounts of sweat, even when we appear not to be perspiring. In this way they maintain the body temperature at a constant 36.8–37°C.

Apocrine glands are found in the underarm, the nipples and the groin area. This kind of gland is larger than the eccrine gland, and is attached to a hair follicle. Apocrine glands are controlled by hormones, becoming active at puberty. They also increase in activity when we are excited, nervous or stressed. The fluid they secrete is thicker than that from the eccrine glands, and may contain urea, fats, sugars and small amounts of protein. Also present are traces of aromatic molecules called pheromones, which are thought to cause sexual attraction between individuals.

An unpleasant smell – body odour – develops when apocrine sweat is broken down by skin bacteria. Good habits of personal hygiene will prevent this.

Cosmetic perspiration control
To maintain hygiene protection during the day, apply either a deodorant or an antiperspirant. Antiperspirants reduce the amount of sweat that reaches the skin's surface: they have an astringent action which closes the pores. Deodorants contain an active antiseptic ingredient which reduces the skin's bacterial activity, thereby reducing the risk of odour from stale sweat.

Sebaceous glands
The sebaceous gland appears as a minute sac-like organ. Usually it is associated with the hair follicle with which it forms the **pilo-sebaceous unit**, but the two can appear independently.

HEALTH & SAFETY

Antiperspirants The active ingredient in most antiperspirant products is the chemical aluminium chlorohydrate. This is known to cause contact dermatitis in some people, especially if the skin has been damaged by recent removal of unwanted hair. Bear this in mind if you are performing an underarm depilatory wax treatment. (See the aftercare instructions, page 552.)

Sebaceous glands are found all over the body, except on the palms of the hands and the soles of the feet. They are particularly numerous on the scalp, the forehead, and in the back and chest region. The cells of the glands decompose, producing the skin's natural oil, sebum. This empties directly into the hair follicle.

The activity of the sebaceous gland increases at puberty, when stimulated by the male hormone androgen. In adults, activity of the sebaceous gland gradually decreases again. Men secrete slightly more sebum than women; and on black skin the sebaceous glands are larger and more numerous than on white skin.

Emotions and their effect upon the skin

Emotions can affect blood supply to the skin: blood vessels in the dermis may enlarge or constrict. The sebaceous glands may become more active with the skin becoming oilier. This may lead to skin blemishes such as pustules and papules. Tension can lead to muscle fatigue and the appearance of frown lines and lines appearing as a result of tension, e.g. around the mouth. Think of different emotions, and how these might affect the appearance of the skin.

At the consultation, if somebody has had a period of stress the effect of this can often be seen in the appearance of the skin. Stress is often asked about when completing the consultation, e.g. asking the client how stressed they feel on a scale of 1-5, not very, to very stressed.

Many beauty therapy treatments have a relaxation benefit which when linked to good client care and communication will improve the feeling of well-being.

Happy client

Sebum is composed of fatty acids and waxes. These have bactericidal and fungicidal properties, and so discourage the multiplication of microorganisms on the surface of the skin. Sebum also reduces the evaporation of moisture from the skin, and so prevents the skin from drying out.

Acid mantle   Sweat and sebum combine on the skin's surface, creating an acid film. This is known as the **acid mantle** and is beneficial as it discourages the growth of bacteria and fungi.

Acidity and alkalinity are measured by a number called the pH. An *acidic solution* has a pH of 0–6.9; a *neutral solution* has a pH of 7; and an *alkaline solution* has a pH of 7.1–14. The acid mantle of the skin has a pH of 5.5–5.6.

Subcutaneous layer   Beneath the dermis lies the subcutaneous layer made up of adipose (fat) tissue. It is supplied with a network of arteries that run parallel to the skin's surface. Fat cells are called adipocytes and contain droplets of fat.

HEALTH & SAFETY

Moisture balance Excessive sweating, which can occur through exposure to high temperatures or during illness, can lead to *skin dehydration* – insufficient water content. Fluid intake must be increased to rebalance the body fluids. Skincare products and routines should be changed to ensure that the skin is rehydrated.

HEALTH & SAFETY

Skin problems are common at puberty when changes in hormone levels cause sebaceous glands to produce excess sebum and the skin's surface becomes oily. Growth of skin bacteria can increase in the sebum causing inflammation of the surrounding tissues. This can lead to the skin disorder acne vulgaris see page 54. The skin should always be kept clean and handled with clean hands.

HEALTH & SAFETY

The lips Sebaceous glands are not present on the surface of the lips. For this reason in all seasons the lips should be protected with a lip emollient preparation to prevent them from becoming dry and chapped. To reduce the effect of premature skin ageing it is beneficial for the product to also contain UV SPF ingredients.

HEALTH & SAFETY

Care using alkaline products
Because the skin has an acid pH, if alkaline products are used on it the acid mantle will be disturbed. It will take several hours for this protective film to be restored; during this time, the skin will be irritated and sensitive.

The fatty layer has a protective function and:

◆ acts as an insulator to conserve body heat, keeping you warm

◆ cushions muscles and bones below from injury

◆ acts as an energy source, as excess fat is stored in this layer.

Knowledge Check

Name each part of the skin's structure shown in the figure. Refer to page 37 & 38 to help you.

Knowledge Check

How do the following structures help to defend the skin from harm?

◆ Mast cells

◆ Macrophages

Refer to pages 43–44 to help you.

Skin diseases and disorders

Having learnt about the skin, hair and nails, the beauty therapist must be able to distinguish healthy skin, hair and nails, from those suffering from disease, disorder or a parasitic condition. Certain disorders, diseases and parasitic conditions prevent treatment: going ahead, would put the beauty therapist and clients at risk of cross-infection through direct or indirect contact. It is therefore necessary that you are familiar with the appearance of skin, hair and nail diseases and disorders which you might come into contact with in the workplace, both those that are a risk and those that are not, and the correct action to take. These are discussed here with relevant diseases, disorders and parasitic conditions also discussed in each treatment chapter.

TOP TIP

Did you know?

The visible changes to the skin which are caused by injury or disease affecting its texture, colour or shape are often referred to as lesions. Examples of lesions include blisters, scales, crust, pustules and papules.

It is important to recognize the different types of skin lesions.

Remember, you cannot always see the symptom of a disorder or disease, there are the sensations that can be felt such as itching, heat and pain.

Impetigo

Bacterial infections

Bacteria are minute single-celled organisms of varied shapes. Large numbers of bacteria live on the surface of the skin which are harmless (non-pathogenic); with some playing an important positive role in the health of the skin. Others, however, are harmful, referred to as pathogenic and can cause disease.

Impetigo An inflammatory disease of the surface of the skin, usually appearing on exposed areas.

Infectious? Yes.

Appearance: Initially the skin appears red and feels itchy. Small thin-walled blisters appear; which burst and form honey-coloured crusts. Untreated small pus-filled ulcers can occur with a dark, thick crust which can lead to scarring.

Site: The commonly affected areas are the nose, the mouth and the ears, but impetigo can also occur on the scalp and limbs.

Treatment: Medical – usually an antibiotic or an antibacterial ointment is prescribed containing corticosteroids such as hydrocortisone as the infection can spread quickly.

Conjunctivitis or pink eye Inflammation of the conjunctiva, the mucous membrane that covers the eye and lines the eyelids.

Infectious? Yes.

Appearance: The skin of the inner conjunctiva of the eye becomes inflamed and the eye becomes very red and feels sore with the sensation of itchiness and as if grit is in the eye. Water and pus may exude from the area leaving a sticky coating on the lashes.

Site: The eyes, either one or both, may be infected.

skin of inner conjunctiva is inflamed

Conjunctivitis or pink eye

eyelash hair follicles become inflamed and contain pus

Hordeolum or styes

Treatment: Medical – usually an antibiotic lotion is prescribed. However, in some cases medical treatment will not be necessary and the infection will heal independently.

Hordeolum or styes

Infection of the sebaceous glands of eyelash hair follicles. It can also be an effect of **blepharitis** (inflammation of the eyelids).

Infectious? Yes.

Appearance: Small red, inflamed lumps containing pus, a sign of infection.

Site: The inner rim of the eyelid.

Treatment: Medical – usually an antibiotic is prescribed.

Furuncles or boils

Infection affecting the hair follicle.

Infectious? Yes.

Appearance: A localized red lump appears around a hair follicle; this then develops a core of pus, yellowish-white fluid formed in infected tissue. Scarring of the skin often remains after the boil has healed.

Site: The back of the neck, the armpits and buttocks and thighs are common areas, but furuncles can occur anywhere.

Treatment: Medical – antibiotics may be prescribed to help control infection.

Carbuncles

Infection of several hair follicles.

Infectious? Yes.

Appearance: A hard, round abscess, larger than a boil, which oozes pus from several points upon its surface. Scarring often occurs after the carbuncle has healed.

Site: In particular occurring where there is friction, such as the back of the neck, or on the thighs. However, they can occur anywhere.

Treatment: Medical – usually involving incision of the skin, drainage of the pus, and a course of antibiotics.

Paronychia

Infection of the skin tissue surrounding the nail (the nail fold). If left untreated, the nail bed may also become infected.

Infectious? Yes.

Appearance: Swelling, redness and pus appears in the nail fold and the area of the nail wall.

Site: The skin surrounding the nail plate.

Treatment: Medical – usually a course of antibiotics, incision and drainage of pus is necessary if it collects in the skin next to the nail plate.

Viral infections

Viruses are minute bodies, too small to see even under an ordinary microscope. They are considered to be parasites, as they require living tissue in order to survive. Viruses invade healthy body cells and multiply within the cell: in due course the cell walls break down, releasing new viral particles to attack further cells, spreading the infection.

localised red lump surrounding a hair follicle indicating infection

Furuncle or boil

HEALTH & SAFETY

Furuncles (boils) Furuncles (boils) occurring on the upper lip or in the nose should be referred immediately to a GP as the infection can be dangerous when near to the eyes or brain.

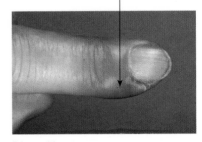

swelling, redness and pus surrounding the nail plate

Paronychia

Herpes simplex

Herpes simplex This is commonly referred to as a cold sore and a recurring skin condition, appearing at times when the skin's resistance is lowered through ill-health or stress. It may also be caused by exposure of the skin to extremes of temperature or to UV light.

Infectious? Yes.

Appearance: Inflammation of the skin occurs in localized areas. As well as being red, the skin becomes itchy and small vesicles (blisters) appear. These are followed by a crust, which may crack and weep tissue fluid.

Site: The mucous membranes of the nose or lips; herpes simplex can also occur on the skin generally.

Treatment: There is no specific treatment, they usually clear in 7–10 days. A proprietary brand of anti-inflammatory antiseptic drying cream is usually prescribed, which must be applied in the early stages of the condition when a tingling, itching sensation is experienced.

Herpes zoster or shingles Caused by the chickenpox virus. In this painful disease, the virus attacks the sensory nerve endings and is thought to lie dormant (inactive) in the body and be triggered when the body's defences are lowered.

Infectious? Yes.

Appearance: Redness of the skin occurs along a line of the affected nerves. Blisters develop and form crusts, leaving purplish-pink pigmentation.

Site: Commonly the chest and the abdomen.

Herpes zoster or shingles

Treatment: Medical – usually including anti-viral medicines. Calamine lotion can soothe the irritation. If there are complications with bacterial infection, antibiotics will be prescribed.

Verrucae or warts Small epidermal skin growths. Warts can be raised or flat, depending upon their position. There are several types of wart: plane, common, plantar and mosaic.

Infectious? Yes.

Appearance: Warts vary in size, shape, texture and colour. Usually they have a rough surface and are raised. If a wart occurs on the sole of the foot it grows inwards, due to the pressure of body weight.

Verruca – plantar wart

A plane wart

Site:

◆ Plane wart (flat wart): the fingers, either surface of the hand, face and legs

◆ Common wart (verruca vulgaris): the hands, elbows and knees

◆ Plantar wart (verrucae): the sole of the foot and toes

◆ Mosaic (palmar warts): hands and feet.

Treatment: Medical – using acids, i.e. salicylic acid, solid carbon dioxide (cryotherapy) or electrocautery.

Infestations

An infestation is where animal parasites live off and invade the host's tissue to gain all their nutrients.

Scabies or itch mites (sarcoptes scabiei)
A condition in which an **infestation** of a tiny parasitic mite burrows beneath the skin and invades the hair follicles. The mite feeds on tissue and fluid as it burrows into the skin.

Infectious? Yes.

Appearance: Initially, minute papules and wavy greyish lines appear, where dirt has entered the burrows. Secondary bacterial infection may occur as a result of scratching the skin.

A scabies burrow

Site: Usually seen in warm areas of loose skin, such as the webs of the fingers, under the fingernails and the creases of the elbows.

Treatment: Medical – an anti-scabetic lotion containing an insecticide.

Pediculosis capitis or head lice
A condition in which small lice parasites infest scalp hair.

Infectious? Yes.

Appearance: The lice cling to the hair of the scalp. Eggs are laid, attached to the hair close to the skin. The lice bite the skin to draw nourishment from the blood; this creates irritation and itching of the skin, which may lead to secondary bacterial infection.

Site: The hair of the scalp.

Treatment: Medical – an appropriate medicated insecticide lotion or rinse.

Head lice

Pediculosis pubis or pubic lice
A condition in which small lice parasites infest body hair.

Infectious? Yes.

Appearance: The lice cling to the hair of the body. Eggs are laid, attached to the hair close to the skin. The lice bite the skin to draw nourishment from the blood; this creates irritation and itching of the skin, which may lead to secondary bacterial infection.

Site: Pubic hair, eyebrows and eyelashes.

Treatment: Medical – an appropriate insecticidal lotion.

Tinea pedis or athlete's foot

Pediculosis corporis or body lice A condition in which small parasites live and feed on body skin.

Infectious? Yes.

Appearance: The lice cling to the hair of the body. Eggs are laid, attached to the hair close to the skin. The lice bite the skin to draw nourishment from the blood; this creates irritation and itching of the skin, which may lead to secondary bacterial infection. Where body lice bite the skin, small red marks can be seen.

Site: Body hair.

Treatment: Medical – an appropriate insecticidal lotion.

Fungal diseases

Fungi are microscopic plants. They are parasites, dependent upon a host for their existence. Fungal diseases of the skin feed off the waste products of the skin. Some fungi are found on the skin's surface; others attack the deeper tissues. Reproduction of fungi is by means of simple cell division or by the production of spores.

Tinea pedis or athlete's foot A common fungal foot infection.

Infectious? Yes.

Appearance: The skin can appear white and spongy-looking. Small blisters form, which later burst. The skin in the area can then become dry, crack and peel, giving a scaly appearance.

Site: Commonly affects the webs of skin between the toes.

Treatment: Thorough cleansing of the area. Medical application of fungicides. Untreated, infections such as bacterial infections may occur. It can also lead to infection of the toe and fingernails.

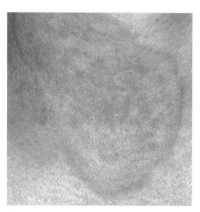

Tinea corporis or body ringworm

Tinea corporis or body ringworm A fungal infection of the skin.

Infectious? Yes.

Appearance: Small scaly red patches, which spread outwards and then heal from the centre, leaving a ring.

Site: The trunk of the body, the limbs and the face.

Treatment: Medical – using a fungicidal cream. Oral anti-fungal medication is necessary if there are several infection sites.

Tinea unguium or onychomycosis Ringworm infection of the fingernails.

Infectious? Yes.

Appearance: The nail plate is white and opaque. Eventually the nail plate becomes brittle, and can crumble and separate from the nail bed.

Tinea unguium

HEALTH & SAFETY

Artificial nails and nail fungus Artificial nails can increase the risk of developing fungal infection due to the natural nail plate being roughened and if not maintained correctly moisture can collect between the artificial nail and the natural nail plate which provides ideal growth for fungi. It is important that the client understands the importance of complying with aftercare advice provided.

Site: The nail plate.

Treatment: Medical application of fungicides.

Sebaceous gland disorders

The sebaceous glands produce sebum, the skin's natural oil which has bactericidal and antifungal properties. This helps to keep the skin healthy and also to prevent the skin from drying out.

They are also the cause of the following disorders:

Milia Keratinization of the skin over the hair follicle occurs, causing sebum to build up in the hair follicle. This condition usually accompanies a dry skin.

Infectious? No.

Appearance: Small, hard, pearly white cysts.

Site: The upper face or close to the eyes.

Treatment: The milium may be removed by a beauty therapist (if qualified to do so) or by a GP, depending on the location. A sterile lancet is used to pierce the skin of the overlying cuticle and thereby free the milium. Micro-dermabrasion may be used to avoid their development. Also retinoid creams may be applied which remove the outer epidermal layers.

Comedones or blackheads Excess sebum and keratinized cells block the mouth or opening of the hair follicle.

Infectious? No.

Site: The skin of the face (the chin, nose and forehead), the upper back and chest.

Treatment: The area should be cleansed and a pre-heating treatment such as an electrical vapour treatment should be given to relax the opening of the hair follicle; a sterile comedo extractor can then be used to remove the blockage. A regular cleansing treatment and use of appropriate skincare products such as exfoliating treatments should be recommended by the beauty therapist to control the production of further comedones.

Seborrhoea Excessive secretion of sebum from the sebaceous gland, resulting in an excessively oily skin. This skin disorder usually occurs during puberty, as a result of hormonal changes occurring in the body.

Infectious? No.

Appearance: The hair follicle openings enlarge and excessive sebum is secreted. The skin appears coarse and oily; comedones, pustules and papules are present.

Site: The face and scalp. Seborrhoea may also affect the back and the chest.

Treatment: The area should be cleansed to remove the excess sebum. Deep cleansing treatments are required, including exfoliation and cleansing **masks**. Medical treatment may be required – this would use locally applied steroid creams.

Steatomas, sebaceous cysts or wens Localized pockets or sacs of sebum, which form in hair follicles or the sebaceous glands in the skin. The outlet becomes blocked and the sebaceous gland becomes enlarged, appearing as a lump on the skin.

Milia on the eyelid

Go to **CHAPTER 7** for more information on extraction.

Comedones or blackheads

Seborrhoeic skin

HEALTH & SAFETY

Open skin lesions If the skin is broken, treatment is contra-indicated as the skin may become infected. This is referred to as secondary infection.

Sebaceous cyst

Scarring shown following
skin healing on a skin
suffering from acne vulgaris

Acne vulgaris

Rosacea

Infectious? No.

Appearance: Semi-globular in shape, and the tissue in the area may feel hard or soft. The cysts are the same colour as the skin, or red if secondary bacterial infection occurs. A comedo can often be seen at the original opening of the hair follicle.

Site: If the cyst appears on the upper eyelid, it is known as a chalazion or meibomian cyst. If it appears on the scalp it is known as a pilar cyst.

Treatment: Medical – often a GP will remove the cyst under local anaesthetic. Small inflamed cysts can be medically treated with steroid medications or antibiotics.

Acne vulgaris
Hormone imbalance in the body at puberty influences the activity of the sebaceous gland, causing an increased production of sebum. The sebum may be retained within the sebaceous ducts causing congestion and possibly leading to bacterial infection of the surrounding tissues.

Infectious? No.

Appearance: Inflammation of the skin, accompanied by comedones, pustules, papules and possibly cysts. Scarring of the skin can be associated with this skin disorder following skin healing after bacterial infection.

Site: Facial acne vulgaris commonly affects the skin on the face, the nose, the chin and the forehead. Acne vulgaris may also occur on other parts of the body such as the chest and back.

Treatment: Medical – oral antibiotics may be prescribed, as well as medicated antibiotic skin preparations. Other preparations which may be prescribed aim to unblock the skin and destroy bacteria. With medical approval, regular salon treatments may be given to cleanse the skin deeply and also to stimulate the blood circulation to promote skin healing.

Rosacea
Excessive sebum secretion combined with a chronic inflammatory condition, caused by dilation of the superficial blood capillaries, their appearance is referred to as telangiectasis.

Infectious? No.

Appearance: The skin becomes coarse, the pores enlarge and the cheek and nose area become inflamed, sometimes swelling and producing a butterfly pattern. Blood circulation slows in the dilated capillaries, creating a purplish appearance. Pustules and papules may also be present in severe cases.

Treatment: Medical – usually including antibiotics.

Pigmentation disorders

Pigmentation of the skin varies, according to each person's genetic characteristics. In general, the darker the skin, the more pigment (melanin) is present, but some abnormal changes in skin pigmentation can occur.

◆ **Hyperpigmentation** – is caused by increased pigment production, seen as darker areas of skin or dark patches.

◆ **Hypopigmentation** – is caused by loss of pigmentation in the skin, seen as lighter areas of skin or white patches.

TOP TIP

Did you know?

Hypopigmentation may result from certain skin injuries, disorders or diseases.

The following disorders relate to changes in pigmentation in the skin:

Ephelides or freckles Multiple, small hyperpigmented areas of the skin. Exposure to UV light (as in sunlight) stimulates the production of melanin, intensifying their appearance.

Infectious? No.

Appearance: Small, flat, pigmented areas, darker than the surrounding skin.

Site: Commonly the nose and cheeks of fair-skinned people. Freckles may also occur on the shoulders, arms, hands and back.

Treatment: Freckles may be concealed with cosmetics if required. A sunblock or high Sun Protection Factor (SPF) sunscreen should be recommended, to prevent them intensifying in colour.

Ephelides or freckles

Lentigo (plural, lentigines) Hyperpigmented areas of skin, slightly larger than freckles. Lentigo simplex occurs in childhood. Actinic (solar) lentigines are related to age and occur in middle age as a result of sun exposure.

Infectious? No.

Appearance: Brown, slightly raised, pigmented patches of skin, of variable size.

Site: The face, hands and shoulders.

Treatment: Application of cosmetic **camouflage products**.

Lentigo

Chloasmata or liver spots Hyperpigmentation in specific areas, stimulated by a skin irritant such as UV light, usually affecting women and darkly pigmented skins. The condition often occurs during pregnancy and usually disappears soon after the birth of the baby. It may also occur as a result of taking the oral contraceptive pill. The female hormone oestrogen is thought to stimulate melanin production.

Infectious? No.

Appearance: Flat, smooth, irregularly shaped, pigmented areas of skin, varying in colour from light tan to dark brown. Chloasmata are larger than ephelides, and of variable size.

Site: The back of the hands, the forearms, the upper part of the chest, the temples and the forehead.

Treatment: A barrier cream or a total sunblock will reduce the risk of the chloasmata increasing in size or number and thereby becoming more apparent.

Chloasmata or liver spots

Dermatosis papulosa nigra Often called flesh moles, these are characterized by multiple benign, small brown to black hyperpigmented papules, common among dark-skinned people.

Infectious? No.

Appearance: Raised pigmented markings resembling moles.

Site: Usually seen on the cheeks and forehead, although they may appear on the neck, upper chest and back.

Treatment: Medical by medication or surgery.

Vitiligo or leucoderma Patches of completely white skin which have lost their pigment, or which were never pigmented.

Infectious? No.

Vitiligo or leucoderma

Appearance: Well-defined patches of white skin, lacking pigment.

Site: The face, the neck, the hands, the lower abdomen and the thighs. If vitiligo occurs over the eyebrows, the hairs in the area will also lose their pigment.

Treatment: Camouflage cosmetic **concealer** can be applied to give even skin colour; or skin-staining preparations can be used in the de-pigmented areas. Care must be taken when the skin is exposed to UV light, as the skin will not have the same protection in the areas lacking pigment.

Albinism   The skin is unable to produce the melanin pigment and the skin, hair and eyes are affected too, and lack colour, but the eyes are often pale blue, as shown.

Albinism

Infectious? No.

Appearance: The skin is usually very pale pink or white and the hair is white. The eyes also are pink in colour and extremely sensitive to light.

Site: The entire skin.

Treatment: There is no effective treatment. Maximum skin protection is necessary when the client is exposed to UV light and sunglasses should be worn to protect the eyes.

Vascular (circulatory) disorders

There are two types of naevus of concern to beauty therapists: vascular and cellular.

Vascular naevi   These are skin conditions in which small or large areas of skin pigmentation are caused by the permanent dilation of blood capillaries.

Cellular naevi   Are skin conditions where changes in the cells of the skin result in skin malformations.

Erythema   An area of skin in which there is an increase in blood to the area, causing the blood capillaries to dilate. The cause can be due either to injury or inflammation as the body's immune system responds to infection or irritation.

Infectious? No.

Appearance: The skin appears red.

Site: Erythema may affect one area (locally) or all of the skin (generally).

Treatment: The cause of the inflammation should be identified. In the case of a **skin allergy**, the client must not be brought into contact with the irritant again. If the cause is unknown, refer the client to their GP.

Dilated capillaries or telangiectasis   Blood capillaries near the surface of the skin that are permanently dilated.

Infectious? No.

Appearance: Small red visible blood capillaries.

Site: Areas where the skin is neglected, dry or fine, such as the cheek area.

TOP TIP

Vascular circulatory disorders

If there is a vascular skin disorder, avoid over-stimulating the skin or the problem will become more noticeable and the treatment may even cause further damage.

Treatment: Dilated capillaries can be concealed using a green corrective camouflage cosmetic, or removed by a qualified beauty therapist using advanced electrologist techniques with diathermy or laser.

Spider naevi or stellate haemangiomas
Dilated blood vessels, with smaller dilated capillaries radiating from them.

Infectious? No.

Appearance: Small red capillaries, radiating like a spider's legs from a central point.

Site: Commonly the cheek area, but may occur on the upper body, the arms and the neck. Spider naevi are usually caused by an injury to the skin.

Treatment: Spider naevi can be concealed using a camouflage cosmetic, or removed by a qualified beauty therapist using advanced electrologist techniques with diathermy or laser.

Spider naevus or stellate haemangiomas

Naevi vasculosis or strawberry marks
Red or purplish raised irregular shaped marks which appear on the skin at birth.

Infectious? No.

Appearance: Red or purplish lobed mark, of any size.

Site: Any area of the skin.

Treatment: About 60 per cent disappear by the age of 6 years. Treatment is not usually necessary; concealing camouflage cosmetics can be applied if desired. A sunblock is also recommended.

Naevi vasculosis or strawberry marks

Capillary naevi or port-wine stains
Large areas of dilated capillaries that contrast noticeably with the surrounding areas.

Infectious? No.

Appearance: The naevus has a smooth flat surface.

Site: Some 75 per cent occur on the head; they are probably formed at the foetal stage. Naevi may also be found on other body areas.

Treatment: Concealing camouflage cosmetic can be applied to disguise the area.

Capillary naevi or port-wine stains

Cellular naevi or moles

Cellular naevi are skin conditions where changes in the cells of the skin result in skin malformations.

Malignant melanomas or malignant moles Rapidly-growing skin cancers, usually occurring in adults.

Infectious? No.

Appearance: Each melanoma commences as a bluish-black mole, which enlarges rapidly, darkening in colour and developing a halo of pigmentation around it. It later becomes raised, bleeds and ulcerates. Secondary growths will develop in internal organs if the melanoma is not treated.

Site: Usually the lower abdomen, legs or feet.

Treatment: Medical – always recommend that a client has a mole checked if it is changing in size, structure or colour, or if it becomes itchy or bleeds.

Junction naevi Localized collections of naevoid cells that arise from the mass production locally of pigment-forming cells (melanocytes).

Infectious? No.

Appearance: In childhood junction naevi appear as smooth or slightly raised pigmented marks. They vary in colour from brown to black.

Site: Any area.

Treatment: None. Camouflage make-up can be used to conceal the area and the application of sunblock can prevent further pigmentation or skin darkening.

Malignant melanoma

Guidance images for moles

Normal Mole	Melanoma	Sign	Characteristic
		Asymmetry	When half of the mole does not match the other half
		Border	When the border (edges) of the mole are ragged or irregular
		Colour	When the colour of the mole varies throughout
		Diameter	If the mole's diameter is larger than a pencil's eraser

Dermal naevi Localized collections of naevoid cells.

Infectious? No.

Appearance: About 1 cm wide, dermal naevi appear smooth and dome-shaped. Their colour ranges from skin tone to dark brown. Frequently one or more hairs may grow from the naevus.

Site: Usually the face.

Treatment: None.

Hairy naevi Moles exhibiting coarse hairs from their surface.

Infectious? No.

Appearance: Slightly raised moles, varying in size from 3 cm to much larger. Colour ranges from fawn to dark brown.

Site: Anywhere on the skin.

Treatment: Hairy naevi may be surgically removed where possible and this is often done for cosmetic reasons. Hair growing from a mole should be cut, not plucked: if plucked, the hair will become coarser and the growth of further hairs may be stimulated.

Skin disorders involving abnormal cellular growth

Psoriasis Patches of itchy, red, flaky skin, the cause of which is unknown.

Infectious? No. Secondary infection with bacteria can occur if the skin becomes broken and dirt enters the skin.

Appearance: Red patches of skin appear, covered in waxy, silvery scales. Bleeding will occur if the area is scratched and scales are removed.

Site: The elbows, the knees, the lower back and the scalp.

Treatment: There is no known **cure**. Medication including steroid creams can bring relief to the symptoms. Medically administered UV treatment is also found to be beneficial.

Benign naevus

Psoriasis

Seborrhoeic or senile warts

Seborrhoeic or senile warts
Raised, pigmented, benign tumours occurring from middle age.

Infectious? No.

Appearance: Slightly raised, brown or black, rough patches of skin. Such warts can be confused with pigmented moles.

Site: The trunk, the scalp and the temples.

Treatment: Medical – the warts can be cauterized where the tissue is destroyed using heat or cold by a GP.

Verrucae filliformis or skin tags

Verrucae filliformis or skin tags
These verrucae appear as threads projecting from the skin.

Infectious? No.

Appearance: Skin-coloured threads of skin 3–6 mm long.

Site: Mainly seen on the neck and the eyelids, but may occur in other areas such as under the arms.

Treatment: Medical – removal using cauterization with advanced electrologist technique using diathermy, either by a GP or by a qualified electrologist.

Xanthomas
Small yellow growths appearing upon the surface of the skin made up of cholesterol deposits.

Infectious? No.

Appearance: A yellow flat or raised area of skin with distinct edges.

Site: Common on the eyelids, but can appear anywhere on the body.

Treatment: Medical – the growth is thought to be connected with certain medical diseases, such as diabetes or high or low blood pressure. Sometimes a low-fat diet can correct the condition.

Keloid

Keloids
Keloids occur following skin injury and are overgrown abnormal scar tissue which spreads, characterized by excess deposits of collagen. To avoid skin discoloration the keloid must be protected from UV exposure.

Infectious? No.

Appearance: The skin tends to be red, raised, shiny and ridged.

Site: Located over the site of a wound or other lesion.

Treatment: Medical by drug therapy, such as cortisone injection, or surgery.

Malignant tumours

Squamous cell carcinomas or prickle-cell cancers
Malignant growths originating in the epidermis.

Infectious? No.

Appearance: When fully formed, the carcinoma appears as a raised area of skin.

Squamous cell carcinoma

Site: Anywhere on the skin.

Treatment: Includes surgical removal, also radiotherapy (treatment with X-ray) or treatment with drugs as necessary.

Basal cell carcinomas or rodent ulcers Slow-growing malignant tumours, occurring in middle age.

Infectious? No.

Appearance: A small, shiny, waxy nodule with a depressed centre. The disease extends, with more nodules appearing on the border of the original ulcer.

Site: Usually on the face.

Treatment: Includes surgical removal, also radiotherapy (treatment with X-ray) or treatment with drugs as necessary.

Basal cell carcinomas

Skin allergies

The skin can protect itself to some degree from damage or invasion. Mast cells detect damage to the skin; if damage occurs, the mast cells burst, releasing the chemical histamine into the tissues. Histamine causes the blood capillaries to dilate, giving the reddening we call 'erythema'. The increased blood flow transports materials in blood which tend to limit the damage and begin repair.

If the skin is sensitive and becomes inflamed on contact with a particular substance, this substance is called an allergen. Allergens may be animal, chemical or vegetable substances, and they can be inhaled, eaten or absorbed following contact with the skin. An allergic skin reaction appears as irritation, itching and discomfort, with reddening and swelling (as with nettle rash). If the allergen is removed, the allergic reaction subsides.

Allergic reaction to nickel body jewellery

Each individual has different tolerances to the various substances we encounter in daily life. What causes an allergic reaction in one individual may be perfectly harmless to another.

Allergic reaction to an ingredient in hair dye

Allergic reaction to an antiperspirant

Contact dermatitis

Here are just a few examples of allergens known to cause allergic skin reactions in some people:

◆ metal objects containing nickel

◆ sticking plaster

◆ rubber

◆ lipstick containing eosin dye

◆ nail polish containing formaldehyde resin

◆ hair and eyelash dyes

◆ lanolin, a skin moisturizing agent

◆ detergents that dry the skin

◆ foods – well-known examples are nut oils, cow's milk, lobster, shellfish and strawberries

◆ plants such as tulips and chrysanthemums.

Dermatitis

Dermatitis An inflammatory skin disorder in which the skin become red, itchy and swollen. There are two types of dermatitis. In *primary dermatitis* the skin is irritated by the action of a substance on the skin, and this leads to skin inflammation. In *allergic contact dermatitis*, the problem is caused by intolerance of the skin to a particular substance or groups of substances. On exposure to the substance the skin quickly becomes irritated and an allergic reaction occurs.

Infectious? No.

Appearance: Reddening and swelling of the skin, with the possible appearance of blisters.

Site: If the skin reacts to a skin irritant outside the body, the reaction is localized. Repeated contact with the allergen will lead to a general hypersensitivity. If the irritant gains entry to the body it will be transported in the bloodstream and may cause a general allergic skin reaction.

Treatment: Moisturizing cream can be used to help prevent drying of the skin. Personal protective equipment should be worn in the case of occupational hazards, i.e. gloves should be worn by a hairdresser (non-latex as this can cause allergic reactions), to avoid developing contact dermatitis due to the hazards in the nature of the work, like contact with water for long periods. When an allergic dermatitis reaction occurs, the only '**cure**' is the absolute avoidance of the substance. Steroid creams such as hydrocortisone are usually prescribed, to soothe the damaged skin and reduce the irritation.

Eczema Inflammation of the skin caused by contact, internally or externally, with an irritant.

Infectious? No.

Appearance: Reddening of the skin, with swelling and blisters. The blisters leak tissue fluid which later hardens, forming scabs.

Site: The face, the neck and the skin, particularly at the inner creases of the elbows and behind the knees.

Eczema

Treatment: If the area is small and the skin unbroken, treatment may go ahead, just avoid contact with the area. Refer the client to their GP. **Eczema** may disappear if the source of irritation is identified and removed. Steroid cream may be prescribed by the GP and special diets may help.

Urticaria (nettle rash) or hives A minor skin disorder caused by contact with an allergen, either internally (food or drugs) or externally (insect bites).

Infectious? No.

Appearance: Erythema with raised round whitish skin wheals. In some cases the lesions can cause intense burning or itching, a condition known as pruritis. Pruritis is a symptom of a disease (such as diabetes), not a disease itself.

Site: At the point of contact.

Treatment: Antihistamines may be prescribed to reduce the itching. The visible skin reaction usually disappears quickly leaving no trace. Complete avoidance of the allergen 'cures' the problem.

Urticaria (nettle rash) or hives

HEALTH & SAFETY

Hypoallergenic products The use of hypoallergenic products minimizes the risk of skin contact with likely irritants. Select these products for clients with skin allergies and hypersensitive skin.

Allergies You may suddenly become allergic to a substance that has previously been perfectly harmless. Equally, you may over time cease to be allergic to something.

Infection following allergy Following an allergic skin reaction in which the skin's surface has become itchy and broken, scratching may cause the skin to become infected with bacteria. This is referred to as a secondary infection.

The ears

The structure and function of the earlobe

The **external ear** collects sound waves and directs these to the inner ear. The part of the ear that is commonly seen pierced is called the pinna, which comprises the helix and lobule. The helix is composed of cartilage, which does not heal quickly, can be painful and can form lumpy, keloid type scar tissue; it is therefore considered unsuitable for piercing. The lobule, in contrast, consists of fibrous and fatty tissue with no cartilage, and is therefore suitable for piercing.

pinna

helix

lobule

The earlobe

The hair

The structure and function of hair and the surrounding tissues

A hair is a long, slender structure which grows out of, and is part of, the skin. Each hair is made up of dead skin cells, which contain the protein called keratin. Hairs cover the whole body, except for the palms of the hands, the soles of the feet, the lips and parts of the sex organs.

Hair has many functions:

◆ *scalp hair* insulates the head against cold, protects it from the sun and cushions it against bumps

◆ *eyebrows* cushion the brow bone from bumps, and prevent sweat from running into the eyes

◆ *eyelashes* help to prevent foreign particles entering the eyes

◆ *nostril hair* traps dust particles inhaled with the air

◆ *ear hair* helps to protect the ear canal. Hair cells in the inner ear send signals to the brain when the head moves, this information is used to help the body maintain balance.

◆ *body hair* helps to provide an insulating cover (though this function is almost obsolete in humans), has a valuable sensory function, and is linked with the secretion of sebum onto the surface of the skin. Terminal hair in the pubic and underarm areas has a purpose to protect the underlying glands and organs.

Hair also plays a role in social communication.

The structure of hair Most hairs are made up of three layers of different types of epithelial cells: the medulla, the cortex and the cuticle.

The medulla is the central core of the hair. The cells of the medulla contain soft keratin, and sometimes some pigment granules. Air spaces between the cells allow light to pass through giving a shiny appearance to the hair. The medulla only exists in medium to coarser hair – there is usually no medulla in thinner hair.

TOP TIP

Did you know?

There are approximately 100 000 hairs on the scalp.

TOP TIP

Did you know?

A strand of hair is stronger than an equivalent strand of nylon or copper. However, repeated chemical treatments weaken the hair. Consider this when booking appointments and allow the recommended intervals between each treatment.

The **cortex** is the thickest layer of the hair, and is made up of several layers of closely packed, elongated cells. These contain pigment granules and also hard keratin, giving the hair its strength.

It is the **pigment** in the cortex that gives hair its colour. When this pigment is no longer made, the hair appears white. As the proportion of white hairs rises, the hair seems to go 'grey'; in fact, however, each individual hair is either coloured as before, or white.

The **cuticle** is the protective outer layer of the hair, and is composed of a layer of thin, unpigmented, flat, scale-like cells. These contain hard keratin, and overlap each other from the base to the tip of the hair.

hair cuticle   cortex   medulla

Cross section of the hair

The parts of the hair and related skin

Each hair is recognized by three parts: the root, the bulb and the shaft:

◆ the root is the part of the hair that is in the follicle

◆ the bulb is the enlarged base of the root

◆ the shaft is the part of the hair that can be seen above the skin's surface.

Each hair grows out of a tube-like indentation in the epidermis, the **hair follicle**. The walls of the follicle are a continuation of the epidermal layer of the skin.

The **arrector pili muscle** is attached at an angle to the base of the follicle. Cold, aggression or fright stimulates this muscle to contract, pulling the follicle and the hair upright. This gives the skin a 'bumpy' appearance, often referred to as 'goosebumps'.

The **sebaceous gland** is attached to the upper part of the follicle; from it, the sebaceous duct enters directly into the hair follicle. The gland produces an oily substance, sebum, which is secreted into the follicle. Sebum waterproofs, lubricates and softens the hair and the surface of the skin; it also protects the skin against bacterial and fungal infections. The contraction of the arrector pili muscle aids the secretion of sebum.

ACTIVITY

The function of hair

Humans are not very hairy but their hairs sometimes stand on end! How does the appearance of skin change? What is the purpose of hair standing on end?

hair follicle

medulla (if present)
cortex   } hair shaft
cuticle

epidermis

arrector pili muscle

sebaceous gland

inner epithelial root sheath

outer epithelial root sheath

hair bulb

matrix

dermis

nerve supply

dermal papilla

Cross section of the skin, hair and hair follicle

The hair bulb

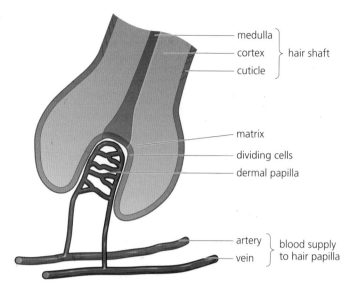

medulla ⎫
cortex ⎬ hair shaft
cuticle ⎭

matrix
dividing cells
dermal papilla

artery ⎫ blood supply
vein ⎭ to hair papilla

The **dermal papilla**, a connective tissue, is surrounded by the hair bulb. It provides an excellent blood supply, necessary to provide nutrition and hormones for the growth of the hair. It is not itself part of the follicle, but a separate tiny organ of blood capillaries which transports blood to the follicle.

The bulb is the expanded base of the hair root. A gap at the base leads to a cavity inside, which houses the dermal papilla. The bulb contains in its lower part the dividing cells that create the hair. The hair continues to develop as it passes through the regions of the upper bulb and the root.

The matrix is the name given to the lower part of the bulb, which comprises actively dividing hair germ cells from which the hair is formed. The hair germ cells grow downwards in a column called the dermal cord. The dermal cord surrounds the dermal papilla and when this occurs cellular changes cause a new hair to grow.

The hair follicle   The hair follicle extends into the dermis, and is made up of three sheaths: *the inner epithelial root sheath,* the *outer epithelial root sheath* and the surrounding *connective-tissue sheath*.

The inner epithelial root sheath grows from the bottom of the follicle at the papilla; both the hair and the inner root sheath grow upwards together. The inner surface of this sheath is covered with cuticle cells, in the same way as the outer surface of the hair: these cells lock together, anchoring the hair firmly in place. The inner root sheath ceases to grow when level with the sebaceous gland.

The outer epithelial root sheath forms the follicle wall. This does not grow up with the hair, but is stationary. It is a continuation of the growing layer of the epidermis of the skin.

Curly	Wavy	Straight
Flat ribbon-like	Oval	Round

Hair shapes

The connective-tissue sheath surrounds the follicle and the sebaceous gland, providing both a sensory supply and a blood supply. The connective-tissue sheath includes, and is a continuation of, the papilla.

The *shape* of the hairs is determined by the shape of the hair follicle – an angled or bent follicle will produce an oval or flat hair, whereas a straight follicle will produce a round hair. Flat hairs are curly, oval hairs are wavy, and round hairs are straight. As a general rule, during waxing curly hairs break off more easily than straight hairs.

The nerve supply The number, size and type of nerve endings associated with hair follicles is related to the size and type of follicle. The follicles of vellus hairs have the fewest nerve endings; those of terminal hairs have the most.

Lanugo hairs

The nerve endings surrounding hair follicles respond mainly to rapid movements when the hair is moved. Nerve endings that respond to touch can also be found around the surface openings of some hair follicles, as well as just below the epidermis.

The three types of hair

There are three main types of hair: *lanugo*, *vellus* and *terminal*.

Lanugo hairs are found on the body prior to birth. They are fine and soft, do not have a medulla, and are often unpigmented. They grow from around the third to the fifth month of pregnancy, and are shed to be replaced by the secondary vellus hairs around the seventh to the eighth month of pregnancy. Lanugo hairs on the scalp, eyebrows and eyelashes are replaced by terminal hairs.

Vellus hairs are fine, downy and soft, and are found on the face and body. They are often unpigmented, rarely longer than 20 mm, and do not have a medulla or a well-formed bulb. The base of these hairs is very close to the skin's surface. If stimulated, the shallow follicle of a vellus hair can grow downwards and become a follicle that produces terminal hairs.

Vellus hairs

Terminal hairs are longer and coarser than vellus hairs, and most are pigmented. They vary greatly in shape, in diameter and length, and in colour and texture. The follicles from which they grow are set deeply in the dermis and have well-defined bulbs. Terminal hair is the coarse hair of the scalp, eyebrows, eyelashes, pubic and underarm regions. It is also present on the face, chest and sometimes the back of males.

Hair growth

All hair has a **cyclical pattern of growth**, which can be divided into three phases: *anagen, catagen* and *telogen*.

Terminal hairs

TOP TIP

Vellus hairs

Vellus hairs grow slowly and take 2 to 3 months to return after waxing. They can remain dormant in the follicle for 6 to 8 months before shedding.

ALWAYS REMEMBER

Waxing terminal hair

Some areas of the body – for example, the bikini line and underarm areas – often have terminal hairs with deep follicles requiring a good blood supply. When these hairs are removed, the resulting tissue damage may cause minor bleeding from the entrance of the follicle. Removal of these deep-seated hairs is obviously more uncomfortable than the removal of shallower, finer hairs.

TOP TIP

Anagen stage

A hair pulled out at the anagen stage will be surrounded by the inner root sheath and have a properly formed bulb.

Anagen is the actively growing stage of the hair – the follicle has reformed; the hair bulb is developing, surrounding the life-giving dermal papilla; and a new hair forms, growing from the matrix in the bulb.

Catagen is the changing stage when the hair follicle shortens and starts to separate from the dermal papilla. The dermal cord maintains contact with the dermal papilla. Over a few days the hair is carried by the movement of the inner root sheath, up the follicle to the base of the sebaceous gland. Here it stays until it either falls out or is pushed out by a new hair growing up behind it. Hairs at this stage are often referred to as 'club' hairs due to the shape of the bulb as it starts to die.

TOP TIP

Catagen stage

A hair pulled out at the catagen or telogen stage can be recognized by the brush-like appearance of the root.

This stage can be very rapid, with a new hair growing straight away; or slower, with the papilla and the follicle below the sebaceous gland degenerating and entering a resting stage, telogen.

Telogen is a resting stage when the hair is shed. Many hair follicles do not undergo this stage, but start to produce a new hair immediately. During resting phases, hairs may still be loosely inserted in the shallow follicles.

The hair growth cycle

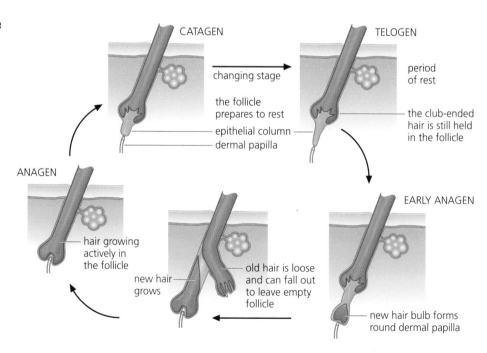

TOP TIP

Hair removal

Because of the cyclical nature of hair growth, the follicles are always at different stages of their growth cycle. When the hair is removed, therefore, the hair will not all grow back at the same time. For this reason, waxing or threading can appear to reduce the quantity of hair growth. This is not so; given time, all the hair will regrow. Waxing and threading are classed as a temporary means of hair removal.

Knowledge Check

Name the different hair types and say where they can be found.

Refer to page 67 to help you.

Speed of growth The anagen, catagen and telogen stages last for different lengths of time in different hair types and in different parts of the body:

◆ *scalp hair* grows for 2 to 7 years, and has a resting stage of 3 to 4 months

◆ *eyebrow hair* grows for 1 to 2 months, and has a resting stage of 3 to 4 months

◆ *eyelashes* grow for 3 to 6 weeks, and have a resting stage of 3 to 4 months.

After a waxing or threading treatment, body hair will take approximately 6 to 8 weeks to return.

Because hair growth cycles are not all in synchronization, we always have hair present at any given time. On the scalp, at any one time for example, 85 per cent of hairs may be in the anagen phase. This is why hair growth after waxing starts within a few days: what is seen is the appearance of hairs that were already developing in the follicle at the time of waxing.

TOP TIP

Hair growth

Male facial hair grows at a rate of approximately 10 mm a month.

Types of hair growth Hirsutism is a term used to describe a pattern of hair growth that is abnormal for that person's sex, such as when a woman's hair growth follows a man's hair-growth pattern. The hair growth is usually terminal when it should be of a vellus type.

Hypertrichosis is an abnormal growth of excess vellus hair for a person's sex, age and race. It is usually due to abnormal conditions brought about by disease or injury.

Superfluous hair (excess hair) is unwanted hair growth. Superfluous hair is considered perfectly normal for the age, sex or gender of the person. For example, at certain periods in a woman's life such as during puberty or pregnancy, terminal hairs can form, usually disappearing once the normal hormonal balance has returned. Those newly formed during the menopause are often permanent unless treated with a permanent method of hair removal, such as electrical epilation or laser treatment.

ALWAYS REMEMBER

Alopecia – loss of hair

This is often caused by a nervous disorder, there are round patches of smooth scalp as the hair follicles are not producing new hairs.

Factors affecting the growth rate and quantity of hair Hair does not always grow uniformly:

◆ *time of day* – Hair grows faster at night than during the day

◆ *weather* – Hairs grow faster in warm weather than in cold

◆ *pregnancy* – In women, hairs grow faster and during mid-pregnancy

◆ *age* – Hairs grow faster between the ages of 16 and 24. The rate of hair growth slows down with age. In women, however, facial hair growth continues to increase in old age, while trunk and limb hair increases into middle age and then decreases

◆ *colour* – Hairs of different colour grow at different speeds – for example, coarse black hair grows more quickly than fine blonde hair

◆ *part of the body* – Hair in different areas of the body grows at different rates, as do different types and thicknesses of hair. The weekly growth rate varies from approximately 1.5 mm (fine hair) to 2.8 mm (coarse hair), when actively growing

◆ *heredity* – Members of a family may have inherited growth patterns, such as excess hair that starts to grow at puberty and increases until the age of 20–25

◆ *health and diet* – Health and a varied, balanced diet are crucial in the rate of hair growth and appearance

◆ *stress* – Emotional stress can cause a temporary hormonal imbalance within the body, which may lead to a temporary growth of excess hair

◆ *medical conditions* – A sudden unexplained increase of body hair growth may indicate a more serious medical problem, such as malfunction of the ovaries, or result from the taking of certain drugs, such as corticosteroids and certain birth control and high blood pressure medications.

The quantity as well as the type of hair present may vary with race:

◆ *people of Latin extraction* tend to possess heavier body, facial and scalp hair, which is relatively coarse and straight

◆ *people of East Asian extraction* tend to possess very little or no body and facial hair growth, and usually their scalp hair growth is relatively coarse and straight. This gives the appearance of greater hair density but they actually have a lower hair density than Caucasian Latin and African–Caribbean people

◆ *people of Northern European white extraction* tend to have light to medium body and facial hair growth, with their scalp hair growth being wavy, loosely curled or straight

◆ *people of African–Caribbean extraction* tend to have little body and facial hair growth, but usually their scalp hair growth is relatively coarse and tightly curled.

HEALTH & SAFETY

African–Caribbean clients The body hair of African–Caribbean clients is prone to break during waxing, and to ingrow after waxing. Skin damage can result in the loss of pigmentation (hypopigmentation).

Knowledge Check

What are the different stages of the hair growth cycle called?

What happens to the hair at each stage?

Refer to page 68 to help you.

The nails

The structure and function of the nail

Nails grow from the ends of the fingers and toes and serve as a form of protection. They also help when picking up small objects. The different components of the nails and surrounding tissues are discussed below.

The nail plate The **nail plate** is composed of compact translucent layers of keratinized epidermal cells: it is this that makes up the main body of the nail. The layers of cells are packed very closely together, with fat but very little moisture.

The nail gradually grows forward over the **nail bed**, until finally it becomes the **free edge**. The underside of the nail plate is grooved by longitudinal ridges and furrows, which help to keep it in place.

In normal health the plate curves in two directions:

◆ **transversely** – from side to side across the nail

◆ **longitudinally** – from the base of the nail to the free edge.

free edge
hyponychium
nail plate
nail wall
nail bed
perionychium
lunula
cuticle
matrix
nail groove
eponychium
nail mantle

The structure of the nail

nail plate

The nail plate

free edge

The free edge

matrix

The matrix

nail bed

The nail bed

There are no blood vessels or nerves in the nail plate: this is why the nails, like hair, can be cut without pain or bleeding. The pink colour of the nail plate derives from the blood vessels that pass beneath it – the nail bed.

Function: To protect the living nail bed of the fingers and toes.

The free edge The free edge is the part of the nail that extends beyond the fingertip; this is the part that is filed. It appears white as there is no nail bed underneath.

Function: To protect the tip of the fingers and toes and the hyponychium (see page 72). The free edge when filed can be shaped into a variety of shapes; find out what these are by turning to page 411.

The matrix The matrix, sometimes called the nail root, is the growing area of the nail. It is formed by the division of cells in this area, called mitosis, and is part of the stratum germinativum layer of the epidermis. It lies under the eponychium (see page 72), at the base of the nail. The process of keratinization takes place in the epidermal cells of the matrix, forming the hardened tissue of the nail plate.

Function: To produce new nail cells.

The nail bed The nail bed is the portion of skin upon which the nail plate rests. It has a pattern of grooves and furrows corresponding to those found on the underside of the nail plate; these interlock, keeping the nail in place, but separate at the end of the nail to form the free edge. The nail bed is liberally supplied with blood vessels, which provide the nourishment necessary for continued growth; and sensory nerves, for protection.

Function: To supply nourishment and protection.

The nail mantle The nail mantle is the layer of epidermis at the base of the nail above the matrix, before the **cuticle**. It appears as a deep fold of skin.

Function: To protect the matrix from physical damage.

The lunula The crescent-shaped lunula is located at the base of the nail. These cells have not fully hardened through the process called keratinization. It is white in comparison to the rest of the nail, and there are two theories to account for this:

◆ newly formed nail plates may be less transparent than mature nail plates

◆ the lunula may indicate the size of the underlying matrix – the matrix is thicker than the epidermis of the nail bed, and the blood capillaries beneath it therefore would not show through as well.

Function: None.

ALWAYS REMEMBER

Nail colour

If the nail bed is pink this means the blood circulation to the nail bed is good. Poor health disorders such as respiratory illness and anaemia can affect the appearance of the nail colour called 'blue nail'.

nail mantle

The nail mantle

lunula

Lunula

Hyponychium Nail grooves Perionychium Nail walls

Eponychium

Cuticle

The hyponychium The hyponychium is part of the epidermis under the free edge of the nail.

Function: To protect the nail bed from infection by preventing dirt and bacteria gathering underneath the nail plate by forming a waterproof barrier.

The nail grooves The nail grooves run alongside the edge of the nail plate.

Function: To guide the body of the nail plate as it grows forward over the nail bed.

The perionychium The perionychium is the collective name given to the cuticle at the sides of the nail.

Function: To protect the nail bed from infection by forming a waterproof barrier which prevents dirt and bacteria getting underneath the nail plate.

The nail walls The nail walls are the folds of skin overlapping the sides of the nails.

Function: To cushion and protect the nail plate and grooves from damage.

The eponychium The eponychium is the extension of the cuticle at the base of the nail plate, under which the nail plate emerges from the matrix.

Function: To protect the nail bed from infection by forming a waterproof barrier which prevents dirt and bacteria getting underneath the nail plate.

The cuticle The cuticle is the overlapping epidermis around and extending onto the base of the nail, developing from the stratum corneum. When in good condition, it is soft and loose.

Function: To protect the nail bed from infection by forming a waterproof barrier which prevents dirt and bacteria getting underneath the nail plate.

TOP TIP

Did you know?

Fingernails grow more quickly than toenails. Fingernails grow about 0.1 mm each day, 3–4 mm per month (4 cm per year), and grow faster in summer than in winter.

Nail growth

When **nail growth** occurs the cells divide in the matrix and the nail grows forward over the nail bed, guided by the nail grooves, until it reaches the end of the finger or toe, where it becomes the free edge. When they first emerge from the matrix the translucent cells are plump and soft, but they get harder and flatter as they move towards the free edge. The top two layers of the epidermis form the nail plate; the remaining three form the nail bed.

The nails' cells die in a process called keratinization where the cells become filled with the protein keratin.

The nail bed has a pattern of grooves and furrows corresponding to those found on the underside of the nail plate: the two surfaces interlock, holding the nail in place.

Fingernails grow at approximately twice the speed of toenails. It takes about 6 months for a fingernail to grow from cuticle to free edge, but about 12 months for a toenail to do so.

The beauty therapist must be able to distinguish a healthy nail and surrounding skin from one suffering from a nail/skin disease or disorder. Certain nail/skin diseases and disorders prevent treatment: proceeding would expose the beauty therapist and other clients to the risk of cross-infection through contact. It is therefore vital that you are familiar with the nail/skin diseases and disorders with which you might come into contact in the workplace, those that are a risk and those that are not, and the correct action to take.

Knowledge Check

In what part of the **nail structure** do the cells divide to form the nail?

As the nail cells grow forward they harden; what is this process called?

How long does it take the fingernails and toenails to grow from cuticle to free edge?

Refer to page 73 to help you.

Knowledge Check

What are the functions of the nails?

Refer to page 71 to help you.

ACTIVITY

Recognizing nail structure

With a colleague, try to identify the structural parts of each other's nails. Write down both the parts that you can see and the parts that you cannot see.

Related nail/skin diseases and disorders are discussed in CHAPTER 11 Manicure Treatments and CHAPTER 12 Pedicure Treatments.

The nervous system

The **nervous system** transmits messages between the brain and other parts of the body and is vast and complex. It controls everything that the body does with another body system, the endocrine system, which secretes hormones which are chemical messengers. The nervous system is made up of a network of nerve cells, called neurones. They transmit messages to and from the central nervous system (CNS) in the form of impulses. The nervous system of the body has two main divisions:

1 The central nervous system.

2 The autonomic nervous system.

The central nervous system

The central nervous system (CNS) is composed of the brain and spinal cord. The CNS co-ordinates the activities of the entire body.

The brain transmits impulses to all parts of the body in order to stimulate other organs to act and is protected by the bones of the cranium. The spinal cord runs along inside the vertebral column and is protected by the bones (vertebrae) of the spinal column. The brain is composed of several parts, each of which performs special functions.

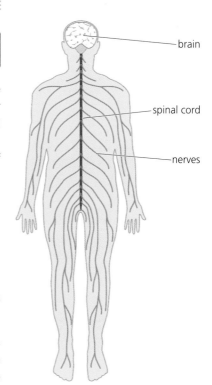

brain

spinal cord

nerves

Central nervous system

Nerves

A **nerve** is a whitish bundle of fibres made up of neurones (nerve cells) that transmits impulses of sensations between the brain or spinal cord and other parts of the body. Nerve cells are long, narrow and delicate. They are made up of a cell body containing a large central nucleus and nerve fibres that transmit messages to other neurones.

Kinds of nerves There are two types of nerve: *sensory nerves* and *motor nerves*. Both are composed of white fibres enclosed in a sheath.

◆ **Sensory or afferent nerves** These receive information from receptors in the sense organs which is passed on to the brain and spinal cord. They are found near to the skin's surface and respond to touch, pressure, temperature and pain.

◆ **Motor or efferent nerves** These are situated in muscle tissue and act on information received from the brain or spinal cord which is passed on to a muscle or gland, causing a particular response, typically muscle movement.

All nerves emerge from the CNS. Sensory (receptor) nerves are linked to sensory receptors, while motor (effector) nerves end in a muscle or gland. Twelve pairs of cranial nerves emerge from the brain associated with our senses of smell, taste, chewing, speech, sight, facial expressions, balance and hearing; 31 pairs of spinal nerves emerge from between the vertebrae of the spinal column supplying all parts of the body affecting our movement.

Nerves of the face and neck These nerves link the brain with the muscles of the head, face and neck.

Cranial nerves control muscles in the head and neck region, or carry nerve impulses from sense organs to the brain. Those of concern to the beauty therapist when performing a facial treatment are as follows:

◆ the 5th cranial nerve, or trigeminal controls the muscles involved in mastication (chewing) and passes on sensory information from the face such as the eyes

◆ the 7th cranial nerve, or facial controls the muscles involved in facial expression

◆ the 11th cranial nerve, or accessory controls muscles involved in moving the head, the sternocleidomastoid and trapezius muscle.

5th cranial nerve This nerve carries messages to the brain from the sensory nerves of the skin, the teeth, the nose and the mouth. It also stimulates the motor nerve to create the chewing action when eating. The 5th cranial nerve has three branches:

◆ the ophthalmic nerve serves the tear glands of the eye, the skin of the forehead, and the upper cheeks

◆ the maxillary nerve serves the upper jaw and the mouth

◆ the mandibular nerve serves the lower jaw muscle, the teeth and the muscle involved with chewing.

7th cranial nerve This nerve passes through the temporal bone and behind the ear, and then divides. It serves the ear muscle and the **muscles of facial expression**, the tongue and the palate.

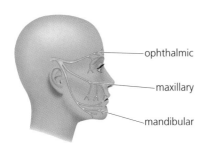

— ophthalmic

— maxillary

— mandibular

5th cranial nerve

TOP TIP

Botox® botulinum toxin A

Botox® has been developed as a cosmetic treatment from its previous use medically to treat eye spasms and disorders of the CNS. A purified protein called botulinum toxin A is injected into the face, where it binds to the nerve endings, preventing the release of the neurotransmitter substance that stimulates the muscle fibres to contract. The result is a paralysis of the muscle preventing expressions that may lead to visible expression lines on the face, such as frown lines.

7th cranial nerve

The 7th cranial nerve has five branches:

◆ the temporal nerve serves the orbicularis oculi and the frontalis muscles

◆ the zygomatic nerve serves the eye muscles

◆ the buccal nerve serves the upper lip and the sides of the nose

◆ the mandibular nerve serves the lower lip and the mentalis muscle of the chin

◆ the cervical nerve serves the platysma muscle of the neck.

11th cranial nerve This nerve serves the sternomastoid and trapezius muscles of the neck, which move the head and shoulders.

Nerve impulses The CNS transmits instructions to organs through nerve impulses – tiny electrical signals – that pass along a neurone. Each nerve consists of a nerve cell and its parts, axons and dendrites. Axons carry nerve impulses away from the cell; dendrites carry impulses towards the cell.

11th cranial nerve

When an impulse reaches the end of a nerve fibre, a chemical called a *neurotransmitter substance* is released. This chemical passes across a tiny gap called a *synapse* and is taken up by an adjacent neurone, generating an electrical impulse in the neurone.

When neurotransmitters land at their receptor sites they can stimulate or inhibit the receiving cell. Both responses are important to relay the correct message through the nervous system.

Neurones can stimulate muscle fibres to contract. The *motor point* is where a motor nerve enters a muscle. When stimulated by a motor nerve, muscle contraction occurs.

TOP TIP

Lifestyle factors affect the nervous system

Caffeine is a stimulant and will increase the release of the neurotransmitter chemical across the synapse between adjacent neurones.

Alcohol is a sedative and will slow the release of the neurotransmitter chemical across the synapse between adjacent neurones.

Can you think of other substances that affect the nervous system?

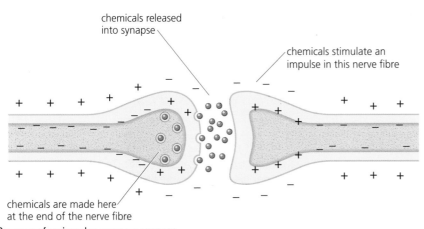

Passage of an impulse across a synapse

TOP TIP

Memory aid

The sympathetic division is associated with stress. The parasympathetic system is associated with peace.

sympathetic = stress

parasympathetic = peace

The autonomic nervous system

The other nervous system division is the autonomic nervous system, the main function being to maintain constant conditions within the body called *homeostasis*.

The autonomic nervous system controls those body structures over which there is no conscious control – the involuntary activities. It regulates the functioning of organs such as the heart, the stomach, the lungs and the secretion of most glands. There are two divisions of the autonomic nervous system – the *sympathetic* and *parasympathetic nervous systems*.

Many organs receive a supply from each division. Fibres from one division stimulate the organ while fibres from the other division inhibit it, thus ensuring balance in the body.

The sympathetic nervous system is stimulated in periods of stress or danger and prepares the body for physical activity. Fibres of the sympathetic division increase blood flow by causing the heart to beat faster and the blood vessels in the muscles to widen. Activities that are not essential in this stressful situation are inhibited.

The parasympathetic nervous system is associated with resting and causes the blood flow to slow by causing the heart to beat slower and the blood vessels in the muscles to contract (become smaller). Fibres of this division stimulate digestion and absorption of food.

The nervous system therefore co-ordinates the activities of the body by responding to stimuli received by sense organs, including the nose, tongue, eyes, ears and skin.

The muscular system

Muscles are responsible for the movement of body parts. Each is made up of a bundle of elastic fibres bound together in a sheath, the fascia. Muscular tissue contracts (shortens) and produces movement. Muscles never completely relax – there are always a few contracted fibres in every muscle. These make the muscles slightly tense and this tension is called **muscle tone**.

Muscle tissue

Muscle tissue has the following properties:

◆ it has the ability to contract

◆ it is extensible (when the extensor muscle in a joint contracts the corresponding flexor muscle will be stretched or lengthened)

◆ it is elastic – following contraction or extension it returns to its original length

◆ it is responsive – it contracts in response to nerve stimulation.

There are different types of muscle which move either involuntarily or voluntarily. Involuntary muscle is made up of smooth or non-striated muscle that we do not control by will, e.g. the part of the eye muscle used when blinking and striated (having a stripy appearance). Voluntary muscles are attached to bones and cause movement which we can control.

A muscle is usually anchored by a strong tendon to one bone: the point of attachment is known as the muscle's origin. The muscle is likewise joined to a second bone: the attachment in this case is called the muscle's insertion. It is this second bone that is moved: the muscle contracts, pulling the two bones towards each other. (A different muscle, on the other side of the bone, has the contrary effect.) Not all muscles attach to bones, however: some insert into an adjacent muscle, or into the skin itself. The muscles with which we are concerned here are those of the face, neck, shoulders, arms, hands, lower legs and feet.

Facial muscles

Many of the muscles located in the face are very small and are attached to (insert into) another small muscle or the facial skin. Muscles also help shape the face. When the muscles contract, they pull the facial skin in a particular way; this creates facial expressions.

With age, the facial expressions that we make every day produce lines on the skin – frown lines or expression lines. The amount of muscle tension, or tone, also decreases with age. When performing treatments such as facial massage, the aim is to improve the general tone of the muscles.

To balance and move the head and facial features the muscles of the head, face and neck work together.

ALWAYS REMEMBER

Nerves of the face

Almost all facial muscles are controlled by the 7th cranial or facial nerve.

TOP TIP

Terminology for action

If a muscle has 'flexor' or 'extensor' in front of the muscle name you will know what the action of the muscle is!

Flexor – bends a joint   *Extensor* – straightens a joint

Abduction – 'move away'   *Adduction* – 'move towards'

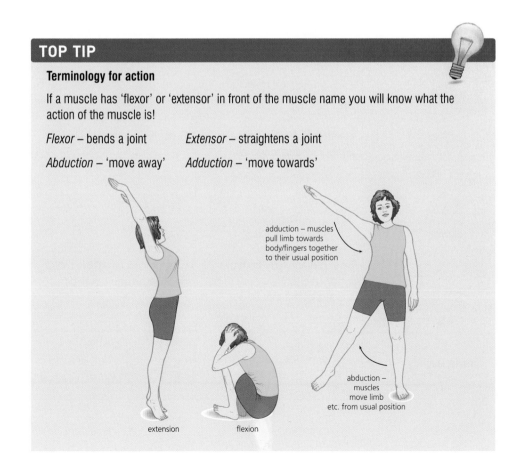

adduction – muscles pull limb towards body/fingers together to their usual position

abduction – muscles move limb etc. from usual position

extension   flexion

Muscles of facial expression

Muscle	Expression	Location	Action
Frontalis	Surprise	The forehead	Raises the eyebrows, causes wrinkling across forehead
Corrugator	Frowning	Between the eyebrows	Draws the eyebrows down and together
Orbicularis oculi	Winking	Surrounds the eyes	Closes the eyelid
Risorius	Smiling, grinning	Extends diagonally from the masseter muscle to the corners of the mouth	Draws mouth corners outwards and backwards in a grinning action
Buccinator	Blowing	Inside the cheeks, between upper jaw and lower jaw	Compresses the cheeks
Zygomaticus (made up of major and minor muscles)	Smiling, laughing	Extend diagonally from the zygomatic (cheekbone) to the corners of the mouth	Lifts the corners of the mouth backwards and upwards

Muscle	Expression	Location	Action
Procerus	Distaste	Covers the bridge of the nose	Draws down eyebrows and wrinkles the skin over the bridge of the nose
Nasalis (made up of several small muscles)	Anger	Covers the front of the nose and surrounds nostrils	Opens and closes the nasal openings
Levator labii	Distaste	Surrounds the upper lip	Raises and draws back the upper lips and nostrils
Depressor labii	Sulking	Surrounds the lower lip	Pulls down the lower lip and draws it slightly to one side
Orbicularis oris	Pout, kiss, doubt	Surrounds the mouth	Purses the lip (as in blowing), closes the mouth
Triangularis	Sadness	The corner of the lower lip extends over the chin	Draws down the mouth's corners

(Continued)

Muscle	Expression	Location	Action
Mentalis	Doubt	Covers the front of the chin	Raises the lower lip, causing the chin to wrinkle
Platysma	Fear, horror	The sides of the neck and chin	Draws the mouth's corners downwards and backwards

Muscles of the face and neck

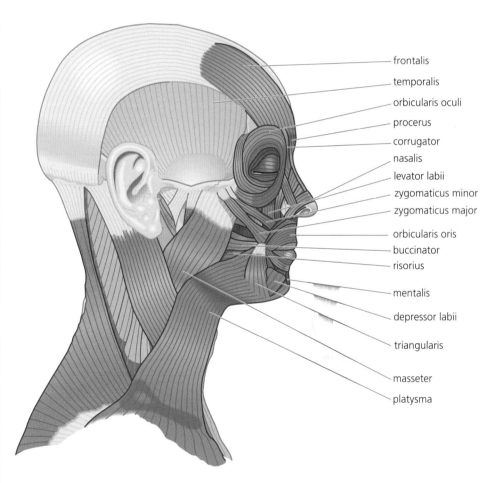

frontalis
temporalis
orbicularis oculi
procerus
corrugator
nasalis
levator labii
zygomaticus minor
zygomaticus major
orbicularis oris
buccinator
risorius
mentalis
depressor labii
triangularis
masseter
platysma

ACTIVITY

Facial expressions

In front of a mirror, move the muscles of your face to create the expressions that you might form each day.

What expressions can you make? Which part or parts of the face are moving? Which facial muscles do you think have contracted to create these expressions?

TOP TIP

Crow's feet

To avoid the premature formation of 'crow's feet':

◆ avoid squinting in bright sunlight – wear sunglasses

◆ have your eyes tested regularly

◆ if you use a visual display unit, ensure that you take regular breaks, and have a protective filter screen to remove glare

◆ use good quality skincare products around the eye.

Muscles of mastication   The muscles responsible for the movement of the lower jawbone (the mandible) when chewing are called the muscles of mastication.

Muscles of the upper body   When massaging the shoulder area you will cover the following **muscles of the upper body**. You will also cover the trapezius muscle that makes up the majority of the upper back (see above).

Muscle	Location	Action
Masseter	The cheek area: extends from the zygomatic bone to the mandible	Clenches the teeth; raises the lower jaw and closes the mouth
Temporalis	Extends from the temple region at the side of the head to the mandible	Raises the jaw and draws it backwards, as in chewing

Muscles that move the head

Muscle	Location	Action
Sternocleidomastoid	Runs from the sternum to the clavicle bone and the temporal bone	Flexes the neck; rotates and bows the head
Trapezius	A large diamond or kite-shaped muscle, covering the back of the neck and the upper back (Also a muscle of the upper-body.)	Draws the head backwards and allows movement at the shoulder
Occipitalis	Covers the back of the head	Draws scalp backwards

TOP TIP

An adult head weighs 5 kg. Strong muscles of the neck and back are required to allow movement of the head.

TOP TIP

Muscles that move the head assist those of facial expression when communicating, e.g. nodding the head.

Muscles that move the head and muscles
of the upper body

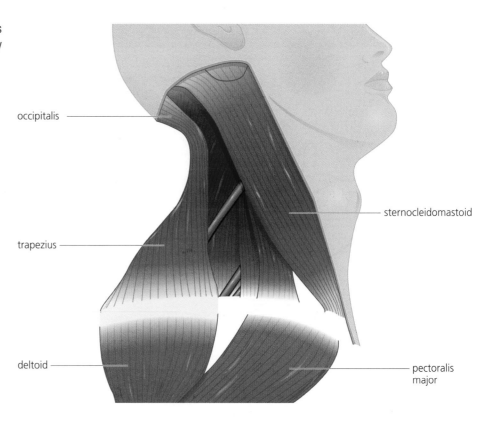

occipitalis

sternocleidomastoid

trapezius

deltoid

pectoralis
major

Muscle	Location	Action
Pectoralis major	The front of the chest	Moves the arm towards the upper body
Deltoid	A thick triangular muscle, covering the shoulder joint	Takes the arm away from the side of the body

The muscles of the hand and arm

The hand and fingers are moved primarily by muscles and tendons in the forearm. These muscles contract, pulling the tendons, and thereby move the fingers much as a puppet is moved by strings.

The **muscles of the hand and arm** that bend the wrist, drawing it towards the forearm, are flexors; other muscles, extensors, straighten the wrist and the hand.

ACTIVITY

Observing the tendons

Tendons are made of strong connective tissue and attach muscle to bone. Hold your palm face upwards, with your sleeve pulled back so that you can see your forearm. Move the fingers individually towards the palm. Can you see the tendons moving?

brachioradialis

flexor carpi radialis

transverse ligaments

thenar muscles

palmaris longus

flexor carpi ulnaris

extensor carpi ulnaris

hypothenar muscles

flexor digitorum tendons

extensor carpi radialis (longus and brevis)

extensor digitorum

transverse ligaments

extensor digitorum tendons

Muscles of the arm and hand

Muscle	Location	Action
Brachioradialis	On the outer (thumb side) of the forearm	Flexes arm at the elbow
Flexor carpi radialis	Middle of the forearm	Flexes and abducts the wrist
Extensor carpi radialis (longus and brevis)	Thumb side of the forearm	Extends and abducts the hand and wrist
Flexor carpi ulnaris	Front of the forearm	Muscle that flexes and adducts the wrist joint in towards the body
Extensor carpi ulnaris	Back of the forearm	Extends and adducts the wrist
Palmaris longus	Middle of the front of the forearm	Flexes the wrist and tenses the palm of the hand
Hypothenar muscle	In the palm of the hand, below the little finger	Flexes the little finger and moves it outwards and inwards
Thenar muscle	In the palm of the hand, below the thumb	Flexes the thumb and moves it outwards and inwards
Flexor digitorum tendons	Front of fingers	Flexes the fingers when contracted
Extensor digitorum tendons	Back of fingers	Extends the fingers when contracted

The muscles of the foot and lower leg

The **muscles of the foot** work together to help move the body when walking and running. In a similar way to the movement of the hand, the foot is moved primarily by **muscles in the lower leg**; these pull on tendons, which in turn move the feet and toes.

Muscles and tendons of the foot

Muscles of the lower leg

anterior aspect

posterior aspect

Muscles and tendons of the lower leg and foot

Muscle	Location	Action
Gastrocnemius	Calf of the leg, inserts through the Achilles tendon into the heel	Flexes the lower leg; plantar flexes the foot (extends and points the toes down)
Tibialis anterior	Front of the lower leg	Inverts the foot (turns sole inwards); dorsi flexes the foot (flexes and points the toes up); rotates foot outwards Supports the medial longitudinal arch of the foot when running or walking
Soleus	Calf of the leg, situated below the gastrocnemius muscle. Inserts through the Achilles tendon into the heel	Plantar flexes the foot (flexes and points toes down). Assists forward motion when walking or running
Peroneus longus	Lateral side of the lower leg	Plantar flexes the foot and everts (turns sole outwards). Supports the foot arches
Extensor digitorum longus	Lateral side of the front of the lower leg	Dorsi flexes the foot up at the ankle and extends the toes

Muscle	Location	Action
Extensor hallucis longus	Arises from the middle front surface of the fibula, passing the transverse aspect of the foot and inserting into the big toe	Extends the big toe
Flexor digitorum longus	Back of the tibia in the lower leg and inserts into the distal four toes	Plantar flexes foot downwards and inverts the foot. Helps the toes to grip. Supports the lateral longitudinal arch of the foot
Flexor hallucis longus	Arises from the back of lower leg and inserts to the plantar aspect of the foot to the base of the big toe	Flexes the big toe and pushes the foot off the ground when walking
Achilles tendon	Attached to the soleus and gastrocnemius down to the heel	Raises the foot when related muscle contracts
Extensor digitorum tendons	Tops of toes	Straightens the toes when related muscle contracts
Flexor digitorum tendons	Underneath the toes	Bends the toes when related muscle contracts

The bones

When carrying out a massage to the face, head, shoulders, arms, hands, legs and feet, you will feel below your hands the underlying bones. Bone is the hardest structure in the body: it is made up of water; non-living (inorganic) material including calcium and phosphorus and living (organic) material such as the cells which form bones called osteoblasts. It protects the underlying structures, gives shape to the body and provides an attachment point for our muscles, thereby allowing movement. There are two main classifications of bone tissue, compact and cancellous (spongy). Bones are made up of both types of tissue which varies according to size and function.

Compact appears to have no visible spaces and is solid in structure making it strong and hardwearing. However, under a microscope it can be seen that it is supplied with blood and lymph vessels and nerves.

Cancellous (spongy) has many spaces which contains red and yellow bone marrow. Red bone marrow produces new red blood cells and yellow bone marrow stores fat cells.

The skeleton is made up of many bones. The average skeleton has 206 bones. It forms a strong framework which supports the softer tissues, maintains the shape of the body and keeps the internal organs anchored in position. Muscles are attached to the bones which contract and relax allowing movement. Together with the muscles and joints, the skeleton allows movement. Many organs are surrounded by a protective cage of bone. Many of the blood cells are made in bone marrow (found inside the bones).

Bones have different shapes, accord to their function. Bones can be classified as: flat; short; irregular; long and sesamoid.

Knowledge Check

Name one muscle located in each of the following: the shoulder, arm and hand.

What are the group of muscles called that bend the wrist, drawing it towards the forearm?

Refer to pages 82–83 to help you.

TOP TIP

Bone acts as a reservoir for important minerals such as calcium and phosphorus and also makes new cells for the blood in certain bones in tissue called bone marrow.

Each bone is connected to its neighbour by *connective tissue*, a structural tissue that supports, surrounds and links different parts of the body. Fibrous connective tissue is used for immovable joints such as those of the cranium. *Fibrocartilage* is used for semi-immovable joints such as those between the bones of the vertebrae. The most common joints – *synovial joints* – are freely moveable and are loosely held together by a form of connective tissue called a *ligament*.

Types of bones

long bones
- head of spongy bone
- marrow cavity
- shaft of compact bone
- covering of articular cartilage

scapula

vertebra bone

phalange

flat bones
- inner layer of cancellous bone
- outer layer of compact bone

irregular bones
- cancellous bone
- very thin layer of compact bone

short bones
- thin layer of compact bone
- spongy bone

Hip
- intracapsular ligament
- socket (pelvis)
- ball (head of femur)

Shoulder
- shallow socket (scapula)
- ball (head of humerus)
- tendon of biceps muscle runs through the joint capsule
- humerus

Knee
- femur
- joint stabilized by internal ligaments and pieces of cartilage
- tibia
- fibula

Elbow
- humerus
- radius
- ulna

Bones of the head, neck, chest and shoulders

The bones which form the head are collectively known as the **skull**. The skull can be divided into two parts, the face and the cranium, which together are made up of 22 bones:

◆ the fourteen **facial bones** form the face

◆ the eight cranial bones form the rest of the head.

As well as forming our facial features, the facial bones support other structures such as the eyes and the teeth. Some of these bones, such as the nasal bone, are made from cartilage, connective tissue, a softer tissue than bone.

The cranium surrounds and protects the brain. The bones are thin and slightly curved, and are held together by connective tissue. After childhood, the joints become immovable, and are called sutures appearing as wavy lines.

Knowledge Check

Name two muscles located in the foot and lower leg and their actions.

Refer to pages 84–85 to help you.

2 malar (zygomatic)

2 lacrimal
2 nasal
2 turbinate
1 vomer
2 maxillae
1 mandible

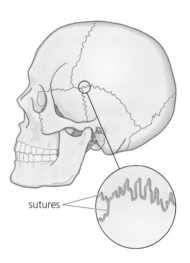

sutures

Bones of the face (14 in total)

*The palatine bones are internal bones

Facial bones

Bone	Number	Location	Function
Nasal	2	The nose	Form the bridge of the nose
Vomer	1	The nose	Forms the dividing bony wall of the nose
Palatine	2	The nose	Form the floor and wall of the nose and the roof of the mouth *internal bones, therefore not illustrated on the diagram above
Turbinate	2	The nose	Form the outer walls of the nose
Lacrimal	2	The eye sockets	Form the inner walls of the eye sockets; contain a small groove for the tear duct
Malar (zygomatic)	2	The cheek	Form the cheekbones
Maxillae	2	The upper jaw	Fused together, to form the upper jaw, which holds the upper teeth
Mandible	1	The lower jaw	The largest and strongest of the facial bones; holds the lower teeth

Cranial bones

Bone	Number	Location	Function
Occipital	1	The lower back of the cranium	Contains a large hole called the foramen magnum: through this pass the spinal cord, the nerves and blood vessels
Parietal	2	The sides of the cranium	Fused together to form the sides and top of the head (the 'crown')
Frontal	1	The forehead	Forms the forehead and the upper walls of the eye sockets
Temporal	2	The sides of the head	Provide two muscle attachment points: the mastoid process and the zygomatic process
Ethmoid	1	Between the eye sockets	Forms part of the nasal cavities
Sphenoid	1	The base of the cranium, the back of the eye sockets	A bat-shaped bone that joins together all the bones of the cranium

Bones of the cranium (8 in total)

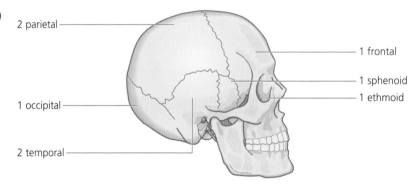

2 parietal

1 occipital

2 temporal

1 frontal

1 sphenoid

1 ethmoid

Knowledge Check

What are the basic functions of bone?

Refer to page 85 to help you.

Sinuses   The sinuses are hollow spaces in the facial and cranial bones containing air and lined with a mucous membrane, producing mucus which drains into the nose and keeps the nasal cavities moist and traps bacteria and dirt. The mucous membrane is continuous with the nasal cavities. They can also get blocked by airborne allergens, e.g. pollen, air pollution and chronic drug misuse. They connect with the inside of the nasal cavity through small openings called ostia. The main sinuses are the:

◆ maxillary, in each cheekbone

◆ frontal, either side of the forehead, above the eyes

◆ sphenoid, between the upper part of the nose and between the eyes

◆ ethmoid, behind the bridge of the nose and between the eyes.

The sinuses contain fibres that slow the flow of lymph fluid through them and which enables macrophages to ingest microorganisms that could lead to infection.

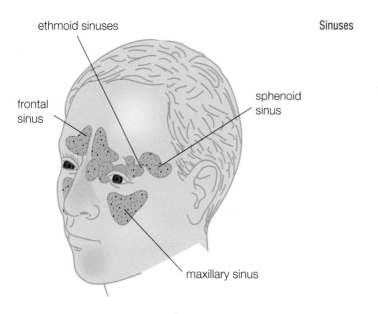

Sinuses

ethmoid sinuses

frontal sinus

sphenoid sinus

maxillary sinus

Bones of the torso

Bone	Number	Location	Function
Cervical vertebra	7	The neck	These vertebrae form the top of the spinal column: the *atlas* is the first vertebra, which supports the skull; the *axis* is the second vertebra, which allows rotation of the head
Thoracic vertebrae	12	Upper and middle back	The rib cage joins to the thoracic vertebra and protects the body's vital organs, i.e. heart and lungs
Hyoid	1	A U-shaped bone at the front of the neck	Supports the tongue
Clavicle	2	Slender long bones at the base of the neck	Commonly called the *collar bones*, these form a joint with the sternum and the scapula bones, allowing movement at the shoulder
Scapula	2	Triangular bones in the upper back	Commonly called the *shoulder blades*, the scapulae provide attachment for muscles which move the arms. The **shoulder girdle**, which allows movement at the shoulder, is composed of the clavicles and the scapulae
Humerus	2	The upper bones of the arms	Form ball-and-socket joints with the scapulae: these joints allow movement in any direction
Sternum	1	The breastbone	Protects the inner organs; provides a surface for muscle attachment and supports muscle movement

Bones of the torso

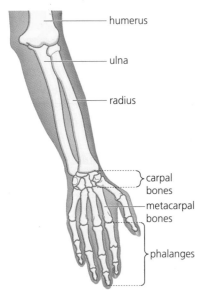

Bones of the arm and hand

Bones of the hands and upper limbs (arms)

The bones of the hand There are 27 **bones of the hand**. The wrist consists of eight small carpal bones, which glide over one another to allow movement. This is called a condyloid or gliding joint.

There are then five metacarpal bones that make up the palm of the hand.

The fingers are made up of 14 individual bones called phalanges – two in the thumb, and three in each of the fingers.

The bones of the arm The **bones of the arm** are three long bones: the humerus is the bone of the upper arm, from the shoulder to the elbow; the radius and ulna lie side by side in the lower arm, from the elbow to the wrist.

ACTIVITY

Identifying bones in the hand

Look very closely at your hand. Can you identify where the bones are? Try feeling the bones with your other hand. How many can you feel?

Having two bones in the lower arm makes it easier for your wrist to rotate. This movement that causes the palm to face downwards is called pronation; the movement that causes it to face upwards is called supination.

Knowledge Check

The wrist is made up of eight small carpal bones, which glide over one another to allow movement. Name them.

Refer to page 91 to help you.

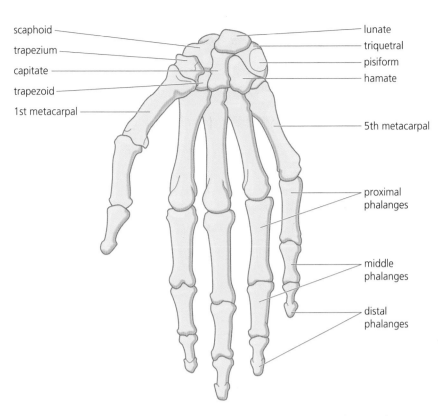

scaphoid
trapezium
capitate
trapezoid
1st metacarpal

lunate
triquetral
pisiform
hamate

5th metacarpal

proximal phalanges

middle phalanges

distal phalanges

Bones of the hand and wrist

Bones of the foot and the lower limbs (legs)

The bones of the foot   There are 26 bones of the foot. They are seven tarsal (ankle) bones, five metatarsal (ball of foot) bones, and 14 phalanges (toes). These bones fit together to form arches, which help to support the foot and to absorb the impact when we walk, run and jump.

3rd phalange (distal)

2nd phalange (middle)

1st phalange

1st metatarsal

medial cuneiform
intermediate cuneiform
lateral cuneiform
navicular

5th metatarsal

cuboid

talus

calcaneus

7 tarsal bones (medial cuneiform, intermediate cuneiform, lateral cuneiform, navicular, talus, cuboid and calcaneus)

Bones of the foot

pronation

supination

Pronation and supination

ACTIVITY

30 bones form each leg and foot, 60 in both! State the location where each bone can be found:

◆ 1 femur
◆ 1 patella
◆ 1 tibia
◆ 1 fibula
◆ 7 tarsal bones
◆ 5 metatarsal bones
◆ 14 phalanges.

TOP TIP

Arches

Footprints made by bare feet show that only part of the foot touches the ground. Weight transfers from the heel to the ball to the big toe when walking. Feet with reduced arches are referred to as 'flat feet', caused by weak ligaments and tendons.

The arches of the foot The arches of the foot are created by the formation of the bones and joints, and supported by ligaments. These arches support the weight of the body and help to preserve balance when we walk on even surfaces.

The longitudinal arch runs longitudinally from the calcaneus to the metatarsals. The arch on the inside aspect of the foot is the medial longitudinal arch, on the outside aspect it is the lateral longitudinal arch. The transverse arch lies perpendicular to this in the metatarsal area, as shown below.

Transverse arch

Medial longitudinal arch

Lateral longitudinal arch

The bones of the leg The **bones of the lower leg** are two long bones, the tibia and the fibula. These bones have joints with the upper leg (at the knee) and with the foot (at the ankle). Having two bones in the lower leg – as with the forearm – allows a greater range of movement to be achieved at the ankle.

ALWAYS REMEMBER

Anatomical definitions

Medial: towards the midline (middle) of the body.

Lateral: away from the median line (middle) of the body. The outer side of the body.

Knowledge Check

Name the bones that form the ankle.

Refer to page 91 to help you.

Bones of the lower leg

femur
patella
tibia
fibula
tarsal bones
metatarsal bones
calcaneus
phalanxes

The circulatory system

Composition and function of blood

Blood is a collection of specialized cells suspended in a liquid called plasma supplying the needs of the body's cells and keeping the body healthy. It is transported around the body by a network of vessels with a length of 90 000 miles.

Blood transports various substances around the body:

◆ carries oxygen from our lungs, and nutrients from our digested food to the cells of the body supply energy – these allow the cells to develop and divide, and the muscles to function

◆ carries waste products and carbon dioxide from the cells and tissues away for elimination from the body

◆ carries various cells and substances which allow the body to prevent or fight disease and heal injuries through blood clotting

◆ transports hormones, the body's chemical messengers, to their target tissue to cause a particular response

◆ helps to maintain the body temperature at 36.8°C: carrying blood flow near to the skin surface increases or diminishes heat loss.

The main constituents of blood

Blood consists of the following:

◆ **Plasma** This constitutes 50 per cent of blood and is a straw-coloured liquid: mainly water (90 per cent), with foods and carbon dioxide.

◆ **Red blood cells (erythrocytes)** These constitute 40–50 per cent of blood. These cells appear red because they contain haemoglobin a protein responsible for their colour. It is this that carries oxygen from the lungs to the body cells.

◆ **White blood cells (leucocytes)** There are several types of white blood cells. Their main role is to protect the body by destroying foreign bodies and dead cells, and carrying away the debris (a process known as phagocytosis).

◆ **Platelets (thrombocytes)** When blood is exposed to air, as happens when the skin is injured, these cells bind together to form a clot. White blood cells and platelets constitute 1–2 per cent of blood.

◆ **Other chemicals** Hormones are also transported in the blood – 'chemical messengers' to target tissues.

Blood cells

Blood circulation

The circulation of blood is under the control of the heart, a powerful muscular organ, the size of a clenched fist, which pumps the blood around the body. The heart requires a constant supply of oxygen and energy from blood.

Blood leaving the heart is carried in large, elastic tubes called arteries. The blood to the head arrives via the carotid arteries, which are connected via other main arteries to the heart. There are two main carotid arteries, one on each side of the neck.

These arteries divide into smaller branches, the *internal carotid* and the *external carotid*. The internal carotid artery passes the temporal bone and enters the head, taking blood to the brain, eyes, eyelids, forehead, nose and internal ears. The external carotid artery stays outside the skull, and divides into branches which supply blood to various regions of the head, face and neck.

- ◆ The occipital branch supplies the back of the head and the scalp.

- ◆ The temporal branch supplies the sides of the face, the head, the scalp and the skin. Some of its important branches are:

  - ◆ frontal: supplies the forehead

  - ◆ parietal: supplies the top and sides of the head

  - ◆ transverse: supplies the masseter muscle

  - ◆ middle temporal supplies the temples and the eyelids

  - ◆ anterior auricular: supplies the front part of the ear.

- ◆ The facial branch, also known as the external maxillary artery, supplies the muscles and tissues of the face.

- ◆ Posterior auricular branch supplies the scalp, back and above the ear.

The blood supply to the head

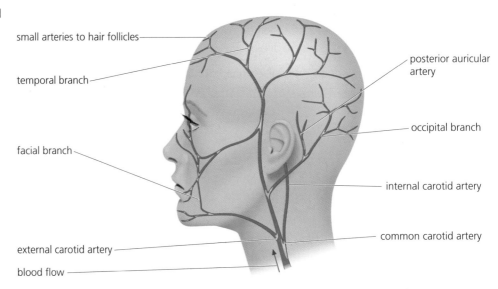

small arteries to hair follicles

temporal branch

facial branch

external carotid artery

blood flow

posterior auricular artery

occipital branch

internal carotid artery

common carotid artery

The blood supply from the head

veins to hair follicles

temporal branch

occipital branch

facial branch

internal jugular vein

external jugular vein

blood flow

These arteries also divide repeatedly, successive vessels becoming smaller and smaller until they form tiny blood capillaries. These vessels are just one cell thick, allowing substances carried in the blood to pass through them into the tissue fluid which bathes and nourishes the cells of the various body tissues.

The blood capillaries begin to join up again, forming first small vessels called venules, then larger vessels called veins. These return the blood to the heart.

Veins are less elastic than arteries, and are closer to the skin's surface. Along their course are valves, which prevent the backflow of blood.

The main veins are the external and internal jugular veins. The internal jugular vein and its main branch, the facial vein, carry blood from the face and head. The external jugular vein carries blood from the scalp and has two branches: the occipital branch and the temporal branch. The jugular veins join to enter the subclavian vein, which lies above the clavicle.

Blood returns to the heart, which pumps it to the lungs, where the red blood cells take on fresh oxygen, and where carbon dioxide is expelled from the blood. The blood returns to the heart, and begins its next journey round the body.

The arteries of the arm and hand

The arm and hand are nourished by a system of arteries that carry oxygen-rich blood to the tissues. You can see the colour of the blood from the capillaries beneath the nail: it is these that give the nail bed its pink colour.

The brachial artery supplies blood to the upper arm. This branches into the ulnar and radial artery which supply the forearm and fingers. The radial and ulnar arteries are connected across the palm by the superficial and deep palmar arches. These arteries divide to form the metacarpal and digital arteries, which supply the palm and fingers.

The veins of the arms and hands Veins deliver deoxygenated blood back to the heart. Blood which has had oxygen removed appears blue. Veins often pass through muscles. Each time muscles contract, veins are squeezed and the blood is pushed along. Massage is particularly beneficial to help this process.

Blood in the digital veins drains blood from the fingers. The palmar venous arches drains blood from the hands. The cephalic and basilic veins drain blood from the forearm.

brachial artery

radial artery

ulnar artery

Arteries of the arm

Arteries of the hand

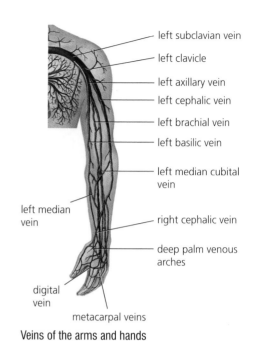

Veins of the arms and hands

HEALTH & SAFETY

Capillaries The strength and elasticity of the capillary walls can be damaged, for example by a blow to the tissues. Broken capillaries are capillaries whose elasticity is damaged and they remain constantly dilated with blood.

The arteries of the foot and leg

The leg and feet are nourished by a system of arteries that carry oxygen-rich blood to the tissues.

In the thigh the external iliac arteries carry blood into the femoral artery. Below the knee the femoral artery branches, forming the posterior and anterior tibial artery.

The anterior and tibial artery supplies blood to the lower leg and foot. The peroneal artery branches off the posterior tibial artery. At the ankle the anterior tibial artery becomes the dorsalis pedis artery. The posterior tibial artery divides at the ankle to form the medial and lateral plantar arteries. The plantar and dorsalis pedis arteries supply the digital arteries of the toes.

When it is cold, and when the circulation is poor, insufficient blood reaches the feet and they feel cold. Severe circulation problems in the feet may lead to **chilblains**.

The veins of the foot and leg The digital veins from the toes drain into the plantar and dorsal venous arch. The dorsalis pedis veins drain to the saphenous vein. The following deep veins drain the lower leg: the posterior tibial vein at the back of the leg, the peroneal vein and the anterior tibial vein at the front of the leg. The deep tibial veins join to form the popliteal vein. Above the knee the popliteal vein continues up the back of the thigh as the femoral vein, which enters into the external iliac vein. The blood from the leg returns to the heart in the inferior vena cava.

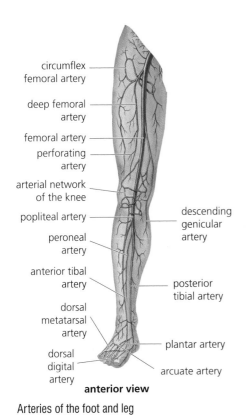

circumflex femoral artery
deep femoral artery
femoral artery
perforating artery
arterial network of the knee
popliteal artery
peroneal artery
anterior tibal artery
dorsal metatarsal artery
dorsal digital artery
descending genicular artery
posterior tibial artery
plantar artery
arcuate artery

anterior view

Arteries of the foot and leg

great saphenous vein
femoral vein
accessory saphenous vein
venous network of the knee
popliteal vein
perforating vein
peroneal vein
anterior tibial vein
posterior tibial vein
small saphenous vein
plantar venous arch
dorsal metatarsal vein
dorsal venous arch
dorsal digital vein

anterior view

Veins of the foot and leg

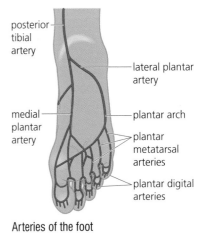

posterior tibial artery
medial plantar artery
lateral plantar artery
plantar arch
plantar metatarsal arteries
plantar digital arteries

Arteries of the foot

The lymphatic system

The **lymphatic system** is closely connected to the blood system, and can be considered as supplementing it. Its primary function is defensive: to remove bacteria and foreign materials, thereby preventing infection. It also drains away excess fluids for elimination from the body.

The lymphatic system consists of the fluid lymph, the **lymph vessels** and the lymph nodes (or glands). You may have experienced swelling of the lymph nodes in the neck when you have been ill, e.g. tonsilitis.

Unlike the blood circulation, the lymphatic system has no muscular pump equivalent to the heart. Instead, the lymph moves through the vessels and around the body because of movements such as contractions of large muscles. Contractions of the body muscles push the lymph through a series of one-way valves. Massage can play an important part in assisting this flow of lymph fluid, thereby encouraging the improved removal of the waste products transported in the lymph.

Lymph

Lymph is a straw-coloured fluid, derived from blood plasma, which has filtered through the walls of the capillaries. Lymph drains into a network of lymph capillaries and then into larger vessels known as lymphatics which contain special filters called nodes or glands. The composition of lymph is similar to that of blood, though less oxygen and fewer nutrients are available. In the spaces between the cells where there are no blood capillaries, lymph provides nourishment. It also carries lymphocytes (a type of white blood cell), which play an important role in the immune system. They can destroy dangerous cells and disease-causing bacteria and viruses directly before they return to the bloodstream.

Lymph travels only in one direction: from body tissues back towards the heart.

Knowledge Check

How are arteries different to veins?
Refer to pages 93–95 to help you.

Lymph vessels and nodes (glands)
in the body

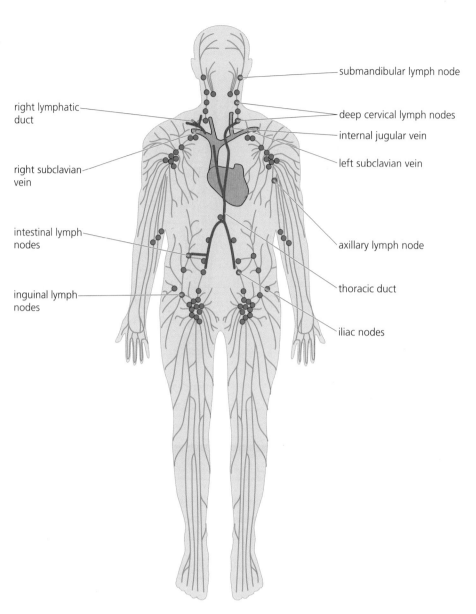

- submandibular lymph node
- right lymphatic duct
- deep cervical lymph nodes
- internal jugular vein
- left subclavian vein
- right subclavian vein
- intestinal lymph nodes
- axillary lymph node
- inguinal lymph nodes
- thoracic duct
- iliac nodes

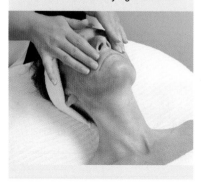

Lymph vessels

Lymph vessels often run very close to veins, forming an extensive network throughout the body. The lymph moves quite slowly, and the valves along the lymph vessels prevent backflow of the lymph.

The lymph vessels join to form larger lymph vessels, which eventually flow into one or other of two large lymphatic vessels: the thoracic duct (or left lymphatic duct) and the right lymphatic duct. The thoracic duct receives lymph from the left side of the head, neck, chest, abdomen and lower body; the right lymphatic duct receives lymph from the right side of the head and upper body.

These principal lymphatic vessels then empty their contents into a vein at the base of the neck, which in turn empties into the vena cava. The lymph is mixed into the venous blood as it is returned to the heart.

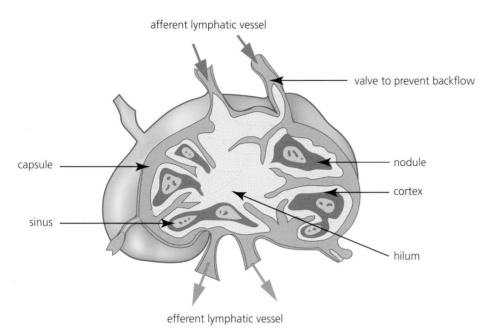

Lymph node

afferent lymphatic vessel

valve to prevent backflow

capsule

nodule

cortex

sinus

hilum

efferent lymphatic vessel

Lymph nodes

Lymph nodes or glands are tiny oval structures between 1 mm and 25 mm in length, made from lymphatic tissue encased in a fibrous capsule which filters the lymph, extracting poisons, pus and bacteria, and thus defending the body against infection by destroying harmful organisms. When we suffer an infection, the lymph nodes closest to the site of infection may swell up and become tender as the white cells attempt to destroy the germs. They are located along the routes of the principal lymphatic vessels. Lymph enters a node through an afferent vessel and leaves through an efferent vessel. Lymphocytes and macrophages, found in the lymph glands, are special cells which produce antibodies which enable us to resist invasion by microorganisms, preventing disease.

Lymph filters through at least one lymph node before returning to the bloodstream.

When performing massage, the hands should be used when appropriate to apply pressure to direct the lymph towards the nearest lymph node: this encourages the speedy removal of waste products. Various groups of lymph nodes drain the lymph of the head and neck.

Knowledge Check

What are the main constituents of lymph?

Refer to page 97 to help you.

Knowledge Check

What are the functions of lymph nodes and glands?

Refer to pages 98–99 to help you.

Lymph nodes of the head and neck

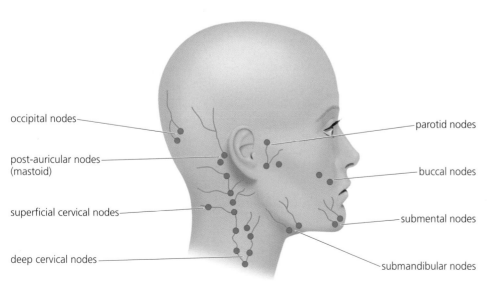

occipital nodes

parotid nodes

post-auricular nodes (mastoid)

buccal nodes

superficial cervical nodes

submental nodes

deep cervical nodes

submandibular nodes

Lymph nodes of the head

◆ The buccal group drains the eyelids, the nose and the skin of the face.

◆ The mandibular group drains the chin, the lips, the nose and the cheeks.

◆ The mastoid group drains the skin of the ear and the temple area.

◆ The occipital group drains the back of the scalp and the upper neck.

◆ The submental group drains the chin and the lower lip.

◆ The parotid group drains the nose, eyelids and ears.

Lymph nodes of the neck

◆ The superficial cervical group drains the back of the head and the neck.

◆ The lower deep cervical group drains the back area of the scalp and the neck.

Lymph nodes of the chest and arms The nodes of the armpit area drain various regions of the arms and chest.

TOP TIP

Frontal–Temporal–Parietal–Occipital–Mandible (mandibular)–Cervical

Learn and remember these names of the main regions of the head and neck. Not only will this assist you in recalling the names and locations of the bones, it will also help you greatly with the names and locations of muscles, arteries, veins, nerves and lymph nodes.

ASSESSMENT OF KNOWLEDGE AND UNDERSTANDING

You have now learnt about anatomy and physiology in the beauty therapy workplace. To test your level of knowledge, answer the following short questions. These will prepare you for your summative (final) assessment.

1. The tissue that contracts and moves the various parts of the body is:

   a. connective   b. epithelial
   c. liquid   d. muscular

2. The muscle attached to the lower surface of the heel which pulls the foot down is the:

   a. gastrocnemius   b. soleus
   c. peroneus brevis   d. peroneus logus

3. The flat bone that protects the inner organs located between the ribs on the anterior view of the body is the _____ bone.

   a. thorax   b. scapula
   c. hyoid   d. sternum

4. List the primary functions of the skeletal system:

   a. Give shape and support to the body
   b. Protect various internal organs
   c. Serve as attachments for muscles
   d. Help produce blood cells

5. Match the following bones of the face with its correct description:

   1) nasal   a) largest and strongest facial forms of the lower jawbone
   2) zygomatic   b) form the cheekbones
   3) maxillae   c) form the bridge of the nose
   4) mandible   d) bones of the upper jaw

6. The system that is also referred to as the cardio-vascular system and controls the steady circulation of the blood flow is:

   a. muscular   b. skeletal
   c. circulatory d. nervous

7. The thick-walled, muscular, flexible tubes that carry oxygenated blood away from the heart are the:

a. capillaries   b.   arteries
c. veins   d.   vessels

8. The arteries that are located on either side of the neck and are the main sources of blood supply to the head, face and neck are the _____ arteries. The internal carotid artery enters the head and supplies blood to the _____. The external carotid artery supplies blood through its branches to the outside of the skull _____. The _____ and _____ arteries are the main blood supply for the arms and hands.

9. Label the parts of the nail.

10. What affects the growth of the nail plate?

11. The appendages of the skin include:

a.   b.
c.   d.

12. What are the sebaceous or oil glands of the skin connected to?

13. The reticular layer contains the following structures within its structure:

a.   d.
b.   e.
c.   f.

14. Label the cross section of the hair follicle.

15. Match the following ear part with its correct description:

1) helix   a) The part of the ear that stands out from the sides of the head

2) pinna   b) Made up of fibrous fatty tissue with no cartilage, it forms the lower part of the earlobe

3) lobule   c) Made up of cartilage tissue, it forms the upper part of the earlobe

16. Label the lymph nodes of the head.

3 Health and Safety

LEARNING OBJECTIVES

There are two learning outcomes to achieve for this mandatory unit:

1 Be able to maintain health, safety and security practices.

2 Be able to follow emergency procedures.

The assessment range applied requires you to:

◆ Deal with hazards within own area of responsibility.

◆ Maintain appropriate level of personal presentation.

◆ Follow salon policy for security.

◆ Use required personal protective equipment (PPE).

◆ Describe and correctly dispose of all types of salon waste.

◆ Outline the main provisions of workplace related health and safety legislation.

◆ State the employers' and employees' health and safety responsibilities.

◆ State the difference between a hazard and a risk.

◆ Describe the methods used in the salon to ensure hygiene.

◆ Identify named emergency personnel.

◆ State the dangers of the incorrect use of fire-fighting equipment on different types of fires.

◆ Describe procedures for dealing with emergencies.

KEY TERMS

accident book

accident form

antiseptic

autoclave

bacteria

behaviour

clinical waste

codes of practice

contra-indicate

Control of Substances
    Hazardous to Health (COSHH)
    Regulations (2002)

Controlled Waste (Amendment)
    Regulations (1993)

cross-infection

disinfectant

Electricity at Work Regulations
    (1989)

Employer's Liability (Compulsory
    Insurance) Act (1969)

evaluation

Fire Precautions Act (1971)

fungi

hazard

Health and Safety (Display
    Screen Equipment)
    Regulations (1992)

Health and Safety (First Aid)
    Regulations (1981)

Health and Safety at Work Act
    (1974)

health and safety policy

Industry Codes of Practice

infection

ingestion

inhalation

legislation

Local Government (Miscellaneous
    Provisions) Act (1982)

Manual Handling Operations
    Regulations (1992)

Personal Protective Equipment
    (PPE) at Work Regulations
    (1992)

posture

Provision and Use of Work
    Equipment Regulations
    (PUWER) (1998)

public liability insurance

Regulatory Reform (Fire Safety)
    Order (2005)

Reporting of Injuries, Diseases
    and Dangerous Occurrences
    Regulations (RIDDOR)
    (1995)

risk

salon requirements

secondary infection

sterilization

systems

tools and equipment

viruses

Waste

Workplace (Health, Safety
    and Welfare) Regulations
    (1992)

workplace policy

workplace practices

workplace policies

Unit Topic

Follow health and safety practice in the salon
This VRQ unit is linked to the Beauty Therapy NOS Unit G20.

INTRODUCTION

This unit is all about knowing what makes a safe working environment and how safe working practices are put in place to ensure the safety of yourself, clients and colleagues. The chapter covers health and safety, security and emergency duties and responsibilities for everyone in the workplace.

You will be assessed whilst carrying out health and safety practice and procedures in the salon. Health and safety should be considered at all times within all work areas and in every action/treatment that takes place. You must be able to show you have the necessary practical skills and underpinning knowledge to comply with all related health and safety practice in the salon.

Outcome 1: Be able to maintain health, safety and security practices

Learn how to maintain health, safety and security practices

PRACTICAL SKILLS

Conduct self in the workplace to meet with health and safety practices and salon policies

Deal with hazards within own area of responsibility following salon policy

Maintain a level of personal presentation, hygiene and conduct to meet legal and salon requirements

Follow salon policy for security

Make sure tools, equipment, materials and work areas meet hygiene requirements

Use required personal protective equipment (PPE)

Position self and the client safely throughout the treatment

Handle, use and store products, materials, tools and equipment safely to meet with manufacturer's instructions

Dispose of all types of salon waste safely and to meet with legal and salon requirements

UNDERPINNING KNOWLEDGE

Explain the difference between legislation, codes of practice and workplace policies

Outline the main provisions of health and safety legislation

State the employers' and employees' health and safety responsibilities

State the difference between a hazard and a risk

Describe hazards that may occur in a salon

State the hazards which need to be referred to an appropriate member of staff

State the purpose of personal protective equipment (PPE) used in a salon during different treatments

State the importance of personal presentation, hygiene and conduct in maintaining health and safety in the salon

State the importance of maintaining the security of belongings

Outline the principles of hygiene and infection control

Describe the methods used in the salon to ensure hygiene

Describe the effectiveness and limitations of different infection control techniques

Describe how to dispose of different types of salon waste

Taking care of all in the workplace

When working in the beauty industry, you are legally required to provide a safe, secure and hygienic environment. This applies wherever you are working: in a hotel, a spa, a department store or a beauty salon. Even when working as a freelance beauty therapist

INDUSTRY ROLE MODEL

WENDY NIXON Health and Safety Consultant to the hair and beauty industry

As an Environmental Health Practitioner, specializing in health and safety enforcement, I have developed health and safety initiatives, including HSE training materials, the Bad Hand Day Campaign and the Health and Safety Award Scheme to raise standards and recognize excellence within this industry.

My current role as a Consultant includes setting standards for both best practice guidance and qualifications. I am involved in government and industry initiatives at both National and European level whilst offering training, guidance and consultancy services to both enforcement officers and industry professionals.

where you are self-employed and don't work for a single employer, you must comply with all related legislation wherever it is you are working at any time.

Legal responsibilities

If you cause harm to your client, or put a client at risk, you will be held responsible and you will be liable for prosecution, with the possibility of being fined or, at worst, imprisoned.

There is a good deal of **legislation** relating to health and safety. You will need to know the laws relating to your work role and you must be aware of your rights and responsibilities.

You will need an awareness and understanding of all of the following legislation:

Health and Safety at Work Act, Personal Protective Equipment at Work Regulations, Workplace (Health, Safety and Welfare) Regulations, Manual Handling Operations Regulations, Control of Substances Hazardous to Health Regulations (COSHH), Provision and Use of Work Equipment Regulations, Electricity at Work Regulations, Reporting Injuries, Diseases and Dangerous Occurrences (RIDDOR), Fire Precautions Act, Health and Safety First Aid Regulations, Health and Safety (Display Screen Equipment) Regulations.

This chapter will outline the main provisions of related health and safety legislation.

Enforcement of health and safety legislation is divided between local authorities (LAs) and the Health and Safety Executive (HSE). It is a good idea to obtain and read all relevant

ACTIVITY

Workplace health and safety policy

Discuss the rules which apply to you in your workplace's health and safety policy. The health and safety policy identifies how health and safety is managed: who does what, when and why.

ACTIVITY

Keep up to date with health and safety

Health and safety information is continually updated. Access information online or write to your local Health and Safety Executive office (www.hse.gov.uk) or Local Authority Environmental Health Department, the bodies appointed to support and enforce health and safety law, to ask for a pack of relevant health and safety information. Legislation relevant to business operations can also be found in the Health and Safety pack for salons.

Visit www.habia.org to research current beauty therapy health and safety legislation and minimum requirements.

publications from your local HSE offices. The HSE is there to support the beauty sector to reduce the incidence of work-related accidents and ill-health, and provides guidance and information on all aspects of health and safety legislation, which can be accessed online.

In addition, as the standards-setting body for beauty therapy, the hair and beauty industry authority, Habia, provide health and safety working guidelines and legislative requirements. **Codes of practice** are available from Habia, sharing best and mandatory working practice approved by both industry experts and health and safety advisors. Approved codes of practice are recognized by the HSE.

Health and safety legislation

The Health and Safety at Work Act (1974) (HASAWA) The **Health and Safety at Work Act (1974)** is continually reviewed and is the main piece of legislation affecting health and safety issues. It was developed from experience gained over 150 years and incorporates any earlier legislation, including the Offices, Shops and Railway Premises Act (1963) and the **Fire Precautions Act (1971)**. It lays down the minimum standards of health, safety and welfare required in each area of the workplace. For example, it requires business premises and equipment to be safe, in good repair and fit to work in. It is the employer's legal responsibility to implement the Act and to ensure, so far as is reasonably practicable, the health and safety at work of the people for whom they are responsible and those who may be affected by the work they do. This will require that staff receive appropriate training for the tasks that they are required to carry out and only work within their responsibility. The requirements of this Act will include providing a safe work environment for clients and any visitors to the workplace.

The HASAWA Act also affects those who operate freelance and do not have a specific workplace base.

The Health and Safety (Information for Employees) Regulations (1989) (HSIER) were amended in April 2009. Employers are required to provide information relating to health, safety and welfare in the workplace by displaying a copy of the approved health and safety poster or providing a copy of the leaflet.

Each employer of more than five employees must formulate a written **health and safety policy** for their business. Habia have resources providing guidance on creating a written policy. The health and safety policy identifies how health and safety is managed for that business, who does what, when and why. The policy must be issued and discussed with each employee at induction and should outline the health and safety responsibilities they should undertake. Temporary staff are to be included and must be made aware of its content. It should also include items such as:

◆ details of the storage of chemical substances

◆ details of the stock cupboard or dispensary

◆ details and records of the checks made by a qualified electrician on specialist electrical equipment

◆ names and addresses of key holders

◆ firefighting equipment and its location

◆ escape routes and emergency evacuation procedures

◆ whom to report emergencies and significant risks to.

HEALTH & SAFETY

Health and safety law information notice Every employer by law is required to display a health and safety law poster in the workplace. The health and safety law poster tells employees what they and their employers need to do in simple terms to comply with the law. An information leaflet is available called 'Your health and safety – a guide for workers'. Both poster and leaflets are available from the HSE.

HEALTH & SAFETY

Lone workers If you are self-employed and work alone, consider your safety. Guidance is provided in the information 'Working alone: health and safety guidance on the risks of lone working', INDG73 (rev2).

HEALTH & SAFETY

Five steps to risk assessment This is an HSE publication providing guidance on the requirements for risk assessment.

The health and safety policy should be reviewed regularly to ensure it continues to meet all relevant legislation guidelines including any updates. Health and safety training should also be carried out regularly and recorded. Regular health and safety checks should be made and procedures reviewed to ensure that safety is being satisfactorily maintained.

Refer to page 118 where health and safety hygiene rules are discussed further.

Hazards and risks

Employees must always co-operate with their employer to provide a safe, secure and healthy workplace. As soon as an employee observes a **hazard** (anything that has potential to cause harm) this must be either dealt with or reported to the relevant responsible person so that the problem can be put right. A **risk** is the likelihood of a hazard's potential being realized. Hazards in the workplace include:

◆ obstructions to walkways, stairways and fire exits (an obstruction is anything that blocks the traffic route, walkways in the salon work environment)

◆ spillages and breakages

◆ trailing wires

◆ faulty electrical equipment.

If there are fewer than five employees, appropriate health and safety arrangements and procedures should be in place. In 1992, European Union (EU) directives updated the legislation on health and safety management. Current legislation (at the time of writing) is outlined below.

The Health and Safety at Work Act covers many other smaller regulations which are also discussed.

Health and safety rules and regulations and examples of compliance to be displayed include:

◆ fire evacuation procedures

◆ public liability insurance certificate

◆ Health and Safety (Information for Employees) Regulations (1989) poster, updated April 2009 (the previous poster can continue to be displayed until 2014)

◆ health and safety policy (dependent upon employee numbers)

◆ risk assessment records and guidance.

Inspection and registration of premises

Inspectors from the HSE or your LA enforce the health and safety laws. They visit the workplace to ensure compliance with government health and safety legislation.

The officer will observe workplace activities and the health and safety management system that the business has in place. If the inspector identifies any hazards, it is the responsibility of the employer to remove the hazard within a designated period of time. The inspector issues an improvement notice. Failure to comply with the notice will lead to prosecution. The inspector also has the authority to close a business or stop a particular activity until they are satisfied that all potential danger to employees and public has been removed. A closure involves the issuing of a prohibition notice.

HEALTH & SAFETY

You should use your initiative and deal with low risk hazards within your responsibility, following workplace policy and legal requirements.

HEALTH & SAFETY

Protective equipment: gloves
If you are to come into contact with body tissue fluids or with chemicals, wear protective disposable surgical gloves. Latex gloves can cause allergic reactions and in some cases the development of asthma, and are not therefore recommended.

An alternative glove that provides adequate protection from contamination should be used, e.g. nitrile or PVC formulation.

HEALTH & SAFETY

Handcare Always wash your hands on glove removal, following the correct hand washing procedure. Dry hands thoroughly and moisturize them regularly.

CourseMate video: Handling Chemicals

Risk Assessments

When writing or reviewing your risk assessments always look for shortcuts staff may take and assess the impact on health and safety, e.g. plugging in electrical appliances before removing protective gloves. Remember that the exterior of the glove is wet and thus you are putting yourself at risk when handling electrical equipment. (The glove is only to protect you from the chemical.)

Wendy Nixon

Any concern about health, safety and welfare in the workplace that is not being addressed can be reported to the LA for advice. Certain beauty therapy treatments, such as ear piercing, are higher risk because they might produce blood and body tissue fluid. Inspection of the premises is necessary before such treatments can be offered to the public. The inspecting officer will visit to make sure that the guidelines listed in the **Local Government (Miscellaneous Provisions) Act (1982)** relating to this area are being complied with in terms of levels of hygiene and training. Good **infection** control systems are essential and the working environment must be suitable. When the inspecting officer is satisfied, a certificate of registration will be awarded.

The Personal Protective Equipment (PPE) at Work Regulations (2002)
The **Personal Protective Equipment (PPE) at Work Regulations (1992)** require employers to identify – through a risk assessment – those activities or processes which require special protective clothing or equipment to be worn. Ear piercing is an example where this will be necessary because of the high risk of contamination with blood or body tissue fluid.

If PPE is required this clothing and equipment must then be made available, and must be suitable and in adequate supplies. PPE includes aprons, gloves and particle masks. Employees are required to wear the protective clothing and use the protective equipment provided, and make employers aware of any shortage so that supplies can be maintained.

The Workplace (Health, Safety and Welfare) Regulations (1992)
The **Workplace (Health, Safety and Welfare) Regulations (1992)** cover a broad range of basic health, safety and welfare issues and require all staff in the workplace to provide and maintain a safe, healthy and secure working environment. Employers and

PPE for handling chemicals

HEALTH & SAFETY

Training should be provided on the correct use of PPE, its application and its removal and disposal. Compliance with PPE requirements should be monitored. If not used the reason why should be investigated as this then becomes a risk.

You should use PPE to protect yourself against potentially hazardous substances such as:

◆ disinfectants – which can cause chemical irritation to the skin, possibly leading to skin disorders such as dermatitis
◆ body tissue fluids – direct contact can lead to skin infections and disease
◆ other harmful products and materials used, such as solvents that can create harmful vapours, acrylic fumes which can cause headaches and nausea and dust created during the application of artificial nails which could lead to respiratory problems.

PPE should be 'CE' marked, which means it complies with the Personal Protective Equipment at Work Regulations 1992 and satisfies basic safety requirements.

Knowledge Check
What is a hazard?

What is a risk?

employees need to be aware of and comply with their responsibilities as required in these regulations. The regulations aim to ensure the workplace meets the health, safety and welfare needs of all the workforce. The Equality Act 2010 requires the access and facilities provided at the business premises must be equal for all regardless of age, disability, gender reassignment, marriage and civil partnerships, pregnancy and maternity, race, religion or belief, sex or sexual orientation. The regulations include legal requirements in relation to the following aspects of the working environment:

◆ maintenance of the workplace and equipment in efficient working order

◆ adequate ventilation is required, ensuring that the air is changed regularly and fumes or strong smells are removed. Fresh air should be drawn from outside the workplace

◆ working temperature should be regulated and determined by how physically demanding the work is

◆ lighting should be adequate to enable people to move safely and perform tasks competently

◆ cleanliness of furniture, equipment, furnishing and fittings and correct handling and disposal of **waste** materials

◆ safe salon layout, dimensions adequate for traffic flow (pedestrian traffic) and nature of the work

◆ safety protection against falls and falling objects, objects should be stored safely

◆ windows, doors, gates and walls should be safe and fit for purpose

◆ floor and traffic routes in good repair without uneven surfaces

◆ escalators and moving walkways should operate safely and have appropriate safety mechanisms

◆ sanitary conveniences for all staff and clients should be suitable and sufficient

◆ washing facilities of hot and cold running water should be available with soap and a means of drying hands

◆ drinking water: adequate high quality supply

◆ facilities for changing and storage of clothing should be adequate and secure

◆ facilities for staff to rest and eat meals should be suitable

◆ fire exits are clearly located and accessible and firefighting equipment is available and maintained.

Manual Handling Operations Regulations (1992)
The **Manual Handling Operations Regulations (1992)** apply in all occupations where manual lifting occurs, the aim being to prevent skeletal and muscular disorders and repetitive strain disorders due to poor working practice. The employer is required to carry out a risk assessment

ACTIVITY

PPE risk assessment

Carry out your own risk assessment on risks of possible cross-infection by contamination in the salon. List the potentially hazardous substances that you may be required to handle. What protective clothing should be available to provide protection?

ACTIVITY

Moving objects in the salon

What types of equipment or objects may you be required to move in the salon? Think of three examples and how best they should be lifted and handled.

TOP TIP

Broken goods

When you unpack a delivery, always make sure that the product packaging is undamaged, to avoid risk from broken goods.

Work equipment

How many of us try to multitask and use more than one piece of work equipment at the same time? This is a common problem amongst beauty receptionists who are required to answer the telephone and make appointments. Trying to balance the telephone on your shoulder whilst writing or typing can cause musculoskeletal problems such as neck and back pain but can be solved easily by providing a headset for the telephone allowing free movement of both hands and encouraging a good posture.

Wendy Nixon

ACTIVITY

European directives

The Workplace (Health, Safety and Welfare) Regulations were implemented following a European Union directive on minimum safety and health requirements for the workplace.

1 Obtain a copy of the *Workplace (Health, Safety and Welfare) Regulations 1992* (available online at www.hse .gov.uk).
2 Look through the publication, and make notes on any information relevant to you in the beauty workplace.

Knowledge Check

What is PPE? Why is it used?

Refer to page 108 to help you.

ALWAYS REMEMBER

Temperature and lighting

The salon temperature should be a minimum of 16°C within 1 hour of employees arriving for work. The salon should be well ventilated, or carbon dioxide levels will increase, which can cause nausea. Many substances used in the salon can become hazardous without adequate ventilation. If the working environment is too warm this can cause heat stress, a condition that is recognized by the HSE. Lighting should be adequate to ensure that treatments can be carried out safely and competently, with the minimum risk of accident.

of all activities undertaken which involve manual lifting. Risk assessment records must be available for audit when required.

The risk assessment should provide evidence that the following have been considered:

◆ risk of injury

◆ the manual movement involved in performing the activity

◆ the physical constraint the load incurs

◆ the environmental constraints imposed by the workplace

◆ workers' individual capabilities

◆ action taken to minimize potential risks.

Manual lifting and handling Always take care of yourself when moving goods around the salon. Assess the risk. Do not struggle or be impatient: get someone else to help. When lifting, reduce the risk; where possible break up larger items into more manageable loads; lift from the knees, not the back. When carrying, balance weights evenly in both hands and carry the heaviest part nearest to your body.

Provision and Use of Work Equipment Regulations (PUWER) (1998)

The Provision and Use of Work Equipment Regulations (PUWER) (1998) lay down the important health and safety controls on the provision and use of work equipment both new and secondhand. They state the duties for employers and employees, including the self-employed. The regulations affect both old and new equipment. They identify the requirements in selecting suitable equipment and in maintaining it so that it is fit for purpose. They also discuss the information provided by equipment manufacturers, and instruction and training requirements in the safe use of equipment. Specific regulations address the dangers and potential risks of injury that could occur during operation of the equipment and not using it for its intended purpose. Suitable safety measures must be in place, including making protective devices available and warning signage as appropriate.

Health and Safety (Display Screen Equipment) Regulations (1992)

The Health and Safety (Display Screen Equipment) Regulations (1992) cover the use of display screen equipment including computer screens. They specify acceptable levels of radiation emissions from the screen and identify correct posture, seating position, permitted working heights and rest periods. Employers have a responsibility to comply with this regulation to ensure the welfare of their employees in avoiding the potential risks of eyestrain, mental stress and muscle fatigue.

HEALTH & SAFETY

COSHH assessment All hazardous substances must be identified when completing the risk assessment. This includes cleaning agents such as a wax equipment cleaner.

High-risk products should, wherever possible, be replaced with lower risk products.

COSHH assessments should be reviewed on a regular basis and updated to include any new products. There should be an identified responsible person to carry out this important procedure.

Everybody must be familiar with the COSHH assessment risk reports so that they actively reduce any risk.

Consider where you are going to move the load to. If too large / heavy can it be made smaller?

Ensure you feel stable before you lift and move the object.

Bend the knees, keep the back straight. Lean slightly forward over the load and ensure you have a good grip of the object. You should be able to move the object smoothly with minimum effort and without twisting.

Carry the heaviest part nearest to your body.

Place one foot slightly forward to support balance.

Best practice for manual handling

Control of Substances Hazardous to Health (COSHH) Regulations (2002)

The **Control of Substances Hazardous to Health (COSHH) Regulations (2002)** were designed to make employers consider the substances used in their workplace and assess the possible risks to health. Many substances that seem quite harmless can

International hazard symbols

prove to be hazardous if used or stored incorrectly. A hazardous substance is anything that can harm your health. All cosmetic products must comply with the Cosmetic Products (Safety) Regulations (2008). This legislation requires that cosmetics and toiletries are safe in their formulation and safe for use for their intended purpose.

Employers are responsible for assessing the risks from hazardous substances and controlling exposure to them to prevent ill-health. Any hazardous substances identified must be formally recorded in writing. Safety precaution procedures should then be implemented and training given to employees to ensure that the procedures are understood and will be followed correctly. Employers must control substances that can harm employees' health. As an employee it is then necessary for you to follow this procedure to avoid exposure to hazard.

Hazardous substances are identified by the use of known symbols which you should recognize, examples of which are shown below. Any substance in the workplace that is hazardous to health must be identified on the packaging and stored, handled and disposed of correctly.

Hazardous substances can enter the body via the:

◆ eyes

◆ skin

◆ nose (**inhalation** – breathing in)

◆ mouth (**ingestion** – swallowing).

Each beauty product supplier is legally required to make guidelines available on the chemical ingredients contained in their products with their hazard rating. Also guidance on how the product should be safely used, stored and disposed of. These are called material safety data sheets (MSDSs) and will be supplied on request.

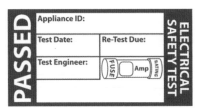

PAT test sticker

REACH (2007) REACH 2007 is a European Union Regulation concerning the:

Registration

Evaluation

Authorization, and restriction of

Chemicals.

It operates alongside COSHH and is designed to improve the information provided by chemical manufacturers through the provision of adequate safety data sheets.

Electricity at Work Regulations (1989) Electricity, if unsafe or used carelessly, can harm and even kill. The **Electricity at Work Regulations (1989)** state that every piece of electrical equipment in the workplace must be tested every 12 months by a qualified electrician to confirm if it is safe to use. This is called portable appliance testing or (PAT). A written record of testing must be retained and made available for inspection. In larger organizations a PAT test sticker is applied which indicates if it has passed the PAT test or not. A list of all salon electrical equipment should be available with its unique serial number and date of purchase/disposal.

In addition to annual testing, a trained member of staff should regularly check all electrical equipment for safety. This is recommended every three months. If you see any of these potential hazards they must be immediately reported:

ACTIVITY

Personal appearance

1 Collect pictures from various suppliers of overalls. Select those that you feel would be most practical for a Level 2 beauty therapist, make-up artist or receptionist. Briefly describe why you feel these are the most suitable.

2 Design various hairstyles, or source pictures, to show how the hair could be smartly worn by a beauty therapist with medium-length to long hair, whilst being hygienic.

◆ exposed wires in flexes

◆ cracked plugs or broken sockets

◆ worn, loose cables

◆ overloaded plug sockets.

Although it is the employer's responsibility to ensure all equipment is safe to use, it is also the responsibility of the employee to check that equipment is safe before use, and never to use it if it is faulty. This complies with the requirements of public liability insurance. Failure to do so could lead to an accident which would be considered negligent. Electrical equipment should only be operated by those qualified to do so.

Any pieces of equipment that appear faulty must be checked immediately and, if necessary, repaired before use. If faulty they must be labelled to ensure that they are not used by accident and a record made of the fault and date.

Personal health, hygiene and presentation

Your appearance enables the client to make an initial judgement about both you and the salon, so make sure that you create the correct impression! Employees in the workplace should always reflect the desired image of the profession that they work in. This is discussed in more detail in Chapter 1 Introduction.

Ethics

Beauty therapy has a code of ethics. This is a code of **behaviour** and expected standards for the professional beauty therapist to follow, which will uphold the reputation of the industry and ensure best working practice for the safety of the industry and members of the public. Beauty therapy professional bodies produce **Industry Codes of Practice** for their members. A business may have its own code of practice. Although not a legal requirement, this code may be used in criminal proceedings as evidence of improper practice.

Lifestyle

A beauty therapist requires stamina and energy. To achieve this you need to eat a healthy, well-balanced diet, drink an adequate amount of water, take regular exercise and have regular sleep – recommended 7–8 hours per night. You can read more about nutritional advice in Chapter 7 Facial Skincare.

Posture

Posture is the way you hold yourself when standing, sitting and walking. *Correct* posture enables you to work longer without becoming tired, it prevents muscle fatigue, repetitive strain injury (RSI) and stiff joints, and it also improves your appearance.

Good standing posture If you are standing with good posture, you will have your:

◆ head up, centrally balanced

◆ shoulders slightly back, and relaxed

◆ chest up and out

◆ abdomen flat

◆ hips level

Personal presentation should show a professional image

Good standing posture

Good sitting posture

◆ fingertips level

◆ bottom in

◆ knees level

◆ feet slightly apart and weight evenly distributed.

Good sitting posture To have good sitting posture, sit on a suitable chair or stool with a good back support and:

◆ sit with the lower back pressed against the chair back

◆ keep the chest up and the shoulders back

◆ distribute the body weight evenly along the thighs

◆ keep the feet together, and flat on the floor

◆ do not slouch, or sit on the edge of your seat.

> **Dermatitis**
>
> Always dry your hands thoroughly using a clean, disposable paper towel or warm-air hand dryer. Remember to dry between the fingers and around the thumb and wrist. I often see beauty therapists drying their hands on damp towels previously used on clients. This is not effective and can lead to skin damage and dermatitis. Your hands are your tools, so take a few minutes to protect your skin and ultimately your career.
>
> *Wendy Nixon*

HEALTH & SAFETY

Repetitive strain injury (RSI) If you do not follow correct postural positional requirements when performing treatments, muscle and ligaments may become overstretched and overused resulting in repetitive strain injury (RSI). This may result in you being unable to work in the short term, and potentially long term in the occupation.

Personal hygiene

It is vital that you have a high standard of personal hygiene. You are going to be working in close contact with people.

Bodily cleanliness is achieved through daily showering or bathing. This removes the stale sweat, dirt and bacteria which cause body odour. An antiperspirant or deodorant may be applied to the underarm area to reduce perspiration and thus the smell of sweat. Clean underwear should be worn each day.

Hands Your hands and everything you touch are covered with germs. Although most are harmless, some can cause ill-health or disease. Wash your hands regularly, especially after you have been to the toilet and before eating food. You must also wash your hands before and after treating each client, and during a treatment if necessary. Washing the hands before treating a client minimizes the risk of cross-infection and presents to the client a hygienic, professional, caring image. Disinfecting hand gel may also be applied to the clean hands before treatments are delivered. See the Step-by-step: How to wash your hands for more information.

Skin on the hands should be regularly checked for dryness or soreness. If this occurs hand maintenance systems should be reviewed including PPE.

Feet Keep your feet fresh and healthy by washing them daily and then drying them thoroughly, especially between the toes to avoid foot disorders developing, such as athlete's foot. Deodorizing foot powder may then be applied.

Oral hygiene Avoid bad breath by brushing your teeth at least twice daily and flossing the teeth frequently. Remember, some foods consumed such as garlic can be present on the breath the following day. Breath fresheners and mouthwashes may be

STEP-BY-STEP: HOW TO WASH YOUR HANDS

1 Wet your hands, wrists and forearms thoroughly using running water

2 Apply around 3 ml to 5 ml of liquid soap

3 Start the lathering process, rubbing palm to palm

4 Interlock fingers and rub, ensuring a good lather

5 Rub right hand over back of left, then left over right hand

6 Rub with fingers locked in palm of hand ensuring fingertips are cleaned

7 Lock thumbs and rotate hands

8 Grasp thumb with hand and rotate, repeat with opposite thumb

9 Rotate hand around wrist, repeat on opposite wrist

10 Rinse hands and wrists thoroughly using running water

11 Dry the hands and wrists thoroughly using a clean, disposable paper towel or warm-air hand dryer

12 Turn off the tap using a clean paper towel to avoid contaminating the hands. Dispose of the paper towel without coming into contact with any part of the waste bin

Personal hygiene for the hands using hand disinfection

used as required to freshen your breath. Visit the dentist regularly to maintain healthy teeth and gums. Avoid eating strong flavoured foods which could cause offence in close proximity.

Hair Your hair should be clean and tidy. Have your hair cut regularly to maintain its healthy appearance, and shampoo and condition your hair as often as needed. If your hair is long, wear it off the face and taken to the crown of the head. Medium-length hair should be clipped back, away from the face, to prevent it falling forwards.

ACTIVITY

Hand hygiene

What further occasions can you think of when it will be necessary to wash your hands when treating a client?

Knowledge Check

Why is good posture important?

Refer to pages 113–114 to help you.

TOP TIP

Fresh breath

When working, avoid eating strong-smelling, highly spiced food.

HEALTH & SAFETY

Long hair and hygienic working practice If long hair is not taken away from the face, the tendency will be to move the hair away from the face repeatedly with the hands, and this in turn will require that the hands be washed repeatedly.

CourseMate video: Clean Up

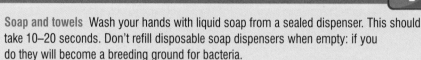

HEALTH & SAFETY

Soap and towels Wash your hands with liquid soap from a sealed dispenser. This should take 10–20 seconds. Don't refill disposable soap dispensers when empty: if you do they will become a breeding ground for bacteria.

Disposable paper towels or warm-air hand dryers should be used to thoroughly dry the hands.

Protecting yourself You will be wise to have the relevant inoculations, including those against tetanus and hepatitis, to protect yourself against ill-health and even death.

Protecting the client If you have any cuts or abrasions on your hands, cover them with a clean dressing to minimize the risk of secondary infection. Disposable gloves may be worn for additional protection.

Certain skin disorders are contagious. Beauty therapists suffering from any such disorder must not work, but must seek medical advice immediately.

Face masks may be worn when working in close proximity to the client.

Hygiene and infection control in the workplace

Infections Effective hygiene and infection control is necessary in the salon to prevent *cross-infection* and *secondary infection*. Infection can occur through poor practice, such as the use of tools that are not sterile. Reusable (as opposed to disposable) **tools and equipment** become contaminated – infected with skin and nail debris. An infection can be recognized by red and inflamed skin, or the presence of pus. All staff must be trained in and carry out effective decontamination procedures to remove and/or destroy the contamination.

Cross-infection occurs because some microorganisms are contagious – they may be transferred through personal contact or by contact with an infected tool that has not been disinfected or sterilized. Cross-infection can occur through blood contamination and skin or nail infections.

Secondary infection can occur as a result of injury to the client during the treatment or, if the client already has an open wound, bacteria can penetrate the skin and cause infection. **Sterilization** and disinfection procedures (see later) are used to minimize or destroy the harmful microorganisms which could cause infection – **bacteria**, **viruses** and **fungi**.

Infectious diseases that are contagious **contra-indicate** beauty treatment: they require medical attention. People with certain other skin disorders, even though these are not contagious, should likewise not be treated by the beauty therapist, as treatment might lead to secondary infection.

Sterilization and disinfection

Sterilization is the total destruction of all living microorganisms from metal tools and equipment. Disinfection is the destruction of most living microorganisms from non-metal tools, equipment and work areas. Disinfection aims to reduce the level of microorganisms to a level that will not lead to infection. Sterilization and disinfection techniques practised in the beauty salon involve the use of *physical* agents such as radiation and heat and *chemical* agents such as antiseptics and disinfectants. Sterilization and disinfection procedures must be performed between each client.

Radiation – a quartz mercury-vapour lamp can be used as the source for UV light, which minimizes harmful microorganisms. However, UV light has limited effectiveness and cannot be relied upon for complete sterilization. Radiation only destroys microorganisms on the surface that the UV rays strike, requiring the object to be turned. For each surface of the object 20 minutes exposure is required. A UV cabinet is a useful place to store previously sterilized objects.

Heat – dry and moist heat can both be used for sterilization.

◆ **Dry heat** One dry heat method is to use a dry hot-air oven. This is similar to a small oven and heats to 150–180°C. It is seldom used in the salon. Available also is a glass bead heater where tiny glass beads are heated in an insulated container to between 190 and 300°C. This is only suitable for small, metal objects.

◆ **Moist heat** The **autoclave** (similar to a pressure cooker) is a popular moist heat method of sterilization where water is boiled and because of the increased pressure, the water reaches a temperature of 121–134°C. Autoclaving is the most effective method and highly recommended for sterilizing objects in the salon.

Disinfectants and antiseptics

If an object *cannot* be sterilized, it should be placed in a chemical **disinfectant** solution. A disinfectant destroys most microorganisms, but not all. Hypochlorite is a disinfectant – bleach is an example of a hypochlorite. Hypochlorite is suitable for cleaning work surfaces but is particularly corrosive and unsuitable for use with metals – use as directed by the manufacturer. Ammonium compound disinfectants such as 'Barbicide' can be used with metal and plastic items. Alcohol-impregnated wipes are a popular way to clean the skin using a disinfectant such as isopropyl alcohol.

A UV light cabinet

An automatic medical autoclave

All sterilization/disinfection techniques must be carried out safely and effectively following the manufacturer's instructions for correct use:

1 Select the appropriate method of sterilization or disinfectant for the object. *Always* follow the manufacturer's guidelines on the use of the sterilizing or disinfecting unit or agent.

2 Always clean the object in clean water and a detergent, such as liquid soap, to remove dirt, debris and grease. This is often referred to as sanitization in the salon. (Dirt left on the object might prevent effective sterilization or disinfection.)

3 Dry it thoroughly with a clean, disposable paper towel.

4 Sterilize or disinfect the object, allowing sufficient time for the process to be completed. Contact with all surfaces of the object must be made.

> ### Hygiene
>
> As an inspector I have seen too many jars of disinfection fluid which have turned black and are full of floating debris. This not only gives a poor visual message to the clients but it will not be effective. Always wash equipment to remove visual contamination prior to disinfection or sterilization. Disinfection fluids must be changed daily in accordance with the manufacturer's instructions. If you use an autoclave run a test strip through the system each morning.
>
> *Wendy Nixon*

5 Following disinfection/sterilization handle the objects with clean tongs or protective gloves. Place objects that have been sterilized or disinfected in a clean, covered container, ideally labelled. After 24 hours the object will be clean but not disinfected.

Keep several sets of the tools you use regularly, so that you can carry out effective sterilization and disinfection.

Workplace policies
Each workplace should have its own workplace policy to identify hygiene rules. This should cover the following:

◆ *Health and safety* Follow the health and safety policies for the workplace.

◆ *Personal hygiene* Maintain a high standard of personal hygiene. Wash your hands with a detergent containing chlorhexidine gluconate, which protects against a wide range of bacteria. The addition of isopropyl alcohol provides a stronger hand disinfectant, removing surface bacteria and fungi.

◆ *Cuts on the hands* Always cover any cuts on your hands with a protective dressing.

◆ *Cross-infection* Take great care to avoid cross-infection in the salon. *Never* treat a client who has a contagious skin disease or disorder, or any other contra-indication. Refer the client tactfully to their GP.

◆ *Use hygienic tools* Never use an implement unless it has been effectively sterilized or disinfected as appropriate.

◆ *Disposable applicators* Wherever possible use disposable applicators, also referred to as 'single use' tools.

◆ *Working surfaces* Disinfect all working surfaces (such as trolleys and couches) with a commercial disinfectant or chlorine preparation, diluted to the manufacturer's instructions. Cover all working surfaces with clean, disposable paper tissue.

◆ *Gowns and towels* Clean gowns and towels must be provided for each client. Towels should be laundered at a temperate of 60°C.

◆ *Laundry* Dirty laundry should be placed in a covered container.

◆ *Waste* Including clinical waste and non-contaminated waste, must be disposed of following the COSHH procedures and guidelines provided by the LA and training by the employer. For contaminated waste comply with the Controlled Waste Regulations (1992). Put waste in a suitable container lined with a disposable waste bag. A yellow 'sharps' container or heavy duty yellow bag, should be available for clinical waste contaminated with blood or tissue fluid. Protective gloves should be worn to avoid risk of contamination.

◆ *Eating and drinking* Never eat or drink in the treatment area of the salon. Not only is it unprofessional, but harmful chemicals may also be ingested.

◆ *Drugs and alcohol* Never carry out treatments in the workplace under the influence of drugs or alcohol. Your competence will be affected putting yourself, clients and possibly colleagues at risk. Any accident as a result would be termed negligent and you would be liable.

Ensure that your behaviour at work is in accordance with your workplace policies and doesn't endanger yourself or others.

Salon security

It is important that adequate precautions are taken to secure the premises against theft (during business hours) and burglary (outside business hours). Insurance companies

A disinfection tray with liquid

ALWAYS REMEMBER

Before sterilization, wash and clean the object requiring sterilization. Surgical spirit or isopropyl impregnated tissues may be applied; clean cotton wool may be used before sterilization to remove debris from small objects.

TOP TIP

HSE advice on cleaning

Advice on cleaning work surfaces and equipment can be found on the COSHH Essentials website: www.coshh-essentials.org.uk

Medi-swabs (sterile isopropyl tissues)

Disinfecting work surfaces

> **COSHH**
>
> When undertaking your COSHH assessments in the salon, don't forget to include the general cleaning or laundry products. Also ensure that you record the precautionary measures to reduce risks to the client as well as the staff, e.g. skin sensitivity tests. Your written procedures should note that you undertake skin sensitivity tests under the heading 'what action should I take' on your assessment forms.
>
> *Wendy Nixon*

HEALTH & SAFETY

Cuts on the hands Open, uncovered cuts provide an easy entry for harmful bacteria, and may therefore lead to infection. Always cover cuts.

HEALTH & SAFETY

Misuse of Drugs Act (1971) This Act categorizes drugs into classes and details the penalties for those caught possessing them. Therefore, you are acting illegally if found in possession of a controlled drug.

HEALTH & SAFETY

Security A Crime Prevention Officer can complete a security check and provide advice on effective ways of securing the business premises.

Some businesses use closed circuit television (CCTV).

will not insure a business where there are inadequate security measures. Staff must be trained in all aspects of security with procedures. Updates should be discussed at staff meetings. All staff at induction should be made aware of the consequences of theft. Theft is often referred to as gross misconduct and may lead to dismissal and prosecution.

The employer should have a formal policy and procedures to ensure the security of:

◆ people and possessions

◆ premises

◆ tools and equipment

◆ stock

◆ cash and equivalents.

Security concerns should be taken into consideration at all times. **Systems** should be in place to monitor till transactions, stock and personal possessions, including client and staff belongings.

◆ Personal possessions – secure areas such as lockers should be available to staff for storing personal possessions while they are at work. If a treatment requires the removal of clothing and/or jewellery, the client's possessions should be given to the client for safe keeping or kept within view of the client. It is customary to display a notice disclaiming responsibility in the event of theft.

◆ Stock – areas vulnerable to theft, such as the retail area, should be designed so as to be in full view of staff. Only authorized staff should handle and have access to stock. Expensive equipment may be locked away when not in use. Regular and random stock checks will show up any missing stock.

◆ Cash and equivalents – only authorized staff should handle money. Security systems should be in place so that all errors are traceable. There should be a salon policy to deal with fraudulent monetary transactions. In accordance with the Data Protection Act (1998), confidential information about staff or clients must only be recorded and stored if consent has been given. Records must be stored in a secure area.

Accidents

Accidents in the workplace usually occur through negligence by employees or unsafe working conditions.

Outcome 2: Be able to follow emergency procedures

Learn how to follow emergency procedures

PRACTICAL SKILLS

1 Follow emergency procedures

2 Follow accident reporting procedures which meet with salon policy

3 Identify named emergency personnel

4 Locate firefighting equipment

UNDERPINNING KNOWLEDGE

1 Outline the correct use of firefighting equipment for different types of fire

2 State the dangers of the incorrect use of fire-fighting equipment on different types of fires

3 State the importance for reporting and recording accidents

4 Describe the procedure for reporting and recording accidents

5 Describe procedures for dealing with emergencies

Any accidents occurring in the workplace must be dealt with following the workplace policy and details recorded on a report form, and entered into an **accident book**. Incidents in the accident book should be reviewed regularly to see where improvements to working practice can be made. The **accident form** requires more details than the accident book. You must note:

◆ the date and time of the accident

◆ the date of entry into the accident book

◆ the name of the person or people involved

◆ the accident details

◆ the injuries sustained

◆ the action taken

◆ what happened to the person immediately afterwards (e.g. went home or to hospital)

◆ name and address of the person who was providing the treatment

◆ the signature of the person making the entry.

In the instance of an accident, first aid should only be administered by employees qualified to do so.

Breakages and spillage Accidents can damage stock, resulting in breakage of containers and spillage of contents. Breakage of glass can cause cuts; spillages can cause somebody to slip and fall. Any breakages or spillages should therefore be dealt

ALWAYS REMEMBER

Security procedures should be:

◆ current

◆ fit for purpose

◆ implemented

◆ performed by a designated person.

HEALTH & SAFETY

Breakages and spillages
When dealing with hazardous breakages and spillages, the hands should always be protected with gloves. To avoid injury to others, broken glass should be put in a secure container prior to disposing of it in a waste bin, in compliance with waste disposal regulations.

ACTIVITY

Accidents

Discuss potential causes of accidents that could occur in the workplace. How could these accidents be prevented? Who would you report an accident or injury to in the workplace and when?

HEALTH & SAFETY

First aid What is adequate will depend upon each workplace and requires an assessment of first aid needs. Detailed information can be found in the Approved Code of Practice and Guidance: First Aid at Work. The Health and Safety (First Aid) Regulations (1981).

First aid kits

HEALTH & SAFETY

First aid

◆ This should only be given by a qualified first aider.

◆ A first aid certificate is only valid for 3 years after qualifying and must then be renewed. This may mean additional first aid training.

◆ Know what action you can take within your responsibility in the event of an accident occurring.

◆ An accident book should be available to record details of any accident that has occurred.

with immediately and in the correct way. Remember to always deal with a hazard within your responsibility – a hazard is anything that has potential to cause harm.

You must determine whether the spillage is a potential hazard to health and what action is necessary. To whom should you report it? What equipment is required to remove the spillage? Is it necessary to wear PPE? How should the materials be disposed of? Always consider your COSHH data and check to see how the product should be handled and disposed of.

Reporting of Injuries, Diseases and Dangerous Occurrences Regulations (RIDDOR) (1995)

The Reporting of Injuries, Diseases and Dangerous Occurrences Regulations (RIDDOR) (1995) requires the reporting and recording of work-related deaths and serious major injuries, cases of diagnosed industrial disease and certain 'dangerous occurrences' (near miss accidents).

Deaths and serious major injuries occurring in the workplace related to a work activity must be reported. It is a legal requirement to notify the HSE Incident Contact Centre (ICC). This must be immediate, by telephone, followed by a written report on HSE Form F2508, within 10 days of it happening. This action is completed by the person in a position of control for the workplace. If a person is absent from work for 7 consecutive days due to injury this must also be reported, within 15 days of the accident.

In all cases where personal injury occurs, an entry must be made in the workplace accident book. It is a legal requirement to keep an accident book. Occupational diseases such as dermatitis (see page 121) must also be reported. Where visitors to the work premises, such as clients, are injured and taken to hospital, the same reporting systems apply. This information assists the HSE in investigation of serious accidents.

The HSE website provides guidance on what constitutes a reportable major injury, occupational disease and dangerous occurrence.

First aid

The Health and Safety (First Aid) Regulations (1981) state that workplaces must have first aid provision. Employers must have appropriate and adequate first aid arrangements in the event of an accident or illness occurring. It is recommended that at least one person holds an HSE-approved basic first aid qualification.

All employees should be informed of the first aid procedures, including:

◆ where to find the first aid box which should be clearly identifiable and easily accessible

◆ who is responsible for keeping the first aid box well stocked

◆ which member of staff to inform in the event of an accident or illness occurring

◆ the staff member to inform in the event of an emergency.

An adequately stocked first aid box that complies with the Health and Safety (First Aid) Regulations for your workplace must be available.

Basic items include:

◆ basic first aid guidance leaflet (1)

◆ assorted individually wrapped sterile adhesive dressings (20)

◆ individually wrapped sterile triangular bandages (6)

◆ safety pins (6)

◆ sterile eye pads, with attachments (2)

◆ medium-sized individually wrapped sterile unmedicated wound dressings, 10 cm × 8 cm (6)

◆ large individually wrapped sterile unmedicated wound dressings 13 cm × 9 cm (2)

◆ extra large sterile individually wrapped medicated wound dressings 28 cm × 17.5 cm (3)

◆ individually wrapped medical wipes

◆ antiseptic cream

◆ sterile water

◆ disposable non-latex gloves.

Where clean tap water is not readily available, sterile water should be stored in sealed containers for bathing eyes.

TOP TIP

First aid booklet

HSE guidance publication *Basic advice on first aid at work INDG 347 (rev 1)* can be stored in the first aid box.

Examples of first aid procedures

Problem	Action to be taken
Casualty is not breathing	1 Place the casualty on their back. Open and clear their mouth. Shout for help, immediately contact emergency services 2 Tilt head backwards to open airway (maintain this position throughout). Support the jaw 3 Kneel beside casualty, while keeping head backwards. Open mouth and pinch nose 4 Open your mouth and take a deep breath. Seal mouth with yours and breathe firmly into it. Casualty's chest should rise. Remove your mouth and let their chest fall. If chest does not rise, check head is tilted sufficiently. Repeat at a rate of ten times a minute until the casualty is breathing alone 5 Place them in the recovery position
Unconscious	Immediately contact emergency services. Place into recovery position
Severe bleeding	Immediately contact emergency services. Control by direct pressure using fingers and thumb on the bleeding point. Apply a dressing. Raising the bleeding limb (unless it is broken) will reduce the flow of blood
Suspected broken bones	Immediately contact emergency services. Do not move the casualty unless they are in a position which exposes them to immediate danger. Gain expert help
Burns and scalds (due to heat)	Do not remove clothing sticking to the burns or scalds. Do not burst any blisters. If burns and scalds are small, flush them with plenty of clean, cool water for 10 minutes before applying a sterilized dressing. If burns and scalds are large or deep, wash your hands and apply a dry sterilized dressing. The casualty must be immediately professionally attended to

(Continued)

Problem	Action to be taken
Burns (chemicals)	Avoid contaminating yourself with the chemical. Remove any contaminated clothing that is not stuck to skin. Flush with plenty of cool water and apply a sterilized dressing. The casualty must be immediately professionally attended to
Foreign body in eye	Wash out eye with clean cool water. A person with an eye injury should be sent to hospital with the eye covered by an eye pad. Never attempt to remove the foreign body
Chemicals in eyes	Wash out the open eye continuously with clean, cool water gently holding the eye lid open. A person with an eye injury should be sent to hospital with the eye covered with an eye pad
Electric shock	Don't touch the casualty until the current is switched off. If the current cannot be switched off, stand on some dry insulating material and use a wooden or plastic implement to free the casualty from the electrical source. If breathing has stopped, start mouth-to-mouth breathing and continue until the casualty starts to breathe by themselves or until professional help arrives
Gassing	Use suitable protective equipment. Move casualty to fresh air. If breathing has stopped, start mouth-to-mouth breathing and continue until the casualty is breathing by themselves or until professional help arrives. Send to hospital with a note of the gas involved
Minor injuries	Casualties with minor injuries of a nature they would normally attend to themselves may wash their hands, apply disposable gloves if necessary and apply a small sterilized dressing from the first aid box to the area. Keep wounds clean and dry

Sharps container

Find out more about environmentally friendly working practices on page 128.

Disposal of waste

Waste should be sorted and disposed of according to its risk and in an environmentally friendly way. Remember, recycle your waste and packaging wherever possible. Waste which is general, not hazardous, should be disposed of in an enclosed waste bin fitted with a polythene bin liner that is durable enough not to tear. The bin should be regularly cleaned and disinfected in a well-ventilated area; wear protective gloves while doing this. When the bin is full, the liner can be sealed using a wire tie and placed ready for refuse collection. If the bin liner punctures, the damaged liner and waste should be placed inside a second bin liner.

Clinical (contaminated) waste is classed as high risk, hazardous waste containing waste derived from human tissues. This includes blood and body tissue fluids. The microorganisms in clinical waste can cause disease. Hazardous waste must be handled following the COSHH procedures and training by the employer. **Clinical waste**, including items such as wax strips, must be disposed of as recommended by the Environment Agency in accordance with the **Controlled Waste (Amendment) Regulations (1993)**. Items which have been used to pierce the skin, such as disposable micro lances, should be safely discarded in a disposable sharps container. Contact your local environment health department to check on waste disposal arrangements for these items.

Items that could cause injury to others such as broken glass should be put in a secure container, e.g. a heavy duty card box, prior to disposal.

Chemicals that can be disposed of down the sink should be diluted and rinsed away using lots of water. Remember to always handle chemicals correctly, referring to your COSHH data sheets.

Fire

The **Regulatory Reform (Fire Safety) Order (2005)** replaces all previous legislation relating to fire, including fire certificates which no longer have any validity. This law is applicable to England and Wales only. Northern Ireland and Scotland have their own similar legislation.

The Regulatory Reform (Fire Safety) Order (2005) places responsibility for fire safety onto the 'responsible person' which is usually the employer. The 'responsible person' will have a duty to ensure the safety of everyone who uses their premises and those in the immediate vicinity who may be at risk if there is a fire. The 'responsible person' (emergency personnel fire warden) must carry out a fire safety risk assessment.

Fire risk assessments will include:

◆ identifying and removing any obstacles that may hinder fire evacuation

◆ ensuring that suitable fire detection equipment is in place, such as a smoke alarm

◆ making sure that all escape routes are clearly marked and free from obstacles

◆ testing fire alarm systems regularly to ensure they are in full operational condition.

All staff must be trained in fire and emergency evacuation procedures for their workplace. They should be confident in knowing how the alarm is raised. The emergency exit route will be the easiest route by which staff and clients can leave the building safely. Fire action plans should be prominently displayed to show the emergency exit route. There should be a designated fire evacuation assembly point where staff can meet having safely left the building, clients will be requested to assemble here also. Firefighting equipment should be available for use on different types of fire and maintained. Equipment should be used only by those trained to use it.

TOP TIP

Incentive to recycle

Some beauty companies will provide a free product on the return of a used product packaging – check with your manufacturer/supplier.

Fire alarm

HEALTH & SAFETY

Fire safety awareness Training must be given to new staff during their induction. Training for all staff must be regularly updated. Fire drills must be held at regular intervals. Following a fire drill, feedback should be given on any risks that need to be addressed.

Fire exit door

Fire blankets

Firefighting equipment Firefighting equipment must be available, located in a specified area. The equipment includes fire extinguishers, blankets, sand buckets and water hoses. Firefighting equipment should be used only when the cause of the fire has been identified – using the *wrong* fire extinguisher could make the fire worse.

Fire classifications include class A, B and C. Symbols are used to identify these classifications and choice of fire extinguisher as shown below.

Class D Fires involve metals.

Never use firefighting equipment unless you are trained in its use.

Class A Fire – carbonaceous materials such as paper and wood.

Class B Fire – flammable liquids such as petrol, oil and paints.

Class C Fire – flammable gases such as methane and acetylene.

Electrical hazard symbol – for extinguisher products safe on electrical fires.

Fire extinguisher symbols

Fire extinguishers Fire extinguishers are available to tackle different types of fire. These should be located in a set place known to all employees. It is important that these are checked and maintained as required.

Fire blankets are used to smother a small, localized fire or if a person's clothing is on fire. Sand is used to soak up liquids if these are the source of the fire and to smother the fire. Water hoses are used to extinguish large fires caused by paper materials and

Fire extinguisher label colour code

Cause of fire and choice of fire extinguisher

Cause	Extinguisher type	Label colour code
Electrical fire, flammable gases	Carbon dioxide (CO_2) extinguisher	Black
Solid material fire (paper, wood, etc.)	Water extinguisher	Red
Flammable liquid	Foam extinguisher	Cream/yellow
Electrical fire, flammable liquids	Dry-powder extinguisher	Blue
Flammable metal fire	Vaporizing liquid	Green

HEALTH & SAFETY

Fire exits Fire exit doors must be clearly marked, remain unlocked during working hours and be free from obstruction.

ALWAYS REMEMBER

Fire extinguishers

Label colour and symbols indicate the use of particular fire extinguishers. Make sure you know the meaning of each of the colours and symbols.

Knowledge Check

Which set of regulations determines fire safety in the workplace?

Refer to page 125 to help you.

the like – buckets of water can be used to extinguish a small fire. *Remember: turn off the electricity at the mains first!*

Never put yourself at risk – fires can spread quickly. Leave the building at once if in danger and raise the alarm by telephoning the emergency services on the emergency telephone numbers, 999 or 112.

Other emergencies

Other possible emergencies that could occur relate to fumes and flooding. Learn where the water stopcocks and gas stopcocks are located. In the event of a gas leak or a flood, shut off the water stopcock and switch off the mains gas supply, open the windows to increase ventilation. Evacuate the building following the fire drill procedure and contact the appropriate emergency service.

It is a good idea to get a gas detector which sounds when it detects a gas leak.

Never switch on an electric switch as this could cause a spark and ignite the gas!

In the event of a bomb alert staff must be trained in the appropriate emergency procedures. This will involve recognition of a suspect package, how to deal with a bomb threat, evacuation of staff and clients and contacting the emergency services. Your local Crime Prevention Officer (CPO) will advise on bomb security.

Environmentally friendly working practices

Being environmentally friendly, also known as 'eco-friendly' or 'green', means that you consider how you can help to minimize harm to the environment and put this into practice in everyday working practice. Think about how you use and dispose of products within your workplace. Are you always environmentally friendly? Consider the following changes:

◆ use biodegradable packaging for disposal of non-contaminated waste

◆ revert back to cups and glasses that can be washed for hospitality drinks, rather than use disposable plastic cups

◆ dispose of chemicals safely, not down the sinks

◆ use wooden spatulas from sustainable wood sources

◆ use recycled consumable materials where possible, e.g. bed-roll, tissues and cleaning products

◆ use light bulbs that minimize energy use

◆ switch off lights in rooms not being used and also equipment when not in use – if safe to do so

◆ turn down the heating thermostat rather than opening windows (this will save money too)

◆ buy in bulk, reducing trips to the wholesaler, and buy locally

◆ recycle your waste and packaging where possible, use colour-coded waste bags that are of course made from recycled materials

◆ recycle used printer cartridges

◆ some beauty companies will provide a free product on the return of a used product packaging.

Small steps can make a big difference.

Get involved

Keeping up to date with health and safety doesn't have to be hard work. Check out the Habia website regularly and become a member. The HSE website also provides generic information to keep you up to date. Use your local inspector by ringing them for a chat. Inspectors will always work with business.

Get actively involved in daily checks which quickly become part of your routine work and encourage staff to get involved by discussing health and safety issues in staff meetings, report back on findings or promote discussion and recognize good practice.

Wendy Nixon

Control of Noise at Work Regulations (2005) Loud noise can damage hearing. Noise is measured in decibels (db) which have different kinds of weighting. A-weighting is sometimes written as 'dB(A)', which is average noise level. C-weighting is 'dB(C)' – noise which is at its highest point, e.g. explosives.

As an employer a safe working environment should be provided with noise levels kept within safe levels. This does not include low-level noise. As in all **workplace practices**, noise levels can be classified as a **risk.** If a risk is identified, action should be taken to correct it. This could be a PPE hearing protection. Information, instruction and training must be provided and must also be monitored.

Insurance

Insurance must cover all activities in the workplace. **Public Liability Insurance** protects employers and employees against the consequences of death or injury claim by a third party while on the premises. This does not apply to claims by employees. Professional indemnity insurance extends public liability insurance to cover named employees against claims.

Product and treatment liability insurance is usually included with your public liability insurance but this should be checked with the insurance company. Product liability insurance covers you for risks which might occur as a result of the products you are using and/or selling.

It is a legal requirement under the **Employer's Liability (Compulsory Insurance) Act (1969)** that every employer must have employer's liability insurance. This provides financial compensation to an employee should they be injured as a result of an accident in the workplace. A current employee/public liability insurance certificate notice must be displayed in a prominent place indicating that a policy of insurance has been obtained.

ACTIVITY

Causes of fires

Can you think of several potential causes of fire in the salon? How can each of these be prevented?

Knowledge Check

Why is it important to have insurance?

ALWAYS REMEMBER

To avoid potential hazards and risks in the workplace you should:

◆ be aware of the workplace health and safety policy and your responsibility in its implementation

◆ ensure your personal presentation and conduct at work meets health and safety and legislative requirements in accordance with workplace policies

◆ follow the most recent workplace policies for your job role and manufacturer's instructions for the safe use of resources

◆ follow the latest health and safety legislation related to your work

◆ know who is responsible for health and safety in your workplace. Pass on any suggestions for reducing health and safety risks within your job role

◆ report or deal immediately with any risk which could be a hazard, complying with workplace policies and legal requirements

◆ be aware of first aid arrangements in the event of an accident or illness

◆ know the workplace fire evacuation advice and procedure

◆ ensure your working practice minimizes the possible spread of infection or disease.

ASSESSMENT OF KNOWLEDGE AND UNDERSTANDING

You have now learnt about health and safety in the beauty therapy workplace. To test your level of knowledge, answer the following short questions. These will prepare you for your summative (final) assessment.

1. Cleaning agents that are formulated for use on skin are:

   a. disinfectants
   b. antiseptics
   c. sterilizers
   d. sanitizers

2. The hygiene control method of sterilization:

   a. is the destruction of most living organisms
   b. is the cleaning method using a disinfectant cleaning agent
   c. is the total destruction of all living microorganisms
   d. uses UV light to minimize harmful microorganisms

3. What is a disinfectant?

   a. a chemical solution that destroys most microorganisms
   b. a solution that prevents the multiplication of microorganisms
   c. a type of distilled water to avoid damaging the autoclave

   d. a physical agent that destroys most microorganisms

4. How often should the beauty therapist wash their hands?

   a. after each treatment to prevent cross-infection
   b. before each treatment to prevent secondary infection
   c. after eating to maintain personal hygiene
   d. regularly to prevent cross-infection

5. If a towel accidentally dropped onto the floor, what should you do with it?

   a. pick it up, fold it and replace on the work surface to prevent somebody tripping over it
   b. place it in the laundry bin for washing
   c. use it to dry your hands on after washing rather than use it on a client
   d. use it when cleaning to dry the work surfaces before washing

6. What do the Control of Substances Hazardous to Health (COSHH) regulations regulate for health and safety?

   a. those activities or processes that require special protective clothing or equipment to be worn

b. substances used in the workplace that may cause a risk to health

c. the provision and use of work equipment

d. the clinical disposal of contaminated waste

7. When completing a client's record card, you recognize that the client has a contra-indication as the client has an infectious skin disorder. Identify this from the list below:

a. eczema

b. bruising

c. verruca

d. lentigo

8. Which firefighting equipment should be used on an electrical fire?

a. water extinguisher

b. vaporizing liquid

c. foam extinguisher

d. carbon dioxide (CO_2) extinguisher

9. What is a fire drill?

a. fire detection equipment

b. testing the fire alarm system to comply with health and safety procedures

c. a notice to show people to the emergency exit route

d. practice of the fire evacuation procedure

10. A risk is:

a. anything that has the potential to cause harm

b. the likelihood of potential harm from a hazard happening

11. Clients' records should be stored securely in accordance with the:

a. Data Protection Act

b. Provision and Use of Work Equipment Regulations

c. Health and Safety at Work Act

d. Health and Safety (Display Screen Equipment) Regulations

12. If an accident occurs in the workplace:

a. you should provide immediate assistance

b. you would report this to the Health and Safety Executive (HSE) Incident contact centre

c. record the details immediately on the accident report form and enter it into the accident book

d. you would inform the member of staff with a HSE approved basic first aid qualification

4 Selling Skills

LEARNING OBJECTIVES

There is one learning outcome for this mandatory unit which you must achieve:

1 Be able to promote products and treatments to the client.

From the range statement, you must show that you can:

◆ Use appropriate communication and consultation techniques.

◆ Promote treatments and/or products relevant to the clients needs.

◆ Provide accurate and relevant information on the features and benefits of treatments/ products.

◆ Maintain a high level of professional, commercial personal presentation.

◆ Demonstrate the stages of the sales process.

◆ Comply with relevant sales legislation.

◆ Deal with different methods of payment.

KEY TERMS

additional products and treatments	body language	consultation
allergic reaction	code of practice	contra-action
benefit	communication	

Consumer Protection (Distance
    Selling) (Amendment)
    Regulations (2005)
Consumer Protection Act (1987)
Consumer Safety Act (1978)
continuous professional
    development (CPD
contra-action)
contra-indication
Cosmetic Products (Safety)
    Regulations (2004)

Disability Discrimination
    Act (1996)
Data Protection Act (1998)
feature
legislation
methods of payment
moisturizer
personal presentation
Prices Act (1974)
products
promotion

Resale Prices Acts (1964
    and 1976)
Sale and Supply of Goods
    Act (1994)
services
stock-keeping
Trade Descriptions Acts
    (1968 and 1972)

Unit Topic

Promote products and treatments to clients in a salon

This VRQ unit is linked to the Beauty Therapy NOS Unit G18.

INTRODUCTION

Each business requires that their clients are informed of the different products and treatments that are available to meet their ongoing needs and requirements. To ensure you target all client groups, the use of a range of media is required including text messaging, social media and mail drops. Businesses must remain competitive within the marketplace, being aware of and preparing for future trends, ensuring that their staff have the necessary skills to carry these out. Products too are constantly changing, especially make-up and nails which are fashion influenced. It is important for a business, even one without local competitors, to encourage its clients to try new treatments or products to maximize overall treatment results. Obviously this will also increase financial revenue for the business.

This unit is all about your need to keep pace with new developments in the workplace, and for you to pass on your professional knowledge and advise your clients. Clients expect more and more from their beauty treatments and products; their awareness of what is available will give them greater choice to select a product or service that will meet their needs.

You must be able to show you have the necessary practical skills and underpinning knowledge to promote products and treatments to clients.

INDUSTRY ROLE MODEL

SAMANTHA SWEET Co-founder Sweet Squared LLP

"I have literally grown up in the nail industry! From aged 18 I was having my nails enhanced with my mum, global nail legend Gigi Rouse. For 22 years I have represented Creative Nail Design (CND) and in 2006 Samuel and I founded Sweet Squared, the largest most respected nail distributor in the UK, embracing a unique philosophy; we see distribution as a way to connect with our customer. Since 2007 we have won 30 industry awards including 2013 *Scratch*

Stars Best Customer Care, CND Global Distributor of the Year and in 2010 I was awarded Outstanding Contribution to the Nail Industry by BABTAC. I am a member of the HABIA Nails Forum and I'm the Nail Consultant for PHAB Standards.

TOP TIP

Client refreshments

Light refreshments may be promoted as an additional retail opportunity. Increasingly even a glass of champagne may be offered whilst receiving a treatment, making the client's retail beauty experience feel extra special!

The importance of product or treatment promotion

When clients select a beauty therapy treatment or product they do so for one of a number of reasons. This may be:

◆ to improve their appearance, e.g. an eyelash tint or manicure

◆ for a special occasion, e.g. make-up application

◆ for therapeutic reasons, to receive a quality professional treatment in calm, relaxing surroundings, e.g. a de-stress facial massage

◆ for aspirational reasons, e.g. to imitate the appeal of an advertising campaign, achieve a fashion look

◆ to seek professional guidance on what would best suit their needs and requirements, e.g. skincare advice

◆ for performance, the product or treatment has guaranteed results

◆ to maintain the benefits of a particular treatment they have received before, e.g. repeat booking for leg waxing treatment

TOP TIP

Seeking selling opportunities

The client's skincare preparations should change according to the different seasons. As such, the client should be advised on products that are most suitable to maintain skin health and appearance. This gives you the opportunity to educate your clients on the need to change skincare routines and promote additional products, maintaining client interest.

"Don't have a competitive spirit, have a creative one. If you are always worrying about what your competitors are doing then you lack confidence in what YOU are doing! Concentrate on your own business as only that will make you truly successful – when people put prices down – be the one to stand by your convictions and put your prices up!

Samantha Sweet

- for social reasons, they enjoy visiting the salon as much as receiving the treatment

- to give a friend a treatment or product as a gift, e.g. a gift voucher

- value for money – the product or treatment is on promotion at a discounted price.

Whatever the reason, you want the client to feel pleased with their choice, enjoy their experience and inform others of their satisfaction – thus promoting the business. Retail sales are of considerable importance to the beauty business: they are a straightforward way of increasing income without too much extra time and effort. Beauty therapy treatments are time-consuming and labour-intensive; selling a product in addition to providing the treatment will immediately increase profitability. Importantly it can also benefit and support the client to achieve their treatment aim. For example, if the client receives a manicure and has weak, flaking nails recommend a specialized nail treatment and a strengthening retail product.

Clients need to be given ongoing information about further products and treatments available. This will help maintain their interest and awareness of salon treatments and overall satisfaction with the salon. A high standard of **personal presentation**, including personal hygiene, is very important and will encourage the client to initially engage with you. You must inspire confidence and be a positive advertisement for the products and treatments you are selling. Staff knowledge of products and treatments is essential to ensure personal effectiveness and helps in gaining client confidence.

> " Find a brand that you love and believe in. Customers will trust your judgement. Stay on trend and bring things into the salon that will sell. If you're not confident in retailing, LEARN. The extra income retailing can bring into a salon is huge and so many ignore it! When giving advice, always make sure you don't give opinion but that your advice can be backed up by fully fledged fact!
>
> *Samantha Sweet*

If you have got it right the client will maintain their loyalty to you and this helps the business to grow. For example, a facial treatment might take 1 hour and cost the client £40. You might then sell the client a **moisturizer** costing £40, of which £10 might be clear profit. Supposing that you sold eight products each day each yielding £10 profit. That would be a profit of £80 per day or £400 per week, or £1600 each month and thus, £19 200 profit over the whole year: a significant sum.

ACTIVITY

Express treatments

Increasingly, clients are requiring a fast treatment often received in their lunch break. Examples include express artificial lashes for that unexpected special occasion. Find out what other treatments may be offered as an express treatment. Remember, when the client experiences an express treatment this provides the opportunity to explain the benefit of the full treatment.

HEALTH & SAFETY

Contra-indications If the client appears to have a **contra-indication** to a treatment they wish to receive, recommend they seek their GP's approval first. You may require written evidence of this before treatment can proceed. Remember to make a note on the client's record to follow this up.

In **CHAPTER 5** we look at the importance of creating an initial positive impression to the client.

Outcome 1: Promote products and treatments to clients in a salon

Learn how to promote products and treatments to the client

PRACTICAL SKILLS

Establish the client's requirements

Use suitable communication techniques to promote products and treatments

Introduce treatments and/or products to the client at the appropriate time

Give accurate and relevant information to the client

Identify buying signals and interpret the client's intentions correctly

Identify treatments and/or products to meet requirements of the client

UNDERPINNING KNOWLEDGE

Describe the benefits to the salon of promoting treatments and products to the client

Describe the listening and questioning techniques used for promotion and selling

Describe the different consultation techniques used to promote products and treatments

Explain the terms 'features' and 'benefits' as applied to treatments and products

Describe the principles of effective face-to-face communication

State the importance of effective personal presentation

State the importance of good product and treatment knowledge

Outline the stages of the sale process

Describe how to interpret buying signals

Describe how to secure agreement and close the sale

Explain the legislation that affects the selling of treatments and products

Describe methods of payment for treatments and products

When promoting products or treatments, find out first about your client and their needs and expectations. This will help you identify the best treatments or products for them. Carry out a **consultation** – this is a discussion with the client that enables you to assess their needs. This will use your questioning and listening skills. Consider the following:

◆ What is the client's main priority? What would they like to achieve? This information will guide you on selecting and advising them of the most suitable product or treatment.

◆ Is a skin sensitivity test necessary before the treatment? Legally you may be required to carry this out before a treatment can be received, for example, before an eyelash tint treatment. Ensure there will be sufficient time to carry out any necessary tests when promoting a treatment to ensure you can check client suitability before they receive it.

TOP TIP

Testers for products

Encourage your client to try the product testers. You can also take the opportunity to apply the product, explaining its special qualities, to show it at its best effect to suit the client.

◆ Is the client allergic to any particular substance, contact with which should be avoided? Check ingredients if a client identifies an allergy.

◆ Does the client have a skin disorder or nail disease which might contra-indicate use of a particular product? Contra-actions to products must always be noted on your salon records and the appropriate action to take explained to the client.

◆ Is the client planning to use the product over a skin disorder, e.g. eczema? If so, is this safe? Your professional guidance should be given at all times.

◆ Find out what treatments the client has received before. Were they satisfied or disappointed in any way with them? If so, find out why.

◆ How much is the client used to spending on products? You can tactfully find this out by asking about what they are presently using: this will give you an idea of the types of product they have experience with using, and the sort of prices they are used to paying.

Bearing in mind the client's needs, you can now guide them to the most suitable treatment or product. This is where your expertise and knowledge are so important: you can describe fully and accurately the features and benefits of the treatments and products you can offer.

> " Remember – you know way more than your customer (or you most certainly should) and as such must carry the confidence and the courage of your convictions when prescribing the correct treatment for them. If they choose not to listen to professional advice, they must be prepared to sign a ready-made document/waiver to acknowledge that they have chosen to ignore the professional advice given. The responsibility of their chosen treatment now sits on their shoulders!
>
> *Samantha Sweet*

Skincare retail products

Retail product display

TOP TIP

Features and benefits

A feature is the product's specialist ingredients and the effects they can achieve.

A benefit is what the client can expect from buying the product.

ACTIVITY

Features and benefits

Discuss and write down the features and benefits of a product or treatment sold in your workplace.

Knowledge Check

Why are retail sales important to the beauty business?

Refer to page 135 to help you.

Features and benefits

This can be repeated again later to help the client make a purchase decision when there may be several items to consider.

A **feature** is the uniqueness or individuality of a product or treatment, e.g. new technology used in the ingredient formulation of a product or the design technology of a piece of equipment.

A **benefit** is the gain to be made by the client from using the product or treatment.

Selling products

The products themselves must be presented to the client in such a way that they seem both attractive and desirable: the presentation should further encourage the client to purchase them. The packaging and the product should be clean and in good condition, and testers/samples to take away should be available wherever possible so that the client can try the product before purchasing it.

The final choice of product is with the client, of course, but often the client will ask for a recommendation, for example if they cannot decide between two possibilities. It is in these circumstances that your ability to answer technical questions fully, from a complete knowledge of the product, will help in closing the sale. Speaking with confidence and authority on the one product that will particularly suit the client's requirements may well persuade them to buy it.

Product suitability

If the client has not used the product or received the treatment before there is always a possibility of an allergic reaction.

HEALTH & SAFETY

Skin sensitivity tests If the client has not tried a product before, or if there is doubt as to how their skin will react, a skin sensitivity patch test must always be carried out. Also, always check your manufacturer's guidelines to confirm if a skin test is required. Failure to comply with requirement in the use of a product could lead to future non-compliance legal issues in the result of a client contra-action.

1 Select either the inner elbow or the area behind the ear. The skin here is thinner, more sensitive and less tolerant.

2 Make sure the skin is clean.

3 Apply a little of the product to the skin, using a clean applicator.

4 Leave the area alone for 24 hours.

5 If there is no reaction (referred to as a negative reaction) after 24 hours, the client is not allergic to the product: they can go ahead and use it. If there has been any itching, soreness, erythema, or swelling in the area where the product has been applied, the client is allergic to it and should not use it (referred to as a positive reaction).

Allergic reaction to a cosmetic product that has affected the eyes

If the client does not know what an **allergic reaction** is – or how to recognize an allergy – it is important that you describe it to them (red, itchy, flaking and even swollen skin). If they experience this following a treatment, termed professionally as a **contra-action,** they should contact you immediately for further advice, or, in the case of product intolerance, stop applying the product the client suspects is producing it.

Techniques in selling

The first rule of selling is *know your products*. This applies to all retail products and to all salon treatments.

Staff training

It is important that everybody is knowledgeable and able to answer the client's questions – this also includes the receptionist, who is often the first and last member of staff the client comes into contact with in a salon. In conversation, especially during quieter periods, they have opportunities to discuss products and treatments informally.

> Great nails start with great education! Do education updates at least twice a year. Updating skills and mastering new ones is what will always keep you ahead of the pack – ALWAYS! Whenever you do update your skills it gives you added confidence which soaks through the salon. A guess what? You get more business which equals more income! Practise does NOT make perfect! PERFECT Practise makes perfect!
>
> *Samantha Sweet*

Often product companies provide training either at the business or at another venue. This is a great opportunity to update your knowledge and skills, which you will be able to share enthusiastically with your clients. Certificates to recognise the training achieved are usually provided and these should be professionally displayed in the salon.

It is not always possible for all staff to take part in training unless it is on a day when the business is closed. It is important that any new information is passed on to these colleagues. Team meetings are a good opportunity to discuss workplace policy and new products and promotions.

Information on products and treatments must be available for clients to read, and eye-catching displays should be set up to gain attention. Be aware of your competitors and their current advertising displays and campaigns.

If your business has a website, ensure it is kept updated. It is a great resource for keeping clients updated with details of sharing product/treatment promotions. If you have the software facility, clients may be able to purchase products or treatments online also.

Methods of promoting products and treatments

When promoting products and **services** it is good to raise client interest and awareness by considering the points listed on the following page.

◆ eye-catching promotional material (usually provided by the product supplier): displays in the window will encourage new clients! This should be changed regularly to maintain interest. Think of all the special dates in the calendar year, there are lots of great marketing occasions that should not be missed

◆ updated salon literature discussing benefits and costs of products and treatments may be provided. These may be available as hard copies and duplicated online, available for download wherever possible

◆ a promotional launch event, where clients can enjoy a social event and perhaps book treatments or buy products at discounted prices, may be held

◆ promotional packages may be presented at reduced cost or limited edition products can be purchased

◆ sample products may be given following a treatment for the client to try at home. Client feedback can be followed up when you next meet with the client

◆ products to enhance the treatment may be promoted, e.g. specially formulated mascara to wear with individual false lashes that enhance the overall result, ensuring client satisfaction. Always spot and make use of a selling opportunity without being 'too pushy', which may be off-putting to the client

◆ if you have a website you may wish to promote products and treatments on your home page. Special offers may be featured and you may have the facility for clients to book online

◆ special events or occasions, e.g. if the client is going on holiday, recommend travel-size products

◆ finally, remember: if promoting a particular treatment or product such as nails – your nails should look great!

Know your products and treatments

Product usage must be discussed with clients, as necessary, and advice given on which product and treatment will best suit each of them. The only way to be able to do this is to memorize the complete range: all your products and treatments, including for example which skin types or treatment conditions each is for, what the active ingredients are, when and how each should be used, and its cost. Any questions asked must be answered with authority and confidence. Clients expect the staff in a beauty salon to be professionals, able to provide expert advice:

◆ speak with confidence and enthusiasm

◆ avoid confusing technical words

◆ explain the features and benefits and personalize these, matching them to the needs of each client.

Always give accurate and relevant information to the client. If the client requests advice on products or treatments that are outside of your responsibility, refer them to the relevant colleague who has the expertise. You may have information literature you are able to provide to your client to find out more that will prevent possible loss of a sale, so pass it on.

Information to read The information available to clients may start from the salon window display. If available, use the window adverts supplied with product ranges, and promote information that advertises the salon's treatments. Wherever you are situated it is important that potential customers know you are there.

Promotional posters are supplied with good-quality product and treatment ranges, and most suppliers provide information leaflets for clients. Use the posters and display leaflets in the reception area; clients can then help themselves, and read about the products and their benefits. This will generate questions – and sales.

Product and retail displays Two types of display can be used in the beauty salon. In the first, the display is there simply to be looked at, and seen as part of the decor. It should be attractive and artistically arranged, and can use dummy containers. It is not meant to be touched or sold from, so it can be behind glass or in a window display.

On the other hand, in the second, products are there to be sold. In this case products must be attractive but also accessible. The display should include testers so that clients can freely smell and touch. Each product must be clearly priced, and small signs placed beside the products or on the edge of the shelves to describe the unique selling points of each product.

This sort of active display must always be in the part of the salon where most people will see and walk past it – the area of 'highest traffic'. A large proportion of cosmetic and perfume sales are impulse buys. It is no accident that perfumery departments are beside the main entrances to department stores, or right beside access points such as escalators. Product displays must also feature in the beauty treatment area. As the beauty therapist uses the products, they can discuss and recommend them for the client. If displays are there to see and to take from, the sale can be closed even before the client returns to reception. Although in theory clients can of course change their minds between the treatment area and actually paying, in practice once they have the product in their hands they will go on to buy it.

Most small salons will design and create their own displays using the counter display packs provided by the product companies. Some larger businesses will have a professional window dresser to regularly change the window displays for the best effect.

A promotional poster for self-tanning products

ACTIVITY

Learning the product range

Learn about and memorize the product range sold in the training establishment you attend. Once you have learnt about the range, memorize the cost of the products.

Promotional product display for self-tanning products

Knowledge Check

How do you think speaking with confidence and authority about a product will influence the client to buy?

Refer to page 140 to help you.

HEALTH & SAFETY

Testing products To prevent contamination, spatulas must be used so customers do not put their fingers into the pots either when testing or during home use. You may also like to sell spatulas for clients to use at home.

ACTIVITY

Collecting information

Collect information about products and treatments from local beauty salons and beauty product counters in department stores. Is this literature attractive? Does the presentation encourage sales? What makes information appealing in its presentation? If not, why not?

Email wholesalers and product companies for information about the display packs they supply with their products.

Look at websites also. What are the features of a good business website?

Displays should always be well stocked, with smart undamaged packaging. Eye-level displays are best and ideally should be accessible. Change the display regularly according to the **promotion**, for example UV skin protection products in summer.

Displays must be checked and cleaned regularly – in busy salons this will usually mean daily. A window display will need to be dusted, straightened, and looked at from outside to make sure that it looks its best. The display from which products are being sold will also need to be dusted, perhaps wiped over (if testers have dripped), and straightened up. Testers need to be checked to make sure they are not sticky and spilt, and that no one has left dirty fingerprints on them.

The range of products

It is not enough to stock just a few items and expect clients to fit in with the range you carry: different ranges must be available for each skin type, and a number of specialist products – such as eye gel, skin serums or creams – that will suit all skin types. Make-up and nail polish should be attractive to all ages and diversity of customer. Sales must not be lost because of a lack of product range.

Information provided to the client should be accurate and not false or misleading. Legal action could follow in the case of non-compliance with consumer protection **legislation**.

A cosmetic product range

BEAUTY TREATMENT CLIENT CONSULTATION CARD

Surname _____ Forename _____ Date of Birth __ / __ / ____

Street _____

Town _____ County _____ Postcode _____

Telephone (Home) _____ Work _____

Products used _____

Treatment completed _____ Date _____

STATISTICS   Height _____ Weight _____ Chest _____ Waist _____ Hips _____

PRESCRIBED MEDICATION   SKIN ANALYSIS

Yes ☐ No ☐ Details _____   Dry ☐   Combination ☐
                                              Oily ☐   Sensitive ☐
SURGERY   Fair ☐   Dark ☐
Yes ☐ No ☐ Details _____

AILMENTS   ALLERGIC REACTIONS TO ANY PREVIOUS TREATMENT

Yes ☐ No ☐ Details _____   Yes ☐ No ☐ Details _____

Knowing when to promote the product or treatment

Choose the most appropriate time to inform the client about **additional products and treatments**. Present information on the product or treatment at a pace relevant to the client's knowledge and experience. If the information is new this may be slower and detailed. If the client is receiving a treatment this may be at the consultation, when discussing the treatment objectives, during treatment delivery when you have the opportunity to recommend and share advice, or when discussing aftercare. Here you will be able to reinforce the importance of further products and treatments to enhance the treatment benefits gained. Establish the client's requirements. This may be further use of products or treatments that the client has used before or of those that are new to the client.

Using good communication techniques

Good communication with clients, both verbal and non-verbal, is important. Establish a rapport with your client and give your attention fully to the client above any other tasks. Use your client's name: this increases their sense of self-importance and value.

◆ At all times remain polite, friendly and respect the client's individual opinions and preference. Never be critical; this may lose a sale.

◆ A client may be already considering purchasing a product or treatment and the type of questions they ask will signal this. The most common question is 'How much is it?'

◆ Make eye contact, observe the client's **body language**: are they interested in what you are telling them? If the client is interested, they will agree with you and their body language will be relaxed yet attentive. There are many customer types: those that are decisive, indecisive, chatty, quiet, opinionated, awkward and disbelieving. This should be considered in your approach: it is important that the client gains confidence in you and ultimately your products or treatment. This will be secured through your appearance, communication, style and manner.

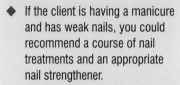

TOP TIP

Create your own selling opportunity

◆ If the client is having a manicure and has weak nails, you could recommend a course of nail treatments and an appropriate nail strengthener.

◆ If the client is going away on holiday tell them about the special 'holiday package promotion'.

◆ If the client is having an eyelash tint, tell them how quick and simple an eyebrow wax is and the difference it can make!

TOP TIP

Always pay careful attention to your client and their responses. Remember: question, listen, answer.

◆ *Question* your client as to their needs.
◆ *Listen* to the answer.
◆ *Answer* with the relevant information.

◆ Questions must be accurate and detailed. You are the expert: show your knowledge. Do not ask the client what sort of skin they have – they are not the expert, and will probably give the wrong answer. Instead, ask more detailed questions, such as 'Does your skin feel tight?' (which may indicate dryness), or 'Do you have spots in a particular area?' (which may indicate an oily area). Use open questions. These are questions that may not be answered with yes or no. Open questions usually start with 'why', 'how', 'when', 'what' and 'which'.

◆ Listening is a skill. Listen to your client; this will help you to identify their treatment or product needs. Always listen carefully to the answers your client gives: do not talk over their answer or interrupt. Only when they have finished talking should you give a considered, informed reply. Summarize simply and repeat what they have said to show you understand – this is called reflective listening. You may need to ask another question, or you may be able straightaway to direct them to the best product or treatment for their needs based upon your conversation.

◆ Ensure that the client receives adequate attention whilst providing them with the products that they have agreed to purchase. Present the products to them and explain any specific requirements in their use in order that they gain maximum benefit from their use.

◆ Allow time for the client to think about the purchase.

◆ In the case of a treatment, make an appointment and provide the client with an appointment card and relevant literature relating to the treatment. If the client has made a decision to receive a treatment or purchase a product, you may find there is a delay in its availability. Ensure any delay is minimal. Do not be tempted to offer unsuitable alternatives, which are not as suited to the client's needs or treatment requirements. Inform the client honestly and realistically of their availability. In the case of a product you may be able to give the client a sample to use until the product is available.

◆ Ensure that the client has sufficient information to make a confident selection in their treatment or product choice.

◆ Give the client an opportunity to ask questions and answer these confidently.

◆ Questions may lead to the opportunity to increase the sale of more products or treatments.

◆ Ensure the environment is conducive to all clients feeling comfortable to ask questions.

> Remember, it's about the client in front of you – she is paying for her time so become a good LISTENER! As a nail professional you get to be privy to personal information from your customers. Never gossip! With anyone! That info is private and should remain as such.
>
> Never bring your personal baggage into work! It will still be waiting for you at the end of the day and it's not professional. Put it aside and get on with the job in hand!
>
> *Samantha Sweet*

TOP TIP

Competitions, loyalty cards and free gifts are a popular incentive for clients to purchase products. Make your client aware of any incentives.

TOP TIP

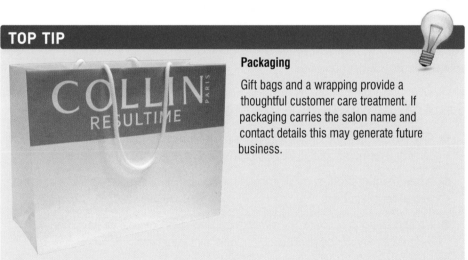

Packaging

Gift bags and a wrapping provide a thoughtful customer care treatment. If packaging carries the salon name and contact details this may generate future business.

◆ If a sale is achieved, be positive – smile, this will help to make the client feel they have made a good decision.

◆ Ask the client if there is anything else they need when closing the sale on the product. Confirm the size of product the client wishes to purchase, explaining any financial benefit to their selection.

◆ Explain any policies that relates to the sale of the treatments/products, e.g. the salon's policy on the return/exchange of products or when a gift voucher expires.

◆ Be appreciative, and thank the client when they are about to leave even if an enquiry has not resulted in a purchase.

◆ Record all sales on the client's record card. This is a useful reference point for the beauty therapist and client to refer back to.

Knowledge Check

How can you interpret buying signals?

Refer to pages 143–144 to help you.

These payment methods are discussed in more detail in **CHAPTER 6** Salon Reception.

TOP TIP

Effective stock control

It is important that you try to always have the range of retail stock available so effective stock-keeping is important. It is disappointing for the client if they are unable to purchase a retail item and this could potentially result in the loss of a sale – especially if they source an alternative elsewhere.

TOP TIP

Promotion

All staff should be aware of any promotions that their business is offering so that they can build on a client's initial interest in a product or treatment and turn it into a sale. Always know about your products and treatments.

TOP TIP

Demonstrations

An effective demonstration will always create sales. Have the product ready to sell, or give out vouchers to encourage clients to purchase the product or treatment at a discounted rate.

Client suitability

If the client is not interested, they will probably not engage with you, and will appear disinterested in what you are saying. If this occurs go back to the beginning and suggest alternatives to attempt to regain their interest, but avoid pressuring the client. Following discussion about a product or treatment, you may feel that the client is unsuitable. Tactfully explain to the client why this is. If it is for medical reasons, ask them to seek permission from their GP before the product or treatment is provided. The expectations of some clients may be unrealistic. If this is the case, patiently and diplomatically explain why and aim to agree to a realistic treatment programme. Remember your legal duty under the Health and Safety at Work Act (1974) to take reasonable care to avoid harm to yourself or others.

Methods of payment for products and treatments

When the sale of products/treatments is closed and the client is satisfied, the final stage is payment. There are different methods of payment including cash, cheque, credit card, debit card and vouchers.

Promotion

Promotions are another way of informing your clients about products or treatments that are currently available. They are also a great way of gaining interest in a product or treatment from a wider audience.

General benefits of a promotion

◆ Clients may take the opportunity of using a product or treatment because it is on offer at a reduced cost. If they do not like it, it is less of a costly mistake.

◆ A treatment or product on promotion may cost less and therefore be accessible to a wider client base.

◆ Limited editions or offers are a way of gaining client interest as the product or treatment may not be available or on offer at a later date.

◆ The enthusiasm of some clients will motivate others to purchase.

Demonstration

Demonstrating to an audience needs particularly careful planning if the demonstration is to achieve the maximum benefit. Everything required must be available, and all the relevant literature to be given out to the audience or clients.

Consider all possibilities in your planning. What type of demonstration is required? Will you be working on one client, to demonstrate and sell a product, or demonstrating to a group? Is a range of products or treatments to be demonstrated, or just one item?

Single client Demonstrations may be used to discuss facial skincare, make-up application and false strip lash extension and removal techniques. When demonstrating on a client, have a mirror in front of them so that you can explain as you go along and the client can watch. They can then see the benefit of the product and learn how to use it at the same time. This is a simple but effective way to sell products.

Trade demonstration

TOP TIP

Visual promotional resources

You may wish to have the demonstration professionally recorded. This may then be used as a video on your website (if available) or in reception to capture clients' interest and generate questions from those who did not attend.

Knowledge Check

Describe three different methods of payment that may be used for products and treatments.

A group The presentation should include an introduction to the demonstrator and the product, the demonstration itself, and a conclusion, with thanks to the audience and model. Written promotional material can be placed on the seats before the audience arrives, or handed out at an appropriate point during the demonstration; samples can be handed around for the audience to try while the product is being discussed.

The demonstration itself must be clear, simple and not too long. The audience *must* be able to see what is being done and hear the commentary. Maximize the impact of the demonstration by giving the audience the opportunity to buy the product immediately. If this is not possible – because the demonstration is in another room, away from the products or at another venue, not the salon business premises – ensure that members of the audience leave with a voucher to exchange for the product. This should offer some incentive, such as a discount, to encourage potential buyers to make the effort to come to the salon and buy. Never sell the features and benefits to potential customers, creating the desire for the product, without also giving them the chance to buy it.

ACTIVITY

Siting of product displays

In your nearest large town, go into the big department stores and note where the cosmetic and perfumery department displays are situated. Research and list why this is a good place to site these products.

Consumer protection legislation

The salon has a legal obligation to implement and/or abide by the following legislation, designed to protect the rights of clients.

Consumer Safety Act (1978)

The **Consumer Safety Act (1978)** aims to reduce risk to consumers from potentially dangerous products. It outlines the minimum safety standards to be met. Amendments to this Act includes the Consumer Protection Act 1987.

Consumer Protection Act (1987)

The **Consumer Protection Act (1987)** follows European Union (EU) directives to protect the customer from unsafe, defective treatments and products that do not reach safety standards. It is important, therefore, to only use reputable products, purchased from a reliable source and that adequate information is provided to the client on their correct use. All staff should be trained in using products and maintaining them so they are in consistently good condition. It also covers misleading price indications about goods or treatments available from a business. Up-to-date prices for products and services must be available. Local authorities are responsible for protecting consumers. Trading Standards or Consumer Protection Departments check that trading standards and laws are adhered to and investigate any complaint. This Act makes provisions with respect to the liability of persons for the damage caused by defective products. If proven to be at fault and an offence has occurred the business may face legal action. For more information visit **www.ico.gov.uk**

Prices Act (1974)

The Prices Act (1974) states that the price of products or services has to be displayed in order to prevent the buyer being misguided.

Trade Descriptions Acts (1968 and 1972)

The Trade Descriptions Acts (1968 and 1972) prohibit the use of false descriptions of goods and services provided by a business. Products must be clearly labelled. When retailing, the information supplied both in written and verbal form must always be accurate. The supplier must not:

◆ supply misleading information

◆ describe products falsely

◆ make false statements.

In addition they must not:

◆ make false comparisons between past and present services

◆ offer products at what is said to be a 'reduced' price, unless they have previously been on sale at the full price quoted for a 28-day minimum

◆ make misleading price comparisons.

The Acts also require accurate information to be included in advertisements.

Resale Prices Acts (1964 and 1976)

Under the provisions of the **Resale Prices Acts (1964 and 1976)** the manufacturer can supply a recommended retail price (MRRP), but the seller is not obliged to sell at the recommended price.

Sale and Supply of Goods Act (1994)

This Act amended the previous Sale of Goods Act (1979) but the customers' rights as outlined in 1979 remain unchanged. The **Sale and Supply of Goods Act (1994)** provides that goods must be as described, of satisfactory quality including fit for their intended purpose, in appearance and finish, free from minor defects and safe and durable. The Act also covers

Knowledge Check

Name three pieces of legislation/ regulations relating to the way products or services are delivered to clients which protect legal rights.

Refer to pages 147–149 to help you.

A range of eye cosmetics for make-up services

the conditions under which customers can return goods. It is the responsibility of the retailer to correct a problem where the goods are not as described. This may be by refund, credit note, repair or replacement.

Cosmetic Products (Safety) Regulations (2004)

The **Cosmetic Products (Safety) Regulations (2004)** consolidates earlier regulations and incorporates current EU directives. Part of consumer protection legislation, it requires that cosmetics and toiletries are safe in their formulation and are safe for use for their intended purpose as a cosmetic and comply with labelling requirements.

> Be happy! Be grateful and thankful for your customers. They are your bread and butter and should be treated as such! Remember the little things – how they take their coffee; have it waiting for them – such a little thing but one that they appreciate because it shows you care! Make their every treatment experience special because that is what will keep them coming back – that and great nails that last!
>
> *Samantha Sweet*

Data Protection Act (DPA) (1998)

The **Data Protection Act (1998)** applies to any business that uses computers or paper-based systems to store information about its clients and staff.

Through **communication** with your client it is necessary to ask clients a series of questions before the service plan can be finalized. Client details are recorded on the client record card. This information is confidential and should be stored in a secure area. The client should understand the reason behind the questions asked of them and how the information will be used. Confidential information on staff or clients should only be made available to persons to whom consent has been given.

Clients who have given information need to know how it will be used; otherwise they have a right to withhold it. Information stored must be accurate and up to date. It is necessary to register with the Data Protection Registrar, who will place the business on a public register of data users. A **code of practice** is provided, which must be complied with. For more information visit **www.ico.gov.uk**

Consumer Protection Act (1987)

This Act follows European laws to protect the customer from unsafe, defective services and products that do not reach safety standards. It also covers misleading price indications about goods or services available from a business.

Consumer Protection (Distance Selling) Regulations (2000)

These regulations, as amended by the **Consumer Protection (Distance Selling) (Amendment) Regulations (2005)** are derived from a EU directive and cover the supply of goods/services made between suppliers, acting in a commercial capacity,

Knowledge Check

Clients have consumer rights. Why is it important to give accurate information about products or treatments?

Refer to pages 147–148 to help you.

and consumers. They are concerned with purchases made where there is no face-to-face contact, that is, by telephone, fax, Internet, digital television or mail order, including catalogue shopping.

Consumers must receive clear information on goods or services, including delivery arrangements and payment, suppliers' details and consumers' cancellation rights, which should be made available in writing. The consumer also has a 7 working-day cool-off period where they may cancel their purchase. The point at which the right to cancel services is reached is detailed in the 2005 amendment to the 2000 Regulations.

Beauty therapist recommending retail products to a client

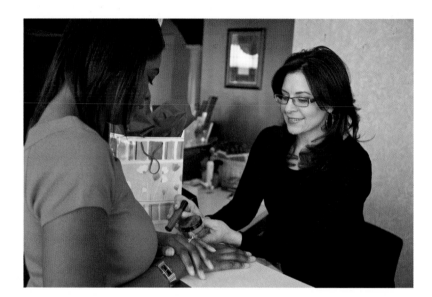

ASSESSMENT OF KNOWLEDGE AND UNDERSTANDING

You have now learnt about selling skills in the beauty therapy workplace. To test your level of knowledge, answer the following short questions. These will prepare you for your summative (final) assessment.

1. Which piece of consumer legislation states that goods must be as described, of merchantable quality and fit for their intended purpose?

   a. **Disability Discrimination Act (1996)**
   b. Sales and Supply of Goods Act (1994)
   c. Resale Prices Acts (1964 and 1976)
   d. Trade Descriptions Acts (1968 and 1972)

2. The feature of a product or treatment is described as:

   a. the individuality of a product or treatment
   b. the gain to be made from using a product or treatment

3. Body language is important when selling, and is also known as:

   a. non-verbal communication
   b. non-verbal questioning techniques
   c. observation techniques
   d. eye contact

4. To provide accurate information to the client when making recommendations you should:

   a. write down information about the products/treatments that you are recommending
   b. use technical words
   c. explain the features and benefits of all products/treatments
   d. ask the client if they have any questions

5. Client record keeping is important as it helps you:

   a. remember recommendations made on a previous salon visit
   b. refer to previous products/treatments used when recommending other suitable products/treatments

   c. provide advice in the instance of a contra-action to product/treatment
   d. all of the above

6. When selling, it is important to:

   a. recommend products/treatments based upon your client's needs
   b. use effective questioning techniques to find out the client's needs
   c. explain the features and benefits of the products/treatments
   d. all of the above

7. Before most clients will purchase products/treatments from you they must:

   a. have received a beauty treatment previously
   b. have confidence in you
   c. observe that your salon is busy
   d. have a specific treatment requirement

8. If a client is undecided on what product to use:

   a. advise them to go away and do some research
   b. recommend that they purchase all the products/treatments recommended
   c. suggest they to go away and think about it
   d. guide the client as to the most suitable choice following your consultation

9. When are the client's needs identified when promoting products and treatments?

   a. following the consultation
   b. following treatment aftercare
   c. after skin analysis
   d. when demonstrating the products/treatments

5 Client Care and Communication

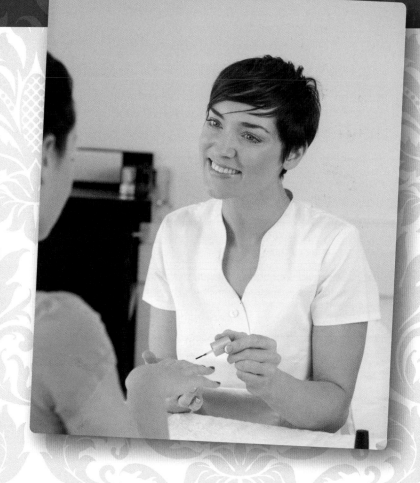

LEARNING OBJECTIVES

There are two learning outcomes to achieve for this mandatory unit:

1 Be able to communicate with clients.

2 Be able to provide client care.

The assessment range applied requires you to:

◆ Use communication and consultation techniques.

◆ Provide clear advice and recommendations understood by the client.

◆ Comply with all related legislation.

◆ When required refer a complaint to the relevant person.

KEY TERMS

assistance	induction	relevant person
code of conduct	job description	targets
confidentiality	legislation	teamwork
complaints procedure	verbal and non-verbal communication	treatment plan
consultation	personal space	visual aids
customer care statement	record card	questioning techniques

Unit Topic

Client care and communication when working in beauty related industries.

INTRODUCTION

This unit is all about taking personal responsibility to improve your communication skills and the overall care you provide when working with your clients.

Delivering a consistently high standard of client care and having excellent communication skills is very important, ensuring a positive, professional image is made with all people coming into contact with you in the workplace. This includes not only clients but visitors to the organization and the team of people you work with – your work colleagues. This will contribute to the overall effectiveness and in the end to the success of the business.

Your communication skills will be developed and adapted to suit the range of situations and different salon-based activities which you will be required to carry out. These include dealing with different enquiries; promoting and selling products and treatments; correctly dealing with difficult situations such as client dissatisfaction; and carrying out client consultations to identify the most appropriate treatment and/or product to meet your clients' needs.

You must be able to demonstrate and will be assessed to prove that you have the necessary practical skills and underpinning knowledge to communicate with clients and provide client care.

INDUSTRY ROLE MODEL

GILL MORRIS Managing Director of GMT Business Training

"I am a Chartered Marketer, Fellow of the RSA, Member of the Professional Speaking Association and a well-known and respected beauty industry professional. I have worked in this industry for many years, starting my career as a therapist, salon manager, then owner of two salons. After a time away from beauty, in corporate sales, I returned as the Technical Sales and Marketing Manager for Ellisons, and then as Director of PR and Training for Sterex. Since 1999 I have run my own highly successful training, coaching and mentoring business assisting salon owners, managers and therapists to reach their full potential.

Outcome 1: Be able to communicate with clients

Learn how to communicate with clients

PRACTICAL SKILLS

Use effective communication techniques

Use client consultation techniques to identify treatment objectives

Provide the client with clear advice and recommendations

UNDERPINNING KNOWLEDGE

Outline different forms of communication used to deal with clients

Describe how to use consultation techniques to identify treatment objectives

State the importance of using effective communication to identify client needs and expectations

Describe the term 'personal space'

State the importance of providing the client with clear advice and recommendations

What is communication?

Communication can be described as the exchange of information between two people or groups of people that is effectively understood.

Communication occurs in different ways and should differ depending upon each workplace and client situation.

ACTIVITY

Do you have good employability 'soft skills'? If you have these they should be promoted on your CV and discussed at any job interview at the appropriate moment.

Some examples of 'soft skills' are listed below:

◆ commitment and attitude to work, i.e. your keenness to complete a task well and to meet any set deadline

◆ positive attitude, i.e. when faced with a problem, this is your confidence that whatever the problem is, it is surmountable – it can be overcome

◆ managing time well – do you ensure that with the time available to you, you manage your workload well? This will often require you prioritizing tasks in order of importance and not putting off tasks that require completion. Your ability to break down one big task into a number of smaller tasks is important and can help to ensure you are realistic about the time you have available to complete it

◆ flexible approach to change or to support a need – this is how you respond when there is a requirement to change something in the workplace or respond to a need. This could be something as simple as changing your lunch to accommodate the treatment of a client.

Being a good team player – do you consider, appreciate and support your colleagues knowing that you all bring different qualities to the workplace?

TOP TIP

The impact of good communication

Good communication creates confidence in your clients. They will trust an organization when communicated with in a certain way – both professionally and with respect.

Communication is often referred to as an employment 'soft skill'. When recruiting staff, employers rank soft skills as highly as the actual qualification. This is because possession of these makes somebody a good employee. 'Soft skills' can be described as an individual's personal qualities. This includes their attitude and ethics (principles, morals, beliefs).

Communication skills will help you to:

◆ gain the client's confidence in your professionalism and technical knowledge

◆ develop a professional relationship or rapport with the client

◆ correctly identify the client's treatment/product needs

◆ confidently and enthusiastically promote the different treatments and products

◆ resolve quickly any misunderstandings, complaints or disputes.

Communication skills

Communication can be verbal or non-verbal. Conclusions about how we see other people are based upon both spoken and unspoken communication.

Verbal communication

Verbal communication occurs when you talk directly to another person, either face to face or over the telephone. To assist effective communication, always speak clearly, slowly and precisely. Your tone of voice is important, you should always sound calm, cheerful and helpful. This will help gain client confidence. Avoid chattering constantly, allow others the opportunity to speak. Avoid interrupting the client while they are speaking, this can appear rude and you may miss important information. Always listen carefully and be patient.

2

ACTIVITY

Telephone communication

A telephone call is often the first contact the client has with the salon and is an important method of communication.

◆ How should the phone be answered?

◆ What action would you take if there was not sufficient time for the appointment at the time requested?

◆ When booking a treatment why would you need to check if the client has been to the salon before, if the client is not known to you?

◆ What information would you need to find out when handling a complaint about a treatment?

◆ How should you close a telephone booking with your client?

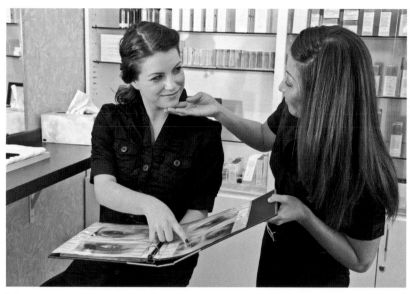

It is important to communicate a desired look with your client

Avoid slang and informal phrases such as 'hang on a minute' when speaking with a client on the telephone.

Having developed a rapport with your client, centre the conversation on them, they should be made to feel important. Consider the client's needs, a nervous client may need to be reassured.

Non-verbal communication

Clients can be made to feel intimidated, uncomfortable or ignored – without even saying anything! This is because you also communicate with your eyes, face and body, transmitting your feelings called body language. This is called **non-verbal communication**. Therefore, how you look and how you behave in front of your clients is very important too. Interpreting your client's body language is an important skill to develop. Learn to notice your client's behaviour, observe their eyes, body, arm and hand movements. An instinctive 'feel' for client's behaviour can be developed with experience.

An example of negative body language

A professional beauty therapist greets a new client

TOP TIP

First impressions count!
On meeting a client, always
smile, make eye contact and greet
them cheerfully – however bad your
own day is!

Knowledge Check

What are listening skills? Why are
they important when deciding upon
the client's needs?

Listening skills when listening to your client give them your undivided attention; this lets them know you are listening. If you are face to face with the client, make eye contact. You must ensure that you *hear* what the other person is saying and you *understand* what they are saying. Then you will be able to *respond* appropriately to what they have said or asked. Do not be afraid of silence, allow the other person to think and consider when listening.

Become a good listener: this will help you identify your client's treatment requirements, expectations and consider if these are realistic. You can then guide the conversation appropriately.

Questioning skills asking your client a question allows you to find out the information you need to know and learn more to help you make decisions. When asking questions never interrogate your client or talk down to them, and avoid technical jargon which can be off-putting – instead, use commonly understood words.

Ask open questions; those that encourage the client to talk and cannot be answered with just *yes* or *no* (these are called closed questions). Open questions start with 'how', 'why',

A beauty therapist listening to a client talking

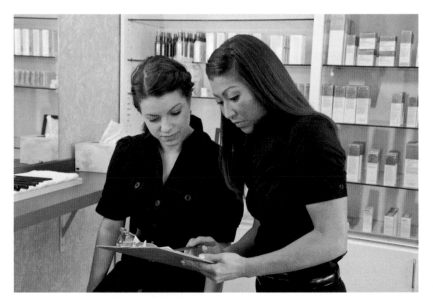

A beauty therapist completing a consultation form before beginning a service

TOP TIP

Dealing with client confusion

If a client appears confused about the information you have given them, try to identify which part is confusing.

Repeat the information clearly and logically, checking for understanding.

Always allow time for clients to consider your response and provide further explanation as necessary.

Confirm client understanding with them and ensure that they are now clear and satisfied.:

'what', 'when', and 'which'. Probing questions can be used and are necessary when you need to gain further information. You may need to use these when specific information is required to assist you in making a decision, e.g. 'How long exactly do you want to wear your artificial eyelashes for?' when deciding which type to apply.

Professional conversation

At all times communication should be professional and relevant to your job role. Avoid all the usual controversial topics, such as sex, religion and politics! This applies to personal topics of conversation too.

> It's important to realize clients do not come to a salon because they need a friend. Clients come to you because you are a skilled professional and they need your knowledge and treatments, just like you when you visit your doctor. They come to you because they want or need something that they can't achieve for themselves.
>
> *Gill Morris*

Conversation should be polite and courteous at all times. Although obvious, never lose your temper, or swear in front of a client.

When you have developed a professional relationship with your client, value it. Clients often share confidences with you. Always remain discreet and tactful. Never pass judgement, and ensure that you deserve your client's trust by maintaining their **confidentiality**.

> **Providing clear advice**
> Always check any advice you have provided is understood by the client. Certain technical information may not appear complicated, but if, for example, a client has bought several skincare products, it is important that they know how to use each safely and efficiently. Always check tactfully with the client to ensure that they have fully understood the information you have provided. You may need to use 'open questions' to confirm this.
>
> *Gill Morris*

Providing accurate advice and recommendations

It may be that the client requests information that you are unable to help with or which lies outside your responsibility. If this occurs, politely inform them that you are not able or qualified to deal with their request but will get somebody else to assist. Always indicate how long this will take if it will not be immediately.

Keeping a client informed is reassuring and important to avoid dissatisfaction with the client care experienced.

TOP TIP

Conversation topics

Make notes on the client's record of topics that interest them. You can introduce these topics in conversation next time the client receives a treatment, and they will be pleased that you have taken the trouble to remember.

Knowledge Check

How could you explain the term communication?

Refer to pages 155–156 to help you.

TOP TIP

Never guess or assume what a client wants or needs or what a client can afford.

Consultation techniques using your communication skills to help identify the client treatment requirements

When you carry out a consultation you will use all your communication skills and techniques to correctly identify the treatment objectives. Through the consultation process you will assess the needs of the client and identify their treatment /product needs.

Client consultation using equipment

 There is only one person who knows what a client wants from you and that's them. It is your job to uncover what they want and need, and you do that during the consultation which should be like a private, confidential conversation.

Gill Morris

It is necessary to ask the client a series of questions before the **treatment plan/** product selection can be finalized. This should ideally be carried out in a private area to maintain client confidentiality and the details should be recorded on the client **record card**. Remember at all times to ensure that the client feels comfortable; ensure that there is sufficient space between yourself and them. This is especially important when communicating with a client you have never met before. If the client feels uncomfortable they may feel you have invaded their **personal space**. Personal space is the space around a person that they see as theirs. Intrusion of this can make them feel uncomfortable. A common reaction will be that they will move away from you, put up a personal barrier by folding their arms, avoiding eye contact. A good seating position is to sit next to the client whilst you carry out the consultation so there is no barrier between yourself and the client.

Ensure that you explain fully the purpose of the consultation and what it will involve, including assessment techniques to be used, in order that the client feels confident

Personal space. There is sufficient space between the client and nail technician and good eye contact, showing the client is comfortable

about its function. Avoid touching the client unnecessarily, as this is an invasion of their personal space. Always observe and read your client's body language.

Open questions help you find out the information you need to recommend a product or treatment to meet the client's needs. Use **visual aids** to assist understanding if necessary. An example may be the use of 'before and after' images to show the benefit of using a nail treatment product.

The information recorded on the record card is confidential and should be stored in a secure area following client treatment. This is enforced through the Data Protection Act (1998).

The client should understand the reason behind the questions asked and feel comfortable when answering them. As such, they should be asked in a sensitive and supportive manner. Avoid technical terms, choosing commonly understood words to ensure client understanding. Ask 'open' questions, which will encourage the client to give more than a one word response of 'yes' or 'no' and will help you to make informed decisions based on the information provided.

> " A new client may be nervous about what happens in a salon and about what you are like. Always consider how they might be feeling and remember what it's like not to know what happens.
>
> *Gill Morris*

Knowledge Check

What is the purpose of the client consultation?

Refer to page 159 to help you.

If, after the consultation, you are unsure of the client's suitability for treatment or use of a product, tactfully explain to the client why this is and ask them to seek permission from their GP if relevant before the treatment is given. Some clients' expectations may be unrealistic and unachievable. If this is the case, tactfully explain why and aim to agree to a realistic treatment plan.

Designing an effective treatment plan includes:

◆ completion of the client record card

◆ checking for client suitability to identified treatments /products

◆ providing clear advice and recommendations

◆ design of a suitable, realistic treatment plan

◆ agreeing the treatment plan with the client.

> " You need to demonstrate to your clients, both existing and new, your knowledge, skills and ability as this demonstrates you are an expert in your field and any advice you give and recommendations you make will be of benefit. After all, if you don't share knowledge with them they'll never know how much of an expert you are. Do not concentrate so much on the treatment that you ignore the client.
>
> *Gill Morris*

Outcome 2: Be able to provide client care

Learn how to provide client care

PRACTICAL SKILLS

Maintain client confidentiality in accordance with legislation

Gain feedback from clients on client care

Respond to feedback in a constructive way

Refer client complaints to the relevant person

Assist in client complaints being resolved

UNDERPINNING KNOWLEDGE

Describe client confidentiality in line with the Data Protection Act

Explain the importance of communication techniques to support retail opportunities

State the importance of client feedback and responding constructively

Outline how to refer and assist in client complaints

Providing client care

Clients want to enjoy their visit to the beauty salon. An important part of this experience is the service which they are paying for. It is essential that during every visit they are made to feel welcome and comfortable whilst in the salon environment with their expectations met. Good communication as discussed previously helps greatly towards achieving this.

Many organizations have a **customer care statement**, which informs customers of the standards of service they can expect. These standards can be used to measure client satisfaction periodically, monitoring if the service standard is being met and if not why.

An important factor for the success of any beauty therapy business is the commitment of each employee to provide a consistently high standard of client care.

For this to occur it is important that all staff are confident and effective in their job role. Carrying out treatments to the highest standard, whilst maintaining positive working relationships with colleagues, creates a happy, productive work environment which is obvious to the clients.

ACTIVITY

Client care

Find out whether your organization has a customer care statement. If so, how well do you do in providing that level of client care? Monitor yourself against the statement, and ask colleagues for feedback too.

ACTIVITY

Dealing with the unexpected

How would you explain the unexpected situations listed below to client(s)? With colleagues, discuss your experiences and record your ideas.

◆ Clients arriving late for appointments.

◆ Double bookings, two clients requiring their treatment at the same time.

◆ Changes required to bookings.

Gaining client feedback

To check the quality of client care you should capture your client's views. Client feedback can be gathered in a variety of ways, both formally and informally.

◆ Client questionnaires can be used formally to measure performance against the service standards. They can also be used at random to evaluate performance, for example following a promotion. The results should be analyzed and appropriate action taken to improve areas of weakness, build on strengths and investigate potential areas of development.

◆ Simply asking the client if they have enjoyed or have been satisfied with the service received is another method of service evaluation.

It is important for all staff to be involved in evaluating feedback and being aware of their part in any actions for improvement. If you are made aware of any poor client feedback it is necessary to pass this on to the relevant person to action.

ACTIVITY

How good are we?

A questionnaire may be useful in monitoring client satisfaction. Questionnaires can be anonymous, and collected at a central point.

Identify several questions to ask your clients. The findings will be important to the team and the business. Collate the findings and use them to evaluate effectiveness and identify areas requiring development. Simple changes can make all the difference!

Client's needs

Always remember the diversity of the range of people you will come into contact with. Diversity includes:

◆ personality

◆ beliefs and attitudes

◆ age

◆ religion, morality

◆ background and culture.

TOP TIP

Eye contact communication

In some cultures eye contact is considered to be disturbing or inappropriate. Always consider client diversity.

Some clients may have physical disabilities including hearing and visual impairment. It is important to behave naturally with such clients.

If visually impaired, introduce yourself and explain the treatment before delivering it. Discuss physical sensations that the client may experience and explain noises that may be heard and what they are. Provide **assistance** as requested . If the client has a guide dog accommodate this in the work area.

If hearing impaired agree with the client how they wish to communicate. This will include body gestures, lip reading and writing information. Always reduce any background noise if the client has hearing impairment. Maintain good facial contact with the client, using facial expressions to reinforce understanding. Write important information if this is a way the client communicates. Point to objects, i.e. nail polishes to select colour and use simple gestures to further assist understanding.

Each client is different with different treatment needs, requiring an individual client care/ treatment approach. Always consider if you have dealt with each client adequately and responded to their needs appropriately. If you identify a skills gap, request the relevant staff for support.

All staff at their workplace **induction** should be informed of the business goals, and their role in achieving them. An induction should occur as soon as an employee starts work, or progresses into a new job role. It should provide general and essential information, such as a description of the work environment facilities, health and safety, security, the staffing structure, roles and responsibilities of colleagues in the organization. For example, who to report to if advice is required outside of the employee's responsibility or if they have a concern. The induction should leave staff feeling more confident about the expectations required from them and how they will be supported, and by whom. Responsibilities should be clearly defined in a written **job description**.

As well as treatment standards, there may also be a staff **code of conduct** which states the expected employee standards to perform successfully in the job role.

Legal requirements

The salon has a legal obligation to implement legislation designed to protect clients' rights. Relevant legislation is discussed below.

Health and safety Following the consultation you may feel that the client is unsuitable for treatment. Explain tactfully why this is and ask them to seek permission from their GP before the treatment is given. Some clients may have unrealistic expectations. If this is the case, tactfully explain why and aim to agree to a realistic treatment programme.

Remember your legal duty under the Health and Safety at Work Act (1974) to take reasonable care to avoid harm to yourself and others. Refer to Chapter 3 Health and Safety for more information.

Data Protection Act (1998) Before treating your client it is necessary to ask them a series of questions so that the treatment plan can be finalized.

Client details are recorded on the client record card. This information is confidential and should be stored in a secure area. The client should understand the reason behind the questions asked of them.

Confidential information on staff or clients should only be made available to persons to whom consent has been given.

TOP TIP

Referring to a client by their preferred title

It is important that a client is greeted appropriately according to their expectations.

Avoid using general informal titles such as 'love'. Never use a client's first name unless invited to do so. If in doubt ask the client how they would like to be referred to.

Consumer protection legislation This legislation referred to as fair trading legislation is designed to both protect the client from harm from products/treatments and protects their rights when purchasing products/treatments. Refer to page 147 to find out more.

ALWAYS REMEMBER

Legislation

Important legislation relating to communication and supply of products/treatments includes:

◆ Data Protection Act 1998

◆ Sale and Supply of Goods Act 1994

◆ Consumer Protection Act 1987

◆ Trade Descriptions Act 1968 and 1972.

You need to be able to describe the importance of each piece of legislation, see chapter 4, Pages 147–149 for more information.

Handling complaints

ACTIVITY

Handling customer complaints

The client is unhappy about how long she has been waiting. What action would you take? List five other complaints that might be made by a client. How would you handle each situation to ensure a positive outcome?

Sometimes clients are unhappy with an aspect of the treatment received or a product they purchased. Occasionally problems arise in which the client cannot be appeased or satisfied. Many complaints are easily resolved but require a procedure to deal with them. A **complaints procedure** is a formal, standardized approach adopted by the organization to handle any complaints. It should also be used to handle complaints related to discrimination.

Whatever the procedure for handling a complaint, all employees should be familiar with it. You should play your part when aware of a client complaint in ensuring that it is quickly resolved.

Clients should be advised of the standard complaint procedure and if not able to be dealt with immediately, they should be left with confidence knowing how it is to be dealt with, and how and when they will be contacted with an update or outcome.

ACTIVITY

In your organization do you know:

◆ who to report a client complaint to?

◆ who you would refer to if information requested was outside your area of responsibility?

Dealing with client dissatisfaction or complaint

If a client is dissatisfied, they may appear angry and complain or they may say nothing. However they react, remember that a dissatisfied client is bad for business.

You may be required to deal with a dissatisfied client:

◆ stay calm and listen to the client's complaint

◆ if you are unable to handle it, refer it as quickly as possible to somebody who can. Inform the client of your actions at all times. (It is important that you know the limits of your authority when handling a complaint.) Inform the relevant person. This may be the manager, receptionist or senior beauty therapist depending upon the nature of the complaint

◆ establish the facts and take appropriate action as laid down in your client complaints procedure.

ALWAYS REMEMBER

Handling and monitoring complaints

A complaint from a dissatisfied client provides the opportunity to put things right and turn a negative into a positive!

Complaints received should be logged, however minor, and reviewed at staff team meetings. There may be patterns to the complaints which if not fixed could affect long-term customer satisfaction.

Knowledge Check

If a client was dissatisfied or had a complaint with a product or treatment, how could you assist in resolving this?

Refer to page 164 to help you.

◆ always aim to repair the relationship, although at times this may not be possible

◆ not all clients are always genuine in their complaint – establish the facts and tactfully advise the client of the outcome

◆ always remain courteous, professional and create a positive impression.

Avoiding client dissatisfaction

Some dissatisfied clients will voice their dissatisfaction; others will remain silent and simply not return to the salon. This situation can often be prevented through good client care and effective communication.

◆ Always ensure that the client has a thorough consultation before any new treatment. This should be carried out by an employee with the appropriate technical expertise.

◆ Regularly check the client's satisfaction. If there is any concern that you cannot handle, inform the **relevant person** of this immediately.

◆ Inform the client of any disruption to treatment – do not leave them wondering what the problem may be. Politely inform them of the situation, for example 'I'm sorry but we are running 10 minutes late – are you able to wait?' If your salon has the facilities, you may offer them a drink.

◆ Inconvenience caused by disruption to treatment can usually be compensated in some way. It is important to resolve problems and keep clients satisfied.

Client care is vital: clients provide the salon's income and your wages. The success of the business depends upon satisfied clients.

Improving your performance

In order to develop personally and to improve your skills professionally, it is important to set yourself **targets** against which you can measure your achievement.

To an employer it is important that you are *consistent*. You must always perform your skills to the highest standard, and present and promote a positive image of the industry and the organization in which you are employed and which you represent.

Developing your communication and client care skills

There will be many opportunities to develop your communication and client care skills and experience, some of these are listed on the following page.

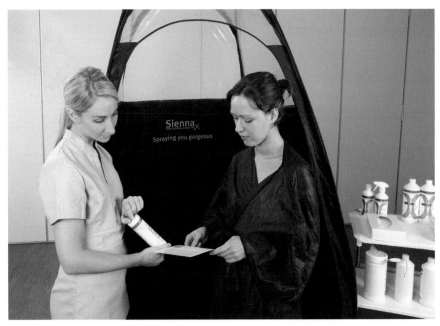

Beauty therapist offering aftercare advice to a client

Opportunities to develop your communication skills include:

◆ active participation in training and development activities

◆ watching and talking to colleagues who have more advanced qualifications or experience

◆ using time effectively, and by practising – all skills take time to master. The more you practise, the more skilled and confident you will become.

Using your communication skills to support retail opportunities

Understanding a client's verbal and non-verbal communication will help you when selling. You must be able to adapt your communication in response to the client.

Be aware that conflicting signals may be given. A client may show interest in a product or treatment, they may smile and nod as if interested but may, in fact, not be. On the other hand, if the client makes the first approach about the product or treatment then they obviously have an active interest already.

> Clients normally always need some help and advice regarding their home care, so don't forget to discuss their regimes at home and see where you can help them. After all, being a good beauty therapist is not just about the great care you give them when they are with you, it's also about how you look after them when they are at home through your advice and the products you have recommended.
>
> *Gill Morris*

Female beauty therapist supporting her male colleague with practical skills training

Initially a client may have a reserved manner and have a stiff body posture. If they become more interested, however, their posture will relax: they may begin to lean forward. It will become obvious at this stage that they are interested, and they then will go on to nod and agree, and to listen actively.

You must use your own body language to good effect too. You must be relaxed but attentive, and listen actively – nodding and shaking your head, and smiling in agreement as they talk. Use relaxed, gentle hand movements: do not twitch or turn away from the client.

If the client is not agreeing with you, or is not interested, they may look bored, tap their fingers, fiddle, look away, or even look at their watch. If these signs are evident, go back to the beginning and try to find out why they are not interested. This is important when selling. Perhaps they do not want the product you have recommended? Or perhaps it is too expensive? Suggest alternatives and see whether you can get their interest again.

When the client has decided to buy, smile – help them to feel that they have made an excellent decision. They should leave feeling proud to have purchased the product.

Communicate effectively as part of a team

There can be no place in a customer care industry for poor working relationships. A great portion of your time is spent in the workplace alongside your colleagues, and if the environment becomes stressful this will affect your effectiveness. It will also be apparent to clients, and relationships between staff members should not trouble them. Disputes must be resolved immediately.

If the dispute cannot be resolved, report this to a senior colleague who has the responsibility to deal with such personnel issues.

Personnel problems may occur when there are ineffective communication systems. It is important that you understand the salon's staffing structure. You need to know who is responsible for what, and who you should approach in various circumstances.

Working under pressure

Sometimes you will be extremely busy and you may be feeling tired and weary. This is not the client's problem! Remain cheerful, courteous and helpful. You should also use your initiative in helping others, for example by preparing a colleague's work area when you are free and they are busy.

You must be able to cope with the unexpected such as:

◆ clients arriving late for appointments
◆ clients' treatments overrunning the allocated treatment times
◆ double bookings, with two clients requiring treatment at the same time
◆ the arrival of unscheduled clients
◆ changes to the bookings.

With effective **teamwork** such situations can usually be overcome.

ASSESSMENT OF KNOWLEDGE AND UNDERSTANDING

You have now learnt about client care and communication in the beauty therapy workplace. To test your level of knowledge, answer the following short questions. These will prepare you for your summative (final) assessment.

1. The first time you meet a client you should be:
   a. polite, friendly, aloof
   b. polite, friendly, chatty
   c. friendly, inviting, distant
   d. casual, friendly, distant

2. The client consultation is the most import part of any treatment:
   a. true
   b. false

3. When an appointment scheduling mix-up occurs, you should:
   a. not admit that you or anyone in the salon made a mistake
   b. argue with the client who wrote the appointment down wrongly
   c. be polite and never argue to see which one of you is correct
   d. blame the salon receptionist and call the manager

4. Which of the following are appropriate ways of dealing with unhappy clients?
   a. find out why the client is unhappy
   b. do not change what the client dislikes until their next visit
   c. tactfully explain the reasons why you cannot make changes
   d. argue with the client to inform them of your opinion
   e. call on the advice of the relevant person to help

5. The legislation designed to protect client privacy and confidentiality is:
   a. Data Protection Act
   b. Workplace Regulations
   c. Health and Safety at Work Act
   d. Provision and use of Work Equipment Regulations

6. Non-verbal communication is:

   a. communicating using the telephone
   b. communicating using body gestures
   c. completion of the client record card
   d. the tone of voice used when talking to the client

7. Personal space is:

   a. the space around a person that they see as theirs
   b. the appointment space booked for each client
   c. where the client's details are recorded
   d. where the client can store their personal belongings

8. A consultation should be provided:

   a. at every treatment
   b. if the client is new to you
   c. each time the client receives a different treatment
   d. at every other appointment

9. The consultation uses the following:

   a. verbal communication
   b. non-verbal communication
   c. listening techniques
   d. verbal and non-verbal communication

10. Verbal **questioning techniques** used to find out your client's needs at consultation use:

    a. open questions
    b. closed questions
    c. a record card to tick the correct answer to a question
    d. a list of set questions that the client provides short answers to

6 Salon Reception

LEARNING OBJECTIVES

There are three learning outcomes for this optional unit which you must achieve:

1 Be able to carry out reception duties.

2 Be able to book appointments.

3 Be able to deal with payments.

From the range statement, you must show that you can:

◆ Deal with a variety of enquiries using a variety of techniques.

◆ Communicate and behave in an appropriate and professional manner with others.

◆ Identify the nature of all enquiries.

◆ Observe all legislation when handling client details.

◆ Deal with the different methods of payment.

◆ Deal with all types of payment problems

KEY TERMS

appointment

behaviour

charge cards

cheques

communication

credit cards

debit cards

discrepancies

enquiries

external client

gift voucher

hospitality

internal client

legislation

messages

method of payment

payment problems

reception

receptionist

salon policy

skin sensitivity (patch) tests

traveller's cheques

verbal communication

Unit Topic

Salon reception duties.

This unit is linked to the Beauty Therapy NOS Unit G4.

INTRODUCTION

The reception is where you receive clients and should feel welcoming and well-organized to clients on their arrival, with their needs prioritized in all circumstances.

This chapter explains how to carry out the important reception skills of welcoming and receiving people entering the beauty therapy business, handling their enquiries, making appointments, dealing with client payments and generally maintaining the appearance and organization of the reception area. Dealing with all visitors in a polite, efficient manner while questioning them to find out what they require, forms an important part of this unit. Excellent organizational and people skills are essential to ensure the smooth running of the reception area. You must be able to show you have the necessary practical skills and underpinning knowledge to fulfil salon reception duties.

INDUSTRY ROLE MODEL

TINA ROOK Head of Saks Education

I joined Saks in 1999 with the task of creating NVQ training programmes in hairdressing and beauty therapy, so that apprentices could learn their trade while working in Saks salons. I am proud to have helped the company achieve Beacon Status and we have also been awarded all Grade 1s by the Adult Learning Inspectorate for providing outstanding training.

Prior to joining Saks, I worked as a beauty therapist for big industry names, including Steiner and Regis. I have run my own business, and have worked at Habia where I was instrumental in the development of NVQs and creating the first ever apprenticeship in beauty therapy – an industry first!

The reception

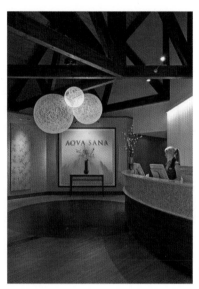

Spa reception

The **reception** is a client's first and also final impression of the business, whether this is on the telephone or in person when they visit. Great receptionists should provide all clients and visitors with an excellent first and last impression. It is becoming increasingly popular to book appointments online. If your salon has an online facility this must be handled smoothly and efficiently. Clients observe and remember the quality of service, making judgements through every contact they have with the business and its staff. It is important that the attitude of the **receptionist** and their response to any query is knowledgeable and extremely helpful. The reception area must be kept clean and tidy at all times. First impressions count, so ensure that the client gets the *right* impression!

You only get one chance to make a good first impression and it only takes a few seconds for a client to form a judgement whether they like you or not! You never get a second chance to make a first impression!

Tina Rooks

Clients need to feel valued. Good interpersonal skills are essential in a receptionist. Interpersonal skills are behaviours – everything you say and do. Clients will reach conclusions based upon your **behaviour**. Always:

◆ act positively and confidently
◆ speak clearly
◆ be friendly, and smile
◆ look at the client and maintain appropriate eye contact, which does not make the client feel uncomfortable
◆ use good listening skills

◆ be interested in everything that is going on around the reception area

◆ give each client individual attention and respect to meet their individuality.

Outcome 1: Be able to carry out reception duties

Learn how to carry out reception duties

PRACTICAL SKILLS

Deal with a variety of enquiries

Communicate and behave in a professional manner

Identify the nature of the enquiry

Maintain appropriate levels of reception stationery

Maintain a hygienic and tidy reception area

UNDERPINNING KNOWLEDGE

Describe procedures for taking messages for a variety of enquiries

State how to communicate and behave within a salon environment

List salon treatments available, their duration and cost

Outline the importance of dealing with enquiries promptly and politely

Explain how to deal with enquiries that cannot be dealt with promptly

Reception area

Location Reception is usually situated at the front of a beauty salon; in a large department store, reception may be a cosmetic counter. It should be clean, tidy and inviting.

If the beauty salon has a window this can be used to attract and capture the attention and interest of potential clients passing by. Clients who are waiting in reception, however, may seek privacy, so if there is a window this should be attractively screened and the seating should be situated away from the view of the main window if possible.

Size The entrance to reception should wherever possible enable wheelchair access. There should be adequate seating, and an area in which to hang clients' coats and wet umbrellas. If the entrance floor becomes wet for any reason, all necessary action should be taken immediately to avoid slippage.

It may be that small treatments, such as manicures, are carried out at reception. These treatments can then be seen by others, and may attract further clients.

Hospitality is important and shows the salon's commitment to client care. If the client arrives early or their treatment is likely to be delayed, offer magazines or refreshments such as coffee, herbal teas or water. Clients may also like refreshments following their treatment, for example, while waiting for their nail polish to dry or while waiting between different treatments. If your salon has a relaxation area ensure this is kept tidy with refreshments available if provided. This is also used as a type of reception area where clients wait for their treatments.

Magazines should be stored in an area of the reception. They should be collected as necessary and returned to this area. Magazines should be renewed regularly and disposed of if in poor condition.

TOP TIP

Cleanliness

An attractive heavy-duty foot mat at the entrance to reception will protect the main floor covering from becoming marked. This may be embossed with the salon logo. Keep the entrance clean and smart at all times and reduce possible accidents from slipping on wet flooring.

ACTIVITY

Magazines

What magazines do you think would be appropriate for the beauty salon? Consider the range and diversity of your clientele.

Smoking prohibited in this area

No smoking sign

Smoking It is illegal to smoke on enclosed or partially enclosed business premises and you are required by law to display a mandatory sign stating this. Out of courtesy if you have an area where clients are able to smoke outside you may inform them of this. Clearly signpost where clients can and cannot smoke.

Decoration The reception area should be decorated tastefully in keeping with the décor in the rest of the salon. Attractive posters promoting proprietary cosmetic ranges/treatments may be displayed on the walls. These should be renewed regularly to keep a fresh feel. Framed certificates of the staff's professional qualifications can be displayed, as well as health **legislation** registration and insurance certificates.

Decorative plants or fresh flowers displayed on reception are attractive. Avoid heavily fragranced flowers which could cause irritation to some people.

Reception resources The reception area should be uncluttered. The main equipment and furnishings required for an efficient reception include the following:

◆ *A reception desk* The size of the desk will depend on the size of the salon; some salons may have several receptionists. The desk should include shelves and drawers; some have an in-built lockable cash or security drawer. The desk should be at a convenient height for the client to make a payment, note down the appointment time etc. It should also be large enough to house the **appointment** book or computer (or both). Consider clients who may be in a wheelchair – the desk must be accessible to them so you can communicate effectively with them and handle their payments.

◆ *A comfortable receptionist chair* The receptionist's chair should provide adequate back support and be the correct height for working at a computer screen.

◆ *A computer* Computers can be used to store data about clients, to book appointment schedules, handle electronic **communication** (e.g. email), to carry out automatic stock control, and to record business details such as accounts and marketing information. They can also be programmed to recommend specific treatments on the basis of personal data about the client! Space should be provided for a printer if required. A shredder is useful to dispose of confidential information when necessary.

◆ *A calculator* This is used for simple financial calculations, especially if the salon does not have a computer.

◆ *Stationery* This should include price lists, paper-based gift vouchers, appointment cards and a receipt pad. Keep a supply available in line with your salon policy.

◆ *A notepad* This is for taking notes and recording **messages**.

◆ *Address and telephone contact details* All frequently used telephone numbers should be available in an electronic or non-electronic format.

◆ *Sales-related equipment* Items such as till rolls, credit card related equipment and resources and a cash book if used.

◆ *A telephone with voicemail facility* The voicemail facility allows clients to notify you, even when the salon is closed, of an appointment request, or an unavoidable change or cancellation. You can then reschedule appointments as quickly as possible. If you are working on your own, this voicemail facility avoids interruptions during a treatment, yet without losing custom.

◆ *A fax machine* This is becoming less popular as a communication system but may be available at reception. The fax is capable of transmitting text and image via a telephone line to another fax machine. This is useful when information needs to be passed on quickly.

◆ *Record cards* Record cards are confidential cards that record the personal details of each client registered at the salon. They should be kept in alphabetical order in a filing cabinet or a card index box, and should be ready for collection by the beauty therapist when treating new or existing clients. See the general beauty therapy units of this book for complete unit-specific examples of record cards. Each card records:

A receptionist booking an appointment

- ◆ the client's name, address and telephone number
- ◆ any medical details
- ◆ any contra-indications (such as allergies) and contra-actions
- ◆ results and dates of any skin tests carried out
- ◆ treatments' aims and outcomes
- ◆ consultation outcomes related to the client which will assist in planning future treatments
- ◆ treatments received, products used and purchased.

These records may be updated by the receptionist at a later stage following the client's treatment. It might be that an electronic database is used to keep client records which makes updating client data easier to carry out.

◆ *Pens, pencils and a rubber* Make sure these stay at the desk and are in good condition.

◆ *A display cabinet* This may be used to store proprietary skincare and cosmetic products, and any other retail products/items sold by the salon.

HEALTH & SAFETY

Eating and drinking

The receptionist and other employees should not eat or drink at reception for reasons of hygiene and to maintain a professional appearance.

TOP TIP

Client/visitor attention at reception

It is important to give the right amount of attention to all clients according to their specific requirements, to ensure client satisfaction. This must always be considered in a busy situation where a client may be kept waiting. Always acknowledge their arrival. It may be necessary for visitors to sign in depending upon the workplace policy. For health and safety it is vital that you are aware of who is on the premises. Have a sign-in book available for this purpose.

ALWAYS REMEMBER

Data Protection Act (1998)
Client records The record card records confidential information about your client. Ensure that how client information is stored and used complies with the Data Protection Act (1998).

Receptionist greeting a client on their arrival

◆ *Retail displays* Available for the client to try and purchase products.

◆ *Waste bin* A covered, lined waste bin may be provided at the reception area. Ensure this is emptied regularly following salon policy.

Data Protection Act (DPA) (1998)

The Data Protection Act (1998) was passed by Parliament to control the way information is handled and to give legal rights to people who have information stored about them. With more and more businesses using computers to store and process personal data, access to confidential information has become increasingly possible.

This legislation is designed to protect the client's privacy and confidentiality. It is necessary to ask the client questions before the treatment plan can be finalized. The relevant information gathered on the client is confidential and should be stored in a safe and secure area following client treatment, whether on a computer or organized paper filing system. Inform the client that their personal details are being stored and will only be accessed by those individuals who are authorized to do so. Remember also, do not provide confidential information over the telephone or in email correspondence.

Receptionists' duties

Receptionists should have a smart appearance and be able to communicate effectively and professionally, creating the right impression.

Receptionist providing hospitality

> Remember as the front of house receptionist you are the first person that a client will see when they walk through the door. You are an advert for your salon and as such your hair, make-up and dress should reflect this. You are a walking advertisement for the services on offer!
>
> *Tina Rooks*

The receptionist's duties include:

- maintaining the reception area including product displays
- looking after clients and visitors on their arrival, sometimes during their time in the salon and on departure
- providing **hospitality**
- answering telephone calls
- dealing with **enquiries** face to face, by telephone, fax, email or possibly text
- scheduling and cancelling appointments
- dealing with complaints and compliments
- telling the appropriate beauty therapist that a client or visitor has arrived
- assisting with retail sales
- dealing with deliveries
- operating the payment point and handling different types of payments
- filing client records (increasingly this is performed electronically).

The receptionist should know:

- the name of each member of staff, their role and their area of responsibility
- the salon's hours of opening, and the days and times when each beauty therapist is available
- the range of treatments or products offered by the salon, their duration and their cost
- any booking treatment restrictions such as skin testing requirements
- who to refer different types of enquiries to
- the person in your salon to whom you should refer reception problems
- any current discounts and special offers that the salon is promoting
- the benefits of each treatment and each retail product
- the approximate time taken to complete each treatment
- how to schedule follow-up treatments.

Skin sensitivity (patch) tests Before clients receive certain treatments, it may be necessary to carry out **skin sensitivity tests** to test skin sensitivity. The skin sensitivity test is often carried out at reception, and the receptionist will be able to perform the test once they have been trained. Every client should undergo a skin test before a permanent

TOP TIP

Business cards

Visitors to the salon may leave a business card, stating the name of the company, and the representative's name, address and telephone number. These cards should be filed by the receptionist for future reference. At a convenient time, store these electronically for ease of reference in the future.

HEALTH & SAFETY

Deliveries to reception You may have to receive and sign for deliveries at reception, confirming their arrival. These should be dealt with at the earliest possibility to avoid them causing an obstruction, for security and for checking accuracy against the delivery note.

TOP TIP

Electronic mail (email)

Email is a popular method of telecommunication. If your salon has an email address this should be provided to your clients. Also, collect your clients' email addresses as an alternative method of communicating if preferred.

TOP TIP

Opportunities for promoting products and treatments

Within your area of training and responsibility, bring to the attention of clients waiting in the reception area any new products, treatments or promotions.

HEALTH & SAFETY

Client well-being Just in case a client should become ill while in the salon, a contact number should be recorded on the client's card. The receptionist should also know who the qualified first aider is and emergency service numbers if required.

ACTIVITY

Designing record card/salon treatment menu

Design a record card to be used to record the client's treatment details. Alternatively, you could design a salon treatment information menu, explaining the different treatments available and their costs. Be creative, and include a business name you may wish to use in the future.

TOP TIP

Useful contact numbers

It is useful to have the contact details of other service providers that a client may ask for that you could personally recommend. Examples include local taxi companies, hairdressers and florists. You may work collaboratively with these businesses, displaying their business cards.

tinting treatment to the eyelashes or eyebrows. Further tests may be necessary, depending on the sensitivity of the client, before treatments such as those for artificial eyelashes or wax depilation.

As a reception duty it may be your responsibility to check that the necessary test has been received on client arrival following the salon policy for this.

The importance of good communication

As discussed previously, clients make quality judgements based on their contact with the business. Effective communication is important to the success of the business. This may be **verbal communication**, that is face to face, over the telephone or written communication, including email, and remember non-verbal communication – we speak through our bodies' gestures. Conclusions about how we see other people are based on their behaviour both spoken and unspoken.

Refer to the relevant chapters to familiarize yourself with the different skin tolerance tests required.

ACTIVITY

Planning a reception area

Design a reception area, to scale, appropriate to a small or large beauty salon. Discuss the choice of wall and floor coverings, furnishings and equipment, and give the reasons for their selection and the image you want to create. Consider clients' comfort, and health and safety.

To help you plan this you may refer to a specialist beauty therapy equipment suppliers' brochure or online information.

Refer to **CHAPTER 5** Client Care and Communication to learn more about good communication skills

HEALTH & SAFETY

Cleaning In a large salon a professional cleaner may be employed to maintain the hygiene of the reception area. In a smaller salon this may be the responsibility of the receptionist. Reception must be maintained to a high standard at all times. Use quieter periods for this purpose and to check stock levels etc.

Always remember the diversity or range of people you will come into contact with.

Your voice and manner should inspire confidence and trust.

Adopting good posture will also positively affect your speech and professional appearance. You will sound and look more energized.

Non-verbal communication
This is often referred to as body language and is how we communicate using our face, body movements and gestures.

Often we do this unconsciously and our body language may contradict what we are actually saying. It is an important skill to be able to interpret body language and the mood of clients. Observing clients' behaviour will help you to recognize their needs and expectations. Your body language should also show you to be attentive; examples include nodding your head and smiling in agreement.

> " Remember there are different ways in which you can communicate with clients. Always be aware of your body language and how this can be interpreted by others, be cautious when sending written communications and how this can be translated! The way you say things can be interpreted differently depending on the tone of your voice, eye contact and your facial expresssions.
>
> *Tina Rooks*

Asking questions It is important to ask verbal questions to ensure, for example, that you are confident and understand what the client has asked you, do not be embarrassed to do this. It will ensure you give an appropriate answer, make the correct decision and that client satisfaction will be achieved. You may ask 'open' or 'closed' questions. Always ask open questions if you need more information as these questions cannot be answered with 'yes' or 'no'. Open questions start with 'what', 'when', 'who' and 'why', etc. Closed questions are used when you need to confirm something quickly. These are answered 'yes' or 'no'.

> **TOP TIP**
>
> **Eye contact**
>
> In some cultures eye contact is considered to be disturbing or inappropriate. Always consider client diversity.

Telephone calls: communication

A good telephone technique can gain clients; a poor technique can lose them. Here are some guidelines for good technique:

◆ *Answer quickly* On average, a person may be willing to wait up to nine rings: try to respond to the call within six rings.

◆ *Build a rapport* Do this by introducing yourself when you answer the telephone.

◆ *Be prepared* Have information and writing materials ready to hand in the event you need to write down a message or record an instruction. It should not normally be necessary to leave the caller waiting while you find something.

◆ *Be welcoming and attentive* Speak clearly without mumbling, at the right speed. Pronounce your words clearly, and vary your tone. Sound interested, and never abrupt.

> **TOP TIP**
>
> **Client care**
>
> If you are engaged on the telephone when a client arrives, look up and acknowledge their presence. This is positive body language and an example of good interpersonal skills, which makes the client feel welcome.

ACTIVITY

Listening to yourself

A pleasant speaking voice is an asset. Do you think you could improve your speech or manner? Record your voice as you answer a telephone enquiry, then play it back. How did you sound? This is how others hear you!

Remember: the caller may be a new client ringing several salons, and their decision whether to visit your salon may depend on your attitude and the way you respond to their call.

Here are some more ideas about good telephone technique:

◆ *Smile* – this will help you put across a warm, friendly response to the caller.

◆ *Alter the pitch of your voice* as you speak, to create interest.

> " Smile when you answer the phone! A smile can be heard in your voice and speaks a thousand words. As a receptionist you cannot have a bad day as you are always in view of your customer either face to face or on the phone! The person on the end of the phone cannot see how busy or harassed you are. So always speak clearly and politely.
>
> *Tina Rooks*

◆ *As you answer give the standard greeting for the salon* – for example: 'Good morning, Visage Beauty Salon, Susan speaking. How may I help you?'

◆ *Listen attentively* to the caller's questions or requests. You will be speaking to a variety of clients: you must respond appropriately and helpfully to each caller.

◆ *Evaluate the information* given by the caller, and be sure to respond to what they have said or asked.

◆ *Use the client's name* if you know it; this personalizes the call.

◆ *In your mind summarize the main requests from the call.* Ask for further information if you need it.

◆ *If you have an enquiry that you cannot deal with yourself* refer to the relevant person promptly for assistance. Tell the client what you are doing.

◆ *At the end* repeat the main points of the conversation clearly to check that you and the client have understood each other.

◆ *Close the call pleasantly* – for example, 'Thank you for calling, Mrs Smith. Goodbye.'

If you receive a business call, or a call from a person seeking employment, always take the caller's name and telephone number. Your supervisor can then deal with the call as soon as they are free to do so.

Transferring calls

If you transfer a telephone call to another extension, explain to the caller what you are doing and thank them for waiting. If the extension to which you have transferred the call is not answered within nine rings, apologize and explain to the caller that you will ask the person concerned to ring back as soon as possible. Take the caller's name and telephone number and offer to take a message. Always make sure the person gets the message.

Taking messages

Messages should be recorded neatly on a memorandum ('memo') pad. Each message should record:

◆ who the message is for

◆ who the message was from

◆ the date and the time the message was received

◆ accurate details of the message including the reason for the call, details of information requested or to be passed on

◆ the telephone number or address of the caller

◆ the signature of the person who took the message.

When taking a message, listen actively and attentively. Repeat the details you have recorded so that the caller can check that you've got it right. Pass the message directly to the correct person as soon as possible. This may be via memo note, telephone, in person or electronically via text or email as appropriate. The important thing is that the message should be received in time to be acted upon.

TELEPHONE MESSAGE RECEIVED			
To	Angela	Date	10.7.13
From	Jenny Heron	Time	9.30 am
Number	273451	Taken by	Sandra

Please ring Jenny Heron regarding her appointment on Saturday

A memo

Listening skills

It is important to listen closely to what people are saying to you in your role as receptionist, to ensure you correctly identify the purpose of any enquiry in order to choose the correct response when dealing with it.

Listening skills include:

◆ being focused on the other person, paying them your full attention

◆ ensuring that your facial expressions show your interest

◆ not interrupting the other person speaking

◆ using positive body language to show your interest; maintain eye contact; nod your head and lean forward

◆ observing the other person's body language, reading what it is telling you while you listen

◆ summarizing what the other person has said to confirm understanding

◆ asking further questions as necessary if unsure in order to give the right response

◆ asking a client to rephrase what you have said in their own words if they appear confused.

How to deal with a dissatisfied client or complaint

Occasionally a client may be dissatisfied and wish to complain. The receptionist is usually the first contact with the client (either face to face or through telephone contact) and may have to deal with dissatisfied, angry or awkward customers. Considerable skill is needed if you are to deal constructively with a potentially damaging situation.

If your business has a procedure for handling complaints this should be followed. Procedures are useful as these can be audited to identify emerging problems that may require correction. If ignored these problems could be harmful to the business.

Never become angry or awkward yourself. Always remain courteous and diplomatic, and communicate confidently and politely.

1   Listen to the client as they describe their problems, without making judgements. Do not make excuses for yourself or for colleagues. Do not interrupt.

2   Ask questions to check that you have the full background details. Summarize the client's concerns to confirm this.

3   If possible, agree on a course of action, offering a solution if you can. Check that the client has agreed to the proposed course of action. It may be necessary to consult the salon supervisor before proposing a solution to the client: if you're not sure, always check first.

4   Log the complaint: the date, the time, the client's name, the nature of the complaint and the course of action agreed.

5   There should also be a system for handling compliments. Again it is good to see those aspects of the business that are particularly successful. This can also be rewarding and motivational for staff to hear. Such compliments can be used in marketing materials.

> " The client is always right! Even when they are wrong! On occasions when a client is being difficult they may be unhappy with some aspect of the service or products they have received. With careful communication and listening skills as well as observing their body language you can easily diffuse the situation and solve the client's problem before things escalate.
>
> *Tina Rooks*

Appointments

Outcome 2: Be able to book appointments

Learn how to book appointments

PRACTICAL SKILLS

Schedule appointments to meet with salon policy and client requirements

Confirm and record client appointment details

Deal with confidential information to meet salon and legal requirements

UNDERPINNING KNOWLEDGE

Describe how to make and record appointments

State the potential consequences of failing to record appointments or messages accurately

State the importance of passing on messages and appointment details to the appropriate colleagues

Outline the legislation designed to protect the privacy of client details

State the possible consequences of a breach of confidentiality

Making correct entries in the appointment book or salon computer is one of the most important duties of the receptionist. The way you handle client records and the information held on them must conform with the Data Protection Act (see page 176). Always handle confidential information in line with both salon policies and legal requirements. Failure to do so is unprofessional and also breaks the law. If the Data Protection Act is not complied with the client may have the legal right to take action. All staff have a responsibility to maintain client confidentiality at all times.

As receptionist you must familiarize yourself with the salon's appointment system, column headings, treatment times and any abbreviations used.

Each beauty therapist will usually have their name at the head of a column. Entries in columns must not be reallocated without the consent of the beauty therapist or supervisor, unless they are absent.

Appointment bookings

When a client calls to make an appointment, record the client's name, confirm the correct spelling of their name, and the treatment they want. Allow adequate time to carry out the required treatment. Inform the client how long the treatment will take. Take the client's telephone number or other contact details in case the beauty therapist falls ill or is unable to keep the appointment for some other reason. If the client requests a particular beauty therapist, be sure to enter the client's name in the correct column.

In addition, software enabling online appointment booking and scheduling is becoming more popular. This is accessed through the business website and clients can book appointments and view the business's information (treatments offered, specials offers, etc.) at any time. The business can make the final decision to accept or reject the appointment. As receptionist this may be your responsibility. Always spellcheck any electronic communication forwarded to clients – it is important that salon correspondence is of a professional standard.

Finally, the hours of the day are recorded along the left-hand side of the appointment page, divided into 15-minute intervals. You must know how long each treatment takes so that you can allow sufficient time for the beauty therapist to carry out the treatment

ACTIVITY

Reception role play

With colleagues, act out the following situations, which may occur when working as a receptionist. You may wish to video the role plays for review and discussion later.

1 A client arrives very late for an appointment but insists that they be treated.
2 A client questions the bill.
3 A client comes in to complain about a treatment given previously (choose a particular treatment).

Alternatively you may choose to do this as a written activity with a discussion of your answers.

Treatment	Abbreviation	Treatment time allowed*
Cleanse and make-up: day / special occasion	C/M/up day / C/M/up special	30 mins / 45 mins
Eyebrow shaping	E/B reshape or trim	15 mins
Eyebrow tint	EBT	10 mins
Eyelash tint	ELT	20 mins
Manicure	Man	45 mins
Pedicure	Ped	50 mins
Leg wax: half / three-quarter / full	½ leg wax / ¾ leg wax / Full leg wax	30 mins / 30–40 mins / 50 mins
Bikini wax	B/wax	15 mins
Underarm wax	U/arm wax	15 mins
Arm wax	F/arm wax	30 mins
Facial wax	F/wax	10–15 mins
Eyebrow wax	E/B wax	15 mins
Threading	EB/Thread / F/Thread	10–15 mins / 10–15 mins
Ear pierce	E/P	15 mins
Facial	F	60 mins
Artificial eye lashes strip/false individual flare	F/Lash	10–20 mins
Artificial nails: full set / nail maintenance / removal	N/ext F/S / N/Infill / N/rem	120 mins / 90 mins / 60 mins
Natural nail overlays	N/O'lays	75 mins
Nail art	N/art	30 mins
Manual tan – full body	Man/tan	60 mins

*Treatment time does not include preparation for treatment and consultation.

TOP TIP

Gaining client satisfaction

Occasionally you will have to disappoint a client such as when cancelling their appointment or explaining they cannot proceed with a treatment for reasons of health and safety. This you should be able to do without offending or upsetting the client. Consider your tone of voice, how you are going to present the information and what alternative options there may be. Through your words and tone you should be able to demonstrate genuine empathy and resolve to recover the situation.

in a safe, competent, professional manner. If you don't allow sufficient time, the beauty therapist will run late, and this will affect all later appointments. On the other hand, if you allow too much time, the beauty therapist's time will be wasted and the salon's earnings will be less than they could be. Suggested times to be allowed for each treatment are given in the treatment chapters.

Ensure that you regularly check scheduled appointments and plan ahead where you can see any potential problem – put a strategy in place to rectify it. This may involve asking others to help you.

Confirm the name of the beauty therapist who will be carrying out the treatment, the date and the time.

Finally, confirm or estimate the cost of the treatment to the client.

Treatments are usually recorded in an abbreviated form. All those who use the appointment page must be familiar with these abbreviations.

If an appointment book is used, write each entry neatly and accurately. It is preferable to write in pencil: appointments can be amended by erasing and rewriting, keeping the book clean and clear.

Electronic appointment booking systems, if used, allow you to read the appointment schedule and add or edit appointments immediately.

Appointment cards May be offered to the client, to confirm the client's appointment. The card should record the treatment, the date, the day and the time. The beauty therapist's name may also be recorded.

HEALTH & SAFETY

Health and Safety (Display Screen Equipment) Regulations (1992) These regulations cover the use of visual display units and computer screens. They specify acceptable levels of radiation emissions from the screen, and identify correct posture, seating position, permitted working heights and rest periods.

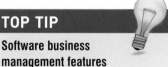

TOP TIP

Software business management features

The software which can be used for booking and scheduling appointments often has the benefits of stock control and ordering, managing client data, and issuing gift cards.

TOP TIP

Appointment reminder

Some software can email or text your clients an appointment reminder directly to their mobile phone.

TOP TIP

Treatment time allowed

Dependent upon the manufacturers' guidelines and the treatment needs of the client including any procedure modifications required, the treatments may take less or more time.

DAY SATURDAY		DATE 15th JANUARY	
THERAPIST	JAYNE	SUE	LIZ
9.00	Mrs Young	DNA	
9.15	1/2 leg wax	Jenny Newley	
9.30	Carol Kreen	EL T/EBT	
9.45	Full leg wax	EB trim	
10.00	B / Wax		
10.15		Sandra Smith	Fiona Smith
10.30	Ms Lord E/B wax	C / M / up	C / M / up
10.45			Strip / lash
11.00		Mrs Jones	
11.15		U/arm wax	
11.30		F/arm wax	Carol Brown
11.45			E/P
12.00			
12.15			
12.30	Nina Farrel		
12.45	Man		
1.00	Ped		
1.15		Sue Uip E/P	
1.30	1/2 leg wax	T Scott	
1.45		3/4 leg wax	
2.00	Karen Davies	U/arm wax	
2.15	Facial		
2.30			
2.45			Pat king
3.00			C / M / up
3.15	Anne Wood		Man
3.30	Man		
3.45	E/B Reshape		
4.00			

Appointment book sample

When the client arrives for their treatment, draw a line or checkmark through their name to indicate that they have arrived.

If the client cancels, indicate this on the appointment page *immediately*, usually with a large C, placed through the booking. This enables another client to take the appointment.

If a client fails to arrive, the abbreviation DNA ('did not arrive') is usually written over the booking. The client's telephone number should then be used to see if a rebooking is required.

Use the relevant recording icon if using an online appointment booking system.

Some salons will have a policy to charge for a missed appointment.

Online appointments page

[Screenshot of salon appointment booking software showing a day view for Saturday 22 December 2007 with columns for Maeve D, Louise S, Debbie D, Steph M, Sarah W, and Res: Sun Bed 1, each containing appointment entries throughout the day.]

Dealing with appointment problems

You are often required to use your initiative in helping colleagues and clients and be able to cope with the unexpected such as:

◆ **Clients arriving late for appointments** – discuss the options, reassure the client that you will always try to accommodate them. It may not be their fault and if arriving for a relaxation treatment the receptionist will have an important role in helping the client to relax. A client can always have the option to rebook the treatment if necessary. If a client's treatment cannot be completed to the correct standard due to lack of time it is preferable to explain this to the client and rebook. Where a client is always late, you will need to discuss this with a supervisor and appropriate action taken to deal with this. Perhaps offer a later appointment. Tact is essential in all situations.

◆ **Double-bookings, with two clients requiring treatment at the same time** – the important outcome is that the client is not disappointed and will return to the salon. Be honest about the mistake, why it has occurred and try to resolve the situation in order that the client receives the treatment wherever possible. A goodwill complimentary gesture may be offered.

◆ **The arrival of unscheduled clients** – always try to find out why they have chosen to arrive for the treatment. It may be that you ran a promotion and they have responded to it, it could be word of mouth, another client may have recommended the salon or treatment. Ensure the client has a positive experience and capture any marketing intelligence for future planning.

◆ **Staff absence with a column of appointments** – inform the client as early as possible if the appointment has to be cancelled. That is why it is important to always have contact details for your clients. Wherever possible consider how the treatment can be accommodated. Another beauty therapist may be able to carry out the treatment but it is important to confirm with the client if this will be acceptable – some clients may be unhappy to have an alternative beauty therapist allocated.

ALWAYS REMEMBER

Next appointments

Appointments can usually be made up to 6 weeks in advance. Often clients will book their next appointment while still at the salon. How far ahead the receptionist is able to book appointments will vary from salon to salon.

ACTIVITY

How would you deal with the following reception problems:

◆ a client arriving late for a treatment
◆ a double-booking
◆ the arrival of an unscheduled client?

Effective teamwork can usually overcome any of the appointment problems already discussed. Inform your colleagues/supervisor of the problem immediately and, dependent upon your experience, state what action needs to be taken or ask them to support you in identifying a solution. You must always:

◆ aim to accommodate clients

◆ not disadvantage or compromise any clients in terms of quality of treatment

◆ keep the client informed of what action is being taken

◆ state how long any delay to treatment will be and if this is unsuitable offer an alternative future appointment

◆ ensure the client is happy with the treatment they have received

◆ use your excellent communication skills!

Outcome 3: Be able to deal with payments

Learn how to deal with payments

PRACTICAL SKILLS	UNDERPINNING KNOWLEDGE
Calculate treatment costs accurately	State how to process different methods of payment
Deal with payments for treatments and/or products to meet with salon policy	Describe how to deal with problems that may occur with payments
Follow security procedures when handling payments	Explain how to keep payments safe and secure

Knowledge Check

When taking messages what is the important information you should record?

Refer to page 180 to help you.

Every business will have a policy for handling cash and for handling the payment. Clients can choose from a wide range of payment methods. It's important that you handle each payment efficiently and correctly. Not all businesses accept every **method of payment** so this should be checked in your training.

It is important that you have received training and are confident to take payment in the client's preferred method, which may be cash or cash equivalent (e.g., **gift voucher**), cheque or payment card.

Before processing payment confirm what it is the client is paying for, i.e. the treatments received and/or the products to be purchased. Confirm the price; ask how they would like to pay. Gaining client confirmation will reduce **discrepancies** later. Always check for any defects in products as you process a sale, e.g. breakage or leakage. If you are responsible for stock control when a product is found to be defective a replacement product is required.

The payment point

Kinds of payment points

Manual tills With manual tills a lockable drawer or box is used to store cash: this may form part of the reception desk. Each transaction must be recorded by hand.

At the end of the working day, record the total cash register in a book, to ensure that accurate accounts are kept. Records of petty cash, small amounts of monies used for expenditures, e.g. milk for clients' coffee, must also be kept so that the final totals will balance.

Automatic tills Electrical automatic tills use codes, one for each kind of treatment or retail sale. These are identified by keys on the till. Using these with each transaction makes it possible to analyze the salon's business each day or each week.

With each sale during the day a receipt is given to the client; the total is also recorded on the till's audit roll.

Automatic tills also provide subtotals of the amounts taken: these can be cross-checked against the amount in the till, to determine the daily takings:

◆ the X reading provides subtotals throughout the day, as required

◆ the Z reading provides the overall figures at the end of the day. This includes a breakdown of payment types and the time they occurred.

Computerized tills Computerized tills provide the same facilities as automatic tills, with additional features to help with the business, including: trading patterns, record-keeping, client treatment cards and treatment history and stock records to calculate staff takings and commission (payment paid to the beauty therapist as a percentage of their takings) if paid.

Both electronic and computerized tills help calculate the client's bill for you, including change to be given.

Electronic scanning facilities are also available. These use infrared light to read barcodes. In-built electronic circuitry detects the price and sends it to the point of sale equipment, such as a computer or cash register till.

Equipment and materials required

◆ **Calculator** This is useful in totalling large amounts of money or when using a manual till.

◆ **Card processing equipment** Where an electronic payment system is used a special till roll which provides a printout for yourself and a copy for the client is required.

◆ **Cash float** At the start of each day you need a small sum of money comprising coins and perhaps a few notes, to provide change: this is called the float. (At the end of the day there will be money surplus to the float: if no mistakes have been made, this should match the takings.) At the start of the working day the float amount should be checked.

◆ **Till roll** This records the sales and provides a receipt. Keep a spare to hand. If you're using a manual cash drawer, you'll need a receipt book.

TOP TIP

Advertisement vouchers

Sometimes the salon may publish other offers, such as a discount on producing a newspaper advertisement for the salon or a website voucher. The advertisement voucher is a form of payment, and must be collected.

ALWAYS REMEMBER

Sale and Supply of Goods Act (1994)

You have a duty to comply with the responsibilities of this Act, ensuring all products sold are of merchantable quality. They must 'conform to contract'. This means fit for purpose and of satisfactory quality.

Receptionist returning the card to the client

Knowledge Check

Why is it important to pass on messages?

Refer to page 180 to help you.

Knowledge Check

What are the common systems used in salons to make appointments?

Refer to page 183 to help you.

TOP TIP

Tills

If there is too little change in the till, inform the relevant person. Running out of change would disrupt service and spoil the impression clients receive.

ACTIVITY

Fraud

Find out about your salon's policy in the case of fraudulent monetary transactions, using either cash or cards. What actions should you take if you found yourself in this situation?

◆ **Audit roll** The retailer's copy of the till roll.

◆ **Cash book** This is a record of income and expenditure, for a manual till.

◆ **Other stationery** A date stamp and a salon name stamp (for cheques), pens, pencils and an eraser, and a container to hold these.

Security at the payment point

Be aware that the reception is usually entered from the street outside, so security should be foremost in one's thoughts at all times.

Having placed money in the cash drawer and collected change as required, always close the cash drawer firmly – never leave it open. Do not leave the key in the drawer, or lying about reception unattended. Regularly remove money from the till and store in a secure area in line with your workplace policy. Large amounts of money should not be left in the till.

Times should be varied when banking monies to ensure personal safety and security from possible theft.

Some members of staff will be appointed to authorize cheques and credit card payments; one of these should initial each cheque.

Errors may occur when handling cheques or when operating an electronic or computerized payment point. Don't panic! If you can't correct the error yourself, seek assistance – but don't leave the cash drawer unattended and open.

Be aware of stolen cards and forged notes and coins. Check at every payment transaction and follow the salon policy if presented. Remember that this must be handled sensitively as the client may not know they are in receipt of a cash forgery.

You may periodically be informed of cards that are invalid, on a credit card warning list from the service provider. If you receive a card that is on a credit card warning list, politely detain the customer, hold onto the card, and contact your supervisor, who will implement the salon's procedure. If the card is unsigned, do not allow the cardholder to sign the card unless you first get authorization from the credit card company's service provider. (The service provider's telephone number should be kept near the telephone.)

Methods of payment

Cash   Training should be provided on the correct procedure for handling the different cash payments in line with your workplace policy. When receiving payment by cash, follow this sequence:

1   Accurately total the charge for the treatments/products received. If using an electronic payment system subtotal the bill. Inform the client of the amount to be paid.

2   Check that the money offered is legal tender – that is, money you will be able to pay into your bank. (Your salon will probably not accept foreign currency, for example.) Also be aware of counterfeit (fake) money and check the validity of bank notes.

3   Place the customer's money on the till ledge until you have given change, or at least state to the customer verbally the sum of money that they have given you. If using a till press the total button, equal to the sum of cash you have been given.

4   Aloud, count the change as you give it to the client. This will help avoid payment disputes.

Forged note detector

5   Thank the client, and give them a receipt.

6   If a client disputes the change given as too little, ask how much money they are missing. Inform the client that when the takings are cashed at the end of the day if there is a surplus and it matches that amount they will be reimbursed. Ensure that you have the client's details so that you can inform them of the outcome the next day. Always follow your salon policy.

Cheques   Cheques are an alternative form of payment.

Some businesses are no longer accepting a cheque as it is becoming more costly to accept as a form of payment.

When receiving payment by cheque, follow this sequence of checks:

1   The cheque must be correctly completed.

2   The cheque must be made payable to the salon the spelling must be correct (you may have a salon stamp for this). The day, date and month should be correct.

3   The words and figures written on the cheque must match those in the box.

4   Any errors or alterations must have been initialled by the client.

5   The signature on the back of the cheque guarantee card must match that on the cheque – compare these as the customer writes their signature on the cheque.

6   The bank's 'sort code' numbers on the cheque must match those on the cheque guarantee card.

7   The date on the cheque guarantee card must be valid.

8   The value on the cheque must not exceed the cheque guarantee card limit.

9   The cheque must be signed by the client.

A cheque

Correctly dated

Payee spelt correctly (initial any mistakes)

Words and figures for amount to be paid must be the same

Amount must not exceed the cheque guarantee card limit

Cheque signed by client
Check signature against that on the cheque guarantee card

Branch sort code to match cheque guarantee card

If your workplace accepts debit or credit cards it is important to know this. Usually there will be signage displayed stating which will be accepted.

Debit cards The card authorizes immediate debit of the cash amount from the client's account and is an alternative to writing a cheque. You cannot perform this kind of transaction unless your salon has an electronic terminal. This processes payment automatically through a telephone connection (chip and PIN). The **debit card** processing company applies a fixed fee for each transaction made.

Credit cards These can be used only if your business has an arrangement with the relevant **credit card** company. A fixed percentage of the total bill is charged by the card processing company for this arrangement.

As the business is required to pay for every transaction with credit and debit cards there may be a minimum spend applied.

Credit cards allow the client to 'buy goods now and pay later' with interest paid each month on the outstanding balance if not paid off in full.

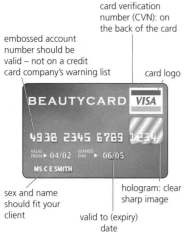

card verification number (CVN): on the back of the card

embossed account number should be valid – not on a credit card company's warning list

card logo

sex and name should fit your client

hologram: clear sharp image

valid to (expiry) date

Credit card checks

Electronic payment systems An electronic computerized terminal may be used for payment by both credit and debit cards. A portable wireless option enables payment from your clients anywhere in the business premises.

TOP TIP

Cards

If cards are accepted as a method of payment, those that are accepted by the business will usually be displayed at the payment point.

VISA   **Maestro**

MasterCard   **Cirrus**   **SWITCH**   **SOLO**

Types of credit and debit card

Knowledge Check

What should you check when receiving payments by cheque?

Refer to page 191 to help you.

Increasingly, credit card terminals also provide an option for processing mail order and telephone order payments from your clients.

1   The card is placed into the chip and PIN machine at the point of sale. The card is verified as genuine.

2   When prompted, use the 'AMOUNT' button on the keypad to input the total sale. (If a mistake is made, you can clear the figures using the CLEAR button.)

3   The client then checks the amount is correct and enters their unique 4 digit Personal Identity Number (PIN). Look away whilst the pin number is entered by the client. The transaction will be declined if the PIN is incorrect. Electronic payment authorization is immediately provided by the bank and transferred electronically.

For security purposes if the PIN number is entered three times incorrectly, the card is declined and deactivated. The client will be required to contact their bank.

Some clients with mobility issues may be unable to use the digital pad and use a chip and signature card system instead. PIN key pads have been designed with raised areas for visually impaired people.

4   A receipt is provided for the client which should be given to the client. A duplicate copy is retained by the business which is used when calculating takings.

5   Place the copies in the till. One copy is for the debit/credit card company, the other is for your records.

Credit card terminal used to process a payment

Mobile card readers are now available which work with mobile phones to process payments. These are convenient for beauty therapists working at different locations.

When receiving payment by debit or credit card, check these points:

1   The card logo for a credit card is at the upper right-hand corner on the front of the card. For a debit card, it should be at the lower right-hand corner of the card.

2   The hologram should have a clear, sharp image and be in the centre right of the card.

3   The date on the card must be valid: if it is out of date ask for another form of payment.

4   The sex (Ms, Miss, Mrs, Mr) and the name of the customer must fit your client.

5   The cardholder's signature on the reverse of the card must match the name on the front of the card.

Knowledge Check

If you make an error when operating the payment point, why must you report this?

Refer to page 190 to help you.

6 The cardholder's card number should be embossed and across the width on the front of the card.

7 The cardholder's card number must not be one of those on the credit card company's warning list.

Traveller's cheques

Traveller's cheques are pre-printed fixed-amount cheques. They may be acceptable, provided they are in particular currencies (usually sterling). Such cheques must be compared with the client's passport for validity. Also available are traveller's cheque cards.

A traveller's cheque

Charge cards

Some businesses accept charge cards such as American Express. These differ from credit cards in that the account holder must repay to the card company the complete amount spent each month. They are considered a more convenient alternative to cash.

Gift vouchers

Gift vouchers are purchased from the salon as pre-payments for beauty therapy treatments or retail sales. Check the following:

◆ there is usually a specific time period in which gift vouchers must be used. Check to see if this is the case and if they are still valid

◆ check the value of the voucher, and remember to request another form of payment if the cost of the treatment is higher than the voucher

◆ for security purposes, some vouchers will have a reference number to reduce the risk of fraudulent copies. The voucher reference number can then be tracked back to the date of purchase and its value, which can be validated.

Cards are also available registered on a database. The value on the card can be read and the credit value debited accordingly.

It is important that all financial transactions are handled competently. However busy you are always follow the guidelines for handling each method of payment.

If you are ever unsure when handling a financial transaction or make a mistake, inform your supervisor immediately. It may be that you have to be discreet when doing this, for example, if a client has handed you a forged bank note! This will also enable a specific financial discrepancy to be justified.

World Of Beauty By Katy

Amount or Treatment
for the value of

SAMPLE

Valid to

WORLD OF BEAUTY by KATY

88 Park Road
Crouch End, London N8 8JQ

A gift voucher

Loyalty cards Increasingly, clients may receive an incentive reward for their customer loyalty and spend with the business. The card records progress towards an agreed target, which may be redeemed against treatments/products as agreed as part of the loyalty scheme.

Financial transactions

It is important that all financial transactions are handled competently. However busy you are always follow the guidelines for handling each method of payment.

If you are ever unsure when handling a financial transaction or make a mistake, inform your supervisor immediately. It may be that you have to be discreet when doing this, for example if a client has handed you a forged bank note!

ASSESSMENT OF KNOWLEDGE AND UNDERSTANDING

You have now learnt about salon reception in the beauty therapy workplace.

To test your level of knowledge, answer the following short questions. These will prepare you for your summative (final) assessment.

1. When a scheduling mix-up occurs, you should:
   a. not admit that you or anyone in the salon made a mistake
   b. argue with the client about who wrote the appointment down wrongly
   c. be polite and never argue the point of which one of you is correct
   d. blame the salon receptionist and call the manager

2. How long should you allow when making an appointment for the following treatments?
   Match the treatment to the correct treatment timing:

   Eyebrow tint   20 mins
   Manicure   60 mins
   Facial   45 mins
   False individual flare lashes   10 mins

3. The reception area should always be:
   a. clean and tidy
   b. clean and noisy
   c. comfortable and messy
   d. dirty and quiet

4. Which important functions does the receptionist handle?
   a. booking appointments
   b. dealing with a variety of enquiries
   c. operating the payment point and handling payments
   d. all of the above

5. If a client disputed the change given as too little following payment what could you do?

6. Which of the following types of card is a debit card?
   a. gift voucher
   b. Switch/Maestro
   c. American Express card
   d. loyalty card

7. What are the important details to record when taking a message?

8. What is the legislation designed to protect the privacy of the client's details?

9. What may be the consequence of non-compliance with privacy legislation?

10. If you were presented with a fraudulent credit card what action should you take?

7 Facial Skincare

LEARNING OBJECTIVES

There are two learning outcomes for this technical unit which you must achieve competently:

1 Be able to prepare for facial skincare treatments.

2 Be able to provide facial skincare treatments.

From the range statement, you must show you can:

◆ Use consultation techniques to identify the client's treatment objectives.

◆ Use products, tools and equipment as appropriate.

◆ Treat all skin types and conditions.

◆ Ensure the environmental conditions are suitable.

◆ Complete a consultation and skin analysis to identify any contra-indications that may affect if and how the treatment can proceed.

◆ Communicate and behave in an appropriate and professional manner.

◆ Follow all health and safety working practices.

◆ Provide relevant aftercare and contra-action advice.

KEY TERMS

aftercare advice	facial products	skin analysis
antioxidant	health and safety	skin condition
antioxidants	masks	skin tone
cleanser	massage	skin types
comedone removal	massage manipulations	specialist skincare treatment
consultation	massage medium	products
contra-action advice	minor	tapotement
contra-actions	moisturizer	toning lotions
effleurage	molecules	treatment objectives
erythema	nutrition	treatment plan
exfoliants	oedema	vapour unit
exfoliation	paraffin-wax mask	vibrations
facial	petrissage	
false eyelashes	pH scale	

Unit Topic

Provide facial skincare

This VRQ unit is linked to the Beauty Therapy NOS Unit B4.

INTRODUCTION

This unit is all about improving and maintaining the health of your client's facial skin, reflected in its appearance. A facial includes the application of facial products, use of associated equipment and facial massage techniques personalized to suit your client's skin type, condition and treatment objectives.

Facials are commonly provided in businesses which offer make-up, beauty therapy and spa services. The objective of each however will slightly differ. A facial offered before make-up will ensure the skin will be in optimum condition showing the make-up at its best effect, with many make-up products serving to enhance the client's skin i.e. providing luminosity and minimizing imperfections such as skin pigmentation. A beauty therapy salon will offer a range of different facials to meet the conditions and possible skin disorders associated with: each skin type; the care the skin has previously received; the racial characteristics; gender and age related requirements. A spa facial will as well as aiming to improve skin condition will use techniques which induce a feeling of tranquility and calmness a theme of the spa environment. You must be able to show you have the necessary practical skills and underpinning knowledge to provide facial skincare.

Dealing with people in a polite, efficient manner and using good communication and questioning skills to find out exactly what they require from the facial forms an important part of this technical service.

INDUSTRY ROLE MODEL

DANIELLA NORMAN Education Operations Manager and Acting Education Department Manager Dermalogica UK and Ireland

" After working as a skin therapist for several years, I joined Dermalogica UK in 2000 as Manager for their flagship skin centre, Leonard Drake. I am passionate about the skincare industry and developing successful businesses, which led me to the Education Department at The International Dermal Institute® in 2005. I have delivered postgraduate training for Dermalogica therapists and also the highly regarded International Dermal Institute®

curriculum. Currently the Education Operations Manager, I am responsible for the overall operations of training centres located across the UK and Ireland and I'm thrilled to have the opportunity to cover maternity leave as the Acting Education Department Manager for UK and Ireland.

> Essential anatomy and physiology knowledge for this unit is identified on the checklist in CHAPTER 2, page 33

Caring for the skin internally and externally

If the skin is to function efficiently it must be cared for both internally and externally. Our lifestyle – the way we care about ourselves – affects the condition and appearance of our skin.

Healthy eating

Internally, a nutritionally balanced diet is vital to the health and appearance of the skin. A number of skin allergies and disorders are in part the result of poor **nutrition**, caused by a poorly balanced diet, including highly processed food, alcohol and a lack of essential nutrients.

Foods contain the chemical substances we need for health and growth, the nutrients: a healthy diet contains all the essential nutrients. The nutrients are carried to the skin in the blood, where they nourish the cells in the processes of growth and repair.

A balanced diet prevents malnutrition (undernourishment) and vitamin/mineral deficiencies. The food triangle diagram on page 199 illustrates the different food groups. The daily recommended amounts to be consumed are:

TOP TIP

Five a day rule

Eat at least the recommended five servings of fruit and fresh vegetables every day. These foods provide vital vitamins and minerals that keep the skin healthy. A serving is:

◆ 1 small glass of pure fruit juice
◆ 3 heaped tablespoons of fruit salad
◆ 4 heaped tablespoons of vegetables
◆ 1 medium fruit (an orange); 2 small fruits (plums)
◆ 1 dessert bowl of salad.

Food group	Recommended daily serving
Fats/oils	1 serving*
Fruit	2–4 servings
Milk and yoghurt	2–3 servings
Proteins	2–3 servings
Starch	6–11 servings
Sugar	1 serving*
Vegetables	3–5 servings
*use scarcely	

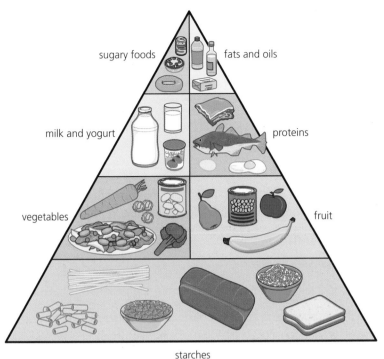

Chart for a balanced diet

Traffic light system food label

A traffic light system of food package labelling shows information on the nutritional content of foods to inform healthy food choices.

There are six principal groups of nutrients:

Carbohydrates

Carbohydrates provide energy quickly. They are either simple sugars or starches that the body can turn into simple sugars.

Food sources: Carbohydrates are found in fruit, vegetables, milk, grains, sugar and honey.

Fats

Fats provide a concentrated source of energy, and are also used in carrying certain vitamins (see below) around the body. Fat is stored in the body around organs and muscles and under the skin. However, if too much fat is deposited under the skin, the elastic fibres there may be damaged by the expansion of the adipose tissue. Fat is also used in the formation of sebum, the skin's natural lubricant.

Food sources: Although this is not always evident, fats are present in almost all foods, from plants and animals.

Proteins

Proteins provide material for the growth and repair of body tissue, and are also a source of energy. Severe protein deficiency in children gives the skin a yellowish appearance, known as jaundice.

Food sources: Proteins are found in meat, fish, eggs, dairy products, grains and nuts.

HEALTH & SAFETY

Vegan diets Proteins are composed of many smaller units called *amino acids*. Animal protein sources contain all the amino acids essential to health. A *vegetarian* consuming dairy food will likewise obtain all the essential amino acids. A *vegan*, however, must be careful to eat an adequate quantity and variety of vegetables and other foods, in order to be sure that they receive all the amino acids they need. Vegans must take vitamin B$_{12}$ as a vitamin supplement as this vitamin occurs naturally only in animal-derived foods.

HEALTH & SAFETY

Special diets Warn your clients about the danger of very low-fat, low-carbohydrate or low-protein diets: these can deprive the body of the nutrients it needs for growth, repair and energy.

Minerals

Minerals provide materials for growth and repair and for regulation of the body processes. The major minerals are calcium, iron, phosphorus, sulphur, sodium, potassium, chlorine and magnesium. Of these, the most important to the skin is iron. A pale, dry skin may indicate anaemia, caused by a shortage of iron.

Food sources: Fruit and vegetables; iron is found in liver, egg yolks and green vegetables.

Vitamins

Vitamins regulate the body's processes and contribute to its resistance to disease. Vitamins are divided into two groups, according to whether they are soluble in water or in fat:

◆ the fat-soluble vitamins are A, D, E and K

◆ the water-soluble vitamins are B and C.

The vitamins most important to the condition of the skin are vitamins A, B_2, B_3, C and E.

Vitamin A Essential for the growth and renewal of skin cells. Insufficient vitamin A in the diet leads to hyperkeratinization (production of too much keratin). This causes blockages in the skin tissue. The skin becomes rough and dry, and eye disorders such as styes may occur.

Food sources: Vitamin A is found in red, yellow and green vegetables, and in egg yolk, butter and cheese.

Vitamin B_2 Vitamin B_2 (also called riboflavin) helps to break down other foodstuffs, releasing energy needed by cells to desquamate and function efficiently. A deficiency of vitamin B_2 causes the skin at the corners of the mouth to crack.

Food sources: Vitamin B_2 is found in brewer's yeast, milk products, leafy vegetables, liver and whole grains.

Vitamin B_3 Vitamin B_3 (also called niacin) has the same function as vitamin B_2, but is also vital in the maintenance of the tissues of the skin.

Food sources: Vitamin B_3 is found in meat, brewer's yeast, nuts and seeds.

Vitamin C Vitamin C (also called ascorbic acid) maintains healthy skin and is important for the production of collagen, providing tone and elasticity. A lack of vitamin C causes the capillaries to become fragile, and haemorrhages of the skin, such as bruising, may occur. Severe deficiency results in scurvy.

Food sources: Vitamin C is found in fruit and vegetables.

Vitamin E Vitamin E is found in most foods. It is an **antioxidant** and helps prevent premature skin ageing. It helps to rehydrate the skin, calms inflammation, helps healing and maintains healthy skin.

Food sources: Vitamin E is found in most foods. The richest sources are vegetable oils, cereal products, eggs and meat.

Water

Water forms about two-thirds of the body's weight, and is an important component both inside and outside the body cells. Water is essential for the body's growth and maintenance. It helps remove waste from the body through urine and sweat and regulates temperature. Water must be regularly replaced through the diet. At least one-and-a-half litres of water should be drunk every day, to avoid dehydration of the body and the skin. Aim to drink 6–8 medium glasses daily.

Food sources: Water is also a constituent of many foods, including fruits and vegetables.

Fibre Fibre is not broken down into nutrients, but it is very important for effective digestion.

Food sources: Fibre is found in fruit, vegetables and cereals

Lifestyle threats to the skin

Internal

Alcohol Alcohol deprives the body of its vitamin reserves, especially vitamins B and C, which are necessary for a healthy skin. Alcohol also tends to dehydrate the body, including the skin. Skin conditions such as acne rosacea, eczema and psoriasis are often aggravated by the consumption of alcohol.

Caffeine Coffee, tea, cocoa and soft fizzy drinks contain a mild stimulant drug called caffeine. In moderate doses, such as two or three cups of coffee per day, caffeine is safe. If you drink too much, however, caffeine can cause nervousness, interfere with digestion, block the absorption of vitamins and minerals, dehydrate and spoil the appearance of the skin, stimulating skin ageing.

Drugs Drugs are chemical substances that affect the way our body performs. When they enter the body they are transported throughout the body in the blood. Recreational drugs are taken because they cause a particular effect or sensation which may feel good initially. Long term, they are harmful and addictive. Most affect blood pressure and heart rate. Stimulants, for example, can cause sweating, shaking and headaches. Heroin, in the class of painkillers called *narcotics*, ravages the skin, causing chronic dryness and premature ageing.

Smoking Smoking interferes with cell respiration and slows down the circulation. This makes it harder for nutrients and oxygen to reach the skin cells and for waste products to be eliminated. Cigarette smoking also releases a chemical that destroys vitamin C. This interferes with the production of collagen, and thereby contributes to premature wrinkling. Nicotine is a toxic substance – a poison!

Medication Certain medicines taken by mouth can cause skin dehydration, oedema – swelling of the tissues – (this may, for example, be caused by steroids) or irregular skin pigmentation (sometimes caused by the contraceptive pill). During the initial consultation with the client, find out whether they are taking any medication – and take this into account in your diagnosis and treatment plan.

Stress Stress is shown in the face as tension lines where the facial muscles are tight. Because blood and lymph cannot circulate properly, this causes a sluggish skin condition and poor facial nutrition. A person suffering from stress usually experiences disturbed sleep or sleeplessness (insomnia). Lack of sleep causes the skin to become dull and puffy, especially the tissue beneath the eyes, where dark circles also appear. Too *much*

HEALTH & SAFETY

Alcohol intake Alcohol intake is measured in units – one unit is one centilitre of pure alcohol and is equivalent to:

◆ 1 single measure of spirits

◆ 1/2 pint lager, beer or cider

◆ 1 small glass of wine.

A maximum of three units a day is recommended for men and a maximum of two units for women. It is increasingly recommended to have two alcohol-free days per week.

TOP TIP

Caffeine

Advise your clients to replace tea with herbal infusions and to drink decaffeinated coffee (in moderation) rather than regular coffee.

Caffeine is a diuretic, causing increased urination and loss of water leading to dehydration.

HEALTH & SAFETY

Smoking Smoking depletes the body of vital nutrients, preventing their absorption.

ACTIVITY

Causes of stress

1 Can you think of everyday situations that may trigger stress?

2 How do you react physically when put in a stressful situation?

3 How can you create a relaxing environment in the salon?

sleep can also cause the facial tissue to become puffy – because the circulation is less active, body fluids collect in the tissues.

If someone is suffering from stress, they may drink more tea, coffee or alcohol, or smoke more cigarettes: this too damages the skin.

Stress and anxiety are often the underlying cause of certain skin disorders. Some skin conditions, such as boils and styes, appear at times of stress; others, such as psoriasis and eczema, may become much worse. At the consultation, try to determine whether the client is suffering from stress: if they are, make sure that the salon treatments promote relaxation.

External

As well as looking after the skin from the *inside*, by diet, it needs care from the *outside* –it must be kept clean, and it must be nourished.

With normal physiological functioning, the skin becomes oily, and sweat is deposited on its surface. The skin's natural oil (sebum) can easily build up and block the natural openings, the hair follicles and pores: this may lead to infection. Facial cosmetics too affect the health of the skin; if not regularly removed, they may cause congestion. Skincare treatments help to maintain and improve the functioning of the skin.

Ultraviolet light Although recently ultraviolet (UV) has been identified as a hazard to skin, it also has some *positive* effects. One of these is its ability to stimulate the production of vitamin D, which is absorbed into the bloodstream and nourishes and helps to maintain bone tissue. UV light also activates the pigment melanin in the skin, and thereby creates a tan. Many people feel better when they have a tan, as it gives a healthy appearance.

UV light is divided into different bands. The most important to skin tanning are UVA and UVB. UVA stimulates the melanin in the skin to produce a rapid tan, which does not last very long. UVA penetrates deep into the dermis where it can cause premature ageing of the skin. Free radicals – highly reactive **molecules** which cause skin cells to degenerate – are also formed. These molecules disrupt production of collagen and elastin, the fibres that give skin its strength and elasticity. Reduced elasticity leads to wrinkling.

UVB stimulates the production of vitamin D. Melanin activation by UVB produces a longer-lasting tan than that produced by UVA. UVB is partially absorbed by the atmosphere – it has a shorter wavelength than UVA – and only 10 per cent reaches the dermis. UVB causes thickening of the stratum corneum layer, which reflects UV away from the skin's surface. UVB causes sunburn: the skin becomes red as the cells are damaged, and the skin may blister. UVB is also implicated in skin cancers, especially malignant melanoma.

The relaxing, warming effect of the sun is caused by the infrared (IR) light. This penetrates the skin to the subcutaneous layer and is thought to speed skin ageing and possibly to cause a cancer called squamous cell carcinoma. The tan is actually a sign of skin damage, therefore, and both UV and IR probably contribute to photo-ageing – the premature ageing of the skin by light.

Although black skin has a high melanin content, which absorbs more UV and allows less to reach the dermis, it is not fully protected against UV and still requires additional protection.

Chemical skin protection, or sunscreens, are designed to absorb UV light (UVA and UVB), reducing the rate of skin ageing in all skin types. Various sunscreens are available, classified by number according to their sun-protection factor (SPF). This is the amount of protection that the sunscreen gives you from the sun. A SPF of at least 15 is recommended in winter and 30 in summer. The application of the sunscreen extends your natural skin protection, allowing you to stay in the sun for longer without burning. For example, if normally you can be in the sun for 10 minutes before the skin begins to go red, a sunscreen with an SPF of 10 will allow you 10 × 10 minutes (i.e. 100 minutes) safe exposure in the sun. Always check the expiry date of sunscreens, they only have a shelf life of 2–3 years.

Artificial UV light produced by sunbeds, used for cosmetic skin tanning, also causes premature ageing. Most sunbeds use concentrated UVA, which causes dermal tissue damage resulting in lines and wrinkles.

It may take years to see the effects of the dermal damage caused by unprotected UV exposure, but once they have occurred the effects are irreversible. UVA rays are present all year round, so to prevent premature ageing, cosmetic preparations containing sunscreens should be worn at all times.

TOP TIP

Hyperpigmentation

Hyperpigmentation marks caused by repeated exposure to UV light eventually remain, even without the exposure to UV. Some clients dislike such marks, and you could advise them on camouflage make-up and daily application of a sunblock skincare product.

HEALTH & SAFETY

Sunbathing Never wear perfume, cosmetic products or deodorants when sunbathing, either in natural sunlight or in artificially produced (sun-canopy) UV. The chemicals in these products can sensitize the skin, causing an allergic skin reaction.

UV can penetrate water to a depth of 1 metre, so even when swimming you need to wear a sunscreen. Special waterproof products are designed for this purpose.

TOP TIP

Fake tanning preparation

To acquire a tan without the damaging effects of the sun or sun-beds, your client can use a *fake tanning* preparation. This treatment is becoming popular in the beauty therapist's salon.

Climate Sebum, the skin's natural grease, provides an oily protective film over the surface of the skin that reduces evaporation. Despite this, unprotected exposure of the skin to the environment allows evaporation from the epidermis which results in a dry, dehydrated skin condition.

The climate has several effects on the skin:

◆ *Sebum production* When the skin is exposed to the cold, less sebum is produced. The skin has reduced protection, allowing moisture to evaporate.

◆ *Perspiration* In very hot weather more moisture is lost as perspiration: perspiration increases to cool the skin and regulate the body's temperature.

◆ *Humidity* Moisture loss from the skin is also affected by the humidity (water content) of the surrounding air. In hot, dry weather humidity will be low, so water loss will be high. In temperate, damp conditions humidity will be high, so water loss will be low.

◆ *Extremes of temperature* Alternating heat and cold often leads to the formation of broken capillaries. These appear as fine red lines on white skin, and as discoloration on black skin.

◆ *Stratum corneum* The cells of the stratum corneum multiply with repeated unprotected exposure to the climate, as the body's natural defence.

The damaging effects caused by the climate can be reduced by using protective skincare preparations such as moisturizers. These spread a layer of oil over the skin's surface, reducing evaporation.

HEALTH & SAFETY

Ashiness A black skin can sometimes appear ashen, with patches of skin becoming grey and flaky. This is caused by sudden changes in temperature combined with low humidity, which can cause the skin to lose moisture. Moisturizers help in alleviating this problem.

ALWAYS REMEMBER

Client's occupation

At the consultation, ask the client their occupation: this will guide you as to their likely skincare requirements. The client who works outdoors, for example, will have different treatment needs from the one who works indoors.

ACTIVITY

Geographical variations

Consider the effects of climate on the skin. Name four different geographical locations, research and state the humidity level and climate you would expect at each location.

Think of the probable effects on the skin. What treatments by a beauty therapist might be needed in each country?

TOP TIP

Dry skin in winter

Central heating creates an environment with humidity similar to that of the desert. Unless you use a moisturizer, the loss of moisture from the skin will cause a dry, dehydrated skin condition.

HEALTH & SAFETY

Effects of water loss   Water loss can sometimes be sufficient to disrupt living cells in the skin to the extent that some actually die. This results in skin irritation and reddening.

ACTIVITY

Environmental factors

It is important that you are aware of all the factors that can affect the health of a client's skin: this knowledge allows you to assess each client's treatment needs. Summarize the different factors you have learnt about.

Environmental stress and pollution   Further causes of moisture loss include harsh alkaline chemicals such as detergents and soaps – which remove sebum from the skin's surface – air conditioning and central heating.

Environmental pollutants such as lead, mercury, cadmium and aluminium can accumulate in the body. One result is the formation of dangerous chemicals that attack proteins in the cells. Such pollutants find their way into food through polluted waters, rain and dust. To protect the body, always wash vegetables thoroughly, and eat a diet rich in vitamins C and E.

Air pollution, involving carbon from smoke, chemical discharges from factories and fumes from car exhausts, should be removed from the skin by effective cleansing. Absorption of these pollutants is reduced by the application of **moisturizer**: this forms a barrier over the skin's surface.

Skincare treatments

The beauty therapist has the professional expertise to help each client improve the appearance and condition of their skin by the application of appropriate skincare treatments and products. The facial skin treatments you may offer include:

◆ consultation and skin analysis

◆ skin cleansing

◆ exfoliation

◆ manual **massage** of the face, neck and shoulders

◆ the application of face **masks**.

The beauty therapist cannot change the underlying skin type, which is genetically determined, but they can keep the physiological characteristics of each skin type in check.

Skin types

The basic structure of the skin does not vary from person to person, but the physiological functioning of its different features does; it is this that gives us **skin types**, recognized by specific visible characteristics and conditions.

The first and most important part of a **facial** treatment is the correct diagnosis of the skin type. This is carried out at the beginning of each facial treatment. The beauty therapist must choose the correct skincare products and facial treatment plan for the client's skin type. This assessment is called a **skin analysis**.

Basic types

There are four main skin types:

◆ normal

◆ dry

◆ oily

◆ combination.

Normal skin Normal skin is often referred to as balanced, the water and oil content is constant, it is neither too oily nor too dry. When young, this skin type seldom has any problems, such as blemishes, and is often neglected. Neglect causes the skin to become dry, especially around the eyes, cheeks and neck, where the skin is thinner.

Normal skin

HEALTH & SAFETY

Air pollution There are many components to air pollution. Car exhaust fumes, for example, release nitrogen oxide and volatile organic compounds. These react with sunlight to form ozone, a highly reactive form of oxygen. This can penetrate deep inside the skin and damage the cells' DNA (their main component), which can lead to skin cancer. Also, accelerated skin ageing is caused by free radical damage caused by unstable molecules, which affect the skin's elasticity. Moisturizers containing antioxidants are essential and should be recommended to neutralize free radicals or repel them from the skin before skin damage is caused.

A normal skin type in adults is very rare. It has these characteristics:

◆ the pore size is small or medium

◆ the moisture content is good

◆ the skin texture is smooth and even, neither too thick nor too thin

◆ the colour is healthy (because of good blood circulation)

◆ the skin elasticity is good, when young

◆ the skin feels firm to the touch

◆ the skin pigmentation is even-coloured

◆ the skin is usually free from blemishes.

Dry skin Dry skin is lacking in either sebum or moisture, or both. Because sebum limits moisture loss by evaporation from the skin, skin with insufficient sebum rapidly loses moisture. The resulting dry skin is often described as dehydrated.

Dry skin has these characteristics:

◆ the pores are small and tight

◆ the moisture content is poor

◆ the skin texture is coarse and thin, with patches of visibly flaking skin

◆ there is a tendency towards sensitivity (broken capillaries often accompany this skin type)

◆ premature ageing is common, resulting in the appearance of fine lines leading to deeper wrinkles, seen especially around the eyes, mouth and neck

◆ skin pigmentation may be uneven, and disorders such as ephelides (freckles) usually accompany this skin type

◆ milia are often found around the cheek and eye area.

ACTIVITY

Recognizing skin types and conditions

Refer to the illustration below. What skin characteristic conditions would you expect to see in each of the numbered areas if performing a skin analysis on a:

◆ dry skin type
◆ oily skin type
◆ combination skin type

Dry skin

Oily skin

ANATOMY & PHYSIOLOGY
See The skin section on page 34

Oily skin In oily skin the sebaceous glands become very active at puberty, when stimulated by the male hormone androgen. An increase in sebum production often causes the appearance of skin blemishes. Sebaceous gland activity begins to decrease when the person is in their twenties.

Oily skin has these characteristics:

◆ the pores are enlarged

◆ the moisture content is high

◆ the skin is coarse and thick

◆ the skin is sallow in colour, as a result of the excess sebum production, dead skin cells become embedded in the sebum, and the skin has sluggish blood and lymph circulation

◆ the **skin tone** is good, due to the protective effect of the sebum

◆ the skin is prone to shininess, due to excess sebum production

◆ there may be uneven pigmentation

◆ certain skin disorders may be apparent – comedones, pustules, papules, milia or sebaceous cysts.

Acne vulgaris and seborrhoea are skin disorders that occur when the skin becomes excessively oily due to the influence of hormones. Treatment of these skin disorders should be carried out to control and reduce sebum flow.

Combination skin Combination skin is partly oily and partly dry. The oily parts are generally the chin, nose and forehead, known as the T-zone. The upper cheeks may show signs of oiliness, but the rest of the face and neck area is usually dry.

Combination skin is the most common skin type. It has these characteristics:

◆ the pores in the T-zone are enlarged, while in the cheek area they are small to medium

◆ the moisture content is high in the oily areas, but poor in the dry areas

◆ the skin is coarse and thick in the oily areas, but thin in the dry areas

◆ the skin is sallow in the oily areas, but shows sensitivity and high colour in the dry areas

◆ the skin tone is good in the oily areas, but poor in the dry areas

◆ there is uneven pigmentation, usually seen as ephelides and lentigines

◆ there may be blemishes such as pustules and comedones on the oily skin at the T-zone

◆ milia and broken capillaries may appear in the dry areas, commonly on the cheeks and near the eyes.

Additional skin conditions

While looking closely at the skin, further **skin conditions** may become obvious. The skin may be:

◆ sensitive

Combination skin

TOP TIP

Skin irritation

In black skin, instead of the redness shown by Caucasian skin, irritation shows up as a darker patch.

◆ dehydrated

◆ moist

◆ oedematous (puffy).

Sensitive skin

Sensitive skin Sensitive skin usually accompanies a dry skin type, but not always. The characteristics of sensitive skin are these:

◆ the skin may show high colouring as it is easily irritated

◆ there are usually broken capillaries in the cheek area

◆ the skin feels warm to the touch

◆ there is superficial flaking of the skin

◆ the skin may show high colouring and tightness after skin cleansing, if it is sensitive to pressure.

Allergic skin Allergic skin is irritated by external allergens, including chemicals in some cosmetics. The allergens inflame the skin and may damage its protective function. At the consultation, always try to discover whether the client has any allergies, and if so, to what.

The allergies of most concern to the beauty therapist are those caused by substances applied to the skin. The beauty therapist must be aware of such substances and avoid their use. Contact with an allergen, especially if repeated, may cause skin disorders such as eczema or dermatitis (see page 61, where skin diseases and disorders are dealt with in more detail).

> **TOP TIP**
>
> **Dehydrated skin**
>
> Encourage clients, especially those with dehydrated skin, to drink six to eight glasses of water a day to replenish the moisture in the body cells.

Dehydrated skin Dehydrated skin is skin that has lost water from the skin tissues. The condition can affect any skin type, but most commonly accompanies dry or combination skin types. The problem may be related to the client's general health. If they have recently been ill with a fever, for example, the skin will have lost fluid through sweating. If they are taking medication, this too may cause dehydration, as may drastic dieting. In many cases the dehydration is caused by working in an environment with a low humidity, or in one that is air-conditioned. You must try to discover the cause, and provide both corrective treatment and advice.

Dehydrated skin

The characteristics of dehydrated skin are as follows:

◆ the skin has a fine orange-peel effect, caused by its lack of moisture

◆ there is superficial flaking

◆ fine, superficial lines are evident on the skin

◆ broken capillaries are common.

Moist skin Moist skin appears moist and feels damp: this is due to the over-secretion of sweat. The beauty therapist cannot correct this skin condition, which is often caused by some internal physiological disturbance such as a hormonal or metabolic imbalance.

Advise the client to use lightweight cleansing preparations. The client should avoid skin-toning preparations with a high alcohol content; these would stimulate the skin, causing yet further perspiration and skin sensitivity. They should avoid highly spiced food, and be aware that alcoholic or hot drinks will cause dilation of the skin capillaries, thereby increasing the skin's temperature.

Puffy skin

Male facial

Oedematous (puffy) skin Oedematous skin is, and appears, swollen and puffy: this is because the tissues are retaining excess water. The condition may be caused by a medical disorder, or may be a side-effect of medication. Hot weather can cause temporary swelling of the tissues, as can local injury to the tissues. Poor blood circulation and lymphatic flow may cause puffy skin, too; this is often seen around the eyes. In this case the condition may benefit from gentle massage around the eye area. Tissue-fluid retention in the facial skin may be caused by an incorrect diet, such as one that includes too much salt or the drinking of too much alcohol, tea or coffee and insufficient water.

Unless you are quite sure about the cause of the oedema, always seek permission from your client's doctor before treating the skin.

The sex of the client

Men have a more acidic skin surface than females and the stratum corneum is thicker on males than females. However, males have coarse facial hair and shaving daily removes cells of the stratum corneum before they are ready to desquamate naturally. This can sensitize and dry the skin, especially if aftershave lotions with a high alcohol content are directly applied. A moisturizer should be applied to protect the skin.

The collagen content of the skin is different in men and women. Collagen and sebum production falls in menopausal women causing skin ageing. Skin does not appear to age as quickly in males as females because collagen, elastin and sebum production remain constant. The skin of males typically feels firmer.

The main reason males choose to have a facial is for relaxation, to improve the appearance of the skin, and increasingly for the anti-ageing benefits.

The age of the skin

Having identified the skin type, the beauty therapist must classify the age of the skin. Age of skin can vary between people of different race because of evolution which may delay the visible signs of ageing due to differences in sebaceous gland and melanin activity in skin.

Often the appearance of the skin in relation to age will relate to skin conditions that are evident. A young client, for example, may have skin blemishes such as comedones, pustules and papules. These disorders are caused by overactivity of the sebaceous gland at puberty, when the body is developing its secondary sexual characteristics. It is at this time that the skin condition acne vulgaris is most likely to occur, due to the hormonal imbalance. The skin of clients aged over 25 years, however, is generally termed mature skin.

The beauty therapist should also consider the client's skin tone and muscle tone in relation to their age. A young skin will probably have good skin tone, and the skin will be supple and elastic. This is because the protein, collagen and elastin fibres in the skin are strong. Poor skin tone, on the other hand, is recognized by the appearance of facial lines and wrinkles.

A healthy young skin will also have good muscle tone, and the facial contours will appear firm. With poor muscle tone, the muscles becomes slack and loose, with the contours of the face less defined.

Poor lifestyle choices and general health will also affect how quickly our skin shows visible signs of ageing.

Mature skin

Mature skin has the following characteristics:

◆ the skin becomes dry, as the sebaceous and sudoriferous glands become less active

◆ the skin loses its elasticity as the elastin fibres harden, and wrinkles appear due to the cross-linking and hardening of collagen fibres

◆ the epidermis grows more slowly and the skin appears thinner, becoming almost transparent in some areas such as around the eyes, where small veins and capillaries show through the skin

◆ broken capillaries appear, especially on the cheek area and around the nose

◆ the facial contours become slack as muscle tone is reduced

◆ the underlying bone structure becomes more obvious, as the fatty layer and the supportive tissue beneath the skin grow thinner

◆ blood circulation becomes poor, which interferes with skin nutrition, and the skin may appear sallow

◆ due to the decrease in metabolic rate, waste products are not removed so quickly, and this leads to puffiness of the skin

◆ patches of irregular pigmentation appear on the surface of the skin, such as lentigines and chloasmata.

The skin may also exhibit the following skin conditions, although these are not truly *characteristic* of an ageing skin:

◆ dermal naevi may be enlarged

◆ seborrhoeic warts may appear on the epidermal layer of the skin

◆ verruca filliformis warts may increase in number

◆ hair growth on the upper lip or chin, or both, may become darker or coarser, due to hormonal imbalance in the body

◆ dark circles and puffiness may occur under the eyes.

ALWAYS REMEMBER

Assessing skin tone

To test skin tone, gently lift the skin at the cheeks between two fingers and then let go. If the skin tone is good, the skin will spring back to its original shape.

TOP TIP

Mature skin

The change in appearance of women's skin during ageing is closely related to the altered production of the hormones oestrogen, progesterone and androgen at the menopause.

Mature skin

ACTIVITY

The ageing process

Collect images showing men and women of different cultures and at various ages.

1 Can you identify the visible characteristics that indicate a person's age?
2 Does ageing occur at the same rate in men and women and in different cultures?
3 Discuss your findings with your colleagues and tutor.

Knowledge Check

How do you identify a client's skin type?

Refer to page 204 to help you.

Differences in skin

Although there is no difference between skin functions such as sweat and sebaceous gland activity in white and black skin, the amount of pigment, called *melanin*, varies, resulting in different skin and hair colour.

There are two forms of the melanin pigment: *eumelanin*, produced in black and brown skin colours, and *phaeomelanin*, found in lighter skins. Both forms of pigment can be present together but the amount of each can vary.

People who originate from hot countries and are nearer the equator have more melanin and a darker skin pigment. This is because the UV is very intense and the skin requires more protection. Those who originate from cooler countries have less melanin and a lighter skin pigment. The pigmentation of the skin is the result of millions of years of evolution.

African-Caribbean skin

African-Caribbean The skin colour ranges in tone to almost black. This is because it has more melanin, which absorbs UV light. As black skin is exposed to UV light it becomes darker and darker.

Care must be taken when dealing with blemishes on darker skins as scars may occur as the skin heals. The scars may become keloids, scarring that becomes enlarged and projects above the skin's surface. Even minor scratches may result in keloid formation.

Hyperpigmentation (uneven patches of skin tone which are darker than the surrounding skin) may also occur with exposure to UV light. It is more common in darker skinned people due to increased melanin. Hyperpigmentation most commonly occurs following skin inflammation, such as acne vulgaris. Keloids may become hyperpigmented if exposed to the sun in the early stages of their formation.

TOP TIP

Skin appearance

As the surface of the skin reflects light and shows the skin colour, the beauty therapist's aim is for the skin surface to be smooth and healthy. This is achieved by the removal of dead skin cells and ensuring it is adequately moisturized.

Asian skin

Vitiligo (a type of hypopigmentation or loss of skin pigment) is a considerable problem when it occurs in dark skin, as it is very obvious. Cosmetics may be applied as a corrective technique.

Male African-Caribbean clients may have a tendency towards *pseudo folliculitis*, an inflammatory skin disorder. This occurs as the hair is coarse and curly and has a tendency as it grows out of the skin to curl back and re-enter it, becoming ingrown. This foreign object in the skin becomes irritated and inflamed. Hyperpigmentation may also accompany this condition.

Dermatosis papulosis nigra, also called flesh moles, can occur. These are brown or black hyperpigmented markings, resembling moles, usually seen on the cheeks. Their cause is unknown but they are sometimes found to be hereditary. They also occur more frequently in women than men.

Hair colour is dark brown to black.

Asian The skin colour has a light to dark tone due to increased melanin, with yellow undertones. There is a tendency towards hyperpigmentation, appearing as dark patches of skin, and scarring can appear following skin inflammation. Dermatosis papulosis nigra can occur. In women there is a normal tendency towards superfluous facial hair.

White skin

Hair colour is dark brown to black.

White The skin colour is pink. This skin has less melanin and so less defence in the presence of UV light; sun damage results in skin burning and premature ageing. Caucasian skin has a tendency to show freckles (ephelides), as a result of uneven melanin distribution in the skin.

Hair colour is usually fair, red or brown.

Oriental The skin colour has more melanin present and has a yellowish tone. Oriental skin is usually oily and prone to hyperpigmentation. Blemishes should be treated with caution as hyperpigmentation and scarring could result due to increased levels of melanin. Female skin generally appears smooth and has little facial hair.

Oriental skin

Hair colour is usually mid-brown to black.

HEALTH & SAFETY

Habia Health and Safety *Hygiene for Hairdressers and Beauty Therapists* booklet is available as a download from www.habia.org providing practical advice on how to avoid infection in the workplace.

ACTIVITY

Which countries do people with the skin types listed below originate from:

◆ Caucasian

◆ Oriental

◆ Asian

◆ African-Caribbean?

Outcome 1: Be able to prepare for facial skincare treatments

Learn how to prepare for facial skincare treatments

PRACTICAL SKILLS

Prepare yourself, client and work area for facial skincare treatment

Use suitable consultation techniques to identify treatment objectives

Carry out a skin analysis

Provide clear recommendations to the client

Select products, tools and equipment to suit client treatment needs, skin types and conditions

UNDERPINNING KNOWLEDGE

Describe salon requirements for preparing yourself, the client and work areas

State the environmental conditions suitable for facial skincare treatments

Describe different consultation techniques used to identify treatment objectives

State the importance of carrying out a detailed skin analysis

Describe how to select products, tools and equipment to suit client treatment needs, skin types and conditions

Identify skin types, conditions and characteristics

Describe the contra-indications which prevent or restrict facial treatments

Chapter 3 **Health and Safety** covers general legal hygiene and safety working practice which you legally have to carry out. You will learn about further specific health and safety.

Remember to always:

◆ give due consideration to general health and safety legislation throughout the treatment

◆ implement hygiene, health and safety requirements as identified in the facial unit practical skills and underpinning knowledge

◆ follow industry hygiene, health and safety working practices throughout the treatment application. Refer to the Habia website to keep up to date with current health and safety practice

◆ dispose of any waste materials safely and correctly.

Preparing the work area

Consideration should be given to the positioning of equipment for ease and safety of use.

Each facial work area should have the following basic equipment: a treatment couch or beauty chair. The couch or chair should be covered with easy-to-clean upholstery; it must withstand daily cleaning with hot water and detergent. It must have an adjustable back rest, for the comfort of both the client and the beauty therapist. If possible, purchase a couch that also has an adjustable leg rest, as this allows treatments such as pedicures to be carried out.

Hydraulic couches are useful as they can be adjusted in height to enable the client to position themself on the couch with ease.

◆ **Equipment trolley** The equipment trolley should be large enough to accommodate all the necessary equipment and products; trolleys are usually of a two- or three-shelf design. Like the chair or couch, the trolley should be made of a material that will withstand regular cleaning. Some models have restraining bars to prevent objects sliding off the trolley. Drawers are useful for storing tools and small consumables. The trolley should have securely fixed easy-glide castors. Some salons may use a large surface work area to display and store equipment and products.

◆ **Beauty stool** The stool should be covered in a fabric similar to that covering the treatment couch. It may or may not have a back rest; in some designs the back rest is removable. For the comfort of the beauty therapist, it should be adjustable in height; to allow mobility, it should be mounted on castors.

◆ **Step-up stool** To assist clients as necessary to position themselves on the couch, have available a step-up stool.

◆ **Magnifying lamp** The magnifying lamp is available in three models: floor-standing, wall-mounted and trolley-mounted.

Treatment couch

Hydraulic treatment couch

Magnifying lamp

A prepared and organized work area

Beauty stools

Step-up stool

◆ **Covered waste bin** A covered waste bin should be placed unobtrusively within easy reach. It should be lined with a disposable bin liner. You should also have a 'sharps' box for the disposal of contaminated equipment.

Arrangements for the collection and disposal of contaminated waste should be made with your local environmental health office.

The following equipment guidelines describe the basic products, tools and equipment for all facial treatments. Further products, tools and equipment relevant to specific facial treatments are discussed later in the chapter.

Products, tools and equipment

◆ **Headband** A clean headband should be provided for each client. Use either a material or disposable headband. Disposables are useful as they can be discarded after the treatment

◆ **Skin-cleansing preparations** The trolley should carry a display of facial skin-cleansing preparations to suit all skin types

◆ **Cotton wool** There should be a plentiful supply of both damp and dry cotton wool, sufficient for the treatment to be carried out. Dry cotton wool should be stored in a covered container; damp cotton wool is usually placed in a clean bowl

◆ **Tissues** Facial tissues should be large and of a high quality. They should be stored in a covered container

◆ **Waste bin** A covered container for waste may be placed on the bottom shelf of the trolley or it can be put into the waste bin at once

◆ **Spatulas** Several clean spatulas (preferably disposable) should be provided for each client. One should be used for tucking any stray hair beneath the headband. Others will be used in removing products from their containers

YOU WILL ALSO NEED:

◆ **Towel drapes** There should be a large towel to cover the client's body, and a small hand towel to drape across the client's chest and shoulders

◆ **Trolley** The surface of each shelf can be protected with a sheet of 500 mm disposable bedroll

◆ **Bowls** To store damp and dry cotton wool

◆ **Steamer** Use to warm the skin for cleansing and skin stimulation, e.g. facial steamer (vapour unit)

◆ **Towel** A clean towel should be placed on the trolley for the beauty therapist to wipe their hands on as necessary

◆ **Gown** A clean gown should be provided for each client as necessary

◆ **Facial sponges, facial mitts or towels** Used to remove facial products from the skin during treatment. They are particularly useful when working on a male client where cotton wool would collect on coarse facial hair

◆ **Mirror** A clean hand mirror should be available for use in consulting with the client before during and after their treatment

◆ **Container for jewellery** A container may be provided in which the client can place their jewellery if they need to remove it prior to treatment – follow your salon procedures in respect of client possessions

On arrival

When the client arrives for the treatment, generally the record card is completed. Record the client's personal details, such as their name and address. Check that there are no contra-indications to facial treatment.

If a client is a **minor**, under the age of 16 years of age, it is necessary to obtain signed written consent before treatment is carried out. It is also necessary that the parent or guardian is present when the treatment is given.

The beauty therapist will add further information to the record card at the consultation and on-going during the treatment.

Clients should not be kept waiting on arrival for their appointment. It is important that the work area is ready to proceed. The work area should always be maintained in a condition suitable for further treatments.

Reception

When a new client telephones to make an appointment for a treatment, always allocate extra time for the consultation beforehand. Explain to the client how long they should allow for the appointment. For example, if a client is seeking a basic skin cleansing and mask treatment, allow 30 minutes; if they are a new client allow 45 minutes so that there is time for the consultation and filling in the record card. If it is necessary to remove facial blockages and to carry out other specialized treatments, allow 45 minutes to 1 hour. For a full facial treatment, allow 1 hour.

Depending on the facial treatment to be carried out, the client may need to remove some clothing. Offer them a gown to wear for modesty. Privacy must be maintained at all times.

Before carrying out *any* facial treatments, the beauty therapist must consult with the client to determine their treatment needs. Consultation is a service that should be offered separately: there should be no pressure on the client to book a treatment following the consultation. Excellent communication skills should be used at consultation to ensure your judgements on the needs of the client are correct.

> " Customers can be more motivated by how you communicate, not necessarily what you are saying. Speak with passion and authenticity. Know your product and have a thorough understanding of how the skin works. Only then can you be credible and give prescriptive treatments and home care that deliver results.
>
> *Danielle Norman*

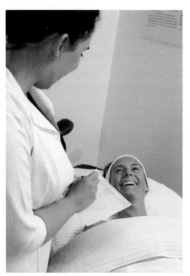

Confirming details following the consultation

The consultation

Carry out the consultation in the privacy of the facial treatment work area. This takes place when the client first meets the beauty therapist and again whenever a new treatment is to be carried out.

The consultation is the time when the beauty therapist can assess whether the client is actually suited to treatment. The beauty therapist must look for contra-indications, and must give no treatment if there are any – this is to safeguard the beauty therapist, the client and, in the case of a client with a contagious skin disorder, other clients who would be at risk of cross-infection. Remember, you are not qualified to diagnose a

ALWAYS REMEMBER

Treatment modification

Always modify your treatment to meet your clients needs. Examples of facial treatment modification include:

◆ altering the pressure or choice of manipulations during massage to suit the client's skin and muscle tone
◆ altering the distance and application of steam heat to take into account skin sensitivity. The more sensitive the skin the greater the distance from the skin.

ALWAYS REMEMBER

Never make assumptions about what the client can afford. Usually the client will indicate to you what they are prepared to spend.

ACTIVITY

Recognizing contra-indications

Think of six skin disorders and six skin diseases. List them in a chart.

Briefly describe how you would recognize each skin condition. Why would it be inappropriate to treat each?

contra-indication. Refer the client to their GP without causing unnecessary cause for concern.

Ask the client specific questions about their present skincare routine and their general health and lifestyle. Listen carefully to their responses to guide you in your assessment.

The beauty therapist's knowledge of facial treatments and advice on skincare will instil confidence in the client. Explain what is involved with the treatment, how long it takes and the aftercare that is recommended. This will demonstrate your professional knowledge and expertise.

The client is likely to ask which is the most suitable product for them, and you must advise them as to which would best meet their needs.

Make the client aware of the cost of the individual treatment – or treatment programme, if necessary – so that they can decide whether or not to undertake the financial commitment involved.

Invite the client to ask questions during the consultation. Visual aids may be used to explain aspects of the treatment. You could demonstrate some of the products, e.g. an exfoliation product, directly on your own skin or theirs, usually the back of the hand. Marketing literature may also be available to refer to. By the end of the consultation, they should understand fully what the proposed treatment involves.

The client may receive the treatment immediately, following the consultation, or go away to consider the proposals.

During the consultation, details are noted on the client's record card. You can fill this in as you speak to them, without diverting your attention away from them.

Contra-indications

The consultation and skin analysis will draw your attention to any contra-indications or conditions that may require special care and attention.

Remember that not all contra-indications are visible. Refer to the checklist of contra-indications on the client's record card.

The following contra-indications are relevant to *all* facial treatments:

◆ **skin disorder**, such as active acne vulgaris (unless medical approval has been sought and given)

◆ **skin disease**, such as impetigo

◆ **bruising** in the area

◆ **haemorrhage**, if recent – wait until the condition has healed

◆ **operation** in the area, if recent – wait for 6 months

◆ **fracture**, if recent – wait for 6 months

◆ **furuncle** (boil)

◆ **inflammation or swelling** of the skin

◆ **scar tissue,** if recent – wait for 6 months

◆ **sebaceous cyst**

◆ **eye disorder**, such as conjunctivitis.

Further information on specific skin diseases and disorders can be found on **CHAPTER 2** pages 47–63.

HEALTH & SAFETY

Herpes simplex (cold sore)
A small skin lesion due to herpes simplex may initially appear to be simply a pustule with a scab. At the consultation, always check whether the client knows if they suffer from any skin disease or disorder.

Herpes simplex

ANATOMY & PHYSIOLOGY
See Skin diseases and disorders
page 47

A sample client record card

Date	Beauty therapist	
Client name		Date of birth (identifying client age group)
Home address		Postcode
Email address	Landline	Mobile phone number
Name of doctor	Doctor's address and phone number	
Related medical history (conditions that may restrict or prohibit treatment application)		
Are you taking any medication? (This may affect the appearance of the skin or skin sensitivity.)		

CONTRA-INDICATIONS REQUIRING MEDICAL REFERRAL (preventing facial treatment application)

☐ bacterial infection (e.g. impetigo)
☐ viral infection (e.g. herpes simplex)
☐ fungal infection (e.g. tinea corporis)
☐ parasitic infection (e.g. pediculosis and scabies)
☐ eye infections (e.g. conjunctivitis)
☐ severe eczema
☐ systemic medical condition
☐ severe skin condition
☐ during chemotherapy or radiotherapy treatment

CONTRA-INDICATIONS WHICH RESTRICT TREATMENT (treatment may require adaptation)

☐ cuts and abrasions
☐ recent scar tissue
☐ skin allergies
☐ styes
☐ bruising and swelling
☐ vitiligo
☐ hyperkeratosis
☐ diabetes
☐ undiagnosed lumps, bumps and swellings
☐ high or low blood pressure
☐ skin disorders
☐ epilepsy
☐ broken bones

SKIN TYPE

☐ oily   ☐ normal
☐ combination   ☐ dry

SKIN CONDITION

☐ sensitive   ☐ mature   ☐ dehydrated

FACIAL PRODUCTS

☐ cleanser
☐ toner
☐ eye cleanser
☐ exfoliant
☐ mask – setting
☐ mask – non-setting
☐ massage medium
☐ moisturizer
☐ specialist skin products (e.g. eye cream/gel)

MASSAGE MEDIUMS

☐ oil   ☐ cream

SKIN CONDITION CHARACTERISTICS

☐ broken capillaries
☐ pustules
☐ open pores
☐ hypopigmentation
☐ keloids
☐ pseudo folliculitis
☐ milia
☐ comedones
☐ papules
☐ hyperpigmentation
☐ dermatitis papulosa nigra
☐ ingrowing hairs
☐ hyperkeratosis

Following skin analysis, identify on the illustration below skin condition characteristics found and in which numbered area they appear.

EQUIPMENT AND MATERIALS

☐ magnifying light
☐ consumables
☐ skin warming devices
☐ facial steamer

MASSAGE TECHNIQUES

☐ effleurage   ☐ petrissage   ☐ vibrations
☐ tapotement   ☐ frictions

Beauty therapist signature (for reference)
Client signature (confirmation of details)

A sample client record card (continued)

TREATMENT ADVICE
Full facial treatment – this treatment will take 60 minutes (1 hour).

TREATMENT PLAN
Record relevant details of your treatment and advice provided for future reference. Ensure the client's records are up-to-date, accurate and fully completed following treatment. Non-compliance may invalidate insurance.

DURING
Find out:

◆ what products the client is currently using to cleanse and care for the skin of the face and neck

◆ how regularly the products are used

◆ satisfaction with their current skincare routine – what they are pleased with and what they don't like.

Explain:

◆ how the products used should be applied and removed by the client.

Note:

◆ any adverse (unwanted) skin reaction, if any occurs.

AFTER
Record:

◆ specific areas treated

◆ any modification to treatment application that was required, e.g. less pressure applied over the cheek area when working on a sensitive skin with broken capillaries in the area

◆ what products have been used in the facial treatment

◆ the effectiveness of treatment – did you achieve what you set out to do?

◆ any samples provided (review their success at the next appointment).

Advise on:

◆ product application and removal in order to gain maximum benefit from product use

◆ where applicable, use of make-up following facial treatment

◆ recommended time intervals between treatments

◆ the importance of a course of treatment to improve the specific skin conditions.

RETAIL OPPORTUNITIES
Advise on:

◆ progression of the treatment plan for future appointments

◆ products that would be suitable for the client to use at home to care for their skin

◆ recommendations for further facial treatments

◆ further products or treatments that you have recommended that the client may or may not have received before.

Note:

◆ any purchase made by the client.

EVALUATION
Record:

◆ comments on the client's satisfaction with the treatment

◆ how you will progress the treatment to maintain and advance the treatment results in the future.

HEALTH AND SAFETY
Advise on:

◆ avoidance of activities or product application that may cause a contra-action

◆ appropriate action necessary to be taken in the event of an unwanted skin reaction.

Knowledge Check

Describe the different communication skills that you would need to use when performing a client consultation.

Refer to pages 156–158 to help you.

Certain contra-indications restrict treatment; that is, the treatment may have to be adapted or delayed until the contra-indication has gone. For example, if eczema is present but the skin is not broken, the treatment can proceed but the area should be avoided as much as possible.

If the client has an allergy to an ingredient in the cosmetic preparations used, treatment cannot proceed until an alternative, non-allergenic product suited to the client is obtained. If the client has a stye, treatment cannot proceed. However, when the eye disorder has gone, treatment may be carried out.

Following the consultation, the client's answers will indicate to the beauty therapist what is required, and what is achievable, from a skincare programme.

When finalizing the most suitable treatment plan:

◆ explain what is involved in each stage of the treatment, how long it takes, and what aftercare and home care are required (if relevant)

◆ assess how much the client is willing to spend, and design a treatment programme within their budget.

This allows the client to:

◆ discover what the beauty therapist can offer to meet their needs

◆ ask questions, and receive honest professional advice concerning the most appropriate choice of skincare treatment

◆ decide how much they are willing to spend.

The beauty therapist should ensure that the client fully understands and is realistic about what the proposed treatment involves and what can be achieved.

When the treatment plan has been agreed, prepare and position the client for treatment.

1 Position the client on the couch. Ensure the client is comfortable and relaxed. Cover the client with the clean, large bath towel or alternative suitable covering. If necessary, drape a small hand towel across their shoulders. Some salons offer a quilt cover to keep the client warm and relaxed.

TOP TIP

Client care

Always give clear instructions to your client. This will help to ensure that they are not embarrassed or uncomfortable at any time.

TOP TIP

Headbands

Check that the headband is comfortable. A tight headband will cause tension and eventually a headache.

Client prepared and positioned for facial treatment

ACTIVITY

Answering questions

You should be able to answer honestly, competently and tactfully any questions related to the beauty treatments you offer. Below are examples of the questions you may be asked at consultation.

◆ 'I have always used soap and water upon my face. Is this a satisfactory way to cleanse my face?'
◆ 'Why do I need to use a separate night cream as well as a day moisturizer?'
◆ 'How often should I have a facial?'
◆ 'I have extremely oily skin. Why do I need to wear a moisturizer?'
◆ 'What can I do to treat these fine lines around my eyes?'

What answers would you give? Think of further questions you might be asked with regard to skincare. A senior beauty therapist will be able to advise you.

2 If facial, neck and shoulder massage is to be given, if applicable ask the client politely to remove their arms from their bra straps in preparation: this avoids disturbance later. All jewellery should be removed from the client in the treatment area and contact lenses may need to be removed to avoid eye irritation.

3 Fasten a clean headband around the client's hairline. Position the headband so that it does not cover the skin of the face. In some cases the head band is not required as a scalp massage may be included as part of the treatment. If using a facial steamer cover the hair to stop it getting damp.

4 After preparing the client, wash your hands: this demonstrates to the client your concern to work hygienically.

The skin should then be cleansed prior to completing a more detailed skin analysis where you can correctly diagnose the skin type and condition.

Choice of facial products selected will be decided upon from the information you have gained so far.

All **facial products** and equipment should be used with due regard to health and safety following manufacturers' instructions.

Skin analysis

Always read the manufacturer's instructions

Cleansing

Skin cleansing is essential in promoting and maintaining a healthy skin. There are various cleansing preparations to choose from; basically their action is the same in each case:

◆ to gently exfoliate dead skin cells from the stratum corneum, exposing younger, fresher cells and improving the skin's appearance

◆ to remove make-up (if worn), dirt and pollutants from the skin's surface, reducing the possibility of blemishes and skin irritation

◆ to remove excess sweat and sebum from the skin's surface, reducing congestion of the skin and the subsequent formation of comedones and pustules

◆ to prepare the skin for further treatments.

Cleansing preparations

A **cleanser** is required that will remove both oil-soluble and water-soluble substances without drying the skin. Oil is capable of dissolving grease; water will dissolve other substances. Usually, therefore, a cleanser is a combination of both oil and water.

Oil and water do not combine: if you simply mix the two together they separate again, with the oil floating on the top of the water. If the two substances are shaken together vigorously, however, one substance will break up and become suspended in the other. The result is known as an emulsion.

Emulsions are used in many cosmetic preparations. They are either:

◆ **oil-in-water** (O/W) – minute droplets of oil, surrounded by water

◆ **water-in-oil** (W/O) – minute droplets of water, surrounded by oil.

CourseMate video: Skin analysis

ALWAYS REMEMBER

Seasonal changes

Seasonal changes affect the skin. You may need to alter the client's basic skincare routine through the year.

HEALTH & SAFETY

Sensitive skin When treating sensitive skin, choose a cleansing product that does not contain common known allergens such as mineral oil, alcohol or lanolin. Such products are usually referred to as *hypoallergenic* or *dermatologically tested*.

Outcome 2: Be able to provide facial skincare treatments

Learn how to provide facial skincare treatments

PRACTICAL SKILLS

Communicate and behave in a professional manner

Follow health and safety working practices

Position yourself and client correctly throughout the treatment

Use products, tools, equipment and techniques to suit client's treatment needs, skin type and condition

Complete the treatment to the satisfaction of the client

Record the results of the treatment

Provide suitable aftercare advice

UNDERPINNING KNOWLEDGE

State how to communicate and behave in a professional manner

State the importance of completing treatment records

Describe health and safety working practices

State the aftercare advice that should be provided

State the importance of positioning yourself and the client correctly throughout the treatment

Describe the structure and functions of the skin

State the importance of using products, tools, equipment and techniques to suit client treatment needs, skin type and conditions

Describe diseases and disorders of the skin

Describe how treatments can be adapted to suit client treatment needs, skin type and condition

Explain how natural ageing, lifestyle and environmental factors affect the condition of the skin and muscle tone

State the contra-actions that may occur during and following treatments and how to respond

State the position and action of the muscles of the head, neck and shoulders

State the importance of completing the treatment to the satisfaction of the client

State the names and position of the bones of the head, neck and shoulders

Describe the structure and function of the blood and lymphatic system for the head, neck and shoulders

Oil-in-water emulsion

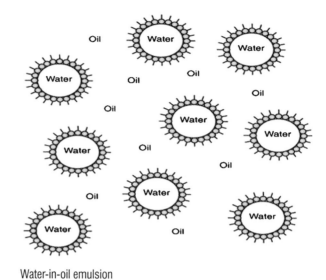

Water-in-oil emulsion

Emulsions

To give the emulsion stability, and to stop it separating out again, an emulsifier is added.

Various cleansing preparations are available to the beauty therapist, with formulations designed to suit the different skin types. They include:

◆ cleansing milks

◆ cleansing creams

◆ cleansing balms

◆ cleansing lotions

◆ facial gel or foaming cleansers

◆ cleansing bars

◆ eye make-up removers.

Whichever cleanser is chosen, it should have the following qualities:

◆ it should cleanse the skin effectively, without causing irritation

◆ it should remove all traces of make-up and grease

◆ it should feel pleasant to use

◆ it should be easy to remove from the skin

◆ ideally, it should be pH-balanced.

The pH scale

The **pH scale** is used to measure the acidity or alkalinity of a substance. Using a numbered scale of 1–14, acids have a pH less than 7; alkalis have a pH greater than 7. Substances with a pH of 7 are neutral.

The skin is naturally slightly acidic: it has an acid mantle. Alkalis strip the skin of its protective film of sebum, making it feel dry and taut. To avoid skin irritation it is preferable to use a product that matches the acid mantle, a product whose pH is 5.5–5.6.

Cleansing preparation cream

ACTIVITY

Acidic or alkaline?

To discover whether a liquid product is acidic or alkaline, carry out a simple test using litmus paper. Litmus changes colour according to the pH:

◆ litmus paper turns *blue* if an *alkali* is present

◆ litmus paper turns *red* if an *acid* is present.

Test the pH of various cleansing preparations.

Cleansing lotion

Facial foaming cleanser being applied

Products for facial skincare treatments

Cleansing milks Cleansing milks are usually oil-in-water emulsions, with a relatively high proportion of water to oil, making the milk quite fluid and light in its consistency.

Cleansing milks have these specific treatment uses:

◆ treating normal to dry skin that is prone to sensitivity

◆ treating sensitive skin.

Cleansing creams Cleansing creams have a relatively high proportion of oil to water, making the emulsion thicker and richer in its consistency than cleansing milks. The high oil content allows the product to be massaged over the skin surface without dragging the tissues. The cream is also more effective in removing grease and oil-based make-up from the skin.

Cleansing creams have these specific treatment uses:

◆ removing facial cosmetics

◆ treating by deep cleansing massage

◆ treating very dry skin.

Cleansing balms Cleansing balms are usually lightweight cleansers which quickly transform from a solid balm to a fluid. They moisturize and improve the texture of the skin while cleansing.

Cleansing balms have these specific treatment uses:

◆ moisturizing, non-drying effect

◆ improvement of skin texture

◆ suitable for all skin types except oily.

Cleansing lotions Cleansing lotions are solutions of detergents in water. They do not usually contain oil, and are therefore unsuitable for the removal of facial cosmetics.

Cleansing lotions have these specific treatment uses:

◆ cleansing a normal to combination skin type

◆ treating oily skin (where a high oil content could aggravate the skin, causing yet further sebum production).

Medicated ingredients may be included in a cleansing formulation: these are only suitable for oily, congested, pustular skin types.

If the client has a mature, normal or combination skin, a cleansing lotion may not be effective because of the reduced oil content. A mature skin benefits from oil content to compensate for reduced sebum production.

Facial gel or foaming cleansers Facial gel or foaming cleansers usually contain a mild detergent which foams when mixed with water. Additional ingredients are selected for the treatment of different skin types. These cleansers are quick to use and afford a suitable alternative for the client who likes to cleanse their face with soap and water. If the client wears an oil-based make-up, advise them to use a cleansing cream first to remove make-up thoroughly before using this cleanser.

Facial foaming cleansers have a general application:

◆ treating most skin types except very dry or sensitive skin

◆ particularly suitable for oily and combination skin due to their formulation which effectively removes sebum without drying the skin.

Cleansing bars Although it is efficient as a cleanser, soap is usually considered unsuitable for use on the skin. It has an alkaline pH, which disturbs the skin's natural acidic pH balance. Soap strips the skin of its protective acid mantle, leaving insoluble salts on the skin's surface. The skin may be left feeling itchy, taut and sensitive.

Cleansing bars are a milder alternative to soap, and are specially formulated to match the skin's acidic pH of 5.5–5.6. They are less likely to dry out the skin.

Cleansing bars have this specific application:

◆ treating oily to normal skin that is not sensitive.

Eye make-up remover Eye tissue is a lot finer than the skin on the rest of the face. It readily puffs if aggravated by oil-based cleansing preparations, and becomes very dry if harsh cleansing preparations are used.

To remove make-up from this area, use an eye make-up remover. This product cleanses the eyelid and lashes, gently emulsifying the make-up. It also conditions the delicate skin. Formulated as a lotion or a gel, it is designed to remove either water-based or oil-based products (or both) from the eye area.

Oily eye make-up removers have these specific treatment uses:

◆ treating clients who wear waterproof mascara

◆ removing wax or oil-based eye shadow.

Non-oily eye make-up removers have these applications:

◆ treating clients with sensitive skin around the eyes

◆ treating clients who wear contact lenses

◆ treating clients who wear individual flare **false eyelashes.**

TOP TIP

Eye treatments

Many eye make-up removers are also eye treatments. If your workplace uses a commercial product in this way apply it to the dampened eye pads used during mask treatment. This may also assist your retail sales, as the client may wish to buy some for home use.

Eye make-up remover

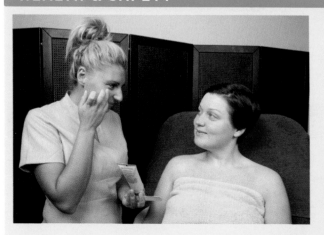

HEALTH & SAFETY

Eye care Never apply pressure over the eyeball when cleansing the eye area.

The ring finger is always used in the eye area when applying products as it provides the least pressure. Discuss this important advice with your client.

TOP TIP

Maintenance of artificial lashes

If the client is wearing semi-permanent false eyelashes avoid the application of high oil content eye make-up removal skincare preparations. These will weaken the adhesive that secures the artificial lashes. Take general care.

Cleansing treatment

There are two manual processes involved in the cleansing routine: *the superficial cleanse* and the *deep cleanse*.

The superficial cleanse uses lightweight cleansing preparations to emulsify surface make-up, dirt and grease. This is followed by the more thorough deep cleanse, in which a heavier cleansing cream is applied to the face. The high percentage of oil contained in the cream formulation allows the cream to be massaged over the skin's surface without evaporation of the product.

HEALTH & SAFETY

Hygiene Never use the reverse side of the cotton wool pad – this is unhygienic.

Never use the same piece of cotton wool to cleanse both eyes, use a separate piece for each eye to avoid cross-infection.

ALWAYS REMEMBER

Unlike the muscles of the body, which attach to bones, most of the facial muscles are attached to the facial skin itself. You should therefore avoid stretching the skin unnecessarily – if you do, you may also stretch the facial muscles and contribute to premature ageing.

TOP TIP

Make-up removal

If there is any make-up left at the base of the lower lashes after eye cleansing, this may be removed with a cotton bud or a thin piece of damp, clean cotton wool. Ask the client to look upwards, support the eye tissue with the other hand and gently draw the cotton wool along the base of the lower lashes, towards the nose.

If the client is wearing facial make-up, it is usual to perform the superficial cleanse twice to ensure all cosmetics are effectively removed.

Superficial cleansing

Each part of the face requires a special technique in the application and removal of the cleansing product. The face is usually cleansed in the following order:

◆ the eye tissue and lashes

◆ the lips

◆ the neck, chin, cheeks and forehead.

Step-by-step: Superficial cleansing

1 Wash your hands. Gloves may be worn if a male client has coarse facial hair that may cause skin irritation to the hands. Ensure that the client's contact lenses are removed if worn.

2 Cleanse the eye area, using a suitable eye make-up remover. If the client is not wearing make-up this product has been formulated for use around the eye area and can still be used. Each eye is cleansed separately. Your non-working hand lifts and supports the eye tissue while the working hand applies the eye make-up remover.

   If eye make-up remover is used, this is applied directly to a clean piece of cotton wool. Stroke down the length of the eyelashes, from base to points. Next, cleanse the eye tissue in a sweeping circle, outwards across the upper eyelid, circling beneath the lower lashes towards the nose. A cotton bud may be used to clean directly under the lower eyelashes. Repeat, regularly changing the cotton wool until the eye area and the cotton wool show clean.

   Sometimes a cleansing milk is used to remove eye make-up. In this case, apply a little of the product to the back of one hand. The ring finger is then used to apply the cleansing milk to the lashes.

   Use damp cotton wool to remove the emulsified product.

   Repeat the cleansing process until the eye area is clean.

3 Cleanse the lips, preferably with a cleansing milk or lotion (as this readily emulsifies the oils or waxes contained in lipstick if worn).

   Apply a little of the product to the back of your non-working hand. Support the left side of the client's mouth with this hand. With the working hand, apply the product in small circular movements across the upper lip, from left to right; and then across the lower lip, from right to left.

   Remove the cleanser from the lips. Support the corner of the mouth; using a clean damp piece of cotton wool wipe across the lips.

   Repeat the cleansing process as necessary, until the lips and the cotton wool show clean.

4 Select a cleansing product to suit your client's skin type.

   Place the product into one hand – sufficient to cover the face and neck – and massage gently over the surface of the skin. Massage the surface of the hands together when using a milk, cream or balm: this warms the product (so that it isn't cold on the client's skin) and distributes it over your hands.

   Clasp the fingers together at the base of the neck, and unlink them as you move up the neck.

   Clasp the fingers together again at the chin, drawing the fingers outwards to the angle of the jawbone.

   Stroke up the face, towards the forehead, with your fingertips pointing downwards and your palms in contact with the skin.

   Using a series of light circular movements with your fingertips, gently massage the product into the skin, beginning at the base of the neck and finishing at the forehead.

5 Remove the cleanser thoroughly with clean damp cotton wool, facial sponges or facial mitts, simultaneously stroking over the skin surface, upwards and outwards. Repeat this process as necessary, using clean cotton wool, if used. Facial sponges and mitts will require regular rinsing with clean, warm water.

STEP-BY-STEP: SUPERFICIAL CLEANSING

2 Cleanse the eye area, using a suitable eye make-up remover. Each eye is cleansed separately. Your non-working hand lifts and supports the eye tissue while the working hand applies the eye make-up remover.

3 Cleanse the lips, preferably with a cleansing milk or lotion (as this readily emulsifies the oils or waxes contained in lipstick if worn).

4 Select a cleansing product to suit your client's skin type and carry out a superficial cleanse

5 Remove the cleanser thoroughly with clean damp cotton wool, facial sponges or facial mitts.

TOP TIP

Effective cleanser removal

Check that the brow hair and the skin beneath the chin are free of grease: it is easy to overlook some cleansing product in these areas.

HEALTH & SAFETY

Careful cleansing When cleansing, be careful that cleanser does not enter the eyes or mouth. When cleansing around the nose, avoid restricting the client's nostrils.

Deep cleansing

The deep cleanse involves a series of **massage manipulations** which reinforce the cleansing achieved with the cleansing product. Blood circulation is increased to the area; this has a warming effect on the skin, which relaxes the skin's natural openings, the hair follicles and pores. This aids the absorption of cleanser into the hair follicles and pores, where it can dissolve make-up if worn, sebum and skin debris.

There are various deep-cleansing sequences; all are acceptable if carried out in a safe, hygienic manner, and all can achieve the desired outcomes. Here is one sequence for deep cleansing.

HEALTH & SAFETY

Safe pressure Reduce pressure when working over the *hyoid bone* at the throat and bony prominences such as the *zygomatic bone* (the cheekbone) and the *frontal bone* (the forehead).

Pressure must always be *upwards* and *outwards*, to avoid stretching the tissues.

STEP-BY-STEP: DEEP CLEANSING

1 Select a cleansing medium to suit your client's skin type. The procedure for application is the same as that for the superficial cleanse.

2 Stroke up either side of the neck, using your fingertips. At the chin, draw the fingers outwards to the angle of the jaw, and lightly stroke back down the neck to the starting position.

3 Apply small circular manipulations over the skin of the neck.

4 Draw the fingertips outwards to the angle of the jaw. Rest each index finger against the jawbone (you will be able to feel the lower teeth in the jaw). Place the middle finger beneath the jawbone. Move the right hand towards the chin where the index finger glides over the chin; return the fingers beneath the jawbone, to the starting position. Repeat with the left hand.

5 Apply small circular manipulations, commencing at the chin working up towards the nose, and finishing at the temples. Slide the fingers from the temples back to the chin.
Repeat step 5 a further five times.

6 Position the ring finger of the right hand at the bridge of the nose. Perform a running movement, sliding the ring, middle and index fingers off the end of the nose. Repeat immediately with the left hand.
Repeat step 6 a further five times with each hand.

7 With the ring fingers, trace a circle around the eye orbits. Begin at the inner corner of the upper brow bone; slide to the outer corners of the brow bone, around and under the eyes, and return to the starting position.
Repeat step 7 a further five times.

▶

8 Using both hands, apply small circular manipulations across the forehead.
Repeat step 8 a further five times.

9 Open the index and middle fingers of each hand and perform a cross-cross stroking movement over the forehead.

10 Slide the index finger upwards slightly, lifting the inner eyebrow. Lift the centre of the eyebrow with the middle finger. Finally, lift the outer corner of the eyebrow with the ring finger. Slide the ring fingers around the outer corner and beneath the eye orbit.
Repeat step 10 a further five times.

11 With the finger pads of each hand, apply slight pressure at the temples. This indicates to the client that the cleansing sequence is complete.

12 Remove the cleansing cream from the skin, using damp cotton wool, facial sponges or facial mitts.

Toning

After the skin has been cleansed it is then toned with an appropriate toning lotion.

Toning preparations

Toning lotions remove from the skin all traces of cleanser, grease and skincare preparations. The toning lotion's main action is as follows:

◆ it produces a cooling effect on the skin when the water or alcohol in the toner evaporates from the skin's surface. (When a liquid evaporates it changes to a gas, which takes energy. In the case of toner, the energy is taken from the skin, which therefore feels cooler.)

◆ it creates a tightening effect on the skin, because of a chemical within the toner called an astringent. This causes the pores to close, thereby reducing the flow of sebum and sweat onto the skin's surface

◆ it helps to restore the acidic pH balance of the skin. Milder skin toners have a pH 4.5–4.6; stronger astringents disturb the pH more severely, and may cause skin irritation and sensitivity.

There are three main types of toning lotions, the main difference being the amounts of alcohol they contain. They include:

◆ bracers and fresheners

◆ tonics

◆ astringents.

Toning lotions

TOP TIP

Toning lotions

All toning lotions have some astringent effect on the skin, but those that contain a relatively high alcohol content are actually marketed as astringents.

Do not use toning lotions that contain more than 20 per cent alcohol on dry skin – they may cause skin irritation.

Avoid the excessive use of astringent on oily skin – the astringent will make the skin dry, and it will then produce more sebum.

Skin bracers and fresheners
Skin bracers and skin fresheners are the mildest toning lotions: they contain little or no alcohol. They consist mainly of purified water, with floral extracts such as rose water for a mild toning effect.

Skin bracers and fresheners are recommended for:

◆ dry, delicate skin

◆ sensitive skin

◆ mature skin.

Skin tonics Skin tonics are slightly stronger toning lotions. Many contain a little of some astringent agent such as orange flower water.

Skin toners are recommended for:

◆ normal skin.

Astringents Astringents are the strongest toning lotions; they have a high proportion of alcohol which can dry out the skin. They may contain antiseptic ingredients such as witch hazel or tea tree oil; these are for use on blemished skin, to reduce the growth of bacteria and promote skin healing. Strong astringents can cause the skin to become dry and irritated if there is any skin sensitivity, so care must be taken.

Astringents are recommended for:

◆ oily skin with no skin sensitivity

◆ mild acne in young skin.

Toning lotions which are suitable for oily skin are becoming increasingly available and rely upon their botanical formulations to control sebum flow and promote skin healing.

Application

Toning lotion may be applied in several ways. Whichever method you choose, it should leave the skin thoroughly clean and free of grease.

The most popular method of application is to apply the toner directly to two pieces of clean damp cotton wool, which are wiped gently upwards and outwards over the neck and face.

Alternatively, the toner may be applied under pressure as a fine spray, using a vaporizer. This produces a fine mist of the toning lotion over the skin. If using this method, always protect the eye tissue with cotton wool pads and hold the vaporizer about 30 cm from the skin, directing the spray across the skin in a sweeping movement. This is preferable when treating a male client, where the cotton wool application technique would be unsuitable.

To produce a stimulating effect, the toning lotion can be applied to dampened cotton wool: hold this firmly at one corner, and gently tap it over the skin.

Blotting the skin

After applying toning lotion, immediately blot the skin dry with a soft facial tissue to prevent the toner evaporating from the skin's surface (which would stimulate the skin). Alternatively, you can make a small tear in the centre of a large facial tissue for the client's nose. Place the tissue over their face and neck, and mould it into position to absorb excess moisture. Alternatively, blot over the face with large facial tissues as shown.

When skin is thoroughly cleansed and toned a thorough skin analysis can occur using a magnifying lamp. If the client is sensitive to light protect the client's eyes with damp cotton wool pads. The skin's surface will be magnified enabling you to comment further and note any characteristics of skin type and skin conditions requiring attention. Record these on a record card.

TOP TIP

Combination skin

When applying toning lotion to a combination skin, you may need to apply different toning lotions to treat separate skin conditions.

TOP TIP

Toning lotion skincare product – home use

For home use, advise the client to apply toning lotion to dampened cotton wool: this is more economical use of the product.

Toning the skin

TOP TIP

Client care using spray toning lotion

Before facial application it is a good idea to spray the mist onto the back of the client's hand: this helps them to relax. Warn the client what to expect. Ask the client to close their eyes and mouth and breathe in, then spray over the face from the forehead downwards as the client breathes out.

Moisturizing

The skin depends on water to keep it soft, supple and resilient. Two-thirds of our body is composed of water and the skin is an important reservoir, containing about 20 per cent of the body's total water content. Most of the fluid is in the lower layers of the dermis, but it circulates to the top layer of the epidermis, where it evaporates.

Removal of products

The skin protects its water content in these ways:

◆ sebum keeps the skin lubricated, and reduces water loss from skin

◆ the skin cells have natural moisturizing factors (NMFs), a complex mix of substances which are able to fix moisture inside the cells

◆ a cement of fats (lipids) between the skin cells forms a watertight barrier.

The natural moisture level is constantly being disturbed. The application of a cosmetic moisturizer helps to maintain the natural oil and moisture balance by locking moisture into the tissues, offering protection and hydration.

 Our body and our hands are vital to how we make a living so take care of them! Ensure you pay special attention to your posture during treatments and commit to doing hand exercises and stretches to avoid injuries and strains.

Danielle Norman

Removal of products

The basic formulation of a moisturizer is oil and water to make an oil-in-water emulsion. The water content helps to return lost moisture to the surface layers; the oil content prevents moisture loss from the surface of the skin. Often a humectant, such as glycerine or sorbitol, is included: this attracts moisture to the skin from the surrounding air and stops the moisturizer from drying out. If a humectant is included, less oil is used in the formulation: this results in a lighter cream.

Moisturizer also has the following benefits:

◆ it protects the skin from external damage caused by the environment

◆ it softens the skin and relieves skin tautness and sensitivity

◆ it plumps the skin tissue with moisture, which minimizes the appearance of fine lines

◆ it provides a barrier between the skin and make-up cosmetics

◆ it may contain additional ingredients which improve the condition of the skin (such as vitamin E, which has a humectant action and is an excellent skin conditioner)

◆ it may contain UV filters, which protect the skin against the age-accelerating sunlight.

Moisturizers are available for wear during the day or the night. These are available in different formulations, to treat all skin types and conditions.

ALWAYS REMEMBER

Oily skin

Even oily skin requires a moisturizer. This skin can become dehydrated by the overuse of harsh cleansers and astringents.

TOP TIP

Tinted moisturizers

If your client likes a natural look for the day, they may wish to wear a moisturizer that is tinted; this gives the skin a healthy appearance.

Antioxidant moisturizers

Antioxidant moisturizers protect against free-radical damage from UV exposure, cigarette smoke, pollution and stress.

Moisturizers are applied at the final stage of the facial when the skin is clean and toned, providing a protective barrier.

Moisturizers for daytime use

Moisturizing lotions Moisturizing lotions contain up to 85–90 per cent water and 10–15 per cent oil. They have a light, liquid formulation, and are ideal for use under make-up.

Moisturizing lotions have these specific applications:

◆ oily skin

◆ young combination skin

◆ dehydrated skin

◆ normal skin.

Moisturizing creams Moisturizing creams contain up to 70–85 per cent water and 15–30 per cent oil. They have a thicker consistency, and cannot be poured.

Moisturizing creams have these specific applications:

◆ mature skin

◆ dry skin.

TOP TIP

Moisturizing creams

Some clients dislike heavier cream, feeling that it is too heavy for their skin. Offer them a suitable moisturizing lotion alternative.

HEALTH & SAFETY

Allergies Hypoallergenic moisturizers are available for clients with sensitive skin. These are screened from all common sensitizing ingredients, such as lanolin and perfume, and they also have soothing properties.

How to apply moisturizer

Moisturizer is applied after the final application of toning lotion. If the moisturizer is being applied before make-up, use a light formulation so that it does not interfere with the adherence of the foundation.

STEP-BY-STEP: HOW TO APPLY MOISTURIZER

1 Remove some moisturizer from the jar, using a disposable spatula or disinfected plastic spatula. Place it on the back of the non-working hand, then take it on the fingertips of your working hand.

2 Apply the moisturizer in small dots to the neck, chin, cheeks, nose and forehead. Quickly and evenly spread it in a fine film over the face, using light upward and outward stroking movements.

3 Blot excess moisturizer from the skin using a facial tissue.

Moisturizers for night-time use

Moisturizers are applied to the skin in the evening, after the skin has been cleansed, toned and blotted dry.

An emulsion night cream with a higher proportion of oil is the most effective for application in the evening: by this time the surrounding air is dry and warm, which encourages water loss from the skin; the oil seals the surface of the skin, preventing this water loss.

A small amount of wax (such as beeswax) may be included in the formulation: this improves the *slip* of the product, making it easier to apply and helping its skin-conditioning effect.

TOP TIP

Fluid moisturizer

If the moisturizer is very fluid, apply it directly to the fingertips of the non-working hand – it would run if applied to the back of the hand.

ACTIVITY

Moisturizers

Collect information on different moisturizers and their specialist ingredients and effects from various skincare suppliers. You could visit local beauty salons, retail stores or beauty wholesale suppliers, or write to professional skincare companies.

ACTIVITY

Eye conditions

Think of different *non-medical* conditions affecting the skin around the eye for which a client might seek your advice. Discuss with colleagues the possible cause of these conditions, and what you could recommend to improve the appearance in each case.

Ampoule products

Specialist skin treatment products

In addition to basic skincare products, **specialist skincare treatment products** are available to target improvement for specific facial areas.

Neck creams The neck can become dry as it is exposed to the weather, often without the protection of a moisturizer. As a client ages, the collagen molecules in the dermis become increasingly cross-linked; they are then unable to retain the same volume of water, and the skin loses its plump appearance.

The formulation for a neck cream is similar to that for a night cream; it also contains various skin conditioning supplements, such as collagen or vitamin E, which help maintain moisture in the stratum corneum.

Encourage your client to include the neck in their cleansing routine, applying facial moisturizer to the neck during the day and either a night cream or specially formulated throat cream in the evening. Recommend that they always apply the throat cream gently in an upward and outward direction, using their fingertips.

To improve the appearance of the neck, good posture is important. If the client is round-shouldered the head often drops forwards, putting strain on the muscles of the neck. This causes tension in the muscles, which become tight and painful. Correct the client's posture, and advise them to massage the neck when applying the throat cream to relieve tension.

Eye creams The eye tissue is very thin and readily becomes very dry, emphasizing fine lines and wrinkles (crow's feet). Special care must be taken when applying products near this area: it contains a large number of mast cells, the cells that respond to contact with an irritant by causing an allergic reaction.

Eye cream is a fine cream formulated specifically for application to the eye area. A small quantity of the product is applied to the eye tissue using the ring finger of one hand, gently stroking around the eye, inwards and towards the nose. Support the eye tissue with the other hand. Do not apply the product too near to the inner eyelid or you will cause irritation to the eye.

Eye gel Eye gel is usually applied in the morning; it has a cooling, soothing, slightly astringent effect. (This is caused partly by the evaporation of the water in the gel, and partly by the inclusion of plant extracts such as cornflower or camomile.)

Eye gel is recommended for all clients, but especially for those suffering with slightly puffy eye tissue. It may also be applied following a facial treatment, to normalize the pH of the skin.

Eye gel may be applied with a light tapping motion, using the pads of the fingers. This will mildly stimulate the lymphatic circulation in the area and help to reduce any slight swelling.

Ampoule treatment Serums are chemicals used to revitalize the skin. They are supplied in ampoules, sealed glass or plastic phials which prevent the content from evaporating and losing their effectiveness. Serums are usually applied for 7–28 days as a skin tonic course for the treatment of different skin types and conditions.

Blemished skincare preparations Professional products are available for the client to apply specifically to blemishes such as pustules and papules.

Benzoyl peroxide is an example of a product ingredient that dries and promotes healing of skin blemishes. The skincare aims to purify the skin while keeping it hydrated.

After cleansing the skin thoroughly the skin is exfoliated.

Exfoliation

The natural physical process of losing dead skin cells from the stratum corneum layer of the epidermis is called desquamation. **Exfoliation** is a salon technique used to accelerate this process. It is normally carried out after the skin has been cleansed and toned, and before further facial treatments.

Exfoliation has the following benefits:

◆ dead skin cells, grease and debris are removed from the surface of the skin

◆ fresh new cells are exposed, improving the appearance of the skin

◆ skin preparations such as moisturizing lotions are more easily absorbed

◆ the blood circulation in the area is mildly stimulated, bringing more oxygen and nutrients to the skin cells and improving the skin colour

◆ hyperpigmentation is improved in appearance by the removal of the pigmented surface skin cells.

Contra-indications

Exfoliation is beneficial for most skin types; however, avoid application if the client has the following:

◆ highly sensitive skin

◆ a vascular skin disorder such as telangiectases or damaged broken veins in the area of treatment application

◆ pustular, blemished skin.

Exfoliants

Various **exfoliants** are available; they may be of chemical or vegetable origin. Alternatively, mechanical exfoliation may be used.

ACTIVITY

Exfoliants

Apply an exfoliant to the back of your own – or a colleague's – hand or arm. Compare the appearance and the feeling of the skin before and after application. This technique produces a particularly marked effect on black skin, as it reduces the greyish appearance of the skin. (This is due to the skin having a thicker stratum corneum.) Pigmented skin will lighten and dehydrated skin will appear smoother in appearance.

TOP TIP

Client advice on rapid weight loss

Advise the client against losing weight quickly, especially when older – the neck tissue can look loose and very wrinkled as the underlying fat is lost.

TOP TIP

Specialist lip products

Products designed to firm the skin around the lips and reduce visible lines are becoming popular. The result aims to smooth and firm and even 'plump' the lip line, reducing the appearance of visible lines caused by lifestyle factors such as smoking and stress.

Exfoliator product

CourseMate video: Face Steamer

TOP TIP

Steaming

Steaming before exfoliation helps to soften the outer skin cells of the epidermis, making them easier to remove. This is particularly beneficial when treating a male client as the skin is thicker.

HEALTH & SAFETY

Exfoliants Avoid exfoliating products that contain sharp grains of nut shells: these can scrape, split and damage the epidermis. Before purchasing, test the exfoliating product on the back of your own hand to feel its action.

TOP TIP

Exfoliation

Exfoliation should be strongly recommended for the mature client. The removal of the surface dead cells has a rejuvenating effect on the skin's appearance.

Teenagers regenerate external skin cells every 14 days. This increases to 30–40 days as a client reaches their forties.

Mechanical exfoliation

TOP TIP

Male skin

A man who shaves exfoliates every day, as shaving removes the top layer of skin. You can recommend that he also uses a cosmetic exfoliating product on areas such as the nose and forehead. If a male client suffers from pseudo folliculitis recommend an electric shave rather than a wet shave which tends to make this disorder worse. Recommend the use of an exfoliant whilst showering, which will facilitate shaving and reduce skin irritation resulting from shaving.

Biochemical skin peel Natural acids (alpha-hydroxy acids – AHAs), derived from fruits, sugar cane and milk, are applied to the skin as a face mask. The natural acids dissolve dead surface cells and stimulate circulation in the underlying skin. These masks are available to suit all skin types.

AHAs may be combined with enzymes derived from fruits such as papaya (papain) to help remove surface dead skin to achieve maximum effect.

When you apply this type of face mask, warn the client that there will be a stinging sensation and then a tightening effect as the mask sets.

Pore grains Pore grains are the most popular exfoliants: a base of cream or liquid containing tiny spheres of polished plastic or crushed nuts is gently massaged over the skin's surface.

Clay exfoliants Gentler clay exfoliants have a clay base which is applied like a face mask. As it dries, the clay absorbs dead skin cells and sebum. The mask is then gently stroked away, using the pads of the fingers. The mask may include enzymes which gently break down the dead skin cells, aiding their removal. A mask style exfoliant is more suitable for a blemished skin accompanying a delicate, sensitive skin type.

Mechanical exfoliation Mechanical exfoliation, or 'facial brushing', softens and cleanses the skin. Dead skin cells and excess sebum are removed as the soft hair bristles rotate over the skin's surface. The rotary action also increases the cleansing action of exfoliation.

If steam is applied before mechanical exfoliation, this will soften the dead skin cells, and skin peeling cream may be applied: together these will maximize the result of exfoliation.

Be careful to avoid over-stimulation and over-exfoliation, resulting in sensitizing the skin's surface, or disturbing the skin's natural protective qualities. Permanent sensitization could result from incorrect exfoliation techniques or over-exfoliation.

> " The skin centre is a professional environment and it's important to conduct ourselves with professional maturity at all times. Each member of staff plays a vital role in the success of the business, so treat each other with respect. Should issues arise, address them immediately, in private, with the individual concerned. You'll spend 70 per cent of your time at work so create the environment you'll enjoy and do what you love.
>
> *Danielle Norman*

STEP-BY-STEP: EXFOLIATION TREATMENT

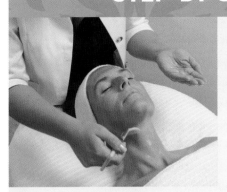

Exfoliant lotion is applied to a dry, sensitive skin type

Plastic film is placed over the exfoliant to speed up the action of the exfoliant lotion

Exfoliation product used in conjunction with a facial brush

1 Facial exfoliant is applied to the skin following cleansing and steaming to warm and soften the skin. The exfoliant containing hydroxy acids is applied, which removes dead skin cells and stimulates skin renewal. Warn the client a mild stinging sensation may be experienced, but will disappear quickly upon removal.

2 A soft facial brush may be used in a rotary action to further enhance the effectiveness of the exfoliant to remove areas of dead skin and sebum. This is particularly beneficial when working on a male client to loosen dead skin and debris surrounding coarse facial hair. A client may purchase the brush to use as part of their home care programme.

Clay exfoliant application

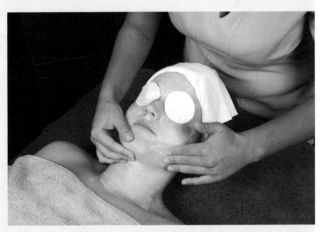

Clay exfoliant removal

3 The clay based exfoliant is ideal for most skin types including delicate skin. It is applied with a brush in a thin layer to the face and neck, application can be applied near to the delicate eye tissue. It is ready to remove when it has lost its damp surface when touched.

4 The mask is gently stroked away, using the pads of the fingers.

ALWAYS REMEMBER

Body exfoliants

Point out to clients that exfoliants designed for use on the *body* are unsuitable for use on the *face* – their action is not as gentle and their ingredients unsuitable unless specifically designed for dual use.

Knowledge Check

What is the purpose of an exfoliant?

Refer to page 237 to help you.

TOP TIP

Exfoliation retail opportunity

To encourage sales of this skincare product, demonstrate the product on the back of one of the client's hands. They will be amazed when they compare the appearance of their hands.

TOP TIP

Steam treatment best practice

Heat the water in the steam unit in advance of its application. This usually takes about 12 minutes and will avoid an unnecessary delay in the facial routine waiting for the water to heat! Ensure that the couch is correctly positioned before treatment when using steam, to allow the steam unit to be positioned at the correct distance from the client's skin.

Advice on home use

The client can be advised to use exfoliants at home as a specialized cleansing treatment after normal cleansing and toning. Exfoliants should be applied once a week for all skin types except oily, for which it may be applied twice a week.

Advise the client to massage the product gently over the skin using their fingertips. Application should always be upwards and outwards to avoid stretching the skin. The application and removal technique will differ according to the exfoliant product type.

After application, any product residue should be thoroughly rinsed from the face using clean, tepid water. The client may then apply a face mask or tone the skin and apply a nourishing skin moisturizer.

A UV sunblock should be used to protect the skin to avoid skin damage.

Following the exfoliation technique applied to suit your client's skin type a suitable skin warming technique is used relevant to the client's needs.

HEALTH & SAFETY

Exfoliants – how and when to use

◆ Tell the client how the skin should look after exfoliation treatment. The skin should be *slightly* increased in colour. Avoid too vigorous a massage application as this may lead to skin irritation and the formation of broken capillaries.

◆ Tell the client to avoid contact with the delicate eye tissue. However, some clay exfoliants are designed for use around the eyes – always instruct the client on the correct use of skincare products.

◆ A client with a pustular skin should not use exfoliant products – they would probably cause discomfort, and any lesions present might burst.

Warming the skin

A steam treatment is the ideal means of producing the required warming effect on the skin to achieve both cleansing and stimulation. Skin warming is often incorporated into a facial treatment after the manual cleansing, so as to stimulate the skin and make it more receptive to subsequent treatments.

The effects are these:

◆ the pores are opened

◆ locally the blood circulation and the lymphatic circulation are stimulated

◆ the surface cells of the epidermis are softened, which helps desquamation

◆ sebaceous gland activity is improved, which benefits a dry mature skin type

◆ skin colour is improved.

Steam is provided by a steam **vapour unit**. Distilled water is heated electrically until it boils to create steam.

The resulting steam is applied as a fine mist over the facial area. As the steam settles upon the skin, it is absorbed by the surface epidermal cells. These cells are softened and can be gently loosened with an exfoliation treatment.

Contra-indications

Although the treatment is suitable for most clients, do not use steam if you discover that the client has any of the following:

◆ *Respiratory problems*, such as asthma or a cold

◆ *Vascular skin disorders* – these would be aggravated by the heating action and increased blood circulation

◆ *Claustrophobia* – fear of enclosure or confined space

◆ *Excessively dilated capillaries*

◆ *Skin with reduced sensitivity*

◆ *Diabetes*, unless the client's GP has given permission

◆ *Rosacea* – a vascular skin disorder, where excess sebum production combined with a chronic inflammatory condition is caused by dilation of the blood capillaries. The skin becomes coarse, the pores enlarge, and the cheek and nose become inflamed

◆ *Dilated capillaries*, where capillaries near the surface of the skin are permanently dilated.

HEALTH & SAFETY

Safe use and care of the steam unit

◆ Always follow manufacturer's instructions on correct usage. Have the unit tested annually by a qualified electrician to ensure its safety in compliance with the Electricity at Work Regulations (1989).

◆ Always use distilled water to avoid limescale build-up in the heating element.

◆ Never fill the water vessel past the recommended level or 'spitting' could occur, where hot droplets of water are ejected and could burn the client's skin.

◆ Never use the equipment if the water vessel is below the recommended level or the heating element could be damaged. Most units have a cut-out feature so that the machine switches off if this occurs.

◆ Never leave the lead trailing across an area where somebody could trip and fall.

Explain to the client:

◆ how long the treatment is to be applied for

◆ the sensations that will be experienced

◆ the physical effect on the skin.

The duration of the application and the distance differ according to the skin type.

HEALTH & SAFETY

Steam application Keep the steam directed away from the client's face until a visible jet of steam can be seen. To avoid skin sensitization, consider carefully where to position the steam so as to ensure even heat distribution.

ANATOMY & PHYSIOLOGY
Chapter 2: Skin diseases and disorders

HEALTH & SAFETY

Ozone Most steam units produce ozone when the oxygen in the steam is passed over a high-intensity quartz mercury arc tube. Ozone is thought to be beneficial in the treatment of blemished skin, as it kills many bacteria, but it may also be carcinogenic (liable to cause cancer) if inhaled. Use a steam vapour unit with ozone selected only in a well-ventilated room, and only for short periods of time.

Blotting the skin following steam vapour treatment

The client should be positioned in a semi-reclined position for facial application.

Before applying steam, protect the client's eyes with damp cotton wool. Areas of delicate skin should be protected with damp cotton wool and if necessary a barrier cream.

The distance between the steam vapour outlet and the client's skin to be treated should be approximately 37–45 cm. The application time will depend on the treatment effect and the type of skin that is being treated. Generally allow:

◆ 5–10 minutes for the face

◆ 10–15 minutes for the body.

Ensure that an even flow of steam covers all the area being treated; reposition as necessary.

If you are using ozone, this is applied following the steam application for the final few minutes, as directed by the manufacturer. The steam will change in appearance to a bluish-white cloud.

After applying steam, blot the skin dry with a soft facial tissue and proceed to remove any blockages.

At the end of the treatment, turn off the machine and unplug it. Check that you have tidied away the trailing lead so that there is no risk of it causing an accident.

Contra-actions

Contra-actions to facial steaming include the following:

◆ *over-stimulation of the skin*, caused by incorrect application distance and duration of the steam

◆ *scalding*, caused by spitting from a faulty steam jet or by the vessel being overfilled

◆ *discomfort*, caused by the steam being too near the skin, leading to breathing difficulties, or by the treatment being applied for too long.

After facial vapour steaming, blot the skin dry with a soft facial tissue and proceed to remove any skin blockages – termed *extraction*.

HEALTH & SAFETY

Steam application Oily skin will tolerate a shorter application distance and a longer application time. For sensitive skin, increase the application distance and reduce the time. What are the manufacturer's guidelines for your equipment? Remember that these are only *guidelines* – observe the skin's reaction and check that the client is comfortable.

HEALTH & SAFETY

Removing skin blockages If the client suffers from severe congestion, do not attempt to carry out all the removals in one session. This would sensitize the skin, making it appear very red, and would be most uncomfortable for the client. Instead they should visit the salon weekly for you to clear the skin gradually as part of an overall treatment programme.

Removing skin blockages

After the skin has been cleansed, you may wish to remove minor skin blemishes such as comedones (blackheads). As discussed, it is preferable to warm up the skin tissues first; this softens the skin and relaxes the openings of the skin that are blocked. Milia (whitehead) extraction pierces the skin and therefore additional advanced training will be required in order to perform this treatment.

Products, tools and equipment

◆ **Disposable non-latex (synthetic) powder-free gloves**

◆ **Medical swabs** Impregnated with isopropyl alcoholic or antiseptic lotion – used to promote skin healing following extraction and prevent secondary infection. Alternatively a mild antiseptic soothing lotion may be applied

◆ **Facial tissues** Soft and white

◆ **Clinical waste sack** For any contaminated waste

◆ **Stainless steel comedone extractor** For manual extraction

HEALTH & SAFETY

Skin blockages Never attempt to remove larger skin blockages such as sebaceous cysts – these should be treated by a GP.

Comedone (blackhead) extraction

Sterilization and disinfection for removal of skin blockages

All contaminated waste material from this treatment (such as facial tissues and gloves) should be disposed of in an identified waste container, as directed by your local health authority.

After use the stainless steel comedone extractor should be cleaned with an alcohol preparation and then sterilized in an autoclave.

Wear disposable gloves while carrying out the treatment to avoid contamination with tissue fluids and to prevent secondary infection.

Comedone extractors

Comedone removal

For **comedone removal** the loop end of the extractor tool is used to apply gentle pressure around the comedone. The comedone should leave the skin, apparent as a plug. You may need to apply gentle pressure with your fingers at the sides of the comedone to ensure that it is effectively removed; when doing this, wrap a tissue around the pads of the index fingers.

Contra-actions

◆ Skin bruising could occur if too much pressure is applied.

◆ Capillary damage could result if too much force is used when squeezing the comedone. The surrounding blood capillaries can rupture, causing permanent skin damage.

Prepare the area of extraction by cleansing the area with a disinfecting lotion or medical swab

Comedone extraction

A mild disinfecting soothing lotion or medical swab may be applied after extraction which will help the skin to heal.

Contra-action If extraction resulted in tissue damage resulting in blood loss, a medical swab should be applied to the area. The contaminated waste should be disposed of as directed by your local authority. The area should then be avoided by the beauty therapist to prevent secondary infection. Inform the client following extraction that the skin may be reddened in the area and to avoid touching the area unnecessarily until the redness subsides. A soothing mild antiseptic lotion is recommended to help avoid secondary infection.

Mask treatment

The face mask is usually a skin-cleansing preparation but may contain a variety of different ingredients selected for their deep cleansing, toning, nourishing or refreshing effect on the skin. The mask achieves this through the following actions. If it contains:

CourseMate video: Face Mask

- ◆ *absorbent* materials, dead skin cells, sebum and debris will adhere to it when it is removed
- ◆ *astringent* ingredients, the pores and the skin will tighten
- ◆ *emollient* ingredients, the skin will be softened and nourished
- ◆ *soothing* ingredients, the skin can be desensitized to reduce skin irritation.

There are basically two types of mask: setting and non-setting. You will need to know when and how to apply each.

Setting masks

Setting masks are applied in a thin layer over the skin and then allowed to dry. The mask need not necessarily set solid – a solid mask can become uncomfortable and be difficult to remove, especially if the client has a sensitive skin condition.

Setting masks come in these varieties:

- ◆ clay masks
- ◆ peel-off masks – including gel, polyvinyl acetate (PVA) and paraffin wax
- ◆ thermal masks.

Clay masks The clay mask absorbs sebum and debris from the skin surface, leaving it cleansed. It can also stimulate or soothe the skin, according to the ingredients chosen. Various clay powders are available – select from these according to the physiological effects you require:

HEALTH & SAFETY

Client comfort

- ◆ Never obstruct the client's nostrils when removing a comedone from the nose area.
- ◆ Never apply pressure on the soft cartilage of the nose.

- ◆ *Calamine* A light pink powder which soothes surface blood capillaries. For sensitive or delicate skin.
- ◆ *Magnesium carbonate* A very light, white powder which creates a temporary astringent and toning effect. For open pores on dry and normal skins.
- ◆ *Kaolin* A cream-coloured powder which has a very stimulating effect on the skin's surface capillaries, thereby helping the skin to remove impurities and waste products. For congested, oily skin.
- ◆ *Fuller's earth* A green, heavy clay powder. It has a very stimulating effect, such that the skin will show slight reddening. It also produces a whitening, brightening

effect. For oily skin with a sluggish circulation. Due to its strong effect, it is not suitable for a client with sensitive skin.

◆ *Flowers of sulphur* A light, yellow clay powder, which has a drying action on pustules and papules. Applied only to specific blemishes (pustules).

To activate these masks it is necessary to add a liquid – an active lotion – which turns the powder to a liquid paste. Active lotions are selected according to the skin type of the client and the mask to be used; they reinforce the action of the mask. Examples are:

◆ *Rose water and orange-flower water* These are very popular; they have a very mild stimulating and toning effect.

◆ *Witch-hazel* This has a soothing effect on blemished skin; it is also an astringent and natural antiseptic and is suitable for use on oily skin.

◆ *Distilled water* This is used on highly sensitive skin.

◆ *Almond oil* This is mildly stimulating. Because it is an oil, it does not allow the mask to dry: it is therefore recommended for highly sensitive skin or dehydrated skin.

◆ *Glycerol* A humectant, which prevents the mask drying and is suitable for dry mature skin.

Clay masks have the disadvantage when treating a black skin in that they tend to leave streaks of white residue when removed. Choose a mask that does not have this effect.

The mask should be kept in place for about 10–15 minutes.

Peel-off masks
Peel-off masks may be made from gel, polyvinyl acetate (PVA) or paraffin wax. Because perspiration cannot escape from the skin's surface, moisture is forced into the stratum corneum. The mask also insulates the skin, causing an increase in temperature.

The gel mask is either a suspension of biological ingredients, such as starches, gums or gelatine, or a mixture of synthetic non-biological resin ingredients. The mask is applied over the skin; on contact with the skin it begins to dry. When dry it is peeled off the face in one piece. Depending on the biological ingredients added, the gel mask can be used to treat all skin types. (If the client has excessive facial hair, such as at the sides of the face, this mask may cause discomfort on removal. To avoid this place a lubricant under the mask, or use a different sort of mask.)

Peel-off masks contain a synthetic resin emulsion such as polyvinyl acetate resin and are used to tighten the skin temporarily, and are suitable for mature skin; they can also be used with dry skin. Algae may be used as an ingredient which causes rapid setting.

HEALTH & SAFETY

Avoiding infection Clay mask ingredients must always be made from sterilized materials, because of the danger from tetanus spores.

Ensure that *all* contents of the skin blockage are removed, or infection may occur.

ALWAYS REMEMBER

Face packs

The term *face pack* is sometimes used instead of face mask: a face pack does not set, but remains soft; a face mask sets and becomes firm.

> At interviews, you are showcasing your understanding and commitment to the industry. Your appearance and trade test are a reflection of this and the type of employee you are likely to be. Attire should be smart and simple. Bring a clean pressed uniform; keep hair up and off the face and nails short and free from polish. It can be nerve wracking working in a foreign environment so focus on your touch and client care.
>
> *Danielle Norman*

Peel off PVA mask

Japanese silk cream mask

The **paraffin-wax mask** is stimulating in its action. The paraffin wax is blended with petroleum jelly or acetyl alcohol which improve its spreading properties. The wax is heated to approximately 37°C and is then applied to the skin as a liquid. It sets on contact, so speed is essential if the mask is to be effective. The wax mask is loosened at the sides and removed in one piece after 15–20 minutes. The paraffin-wax mask is suitable for dry skin. Because of its stimulating action, it is unsuitable for oily skin or highly sensitive skin.

Thermal masks The thermal mask contains various minerals. The ingredients are mixed and applied to the face and neck, avoiding the mouth and eye tissue. The mask warms on contact with the skin: this causes the pores to enlarge, thereby cleansing the skin. As the mask cools it sets, and the pores constrict slightly. The mask is removed from the face in one piece. Thermal masks have a stimulating, cleansing action, suitable for a normal skin or for a congested, oily skin with open pores.

Non-setting masks

Some non-setting masks stay soft on application; others become firm, but they do not tighten like a setting mask. For this reason they do not tone the skin as effectively as setting masks. Non-setting masks include:

- warm oil
- natural masks – fruit, plant and herbal
- cream.

Warm-oil masks A plant oil, typically olive oil or almond oil, is warmed and then applied to the skin. It softens the skin and helps to restore the skin's natural moisture balance. Warm-oil masks are recommended for mature skin and dry or dehydrated skin.

Gauze masks A gauze mask is cut to cover the face and neck, with holes for the eyes, nostrils and lips, e.g. Japanese silk cream mask. This is then soaked in warm oil. A dampened cotton wool eye pad is placed over each eye. The gauze is then placed over the face and neck. It is usually left in place for 10–20 minutes.

Impregnated tissue masks These are placed over the skin and have been impregnated or saturated in active ingredients to achieve specific treatment results, e.g. collagen to hydrate and rejuvenate the skin.

Natural masks Natural masks are made from natural ingredients rich in vitamins and minerals. Fresh fruit and vegetables have a mildly astringent and stimulating effect. Usually the fruit is crushed to a pulp and placed between layers of gauze, which are laid over the face.

Honey is used for its toning, tightening, antiseptic and hydrating effect. Egg white has a tightening effect and is said to clear impurities from the skin. Avocados have a nourishing effect; bananas soften the skin, and are used for sensitive skins.

Cream masks Cream masks are pre-prepared for you. They have a softening and moisturizing effect on the skin. Each mask contains various biological extracts or chemical substances to treat different skin types or conditions. Instructions will be provided with the mask, stating how the product is to be used professionally.

TOP TIP

Gauze or impregnated tissue masks

Ensure that you position the gauze or tissue correctly so that the nose and eye holes are properly placed.

Gauze mask application

Applying a cream face mask

Cream masks are popular in the beauty salon: they often complement a particular facial treatment range used by the salon, and they are available for retail sale to clients.

ACTIVITY

Creating natural masks

Create some masks, listing the ingredients to suit each of the following skin types:

◆ dry
◆ oily
◆ mature, with superficial wrinkling
◆ sensitive.

If possible, arrange to carry out one of the masks on a suitable client. Evaluate the natural face mask. Consider: cost, preparation, application, removal and effectiveness. Remember to ask your client for *their* opinion!

HEALTH & SAFETY

Allergies When using biological masks, always check first whether the client has any food allergies. Avoid contact with any known allergen.

HEALTH & SAFETY

Natural masks Because natural masks are prepared from natural foods, they must be prepared *immediately* before use – they very quickly deteriorate.

Contra-indications

The contra-indications to general skincare apply also to face mask application. In addition, observe the following:

◆ *Allergies* Check whether your client knows if they have allergies. If so, avoid all contact with known allergens.

◆ *Claustrophobia* Do not use a setting mask on a particularly nervous client. Some clients feel claustrophobic under its tightening effect.

◆ *Sensitive skins* Do not use stimulating masks on clients with highly sensitive skin.

HEALTH & SAFETY

Acidic fruit Lemon and grapefruit are generally considered too acidic for use on the face.

Face mask application

Products, tools and equipment

◆ **Clean, dampened and clean, dry cotton wool**

◆ **Cotton wool eye pads (2)** Pre-shaped, round and dampened

◆ **Scissors** To cut cotton wool eye pads (if cotton wool discs are not used)

◆ **Facial tissues (white)** To blot the skin dry after applying toner following mask removal

◆ **Protective headband (clean)**

◆ **Clean spatulas (several)** To mix individual masks (if required) and to remove products from containers

◆ **Face-mask ingredients**

◆ **Gauze** Used in applying certain masks

◆ **Waste bin (covered and lined)** For waste consumables

YOU WILL ALSO NEED:

◆ **Disposable tissue roll** Such as bedroll

◆ **Towels (2)** Freshly laundered for each client

◆ **Flat mask brushes (3)** Disinfected

◆ **Trolley** To display all facial treatment products to be used in the facial treatment

◆ **Client's record card** To record all the details relevant to the client's treatment

◆ **Facial toning lotions (a selection)** To suit various types of skin

◆ **Sterilized mask-removal sponges (2) or facial mitts/ towels** For use when removing the mask using clean warm water

◆ **Large bowl** To hold warm water during removal of the mask

◆ **Lukewarm water** If required for mask removal

◆ **Moisturizers (a range)** To suit different skin types for use after mask removal

◆ **Hand mirror (clean)** To show the client their skin following the facial treatment

TOP TIP

Place a clean facial tissue under the edge of the headband at the forehead, so that it overlaps the headband. This will protect the headband from staining.

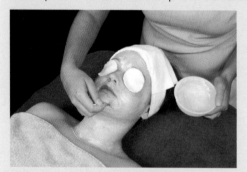

Applying a mask with a brush

Don't mix the mask with the mask brush – if you do, the solid contents will tend to collect in the bristles, the mask won't be mixed effectively, and the brush won't spread the mask evenly.

Sterilization and disinfection for face mask application

After applying the mask, clean the mask brush thoroughly in warm water and detergent. Next, place it in a chemical disinfecting agent; rinse it in clean water; allow it to dry; and then store it in the UV cabinet.

If you use sponges to remove the mask, place them in warm water and detergent. After rinsing them in clean water, place them ready for disinfection in an autoclave. (With repeated disinfection, sponges will begin to break up.)

Thermal mitts should be washed at a temperature of 60°C.

A large high-quality cotton wool disc may be purchased to use in mask removal.

Preparing the work area

Check that you have all the materials you need to carry out the treatment. You may like to place a paper roll at the head of the couch, underneath the client's head, to collect any mask residue on mask removal.

The head of the couch should be flat or slightly elevated. Don't have it in a semi-reclined position during the mask application, as some masks are liquid in consistency and may run into the client's eyes and behind their neck.

Preparing the client

For maximum effect, the mask must be applied on a clean, grease-free surface. If the mask application follows a facial massage, ensure that the **massage medium** has been thoroughly removed.

Select the appropriate mask ingredients to treat the skin type and the facial conditions that require attention.

How to apply and remove the mask

The mask is usually applied as the *final* facial treatment, because of its cleansing, refining and soothing effects upon the skin. The methods of preparation, application and removal are different for the various face mask types, so the guidelines below are a general outline of effective treatment technique.

1   Having determined the client's treatment requirements, select the appropriate mask ingredients. If you use a commercial mask, always read the manufacturer's instructions first.

2   Discuss the treatment procedure with the client, explain:

◆ what the mask will feel like on application

◆ what sensation, if any, they will experience

◆ how long the mask will be left on the skin.

Generally the mask will be left in place for 10–20 minutes, but the exact time depends on the client's skin type, the type of mask, the effect required and the manufacturer's instructions.

3   Prepare the mask ingredients for application.

4   Using the sterilized mask brush or spatula, begin to apply the mask. The usual sequence of mask application is neck, chin, cheeks, nose and forehead.

If you are using more than one mask to treat different skin conditions, apply the one that will need to be on longest first to achieve maximum benefit.

ALWAYS REMEMBER

Brushes

When purchasing mask brushes, note that a plastic-handled brush is preferable to one with a painted wooden handle – the painted one would be likely to peel on immersion in water, which spoils the professional image!

HEALTH & SAFETY

Maintaining hygiene – related mask equipment You need several mask brushes and mask sponges to allow effective disinfection of the tools, and so that you can provide freshly disinfected tools for each client.

HEALTH & SAFETY

Client comfort It is important to check that your client is comfortable while the mask is on their face. (They will suffer discomfort if their skin is intolerant to a particular mask.)

ALWAYS REMEMBER

Ensure that you have plenty of dampened cotton wool – it is used to apply toner to the skin before mask application, to remove the mask or mask residue left on the skin, and to apply toner to the skin after mask removal.

Ideally, buy cotton wool discs to use for the eye pads. This will reduce preparation time and ensure an evenly shaped protective shield for the eye area.

Apply the mask quickly and evenly so that it has maximum effect on the whole face. Don't apply it too thickly; as well as making mask removal difficult, this is wasteful as only the part that is in contact with the skin has any effect.

Keep the mask clear of the nostrils, the lips, the eyebrows and the hairline.

5   To relax the client, apply cotton wool eye pads dampened with clean water.

6   Leave the mask for the recommended time or according to the effect required. Take account also of the sensitivity of the skin and your client's comfort.

7   Wash your hands.

8   When the mask is ready for removal, remove the eye pads.

Explain to the client that you are going to remove the mask. Briefly describe the process, according to whether this is a setting or a non-setting mask.

Remove the mask using an appropriate technique, e.g. mask removal sponges. Some beauty salons use a warm towel method in which towels are steamed to make them hot and damp and then wrapped around the face and used to gently wipe away the mask.

9   When the mask has been completely removed, apply the appropriate toning lotion using dampened cotton wool. Blot the skin dry with a facial tissue.

10 Apply an appropriate moisturizer to the skin.

11 Remove the headband and tidy the client's hair.

12 With a mirror, show the client their skin. Evaluate the treatment.

13 Record the results on their record card.

Contra-actions

Possible contra-actions should be checked for and discussed at various stages of the mask treatment procedure. Before you apply the mask, explain to the client what the action of the mask will feel like on the skin. This will enable them to identify any undesirable skin reaction, evident to them as skin irritation – a burning sensation.

Ask the client initially whether they are comfortable: this will give them the opportunity to tell you if they are experiencing any discomfort. Should there be a contra-action to the mask, remove the mask immediately and apply a soothing skincare product.

If on removal of the mask you can see that there has been an unwanted skin reaction (that is, if you see inflammation), apply a soothing skincare product. In either case, note the skin reaction on the record card, and choose a different mask next time.

Advice on home use

The client may be given a sample of the face mask for use at home. Explain to them the procedure for application and removal, so that they achieve maximum benefit from the mask. Encourage them to purchase a suitable mask for their skin type and condition to apply at home once or twice a week, depending on their skin type, to dislodge dead skin cells and to cleanse and stimulate the skin. The suitability of the mask must be reviewed periodically dependent upon the client's skin needs and environmental and lifestyle factors.

ALWAYS REMEMBER

Paraffin wax

If you are using paraffin wax, remember to heat it in advance.

HEALTH & SAFETY

Allergies When using a commercial mask, try to find out *exactly* what it contains, so that you don't apply a sensitizing ingredient to an allergic skin type.

Setting masks When using a setting mask, ensure that the mask is evenly applied or it will dry unevenly.

Removing the mask with damp towels

Advise the client not to apply the mask directly before a special occasion, in case it causes blemishes, as sometimes happens.

The skin should be toned and moisturized after removing the mask.

Facial massage

Manual massage is the external manipulation, using the hands, of the soft tissues of the face, neck and upper chest. Massage can improve the appearance of the skin and promote a sensation of stimulation or relaxation.

Each massage performed is adapted to the client's physiological and psychological needs. The skin's physiological needs are observed during the skin analysis; the client's psychological needs are usually discovered during the consultation.

The benefits of facial massage include the following:

> Your curriculum vitae can determine whether or not you are considered for a position. Spend time nurturing this document so it's clear and concise with no spelling or grammatical errors. Have a friend proofread it if necessary. Avoid general statements like 'I'm an excellent communicator' unless you're prepared to back it up with examples. Try personalizing statements – 'I'm passionate about communicating with my client to ensure I've understood their skin needs'.
>
> *Danielle Norman*

◆ dead epidermal cells are loosened and shed. This improves the appearance of the skin, exposing fresh, younger cells

◆ the muscles receive an improved supply of oxygenated blood, essential for cell growth. The tone and strength of the muscles are improved, firming the facial contour

◆ the increased blood circulation in the area warms the tissues. This induces a feeling of relaxation, which is particularly beneficial when treating tense muscles

◆ as the blood capillaries dilate and bring blood to the skin's surface, the skin colour improves

◆ the lymphatic circulation and the venous blood circulation increase. These changes speed up the removal of waste products and toxins, and tend therefore to purify the skin. The removal of excess lymph improves the appearance of a puffy oedematous skin (provided that this does not require medical treatment)

◆ the increased temperature of the skin relaxes the pores and follicles. This aids the absorption of the massage product, which in turn softens the skin

◆ sensory nerves can be soothed or stimulated, depending on the massage manipulations selected

◆ massage stimulates the sebaceous and sudoriferous glands and increases the production of sebum and sweat. This increase helps to maintain the skin's natural oil and moisture balance.

Facial massage itself should take approximately 20 minutes, but this may vary according to the client's skin type.

ALWAYS REMEMBER

Mask removal

When using water to remove a mask you may need to renew the water as you work to ensure effective removal.

TOP TIP

During the mask development

While the mask is on the client's face you can tidy the working area and collect together the materials required for mask removal. Do not disturb the client, who will be relaxing at this time. A hand massage may also be offered.

HEALTH & SAFETY

Peel-off masks – removal When using a peel-off mask, make sure that the border of the mask is thick enough – if it isn't, it will be difficult to remove and the client may experience discomfort.

Facial massage

Facial massage is carried out as required, usually once every 4 to 6 weeks. Before the facial massage is given, the skin is cleansed; afterwards it is usual to apply a face mask, which absorbs any excess massage medium from the skin or can enhance further the skin nourishing effect of the treatment.

Warn the client that the skin may appear slightly red and blotchy after the treatment, due to the increase in blood circulation to the area: this reaction will normally subside after 4 to 6 hours. If it does not the client should be advised to contact the salon for further guidance.

Because of the stimulating effect on the skin recommend to the client that they receive this treatment when they do not have to apply any cosmetic products directly afterwards.

Sometimes the skin develops small blemishes after facial massage; this is due to its cleansing action. If the client is preparing for a special occasion, therefore, such as a wedding, make the appointment for at least 5 days in advance.

Massage movements

The facial massage is based on a series of classic massage movements, each with different effects. There are four basic groups of massage movements:

◆ effleurage

◆ petrissage

◆ percussion (also known as tapotement)

◆ vibrations.

STEP-BY-STEP: MASSAGE MOVEMENTS

Effleurage

Effleurage

Petrissage

Petrissage

Percussion

Vibrations

ACTIVITY

Planning a massage

How will your observations from the skin analysis and the client consultation influence the facial massage treatment application?

The beauty therapist can adapt the way each of these movements is applied, according to the needs of the client. Either the *speed of application* or the *depth of pressure* can be altered.

Effleurage   Effleurage is a stroking movement, used to begin the massage, as a link manipulation, and to complete the massage sequence. This manipulation is light, has an even pressure, and is applied in a rhythmical, continuous manner to induce relaxation.

The pressure of application varies according to the underlying structures and the tissue type, but it must *never* be unduly heavy.

Effleurage has these effects:

◆ desquamation is increased

◆ arterial blood circulation is increased, bringing fresh nutrients to the area

◆ venous circulation is improved, aiding the removal of congestion from the veins

◆ lymphatic circulation is increased, improving the absorption of waste products

◆ the underlying muscle fibres are relaxed.

Uses in treatment: to relax tight, contracted muscles.

Petrissage   Petrissage involves a series of movements in which the tissues are lifted away from the underlying structures and compressed. Pressure is intermittent, and should be light yet firm.

Petrissage has these effects:

◆ improvement of muscle tone, through the compression and relaxation of muscle fibres

◆ improvement in blood and lymph circulation, as the application of pressure causes the vessels to empty and fill

◆ increased activity of the sebaceous gland, due to the stimulation.

Movements include picking up, kneading, knuckling, pinching, rolling frictions and scissoring.

Uses in treatment: to stimulate a sluggish circulation; to increase sebaceous gland and sudoriferous gland activity when treating a dry skin condition.

Percussion   Percussion, also known as **tapotement**, is performed in a brisk, stimulating manner. Rhythm is important as the fingers are continually breaking contact with the skin; irritation could occur if the movement were performed incorrectly.

ALWAYS REMEMBER

Client care

The headband can spoil the hair, and the massage medium may enter the hairline. Recommend that the client does not style their hair directly before the facial treatment.

TOP TIP

Neck and shoulder massage

Pressure may be increased when working on larger muscles in the neck or shoulders, especially if the client has tension in this area.

TOP TIP

Stimulation – a requirement of the massage

When a stimulating massage is required, incorporate more petrissage and tapotement into the massage sequence.

Percussion has these effects:

◆ a fast vascular reaction because of the skin's nervous response to the stimulus – this reaction, **erythema**, has a stimulating effect

◆ increased blood supply, which nourishes the tissues

◆ improvement in muscle and skin tone in the area.

Movements include clapping and tapping. In facial massage, only light tapping should be used.

Uses in treatment: to tone areas of loose, crepey skin around the jaw or eyes.

Vibrations

Vibrations are applied on the nerve centre. They are produced by a rapid contraction and relaxation of the muscles of the beauty therapist's arm, resulting in a fine trembling movement.

Vibration has these effects:

◆ stimulation of the nerves, inducing a feeling of well-being

◆ gentle stimulation of the skin.

Movements include *static* vibrations, in which the pads of the fingers are placed on the nerve, and the vibratory effect created by the beauty therapist's arms and hands is applied in one position; and *running* vibrations, in which the vibratory effect is applied along a nerve path.

Uses in treatment: to stimulate a sensitive skin in order to improve the skin's functioning without irritating the surface blood capillaries.

HEALTH & SAFETY

Contra-indications to stimulating massage Do not apply percussion over highly sensitive or vascular skin conditions to avoid excessively increasing blood circulation in the area and over-stimulating the skin.

Equipment and materials

The massage is carried out using a massage medium that acts as a lubricant. A massage cream or oil may be used; these are slightly penetrating, and soften the skin. Choose a product that contains ingredients to suit the client's skin type and the age of the skin.

Whichever product you choose, it should provide sufficient slip while allowing you to control the massage movements.

ACTIVITY

Choosing a massage medium

Compare two professional skincare ranges. Look at:

◆ the choice of available facial-massage preparations to suit the different skin types

◆ the ingredients used in their formulation, and the effects claimed.

TOP TIP

Posture

It is important to maintain good posture during facial massage. If you slouch, you will experience muscle fatigue and long-term postural problems!

STEP-BY-STEP: MASSAGE TREATMENT

There are many different massage sequences, but each uses one or all of the massage manipulations previously discussed. What follows is a basic sequence for facial massage.

1 Effleurage to the neck and shoulders Slide the hands down the neck, across the pectoral muscles around the deltoid muscle, and across the trapezius muscle. Slide the hands up the back of the neck to the base of the skull. *Repeat step 1 a further five times.*

2 Thumb kneading to the shoulders Using the pad of both thumbs, make small circles (frictions) along the trapezius muscle, working towards the spinal vertebrae.
Apply each movement three times; then repeat the sequence (step 2) a further two times.

3 Finger kneading to the shoulders Position the fingers of each hand behind the deltoid, and make large rotary movements along the trapezius.
Apply each rotary movement three times; repeat the sequence (step 3) a further two times.

4 Vibrations Place the hands, cupped, at the base of the neck: perform running vibrations up the neck to the occipital bone. *Repeat step 4 a further six times.*

5 Circular massage to the neck Perform small circular movements over the platysma and the sternomastoid muscle at the neck.

6 Hands cupped to the neck Cup your hands together. Place the hands at the left side of the neck, above the clavicle. Slide the hands up the side of the neck, across the jaw line, and down the right side of the neck; then reverse.
Repeat step 6 a further two times.

▶

7 **Knuckling to the neck** Make a loose fist: rotate the knuckles up and down the neck area. *Repeat step 7 to cover, a further two times.*

8 **Up and under** Place the thumbs on the centre of the chin, and the index and middle fingers under the mandible. Slide the thumbs firmly over the chin. Bring the index finger onto the chin, and place the middle finger under the mandible forming a V shape. Slide along the jaw line to the ear. Replace the index finger with the thumb, and return along the jaw to the chin. *Repeat step 8 a further five times.*

9 **Circling to the mandible** Place the thumbs one above the other on the chin, and proceed with circular kneading along the jaw line towards the ear. Reverse and repeat. *Repeat step 9 a further two times.*

10 **Flick-ups** Place the thumbs at the corners of the mouth. Lift the orbicularis oris muscle, with a flicking action of the thumbs. *Repeat step 10 a further five times.*

11 **Half face brace** Clasp the fingers under the chin; turn the hands so that the fingers point towards the sternum. Unclasp, and slide the hands up the face towards the forehead. *Repeat step 11 a further two times.*

12 **Lifting the eyebrows** Place the right hand on the forehead at the left temple, and stroke upwards from the eyebrow to the hairline. Repeat the movement with the left hand. Alternate each hand; repeat the movement across the forehead. *Repeat step 12 a further two times.*

HEALTH & SAFETY

Massage manipulation 'flick-ups'
Do not flick the lips. Position the thumbs 5 mm from the corner of the mouth to avoid this.

13 **Inner and outer eye circles** Using the ring finger, gently draw three outer circles and three inner circles on each eye, following the fibre direction of the orbicularis oculi muscle.
Repeat step 13 a further two times.

14 **Circling to the chin, the nose and the temples** Apply circular kneading to the chin, the nose and the temples. Return to the starting position.
Repeat step 14 a further two times.

15 **Thumb kneading under the cheeks** Place the thumbs under the zygomatic bones. Carry out a circular kneading over the muscles in the cheek area.
Repeat step 15 a further five times.

16 **Tapping under the mandible** Tap the tissue under the mandible, using the fingers of both hands. Work from the left side of the jaw to the right; then reverse.
Repeat step 16 a further five times.

17 **Lifting the masseter** Cup the hands. Using the hands alternately, lift the masseter muscle.
Repeat step 17 a further five times.

18 **Rolling and pinching** Using a deep rolling movement, draw the muscles of the cheek area towards the thumb in a rolling and pinching movement.
Repeat step 18 a further five times.

19 **Lifting the mandible** Place the pads of the fingers underneath the mandible and pivot diagonally. Lifting the tissues work towards the ear.
Repeat step 19 a further two times.

20 **Knuckling along the jaw line** Knuckle along the jaw line and over the cheek area.
Repeat step 20 a further two times.

21 **Upwards tapping on the face** Using both hands, gently slap along the jaw line from ear to ear, lifting the muscles.
Repeat step 21 a further five times.

22 **Scissor movement to the forehead** Open the index and middle fingers to make a V shape at the outer corner of each eyebrow. Open and close the fingers in a scissor action towards the inner eyebrow.
Repeat step 22 a further two times.

23 **Tapotement movement around the eyes** Using the pads of the fingers, tap gently around the eye area.
Repeat step 23 a further two times.

24 **Eye circling** *Repeat step 12, a further three times.*

25 Apply effleurage to the neck and shoulders to complete the massage treatment.

ALWAYS REMEMBER

Massage medium

If the skin appears to drag during massage, stop and apply more massage medium. If you keep going you may cause skin irritation or discomfort.

HEALTH & SAFETY

Sensitive skin Avoid the use of tapotement over areas of sensitivity.

ACTIVITY

Massage to practise at home

Design a simple massage routine that a client could be taught to use at home.

Which type of massage manipulation is involved in each movement in your sequence? What effect do you wish to achieve by including it?

TOP TIP

During the facial massage, the client's face should relax. If there are evident signs of tension, such as vertical furrows between the eyebrows, check that the client is warm and comfortable.

ACTIVITY

Hand and wrist mobility exercises

Devise ten exercises to increase the strength and mobility of your hands and wrists which will help you when performing facial massage.

TOP TIP

Practise massage manipulations

When learning the facial massage you need to practise. Practise the movements on a Styrofoam® head block with facial features, or mannequin head as used in hairdressing, to perfect the manipulations. If these are unavailable, practise each manipulation on your knee – this will increase the agility and strength of your fingers and wrists.

TOP TIP

Massage medium removal

Massage medium can easily be overlooked in the following areas: the eyebrows; the base of the nostrils; under the chin; in the creases of the neck; behind the ear and on the shoulders. Ensure all massage medium is thoroughly removed.

After the massage

After the facial massage, remove the massage medium thoroughly using clean, damp cotton wool, facial mitts or towels. Check thoroughly that all of the product has been removed.

Apply toner to remove any traces of the massage medium, leaving the skin grease-free. Finally, blot the skin dry.

You may then proceed with further skin treatments, such as a face mask, or simply apply an appropriate moisturizer to conclude the treatment.

Advice on home care

Encourage your client to use massage movements when applying emollient, skin softening skincare products. Show them how to perform such movements correctly.

Facial exercises may be given to the client to practise at home. These should be carried out at least four times per week.

Specialist facial treatments

Specialist treatments should be offered to your client when there is a specific need or if they feel they would like to benefit from such a treatment. Specialist training in these advanced techniques is usually offered by the main product companies.

ACTIVITY

Home care facial products

What products may you recommend a client uses as part of their home care routine?

Home care routine advice

Aftercare

Aftercare and advice is discussed throughout the chapter in relation to each of the facial treatment procedures.

At the conclusion of your facial treatment ensure that you have covered the following in your **aftercare advice**:

◆ checked that the treatment has been completed to the satisfaction of the client

◆ explained what products have been used in the facial treatment and why

◆ advised what products would be suitable for the client to use at home, a basic home care routine, to gain maximum benefit from the treatment

◆ advised on product application and removal, again in order to gain maximum benefit from their use

◆ provided **contra-action advice**, i.e. action to be taken in the event of an unwanted skin reaction for contra-actions (including severe erythema, swelling, allergic reactions to products and tissue damage resulting in blood loss)

◆ suggested lifestyle changes that may improve the overall condition and appearance of the skin, e.g. the importance of a healthy regular diet and adequate water consumption (refer to pages 198–204 for guidance on caring for and avoiding threats to the skin)

◆ discussed the use of make-up if applicable following treatment (only eye and lip make-up should be worn directly after a facial treatment; allow up to 8 hours before make-up application to avoid congestion of the stimulated, cleansed skin)

◆ explained the recommended time intervals between treatments

◆ provided guidance in written or verbal form on what further treatments you would recommend to maintain or improve further the facial skin condition

◆ discussed if product samples are to be provided, when and how they are to be used

◆ provided the opportunity for the client to ask any further questions.

Update and record all details on the client record card, including products purchased. You can discuss their effectiveness at the next facial treatment.

Take the client to the reception to book their next appointment if required.

ASSESSMENT OF KNOWLEDGE AND UNDERSTANDING

You have now learnt how to provide facial skincare in the beauty therapy workplace. To test your level of knowledge and understanding, answer the following short questions. These will prepare you for your summative (final) assessment.

1. The massage manipulation shows finger stroking around the eye. Which muscle of the face is this being specifically applied to?

    a. occipital muscle

    b. orbicularis oris muscle

    c. orbicularis occuli muscle

    d. zygomaticus muscle

2. An oily skin type has increased sebum production caused by overactivity of the:

    a. suderiferous gland

    b. lymph gland

    c. sebaceous gland

    d. sweat gland

3. The following skin condition will restrict facial skincare treatment:

    a. severe psoriasis

    b. allergic skin

    c. sunburn

    d. impetigo

4. The mask type most suitable of cleansing and absorbing dead skin cells and surface skin debris is:

    a. setting mask

    b. non-setting mask

5. An exfoliant improves the appearance of the outer surface layer of the skin, which is the:

    a. stratum granulosum

    b. stratum germinativum

    c. papillary layer

    d. stratum corneum

6. Which massage manipulation can be incorporated to produce a quick erythema of the skin?

    a. effleurage

    b. vibrations

    c. tapotement

    d. petrissage

7. The bone identified is the:

    a. frontal

    b. parietal

    c. ethmoid

    d. occipital

8. The lymph nodes identified are the:

    a. submental nodes

    b. submandibular nodes

    c. occipital nodes

    d. parotid nodes

9. The following skin condition type may often contra-indicate facial steaming:

    a. oily skin type

    b. sensitive skin

    c. dehydrated skin

    d. mature skin

10. Aftercare advice should be provided:

    a. the first time the client receives the facial treatment

    b. following every facial treatment

8 Eyelash and Brow Treatments

LEARNING OBJECTIVES

There are two learning outcomes to achieve for this mandatory technical unit:

1 Be able to prepare for eyelash and eyebrow treatments.

2 Be able to provide eyelash and eyebrow treatments.

The assessment range applied requires you to:

◆ Understand the different eyelash and eyebrow treatments.

◆ Use consultation techniques to identify the treatment objectives.

◆ Conduct skin sensitivity tests where required and understand how the results affect treatment application.

◆ Use the products, tools, equipment and techniques required for each eye treatment.

◆ Ensure the environmental conditions are suitable.

◆ Identify contra-indications that prevent or restrict treatment.

◆ Communicate and behave in an appropriate professional manner.

◆ Follow all health and safety working practices.

◆ Identify normal reaction of the skin and when a contra-action occurs.

◆ Provide relevant aftercare advice.

KEY TERMS

adhesive

aftercare advice

colouring characteristics

consultation

contact dermatitis

contra-action advice

contra-actions

cyst

eyebrow shaping treatment

eyelash adhesive

eyelash and eyebrow tinting

eyelash perming

eye treatment products

false lashes

hair shaft

health and safety

hydrogen peroxide (H$_2$O$_2$)

negative skin sensitivity test

positive skin sensitivity test

salon requirements

solvent

toluenediamine

treatment objectives

treatment plan

tweezers

Unit Topic

Provide eyelash and brow treatments
Shaping and colouring eyebrows
Provide eyelash perming
These VRQ units are linked to the Beauty Therapy NOS Units B15 and B5.

INTRODUCTION

This chapter is about how to enhance and emphasize the appearance of the client's eyebrows and eyelashes using the practical skills of brow shaping, lash and brow tinting and application of false lashes. These services can create an immediate transformation to the client's facial features and overall appearance, including perceived rejuvination! The treatment application will be selected and performed to meet the outcomes required and agreed by the client. Dealing with people in a polite, efficient manner and using good communication and questioning skills to find out exactly what they require from the eye treatment service forms an important part of this technical service.

You must be able to show that you have the necessary practical skills and underpinning knowledge to provide eyelash and eyebrow treatments.

INDUSTRY ROLE MODEL

SHAVATA SINGH Brand Director Shavata UK (encompassing Shavata Brow Studio and Lash Lounge by Shavata)

"Eyebrows have always been a passion of mine. The entire process of creating the perfect arch fascinates me and I am constantly thinking of new ways to make this previously daunting beauty task simpler for my clients. This passion is one of the reasons I founded my first Brow Studio at the Urban Retreat, Harrods. This Brow Studio was my perfect solution for men and women who needed a quick, efficient, effective treatment, that takes just minutes and can transform your look. Shavata Brow Studios and Lash Lounges are now available in selected stores across the UK to help meet the demands of our clients and I have also developed my own range of fabulous products, which can help clients to create the perfect brow in-between their studio appointments.

ANATOMY & PHYSIOLOGY
Essential anatomy and physiology knowledge for this unit is identified on the checklist on page 33.

Purpose of eyelash and brow treatments

The eyebrows and eyelashes protect the eye from moisture and dust as well as define the appearance of the eyes and enhance the facial features. Eyebrows can be shaped and tinted and eyelashes can be tinted and permed. False eyelashes can also be attached to the natural eyelashes to further enhance the appearance of the eyes.

HEALTH & SAFETY

Hygienic working practice A number of pairs of tweezers must be purchased (perhaps five), due to the length of time required for sterilization. Buy good quality stainless steel tweezers: cheaper metals rust after repeated sterilization.

TOP TIP

Purchasing your tweezers

When purchasing tweezers, make sure that the ends meet accurately so they will grasp the hair effectively.

TOP TIP

Mascara wands

Disposable mascara wands are ideal for brushing the hairs during brow shaping.

Eyebrow hair removal

For more information on permanent and temporary hair removal methods, see CHAPTER 9 Threading and CHAPTER 15 Waxing Treatments.

The eyebrows, situated above the bony eye orbits of the face, help to protect the eyes from moisture and dust, and to cushion the skin from physical injury. Misshapen, bushy brows give an untidy appearance to the face, but when correctly shaped, the brows give balance to the facial features and enhance the eyes – the most expressive feature of the face. Eyebrow hair removal can be carried out with temporary or permanent hair removal methods. Permanent methods include the advanced treatments of electrolysis and intense pulsed light (IPL). This section will cover the removal of eyebrow hair using tweezers.

Outcome 1: Be able to prepare for eyelash and brow treatments

Learn how to prepare for eyelash and eyebrow treatments

PRACTICAL SKILLS

Prepare yourself, the client and work area for eyelash and eyebrow treatments

Use suitable consultation techniques to identify treatment objectives

Interpret and accurately record the results of tests carried out prior to treatments

Provide clear recommendations to the client

Select products, tools and equipment to suit client treatment needs

UNDERPINNING KNOWLEDGE

Describe salon requirements for preparing yourself, the client and the work area

Describe the environmental conditions suitable for eyelash and eyebrow treatments

Describe different consultation techniques used to identify treatment objectives

Describe the types of tests that are carried out before providing eyelash and eyebrow treatments

State the importance of carrying out tests prior to the treatment and accurately recording the results

Describe the contra-indications that prevent or restrict eyelash and eyebrow treatments

Describe how to select products, tools and equipment to suit client treatment needs

Describe the types of eyelash and eyebrow treatments available and their benefits

Outline the types of tests that are carried out before providing an eyelash and eyebrow tinting treatment

State the importance of assessing facial characteristics prior to carrying out eyelash and eyebrow treatments

Eyebrow shaping treatments are offered in the workplace as either an eyebrow reshape or eyebrow maintenance – reshape involves removing eyebrow hair to create a new shape, maintenance involves removing only a few stray hairs in order to maintain the existing shape.

Tweezers

There are two sorts of tweezers used to shape the eyebrows. Automatic tweezers are designed to remove the bulk of excess, unwanted hair; they have a spring-loaded action. Manual tweezers are used to remove stray hairs, and to define the brow shape where

Automatic tweezers

Manual tweezers

more accurate care is required. They are available with various ends including slant, claw and pointed; which you use is a matter of personal preference, but slanted ends are generally the most popular choice for eyebrow shaping.

Although many beauty therapists may complete an eyebrow shaping using only automatic or manual tweezers, it is important to be skilled in the use of both these tools.

Preparing the work area for eyebrow shaping treatment

Before the client is shown through to the work area, it should be checked to ensure that the area is clean and tidy. The plastic-covered couch or chair should be clean, having been thoroughly washed with hot soapy water, or wiped thoroughly with a professional disinfectant cleaner. The couch or chair should be protected with a long strip of disposable paper bedroll which may be placed to cover a freshly laundered sheet or bath towel. A small towel should be placed neatly at the head of the couch, for hygiene and protection during treatment. This will be draped across the client's chest; alternatively disposable paper tissue may be used. The tissue will need changing and the towels should be freshly laundered for each client.

When carrying out the treatment the couch should be positioned flat, to avoid the beauty therapist enduring postural fatigue and the chair should be slightly elevated.

Products, tools and equipment

Eyebrow shaping

- **Couch or chair** With sit-up and lie-down positions and an easy-to-clean surface
- **Trolley** On which to place everything
- **Tweezers (stainless steel)** Both automatic and manual
- **Orange sticks** To measure the length and arch of eyebrow when planning hair removal
- **Disposable spatulas** To hygienically remove the product from containers
- **Dry and damp cotton wool** To apply cleansing and soothing agents, and to collect hair removed during treatment
- **Scissors (stainless steel)** For trimming long hairs
- **Facial tissues (white)** For blotting the skin dry in the area
- **Disposable non-latex (synthetic), powder-free gloves** May be worn to prevent cross-infection
- **Disinfectant solution** To store small stainless steel sterilized tools

YOU WILL ALSO NEED:

- **Disposable tissue couch roll** Placed over the couch cover before each treatment for reasons of hygiene
- **Towels (2) (medium sized)** For draping over the client and placing over the top of the couch or chair

- **Eyebrow pencil** Used to mark the skin when measuring brow length and applying temporary brow colour
- **Eyebrow brush or disposable brushes** To comb through the brow hair during and following treatment
- **Headband (clean)** To keep hair away from the brow shaping area if worn
- **Pencil sharpener (stainless steel)** Suitable for use in the autoclave, used to sharpen the eyebrow pencil
- **Skin disinfectant** To cleanse and disinfect the client's skin
- **Cleansing lotion** Used to remove facial make-up from the eye area if worn
- **Soothing lotion or gel** With soothing, healing and antiseptic properties, suitable for use on the skin of the face, e.g. witch hazel liquid/gel

- ◆ **Non-oily eye make-up remover** To cleanse the eye area
- ◆ **Hand mirror (clean)** Used when discussing the brow shaping requirements and to show the client the finished result
- ◆ **Client record card** To record confidential details of each client registered at the salon including personal details, products used and details of the treatment
- ◆ **Light magnifier (cold)** To magnify the area to ensure all hairs have been removed
- ◆ **Disinfectant** For cleaning tweezers and scissors before sterilization
- ◆ **Waste container** This should be a lined metal bin with a lid

The work area should be adequately lit to ensure that the treatment can be given safely, but avoid bright lighting that could cause eye irritation, leading to watery eyes.

Before beginning the eyebrow shaping treatment, check that you have the necessary products, tools and equipment to hand and that they meet the legal hygiene and industry requirements for eyebrow shaping treatment.

Sterilization and disinfection for eyebrow shaping

Sterilize tweezers at an appropriate time during the working day. Ensure that you always have sterile tweezers ready for use with each client. After they have been sterilized in the autoclave, the tweezers should be stored hygienically in a clean, disinfected covered container or in the UV cabinet.

If used, an eyebrow brush should be cleaned in warm, soapy water or brush cleaner following use and, when dry, placed in the UV cabinet. Disposable brushes are effective as they can be thrown away immediately after use.

A fresh disinfectant solution may be used to store a spare pair of tweezers while carrying out an eyebrow treatment. This solution is usually dispensed into a small container stored on the trolley. (Spare tweezers are necessary in case you should accidentally drop the other tweezers during the treatment). After the eyebrow shaping treatment, tweezers must be replaced and resterilized.

Disposable gloves may be worn for protection avoiding cross-infection during the eyebrow shaping treatment – the beauty therapist may come into contact with tissue fluids from the client's skin.

As the waste from the treatment may contain body fluids and pose a health threat, it must be collected and disposed of carefully, in accordance with the local authority Environmental Health Department.

Chemical disinfection of eyebrow shaping tools

Knowledge Check

During an eyebrow shaping treatment when would you select the use of:

- ◆ automatic tweezers?
- ◆ manual tweezers?

Refer to page 267 to help you.

Permanent eyelash and eyebrow tinting

The hair of the eyelashes and eyebrows protects the eyes from moisture and dust, but the lashes and brows also give definition to the eye. Many clients, especially those with fair lashes and brows, feel that without the use of eye cosmetics their eyes lack this definition.

Further definition of the brow and lash hair can be created if a permanent dye is applied to them. Most clients will benefit from **eyelash and eyebrow tinting** because the tips and the bases of these hairs are usually lighter than the body of the hairs, causing the hairs to appear shorter than they actually are. Tinting the length of the lash or brow hair

TOP TIP

Blue tint

When a client requests a blue eyelash tint, make clear that this will not produce an 'electric blue' fashion colour.

makes it appear longer and bolder, whilst the effect created if required can look natural. The appearance to be achieved will be the client's preference.

Because the skin around the eye area is very thin and sensitive, dyes designed for permanently tinting the hair in this area have been specially formulated to avoid any eye or tissue reactions. ***The application of any other dye materials in this area is dangerous and may even lead to blindness.***

Permanent tints are available in different forms, including jelly, liquid and cream tints. The most popular permanent tinting product is the cream tint: this is thicker, so it does not run into the eye and it is easy to control during mixing, application and removal.

Several colours of permanent tint are available, including brown, grey, blue and black.

If the shade you want is not available, you can vary the shade of available tints by leaving the dye on the hair for different lengths of time, or by mixing different colours together. For example, to produce a navy blue colour; leave the tint to process for 3 to 5 minutes. If left to process for 10 minutes, the same tint will produce a raven blue-black colour.

The development of colour

Two products are essential for the permanent tinting treatment:

◆ professional eyelash or eyebrow tint

◆ **hydrogen peroxide (H_2O_2).**

The tint contains small molecules of permanent dye called **toluenediamine**. These need to be 'activated' before their colouring effect becomes permanent: this is achieved by the addition of hydrogen peroxide. The peroxide is said to develop the colour of the tint.

Chemically, hydrogen peroxide is an oxidant, a chemical that contains available oxygen atoms and encourages certain chemical reactions – in this case, tinting.

The hydrogen peroxide container will state either its volume or its percentage strength. To activate the tint and for safe use around the eye area, a 3% or 10-volume strength peroxide is used.

When you add the hydrogen peroxide to the tint, the small dye molecules together form large molecules, which remain trapped in the cortex of the hair. The hair is thus

Small dye molecules are mixed with hydrogen peroxide – they pass through the cuticle layer of the hair into the cortex

Small dye molecules swell and join together, becoming permanently trapped in the cortex of the hair

Permanent hair colouring

permanently coloured, but in time, as it continues to grow, the new hair will show the natural colour.

Preparing the work area

Before the client is shown through to the work area, it should be checked to ensure that the area is clean and tidy. Clean and protect the couch or chair as for the eyebrow-shaping treatment. The couch should be flat and the chair should be slightly elevated.

The work area should be adequately lit to ensure that the treatment can be given safely, but avoid bright lighting that could cause eye irritation and causing the eyes to water. This could lead to tint entering the eye area which must be avoided.

Before beginning the tinting treatment, check that you have the necessary products, tools and equipment to hand and that they meet the legal hygiene and industry requirements for permanent tinting treatment.

Products, tools and equipment

Permanent tinting

◆ **Coloured tints (a selection)** Jelly, liquid or cream, select from blue, black, brown or grey (used as is or mixed to the appropriate colour desired)

◆ **Disposable brushes** To comb through the lash/brow hair following treatment

YOU WILL ALSO NEED:

◆ **Couch or chair** With sit-up and lie-down positions and an easy-to-clean surface

◆ **Trolley** On which to place everything

◆ **Towels (2) (medium-sized)** Freshly laundered for each client

◆ **Headband (clean)** To keep hair away from the brow and eye area and protect long hair or bleached hair from the tint

◆ **Cleansing lotion** Used to remove facial make-up and the skin's natural oils and debris from the eye area

◆ **Eye make-up remover (non-oily)** To cleanse the eye area before treatment application

◆ **Hydrogen peroxide** (10-volume/3%)

◆ **Petroleum jelly** To protect the skin and prevent skin staining

◆ **Brush** To apply the tint

◆ **Damp cotton wool** For cleansing the eye area and for lash and brow tint removal and to soothe the area following eyelash tinting

◆ **Eye shields (commercial)** To prevent skin staining during eyelash tinting

◆ **Facial tissues (white)** For blotting the eye area dry

◆ **Disposable spatulas** For removing the petroleum jelly from its container

◆ **Disposable non-latex (synthetic), powder-free gloves** To be worn if allergic to permanent tint products

◆ **Non-metallic bowl** For mixing the permanent tint (note that some metals cause immediate release of the oxygen from the hydrogen peroxide, causing ineffective processing of the tint)

◆ **Skin stain remover** To remove any accidental staining

◆ **Bowl (clean)** To hold dampened cotton wool

◆ **Waste container** This should be a lined metal bin with a lid

◆ **Hand mirror (clean)** To show the client the finished results

◆ **Client record card** To record confidential details of each client registered at the salon including personal details, products used and details of the treatment.

False eyelashes

HEALTH & SAFETY

Applicator brushes Because it is impossible to sterilize applicator brushes effectively, use disposable brushes for the application of petroleum jelly and permanent tint.

Sterilization and disinfection for eyelash and brow tinting

Hygiene must be maintained in a number of ways:

◆ it is best practice to use disposable applicator brushes for the application of the petroleum jelly and the permanent tint because it is impossible to disinfect brushes effectively. If using a non-disposable brush applicator this should be placed in the UV cabinet after cleaning. Clean brushes should be stored in a clean, covered container.

◆ dispense products from containers using disposable or disinfected plastic spatulas.

ALWAYS REMEMBER

Commercial treatment timing

For false lash application, allow 20 minutes.

ACTIVITY

Choosing lash and brow colours

Which colour do you think would be most suitable for the eyelashes and eyebrows of the following clients:

◆ dark hair

◆ blonde hair

◆ red hair

◆ white/grey hair

◆ elderly client?

False eyelashes

False eyelashes are made from small threads of nylon fibre or real hair. They are attached to the client's natural lash hair imitating natural eyelashes and making the lashes appear longer and thicker, and thereby drawing attention to the eye. There are two main types: semi-permanent false strip lashes and false individual flare lashes.

False lashes are applied for the following reasons:

◆ to create shape and depth in the eye area, when completing corrective eye make-up

◆ simply to add definition to the eye area

◆ to enhance evening or special occasion make-up

◆ to provide thick long lashes for photographic make-up

◆ to provide an alternative eyelash-enhancing effect for a client who is allergic to mascara.

False strip lashes False strip lashes are designed to be worn for a short period, either for a day or an evening. They are attached to the natural eyelashes with a soft, weak adhesive. After removal the strip must be cleaned before reapplication.

False strip and individual lashes

False individual flare lashes False individual flare lashes are attached to the natural lashes with a strong adhesive. They may be worn for approximately 4 to 6 weeks, and are therefore known as false semi-permanent lashes.

Preparing the work area

Before the client is shown through to the work area, check the area is clean and tidy. The plastic-covered couch or chair should be clean, having been thoroughly washed with hot, soapy water or wiped thoroughly with a professional disinfectant cleaner. The couch or chair should be protected with a long strip of disposable-paper bedroll, placed to cover a freshly laundered sheet or bath towel. A small towel should be placed neatly at the head of the couch, ready to be draped across the client's chest for protection during treatment. The tissue will need changing and the towels will need to be laundered for each client.

For this eye treatment the couch or chair should be in a slightly elevated position, to give the optimum position for the beauty therapist when applying the false lashes. In this position, too, the client will not be staring into the overhead light (which might cause the eyes to water).

Before beginning the false eyelash application, check that you have the necessary products, tools and equipment to hand and that they meet the legal, hygiene and industry requirements for false eyelash treatments.

TOP TIP

Retail opportunity

Mascaras are available formulated to be worn with false individual flare lashes. The product is more easily removed than regular non-waterproof mascaras.

ACTIVITY

Position of client

Can you think of further disadvantages of having the client lying flat when applying false lashes?

Products, tools and equipment

False eyelashes

- **Term or chair** With sit-up and lie-down positions and an easy-to-clean surface
- **Trolley** On which to place everything
- **Headband (clean)** To keep hair away from the treatment area. A large clip may be used if the hair has been styled
- **Eye make-up remover (non-oily)** To remove make-up and general skin debris and natural oils from the area
- **Facial tissues (white)** For blotting the eyelashes dry after cleansing
- **Disposable mascara brush** To brush through the lashes after cleansing and before lash application
- **Manual tweezers (2 pairs) (sterilized)** To hold and place the false lash in position. Special tweezers are available, designed specifically to assist in attaching false individual eyelashes
- **False strip eyelash lengths** In a selection of lengths and choice of colours
- **False individual flare eyelashes** In a selection of lengths and choice of colours
- **Sterilized scissors (1 pair)** Used for trimming the length of false strip lashes

YOU WILL ALSO NEED:

- **Solvent** To soften and dissolve the adhesive when removing false lashes

- **Towels (2) (medium-sized)** Freshly laundered for each client
- **Disposable tissue roll** To be placed over the couch cover before each treatment for hygiene reasons
- **Cleansing lotion** Used to remove facial make-up from the eye area
- **Damp cotton wool** For removing cleansing product from the eye area and to protect the skin during false individual flare lash removal
- **Cotton wool buds** To apply solvent when removing false individual flare lashes
- **Surgical spirit** For wiping the points of the tweezers to remove adhesive (on-going)
- **Plastic palette (disinfected)** On which to place the false lashes prior to application (if preferred)
- **Disinfected dish (small)** Lined with foil, in which to place the eyelash adhesive during false individual flare lash application
- **Hand mirror (clean)** To show the client the finished result
- **Client record card** To record confidential details of each client registered at the salon including personal details, products used and details of the service
- **Waste container** Should be a lined metal bin with a lid

HEALTH & SAFETY

Adhesive hygiene In order that you can effectively clean the dish containing the eyelash adhesive after the treatment, you need to line the dish with a disposable lining

Knowledge Check

What is the difference between false strip lashes and false individual flare lashes in their application? What is the recommended duration that they should be worn?

Refer to pages 272–273 to help you.

Sterilization and disinfection for false eyelashes

Hygiene must be maintained in a number of ways:

◆ when preparing to apply false strip lashes, clean the surface of the palette onto which you will stick the lashes (if used) once you have removed them from their packaging. Use disinfectant applied with clean cotton wool for this purpose. The palette may be stored in the UV light cabinet until ready for use. False individual flare lashes come in a special 'contoured' package: you can hold this securely while removing false individual flare lashes, so the lashes can be kept hygienically until required

◆ always have a spare pair of tweezers available during application of the individual or strip false lashes. Should you accidentally drop the tweezers with which you are working, you will need a clean, sterile pair available

◆ scissors, used to trim false strip lashes, should be sterilized before use

◆ dispense products like false lash adhesive hygienically from containers before use

Eyelash perming

Eyelash perming is the process of permanently curling the lashes, which enhances the appearance of the eyes. The lashes immediately appear longer, which suits most clients. The treatment also suits:

◆ short, sparse lashes, to make them appear longer and denser

◆ downward-slanting eyes, as the eyes appear lifted when the outer lashes are curled

◆ special occasions and holidays

◆ clients who are unable to wear eye make-up at work

◆ clients who want a natural effect to enhance the eyes.

The effect lasts as long as the hair growth cycle of the eyelashes.

Chemical process of eyelash perming

Hair maintains its shape and strength by chemical cross bonds in the cortex (the thickest layer of the hair) called disulphide bonds (two sulphur bonds joined together). In the perm processing stage, these bonds must be broken to alter the shape of the hair. When the perm solution is applied to the hair, the chemical cross bonds are broken by the addition

Disulphide bonds

Processing stage: Breaking existing disulphide bonds by the addition of hydrogen

Neutralizing stage oxidation: Forming new disulphide bonds

ALWAYS REMEMBER

Eyelash curling

Mechanical eyelash curling using eyelash curlers as shown creates a temporary curled effect to the eyelashes which is time-consuming and can weaken the lashes, causing breakage of the natural lash. Permanent curling is an ideal alternative.

HEALTH & SAFETY

Storage Store the perm solution in a well-ventilated area, away from direct sources of heat and light. If a spillage occurs, wear gloves while you clean it up, and increase ventilation in the area.

of hydrogen and the hair is softened. The hair then assumes the shape of the rod that it is curled around.

This shape is made permanent by the application of the fixing/neutralizing lotion. This stops the action of the perm lotion. This stage is called the neutralizing stage, where the chemical cross bonds in the cortex are reformed by adding oxygen (known as oxidation) and removing the hydrogen. This stage is completed before the rods are removed. On removal of the rods, the eyelash hair assumes its new shape.

Preparing the work area

Before the client is shown through to the work area, it should be checked to ensure the area is clean and tidy. Clean and protect the couch or chair as for an eyebrow-shaping treatment. The couch or chair should be flat or slightly elevated.

The work area should be adequately lit to ensure that the treatment can be given safely, but avoid bright lighting, which might cause eye irritation, causing the eye to water which would also affect the chemical processing action.

Before beginning the eyelash perming treatment check that you have the necessary products, tools and equipment to hand and that they meet the legal, hygiene and industry requirements for eyelash perming treatment.

Products, tools and equipment

Eyelash perming

- ◆ **Couch or chair** With sit-up and lie-down positions and an easy-to-clean surface
- ◆ **Trolley** On which to place everything
- ◆ **Eye make-up remover (non-oily)** To cleanse the eye area before treatment application
- ◆ **Mild perm solution (usually 6% thioglycollate)** Especially designed for use in the eye area, it is this solution that curls the lash into the desired new shape
- ◆ **Headband (clean)** To protect the hair
- ◆ **Fixing/neutralizing lotion (sodium bromate)** To make the new curl permanent
- ◆ **Eyelash rods (a selection of different sizes)** Small rods are used for fine hair, larger rods for thicker hair
- ◆ **Eyelash adhesive** To secure the lashes to the rods
- ◆ **Lint-free pads** To remove the perm and fixing lotion
- ◆ **Disposable brushes or other recommended applicators** To apply the perm lotion and fixing/neutralizing lotion

YOU WILL ALSO NEED:

- ◆ **Hand mirror** To show the client the results
- ◆ **Towels (medium-sized)** Freshly laundered for each client
- ◆ **Bowls (2, clean)** To hold damp cotton wool or lint-free pads
- ◆ **Timer** To accurately time the curling and fixing processes

- ◆ **Waste container** This should be a lined metal bin with a lid
- ◆ **Disposable wooden sticks or other recommended applicators** To secure the natural lashes to the rods
- ◆ **Damp cotton wool** For cleansing the eye area and to remove excess products
- ◆ **Moisturizing agent** To facilitate removal of the rods
- ◆ **Client record card** To record confidential details of each client registered at the salon including personal details, products used and details of the treatment

Sterilization and disinfection for eyelash perming

Ideally, applicators used for the perming chemical agents should be disposable. Alternatively, several brushes must be available to allow effective disinfection between clients.

TOP TIP

Lash conditioning

A specialized conditioning agent may be applied to the lashes following the chemical processing perming treatment. This would be professionally applied as part of the perming treatment to rehydrate the lashes following manufacturer's instructions.

ALWAYS REMEMBER

Gel lotions

Perm lotions for the eye area are usually of *gel* formulation: this makes the lotion easy to control. Bear this in mind when selecting this product. The bottles are small to reduce the risk of oxidation, which would make the lotion ineffective.

Eyebrow shaping consultation

Reception

When making an appointment it is usual to allow 15 minutes for an eyebrow shaping treatment.

It is wise to have a designated time between treatments so that there is no confusion between the two treatments; a trim or a maintenance treatment and a reshape. For example, under 2 weeks could be regarded as a maintenance, and over 2 weeks as a reshape.

If the client has thick, heavy brows, or if they do not have their brows shaped regularly, they should be encouraged to have them shaped gradually over a period of treatments, until the desired shape is achieved. This will allow the client to become accustomed to the new shape and will minimize any discomfort.

Eyebrow shaping may be carried out as an independent treatment, or combined with other treatments such as permanent tinting of the brows. In the latter case, the brows should be tinted before shaping, to avoid the tint coming into contact with the open follicle and perhaps causing an allergic reaction.

Before brow-shaping treatment commences, carry out a **consultation**. Discuss the shape and the effect that might be achieved. Consider such factors as age, the natural shape of the brow and fashion. It is important that you fully understand the client's requirements because you will be temporarily removing the hair. Ensure that the client agrees the amount of brow hair to be removed and the shape to be achieved.

Remember for all eye treatments, if a client is under the age of 16, it is necessary to obtain parent/guardian permission for the treatment. They will also have to be present when the treatment is received.

Contra-indications

When a client attends for an eyebrow shaping treatment, the beauty therapist should always check that there are no contra-indications that might prevent the treatment.

If, while completing the record card or on visual inspection of the skin, the client is found to have any of the following in the eye area, eyebrow shaping treatment must not be carried out:

- ◆ *hypersensitive skin* – the skin could become excessively red and swollen
- ◆ *any eye disorder*, such as those described in the chart on page 278
- ◆ *inflammation or swelling* – the cause may be medical
- ◆ *skin disease*
- ◆ *skin disorder*, such as severe psoriasis or eczema
- ◆ *bruising* – client discomfort could be caused and the condition made worse
- ◆ *cuts or abrasions* – secondary infection could occur
- ◆ *scar tissue under 6 months old* – the skin lacks elasticity.

The following chart will help you to identify some eye disorders that contra-indicate eyebrow shaping, permanent tinting of the eyebrows and lashes, false eyelash application, eyebrow threading and eyelash perming.

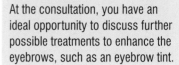

TOP TIP

Positive promotion

At the consultation, you have an ideal opportunity to discuss further possible treatments to enhance the eyebrows, such as an eyebrow tint.

TOP TIP

Communication

At the consultation, identify any peculiarities such as bald patches or scarring in the brow area to avoid any confusion or concern later related to the treatment.

Name	Description	Name	Description
Conjunctivitis or pink eye	Infectious bacterial infection. Inflammation of the mucous membrane that covers the eye and lines the eyelid. The skin of the inner conjunctiva of the eye becomes inflamed, the eye becomes very red, itchy and sore, and pus may exude from the eye area	Watery eye or epiphora	The eye over-secretes tears, which would normally drain into the nasal cavity
Stye or hordeola	Infectious bacterial infection. Infection of the sebaceous glands of the eyelash hair follicles. Small lumps appear on the inner rim of the eyelid containing pus	Blepharitis	Inflammation of the eyelid caused by infection or an allergic reaction
Cyst	Localized pocket of sebum, which forms in the hair follicle or under the sebaceous glands in the skin. Semi-globular in shape, either raised or flat, and hard or soft. The cysts are the same colour as skin, or red if bacterial infection occurs. A cyst appearing on the upper eyelid is known as a chalazion or meibomian cyst	Benign (non-malignant) tumour	Harmless skin-coloured growths. They may appear as a 'thread' of skin on the eyelids growing between the eyelashes. Chemical treatments such as tinting and perming should be avoided to avoid skin irritation. Refer the client to their GP

If you are unsure about the safety of proceeding with treatment – for example, if there is an undiagnosed lump in the area – ask your client to seek medical approval first. Remember, you are not qualified to diagnose a contra-indication. Refer the client to their GP without causing unnecessary cause for concern.

Discuss possible **contra-actions** that may occur during or after the eyebrow shaping treatment with your client at consultation.

Contra-actions

Severe erythema is considered to be a contra-action to the treatment: it is recognized as a marked reddening of the skin seen over the whole area or specifically around one damaged follicle. It is usually accompanied by minor swelling of the area. If this occurs the beauty therapist must try to reduce the redness by applying a cool compress and soothing antiseptic lotion or cream to the area. In extreme cases it may be necessary to apply ice. Record details of any contra-action on the client's record card.

If the reddening reduces in response to your corrective action, you may decide in future to remove only a few stray hairs at each eyebrow-shaping treatment, to minimize the risk of this reaction recurring.

HEALTH & SAFETY

Contra-action: hygiene if using ice
If applying ice to reduce swelling, in order to maintain hygiene, place the ice cube in a new small freezer food bag. Dispose of the bag hygienically after use.

Always discuss possible contra-actions that may occur during or after the eyebrow shaping treatment with your client at consultation.

> " For me, every client is my most important client, so all my staff are trained to the highest standard and customer service is one of the most important components to my business. We also use a combination of techniques to ensure each customer gets the brow shape that suits them best.
>
> *Shavata Singh*

If you accidentally pinch the skin with the tweezers and break the skin, apply a suitable soothing, antiseptic lotion for the skin, whilst wearing gloves. Inform the client not to touch the area and recommend the further application of a suitable antiseptic lotion. The main aim is to avoid secondary infection. All details of action taken must be recorded on the client record card.

Dispose of any contaminated waste according to the local Environmental Health regulations.

Planning the treatment: factors to be considered

Before shaping the brows you must consider the following factors.

The natural shape of the brow The natural brow follows the line of the eye socket. This varies greatly between clients, and affects what is achievable.

If the client has been shaping their own brows, it may be necessary to let them grow for a short period before shaping them professionally. If the brows are very thin or very thick, it may take several sessions before the desired shape is achieved.

If the brows have been plucked over a long period of time, they may not grow back successfully; this should be discussed with the client. In such instances, temporary eyebrow pencil or matt powder eye shadow may be used to achieve the desired effect. Temporary brow colour is useful to apply when growing hairs into a new shape, to create a defined brow shape.

Fashion Each season sees new fashion trends, which also affect eye make-up and eyebrow shapes. This should be considered before using any form of permanent hair removal to shape the brows.

Applying temporary brow colour to emphasise the brow shape

Knowledge Check

Why is it important to have a thorough consultation before you commence the eyebrow shaping treatment?

Refer to page 277 to help you.

TOP TIP

Temporary brow colour

A sharpened eyebrow pencil may be used to simulate brow hairs – apply feathery strokes using the pencil point. To create a natural effect, two different pencil colours may be used, for example brown and grey.

CourseMate video: Male Eyebrows

The age of the client   The brow hair of older clients may include a few coarse, long, discoloured white or grey hairs. These may be removed provided that this does not alter the brow line or leave bald patches or trimmed. Care must be taken to avoid a blunt, spikey appearance to the hair if trimmed.

In general, thick eyebrows can make the client look older, by creating a hooded appearance; and thin eyebrows can make the client look severe. Ideally the brows should therefore be shaped to a medium thickness.

The natural growth pattern   The shape and effect that the client requests may be made impossible by the pattern of the natural growth of the hair, which is genetically determined. When shaping the brows of an Oriental client, for example, you will notice that the eyebrow hair grows in a downward direction. To create an arch it may be necessary to trim the hairs, using a small, sterile pair of sharp nail scissors. Alternatively, you may remove the outer eyebrow length and use a cosmetic eyebrow pencil or powder to create a new brow line. Use your professional judgement to advise the client.

Choosing an eyebrow shape

The eyebrows should be in balance with the rest of the facial features: the right brow shape for each client will depend on the client's facial proportions and natural brow shape.

Practise excellent customer service
◆ Promote great grooming.
◆ Be passionate about eyebrows.
◆ A successful beauty therapist will have a natural talent with people.
◆ Stay level-headed.
◆ Be precise.

Shavata Singh

There is no single ideal brow shape; different brow shapes are shown below.

Oblique eyebrow

Arched eyebrow

Angular eyebrow

Straight eyebrow

Rounded eyebrow

Thin eyebrow

Medium eyebrow

Thick eyebrow

TOP TIP

Semi-permanent make-up for the eyebrows

Suspended pigment particles in a liquid base are inserted into the outer skin using a disposable needle. Many of the popular dyes are based on plant extracts.

The effect gradually fades, lasting up to 3 years.

Before

After

TOP TIP

False eyebrow hair

These are ideal for disguising any bald areas in the natural eyebrow hair using false hair which is attached using adhesive to the skin.

What is achievable? Obviously not all of these brow shapes are achievable for every client, but the skilful application to the eyebrows of temporary cosmetic colour can create the illusion of the desired brow shape.

The quantity of brow hair removed during shaping produces a thin, medium or thick final shape, as illustrated. Other approaches, too, may be used:

◆ *semi-permanent make-up*, also referred to as micro-pigmentation, can be used to add colour permanently to the brows, for example to disguise a bald patch

◆ *hair transplants* are available for a client with sparse eyebrows

◆ *false individual eyebrow hairs* are applied in the same way as false individual flare eyelashes.

Ideally, the distance between the two eyebrows should be the width of one eye. If this is not the case, the illusion may be created by removing hairs or by applying temporary brow colour to create this effect.

Wide-set eyes can be made to appear closer together by extending the brow line beyond the inside corner of the eye; close-set eyes can be made to look further apart by widening the distance between them.

ACTIVITY

Correcting brow shapes through brow-shaping treatment

How would you correct the appearance of the following eye shapes:

◆ wide-set
◆ close-set.

ACTIVITY

Correcting brow shapes

From magazines and the Internet, search and collect pictures of faces showing different eyebrow shapes. Explain which you think are correct and which incorrect for each person.

ALWAYS REMEMBER

Consultation

Accurately record your client's answers to necessary questions asked at the consultation.

ACTIVITY

Recommending brow shapes to suit client face shape

You cannot change the bone structure of the facial features without cosmetic surgery, but brow shaping can create the illusion of improved facial balance and proportion. Discuss why each of the brow shapes below would complement the accompanying face shape.

Face shape	*Recommended brow shape*
Square	Arched — Arched eyebrow
Round	Oblique — Oblique eyebrow
Oblong	Straight — Straight eyebrow
Pear (triangular)	Angular — Angular eyebrow
Heart	Oblique — Oblique eyebrow

Measuring the eyebrow

Measuring the eyebrow: the inner corner of the eye

Measuring the eyebrow: the outer corner of the eye

ALWAYS REMEMBER

Examples of the way eye services may need to be modified include:

Eyebrow shape

◆ Avoiding removing hair that is concealing a bald area, e.g. scar in the area.

◆ Hair removal when shaping a male client's eyebrows.

Eyelash tint

◆ Allowing further processing time to an area where the hair is more resistant (difficult) to colour.

False eyelashes

◆ Selecting an alternative lash length appropriate to the function of the lens, if the client wears glasses.

◆ If long-sighted, the lens will magnify the eye creating an unrealistic look if the false lash length is too long.

Knowledge Check

How can you determine the length of a client's eyebrows that will suit their facial features?

Refer to pages 280–281 to help you.

How to measure the eyebrows to decide length

In order to determine the correct length of the client's eyebrows, there are three main guidelines:

1　Place an orange stick or spatula beside the nose and the inside corner of the eye. This is usually in line with the tear duct. Any hairs that grow between the eyes and beyond this point should be removed. If the client has a very broad nose, however, this guide is inappropriate: tweezing would commence near the middle of the brow. In this instance, use the tear duct at the inside corner of the eye as a guide (as per image above).

2　Place an orange stick or spatula in a line from the base of the nose (to the side of the nostril) to the outer corner of the eye. Any hairs that grow beyond this point should be removed.

3　Place an orange stick or spatula in a vertical line from the centre of the eyelid. This is where the highest point of the arch should be.

Initially these guidelines will be needed to ensure that the correct length and brow shape are achieved, but the experienced beauty therapist will recognize the corrective work to be carried out without the need for measuring.

Following the consultation, record all client details accurately on the client record card. A record card that can be used for the eye treatments follows.

The following record card is designed to record details of all eyelash and brow treatments.

A sample client record card

Date	Beauty therapist name	
Client name		Date of birth (identifying client age group)
Home address		Postcode
Landline phone number	Mobile phone number	Email address
Name of doctor	Doctor's address and phone number	
Related medical history (conditions that may restrict or prohibit treatment application)		
Are you taking any medication? (This may affect the condition of the skin or skin sensitivity)		

CONTRA-INDICATIONS REQUIRING MEDICAL REFERRAL
(preventing eye treatment application)

☐ severe skin conditions, (e.g. severe eczema in area)
☐ eye infections (e.g. conjunctivitis, styes)
☐ eye disease
☐ inflammation of the skin
☐ during chemotherapy and radiotherapy

EYE TREATMENT

☐ shaping eyebrows
☐ tinting eyebrows
☐ tinting eyelashes
☐ false eyelashes
☐ lash perming

BROW SHAPING TECHNIQUES

☐ brow shape selected following measurement of the:
☐ client's natural brow and eye
☐ opening of the pores and hair follicle to facilitate removal
☐ keeping the skin taut
☐ removal of hairs in the direction of hair growth
☐ protection of the eye
☐ hair removed to complement the shape and proportions of client's natural brow, in relation to facial features and shape and to client's satisfaction

TREATMENT AREA

☐ eyebrows
☐ total reshape
☐ maintenance of original shape

CONTRA-INDICATIONS WHICH RESTRICT TREATMENT
(treatment may require adaptation)

☐ recent scar tissue
☐ eye disorders
☐ product allergies
☐ bruising
☐ undiagnosed lumps and swellings

EYELASH OR BROW TINTING

☐ skin sensitivity test carried out
☐ tint colour selection suited to client's colouring characteristics
☐ effectively protecting the surrounding skin
☐ timing, development and removal of tint adapted according
☐ to client's natural colouring characteristics
☐ manufacturer's instructions complied with

COLOURING CHARACTERISTIC

blonde ☐   red ☐   dark ☐   white ☐

FALSE EYELASHES

☐ skin sensitivity test carried out
☐ colour and length of lash type selected to meet agreed
☐ treatment requirement and effect to be achieved
☐ false individual flare lash
☐ false strip lash
☐ manufacturer's instructions complied with

EYELASH PERMING

☐ skin sensitivity test carried out
☐ rod size selected to suit client's lash length and effect to be achieved
☐ treatment application time in accordance with client's eyelash hair and manufacturer's instructions

TREATMENT ADVICE

Eyebrow shape – *allow 15 minutes*
Eyebrow tint – *allow 10 minutes*
Eyelash tint* – *allow 20 minutes*
Eyebrow shape and eyelash tint* – *allow 30 minutes*
Perming* – *allow 45 minutes*

Eyebrow tint, shape and lash tint* – *allow 30 minutes*
False eyelashes – *allow 20 minutes*
*Eyelash tint timing and perming may differ according to the system used. Always follow the manufacturer's instructions.

Beauty therapist signature (for reference)

Client signature (confirmation of details)

A sample client record card (continued)

TREATMENT PLAN

Record relevant details of your treatment and advice provided for future reference. Ensure the client's records are up to date, accurate and fully completed following treatment. Non-compliance may invalidate insurance.

DURING
Find out:

◆ what products the client is currently using to cleanse and care for the skin of the eye area
◆ satisfaction with these products.

Explain:

◆ how the different eye products should be applied and removed.

Note:

◆ any adverse reaction (contra-action), if any occur.

AFTER
Record:

◆ results of treatment
◆ any modification to treatment application that has occurred
◆ what products have been used in the eyelash/eyebrow treatment
◆ the effectiveness of treatment
◆ any samples provided (review their success at the next appointment).

Advise on:

◆ product application and removal in order to gain maximum benefit from product use
◆ use of aftercare products following eye treatment
◆ use of skincare/make-up products following eye treatment
◆ maintenance procedures
◆ recommended time intervals between treatments.

RETAIL OPPORTUNITIES
Advise on:

◆ progression of the **treatment plan** for future appointments
◆ products that would be suitable for the client to use at home to care for the eye area
◆ recommendations for further treatments
◆ further products or treatments that the client may or may not have received before.

Note:

◆ any purchase made by the client.

EVALUATION
Record:

◆ comments on the client's satisfaction with the treatment
◆ if poor results are achieved, the reasons why
◆ how you may alter the treatment plan to achieve the required treatment results in the future, if applicable.

HEALTH AND SAFETY
Advise on:

◆ how to care for the area following treatment to avoid an unwanted reaction
◆ avoidance of any activities or product application that may cause a contra-action
◆ appropriate necessary action to be taken in the event of an unwanted skin or eye irritation.

Tint eyebrow and lashes consultation

Reception

When making an appointment for this treatment, allow 5 minutes for a skin sensitivity test, 10 minutes for an eyebrow tint, and 20 minutes for an eyelash tint. When the client is booking a treatment, ask them:

◆ to visit the salon 24 hours before the appointment for a skin sensitivity test

◆ if they wear contact lenses, to bring their lens container so that they can place the lenses in it during the tinting treatment.

On average, a client will need their lashes tinted every 6 weeks or sooner, if for example, they take a holiday in a climate where sun bleaches them. Eyebrow tinting, on the other hand, should be repeated when the client feels it to be necessary, perhaps every 4 weeks, as eyebrows seem to lose colour intensity more quickly than lash hair.

Skin sensitivity test

Some clients are sensitive to the tint, and produce an allergic reaction immediately on contact with it; others may become allergic later. For this you therefore need to carry out a skin sensitivity test before each lash- or brow-tinting treatment. (For the skin sensitivity test, a hypersensitivity test, or a predisposition test.) A small amount of hydrogen peroxide and permanent dye which is the colour to be applied is mixed together and applied to the skin which has been previously cleaned. This test should be given either on the inside of the elbow or behind the ear. The test should be performed 24–28 hours before the treatment but always follow your manufacturer's instructions for the product used.

Two responses to the skin sensitivity test are possible: positive and negative:

◆ a **positive skin sensitivity test** result is recognized by irritation, swelling or inflammation of the skin – if this occurs, do not proceed with the treatment. The client should be advised to contact the salon in the instance of a positive skin test result and the product should be removed immediately from the skin.

◆ a **negative skin sensitivity test** result produces no skin reaction – in this case you may proceed with the treatment.

The results should be recorded on the client's record card for insurance purposes. Non-compliance with skin testing procedure if required will invalidate your insurance.

Contra-indications

When a client attends for an eyelash or brow tinting treatment, the beauty therapist should always check that there are no contra-indications that might prevent treatment.

After completing the record card and inspecting the eye area, if you have found any of the following in the eye area, do not proceed with the tinting treatment:

◆ *inflammation or swelling* – the cause may be medical

◆ *skin disease*

◆ *skin disorder*, such as severe psoriasis or eczema

◆ *cuts and abrasions* – secondary infection and irritation of the skin could occur

◆ *hypersensitive skin* – the skin could become excessively red and swollen

- **any eye disorders**, such as conjunctivitis, blepharitis, styes or hordeola, watery eye, or cysts
- **a positive (allergic) reaction** to the skin sensitivity test
- **contact lenses** (unless removed).

Refer back to the chart illustrating contra-indications to eye treatments on page 278.

Remember, you are not qualified to diagnose a contra-indication. Refer the client to their GP without causing unnecessary cause for concern.

A particularly nervous client would also be contra-indicated:

- it would be difficult for them to keep their eyes closed for 10 minutes
- they might panic as the tint was applied, creating the possibility of tint entering the eye
- they might blink frequently, making preparation of the eye area and application of the tint both difficult and hazardous.

Inform the client at consultation of any relevant contra-actions that may occur and the action to take.

Contra-actions

If the client complains of discomfort during the treatment, tint may have entered the eye. Take the following action:

1. Remove the tint immediately from the eye area, using clean, damp cotton wool pads in an outward sweep.

2. When you are satisfied that all excess tint has been removed (that is, when the cotton wool shows clean), carefully flush the eye with clean water. Repeat the rinsing process until discomfort has been relieved.

3. Apply a cool compress to cool and soothe the eye area.

If there is a noticeable sensitivity of the eye tissue after eyebrow or eyelash tinting it may be recommended that the client does not receive the treatment again. Alternatively, source another tinting product to test compatibility. Record this on the client's record card so that the offending product may be avoided in the future.

In the event of an allergic contra-action the client should be advised to apply a cool compress and soothing agent to the skin to reduce redness and irritation. If symptoms persist they should seek medical advice.

Planning the treatment

For the eyelashes and eyebrows, select a colour that complements the client's hair **colouring characteristics** (blonde, red, dark and white), the skin colour, age and usual eye cosmetics. Always discuss the choice of colour carefully to discover your client's preference. You may ask certain questions in order to help you in your selection:

- 'What colour mascara do you normally wear?'
- 'How dark would you like your eyelashes/eyebrows?'
- 'Do you normally wear eyebrow pencil? What colour?'
- 'Have you had your eyebrows/lashes tinted before? Were you satisfied with the result?'

ACTIVITY

Allergic reactions

With colleagues, discuss the possible implications that could result from not carrying out a skin sensitivity test and ignoring a positive reaction to the skin test.

ACTIVITY

Explaining poor results

What reasons can you think of to explain why a permanent tint applied to the eyelashes or eyebrows has not coloured the hair successfully? Discuss your answers with your tutor.

HEALTH & SAFETY

Contra-action: allergy to tinting product Source an alternative manufacturer. The client may not be allergic to all products if the cause of the contra-action is allergy.

> " At an interview you don't need to brag, or tell people how fabulous you are; your passion, hard work and the results of your work speak for themselves. Always dress smartly, presentation is key, be willing to work hard, go the extra mile and have attention to detail, these points make ALL the difference.
>
> *Shavata Singh*

False eyelash consultation

Reception

When making an appointment for false eyelash application, find out why the client wants false lashes and determine which type would be most appropriate.

Allow 20 minutes for the application of false individual eyelashes, and again allow a further 45 minutes if applying them in conjunction with a make-up.

Although false individual flare lashes can be worn for up to 6 weeks, they look effective only for approximately 3 weeks. After this time, the appearance of the **false lashes** begins to deteriorate, the lash **adhesive** becomes brittle, and the eyelash area may become irritated.

Due to the cyclic nature of hair replacement, some false individual flare lashes will be lost when the natural lash falls out. These lashes may be replaced each week, as necessary; the client is usually charged a price for each false individual flare lash replaced. The client must be told of this treatment as part of the **aftercare advice**.

When a client makes an appointment for an false lash treatment, they should be asked the following questions:

◆ *Have they had a similar treatment before in this salon?* If they have not, they should visit the salon beforehand for a skin test to assess any sensitivity to the adhesive. Commonly, a small amount of the eyelash adhesive is placed behind the ear. A positive skin reaction where the skin becomes reddened, irritated and swollen means that you cannot proceed with the treatment. A negative skin sensitivity test produces no skin reaction – in this case you may proceed with the treatment. Results should be recorded on the client record card for insurance purposes.

◆ *Are they having the false eyelashes applied for any particular reason, such as a holiday or a special occasion?* In deciding which type of false eyelash would be most appropriate, take into consideration the effect required and for how long the false lashes are to be worn.

If the client wears glasses, the false lashes must not be so long as to touch the lenses. Also, if the lens magnifies the eye, this must be taken into account. Ask the client to bring their glasses with them to the salon.

The client should be shown through to the prepared work area after the record card has been completed.

Consult the record card and check the area for any contra-indications to treatment.

Remember always to provide the opportunity for your client to ask any questions relating to the eye treatment.

False lash adhesive skin sensitivity patch test

Contra-indications

If, following completion of the record card or inspection of the eye area, you have found any of the following, do not apply false eyelashes:

◆ *skin disease*

◆ *skin disorder in the eye area*, such as severe psoriasis or eczema

◆ *inflammation or swelling* around the eye

◆ *hypersensitive skin*

◆ *any eye disorder*, such as styes or hordeola, conjunctivitis, blepharitis, watery eye, or cysts

◆ *a positive (allergic) reaction* to the adhesive skin test

◆ *contact lenses* (unless removed).

A chart is shown on page 278 illustrating some additional contra-indications to eye treatments.

Remember, you are not qualified to diagnose a contra-indication. Refer the client to their GP without causing unnecessary cause for concern.

An unduly nervous client with a tendency to blink could also prove hard to treat in this way. Use your discretion in deciding on the suitability of a client for treatment.

Inform the client at consultation of any relevant contra-actions that may occur and the action to take.

Contra-actions

If, during application of false lashes, the eye starts to water, blot the tears with the corner of a clean tissue. The tears can cause the adhesive to take on an unsightly white crystallized appearance. Any possible irritation of the eyes should therefore be avoided, during both preparation of the eye area and application itself.

Never place eyelashes *underneath* the natural eyelashes – eye irritation would occur.

While practising false individual eyelash application you may find at some point that you have accidentally glued a couple of the lower and upper natural lashes together. Apply adhesive **solvent** to a cotton wool-tipped orange stick, and gently roll this over the lash length to dissolve the adhesive.

If solvent or adhesive should accidentally enter the eye, remove excess product, rinse the eye thoroughly and immediately, using clean water. Repeat this until discomfort is no longer experienced.

The record card should be signed and dated by the client and beauty therapist following the consultation to confirm the suitability and consent with the agreed treatment.

It is important that accurate records are kept and stored in compliance with the Data Protection Act for future reference.

Planning the treatment

A variety of false lashes are available, including lashes intended for corrective work as well as those simply intended to enhance the natural lashes. Lash length may be short, medium or long; their texture may be fine, medium or thick, with differing lash shapes. Strips designed for use on the lower lashes are called partial lashes: here small groups of hairs are placed intermittently along the length of the false-lash base. These may be applied to the upper lashes also to thicken finer lashes, whilst achieving a natural look.

TOP TIP

Fair lashes

If the client has fair lashes, you could promote an eyelash tint treatment before false eyelash application to achieve a more natural, realistic effect.

TOP TIP

Achieve a natural look

False individual flare lashes may be applied in a variety of lengths, short, medium and long, to create a natural look. The longest lashes are applied in the centre of the lashes.

TOP TIP

Streaked lashes

Streaked lashes can be sourced, to give a more subtle effect for the mature client.

Artificial false strip lashes

Heavy, high definition false strip lash

Short and stubby lashes

Sparse lashes

Curly eyelashes

Short and stubby lashes, sparse lashes and curly eyelashes

Partial strip false lash

In a commercial salon, the most popular colours are usually black and brown. For special effects, however, false strip lashes are available in fantasy colours, complete with glitter and jewels!

Factors when choosing false eyelashes

Before applying false lashes the beauty therapist should consider the following points and advise the client accordingly.

The client's age False lashes create a very bold, dramatic effect, which can make an older client look too hard. Remember that the skin colour and the natural hair colour change with age: the lash chosen must enhance the client's appearance.

The client's natural lashes Does the client have short or long, sparse or thick, very curly or straight lashes? Choose an false lash to complement the natural lash. Here are some guidelines:

◆ *Short and stubby lashes* These are commonly seen on older clients who have overhanging eyelids. Choose a medium lash length in a medium thickness at the outer corner of the eyelid; the lashes should become gradually shorter from the centre of the eyelid to the inner corner. Brush the false and natural lashes together after application to ensure that they blend.

◆ *Sparse lashes* Place individual short false lashes along the natural lash line; or, to give a more natural appearance, you may wish to apply partial strip false lashes to the upper eyelid.

◆ *Curly eyelashes* These are very common on African clients. Choose a longer, sweeping strip or individual false lashes, in black. The chosen lashes and colour should give emphasis and depth to the eye.

The natural eyelash colour Select false lashes that complement the hair and skin colour. Natural-hair false eyelashes offer the greatest choice of colour, but these are expensive and may be difficult to source.

Eye shape		Corrective steps
	Small eyes	Place false lashes at the outer corners of the upper eyelid. These should be longer than the natural lashes
	Close-set eyes	Place fine, long, individual or partial lashes at the outer third of the eye. They may be applied to the lower lashes as well as to the upper
	Wide-set eyes	Apply medium-length lashes at the inner corner of the eye and to the centre, becoming slightly shorter towards the outer corner of the upper eyelid. This may be repeated on the lower lash also
	Downward-slanting eyes	Apply longer lashes (individual or partial false strip lashes) to the outer corners of the upper eyelid
	Round eyes	Individual or false strip lashes should be used to lengthen the lash line. Apply the false lashes from the centre of the upper eyelid outwards

Eye shape	Corrective steps
Deep-set eyes	Apply fine lashes to the upper and lower lashes. The upper-lid false lashes should be longer, to draw attention to the eye
Overhanging lids	Apply longer lashes to the upper eyelid, from the outer corner and tapering to a shorter length at the centre of the lid and towards the inner corner

Using false eyelashes for corrective purposes Here are some outlines of corrective techniques for various eye shapes.

On completion, the false lashes should give a balanced and well-proportioned look complementing the client's eye shape, and producing the agreed desired effect.

Eyelash perming consultation

Reception

When making the appointment for eyelash perming, recommend that the client has a skin sensitivity test. Ask them to visit the salon for this 24 hours before the appointment.

If they wear contact lenses, ask them to bring the lens container so that they can place the lenses in it during the eyelash perming treatment.

Advise the client that the treatment requires that they keep their eyes closed for a long time. Some clients may find this uncomfortable, and may choose not to have the treatment.

The client should not have an eyelash tint immediately before perming, as the colour for the lashes will be lightened by the treatment process. However, tinting is effective following eyelash perming and should be promoted. Allow a minimum of 24 hours following the eyelash perming treatment before tinting.

On average, a client will need their eyelashes permed every 2 to 3 months. A treatment takes approximately 45 minutes.

Contra-indications

When a client attends for an eyelash perming treatment, the beauty therapist should always check that there are no contra-indications that might prevent the treatment.

If following completion of the record card or inspection of the eye area you have found any of the following, do not carry out eyelash perming:

◆ *inflammation or swelling* – the cause may be medical

◆ *skin disease*

◆ *skin disorder*, such as psoriasis or eczema

◆ *cuts and abrasions* – secondary infection and irritation of the skin could occur

◆ *hypersensitive skin* – the skin could become excessively red and swollen

◆ *any eye disorders*, such as conjunctivitis, blepharitis, styes or hordeola, watery eye, or cysts

◆ *a positive (allergic) reaction* to the skin sensitivity test

Knowledge Check

Why is a skin sensitivity test needed before every tinting/perming and false individual flare lash treatment?

Refer to page 291 to help you.

ALWAYS REMEMBER

When not to perm the eyelashes

Permanent curling is not advisable if the lashes are:

◆ naturally curly (unnecessary treatment outcome)

◆ very short and sparse (the result will be ineffective)

◆ fragile (hair breakage may occur).

HEALTH & SAFETY

Perm lotion containing lanolin Some eyelash perming lotions contain lanolin. If using such lotions, ask the client before application if they are allergic to lanolin.

◆ *contact lenses* (unless removed)

◆ *considerable nervousness* – a particularly nervous client may make application, fixing and removal hazardous.

Refer to the earlier chart illustrating contra-indications to eye treatments on page 278.

Remember, you are not qualified to diagnose a contra-indication. Refer the client to their GP without causing unnecessary cause for concern.

Inform the client at consultation of any relevant contra-actions that may occur and the action to take.

Skin sensitivity test

Some clients may be sensitive to the perm solution, and may produce an allergic reaction immediately on contact with it; others may become allergic later. For this reason, a skin sensitivity test must be carried out before each eyelash perming treatment. This is essential not just for new clients, but also if there has been a lengthy interval since the previous eyelash perming treatment.

1 Apply a small amount of the perm solution and a small amount of the fixing lotion to the inside of the elbow or behind the ear.

2 Test the client tolerance to the adhesive by applying a small amount of the adhesive to the inside of the elbow or behind the ear.

Avoid immediate contact with clothing.

3 Advise the client how to recognize a positive skin reaction: skin reddening, itching and swelling. Advise them to apply a soothing agent if this occurs and to notify you. This reaction can then be recorded on the client's record card. Non-compliance with skin testing procedure if required will invalidate your insurance.

Never be tempted to cut corners, always strive to be the best you possibly can. Always listen to what your client wants and never be afraid to ask questions. Always be discreet with other staff and clients.

Shavata Singh

Contra-actions

If the client complains of discomfort during the treatment, perm lotion may have entered the eye. Take the following action:

1 Remove the perm lotion immediately from the eye area, using clean, damp cotton wool. Remove the perm rod, using the moisturizing agent if necessary to facilitate.

2 Carefully flush the eye with clean water. Repeat the rinsing process until discomfort has been relieved.

3 Apply a cool compress to sooth the eye area.

Record this information on their record card.

Discuss possible contra-actions that may occur during or after the eyelash perming treatment with your client at consultation.

Undesirable perm results	Possible cause	Preventative action
Hooked end	Incorrect positioning of the point of the eyelash hair around the rod	Ensure that the point of the eyelash is corrected if it appears crooked before application of the perm lotion. Use eyelash adhesive to secure hair into the desired position
Poor curl result	Incorrect preparation of the lashes; oil present on the lashes. Eyelashes too damp before perm lotion application. Uneven application of the perm/fixing/neutralizing lotion. Incorrect rod size for the hair	Ensure that the lashes are clean and excess moisture removed before perm lotion application. Ensure that the lashes are brushed through to separate the ends before rod application. Be methodical in application of perm/fixing neutralizing lotions to ensure effective curl result. Select the correct rod size for the lash length and coarseness of the hair. Use a reliable timing device to ensure accuracy of the timing process
Hairs pointing in different directions	Incorrect placing of the eyelash hair along the eyelash rod	Ensure the hairs are evenly placed and secured along the eyelash rod
Vertical not curled	This tends to occur on short lashes where small rods have been selected and the perm lotion has been applied to the majority of the length of the hair: from the base of the lashes the hair stands vertically	Ensure correct application of the perm lotion
Too curled	Rods too small for the eyelash length	Ensure that the correct rod is chosen for the lash length and thickness

Planning the treatment

The eyelash rod should be selected to suit the natural eyelash hair and length.

The eyelash rod should be measured against the client's eyelid and trimmed to the appropriate length.

Trimming the eyelash curler length

Small rods are suitable for short eyelashes or if a tighter curl is required

Medium rods are suitable for average length lashes and will produce a defined curl

Large rods are suitable for longer lashes and will produce a gently defined curl

Eyebrow shaping

Outcome 2: Provide eyelash and brow treatments

Learn how to provide eyelash and eyebrow treatments

PRACTICAL SKILLS

Communicate and behave in a professional manner

Follow health and safety working practices

Position yourself and the client correctly throughout the treatment

Use products, tools, equipment and techniques to suit client's treatment needs

Complete the treatment to the satisfaction of the client

Record the results of the treatment

Provide suitable aftercare advice

UNDERPINNING KNOWLEDGE

State how to communicate and behave in a professional manner

Describe health and safety working practices

Explain the importance of positioning yourself and the client correctly throughout the treatment

Explain the importance of using products, tools, equipment and techniques to suit client's treatment needs

Describe how treatments can be adapted to suit client treatment needs and facial characteristics

Describe the normal reaction of the skin to eyebrow shaping treatments

State the contra-actions that may occur during and following treatments and how to respond

Describe the chemical reaction which creates the tinting effect

State the importance of completing the treatment to the satisfaction of the client

State the importance of completing treatment records

State the aftercare advice that should be provided

Describe the structure and function of the skin and hair

Describe diseases and disorders of the skin and hair

Eyebrow shaping

1   Position the cold light magnifying lamp to give maximum visibility of the area.

2   Position the client on the couch or chair.

3   Clean your hands using an approved hand cleaning technique.

4   Secure a clean headband in place, to keep client's hair away from treatment area.

5   Working from behind the client, cleanse the eyebrow area, using a lightweight cleansing lotion or eye make-up remover. Apply a mild antiseptic lotion to two damp cotton wool pads, then gently wipe each eyebrow. (This removes all grease from the area, so that the tweezers will not slip.) The brow area should then be blotted dry, using a clean, folded facial tissue.

6   Brush the brow hair with the disposable brush, first *against* the natural hair growth, then with it. This enables you to define the brow shape and to observe the natural line.

7   Measure the brows (using the guidelines on page 283).

8   Place a clean piece of cotton wool in a convenient position for collecting the removed hairs, for instance at the top of the couch next to the client's head.

9   Best practice is to wear disposable gloves, as you may come into contact with body tissue fluid.

10 Begin tweezing, using a sterilized pair of automatic tweezers. These are designed to remove hairs quickly and efficiently, and are therefore used for the bulk of the hair identified for removal. It is usual to start at the bridge of the nose: the skin here is less sensitive than under the brow line.

11 Gently stretch the skin between the index and middle fingers, pressing lightly onto the skin. This will help you to avoid accidentally nipping the skin; it will also open the mouth of the hair follicle and minimize discomfort to the client.

12 Remove the hairs quickly, in the direction of growth. This prevents the hairs from breaking off at the skin's surface. Hair breakage can be seen to have occurred if a stubbly regrowth appears 1 or 2 days after shaping. Incorrect removal may also cause distortion of the hair follicle, or result in the hair becoming trapped under the skin as it starts to regrow (***ingrowing hair*** – see page 538).

Hairs should be removed individually, and the tweezers should be wiped regularly on the pad of clean cotton wool used to collect the removed hairs.

13 Remove the hairs from underneath the outer edge of the brow, working inwards towards the nose. It is advisable to work on each brow alternately. This ensures that the brows are evenly shaped; it also reduces prolonged discomfort in any one area during shaping. Hairs should ideally be removed only from *below* the brow, otherwise the natural line may be lost. It is sometimes necessary, however, to remove the odd stray hair growing *above* the natural line.

During shaping, show the client their brows and avoid removing too much hair.

TOP TIP

Preparing the client for eyebrow shaping

It is often stated that before beginning shaping, the brows should be prepared with warm, damp cotton wool pads, to relax the hair follicles and soften the eyebrow tissue, thus making hair removal easier. During treatment, however, you will be wiping over the area with an antiseptic lotion, which has a cooling, soothing and tightening effect on the skin, so this preparation is often ineffectual but is relaxing for the client.

HEALTH & SAFETY

Cross-infection Use a fresh cotton wool pad for wiping over each eyebrow during eyebrow shaping treatment to avoid cross-infection.

TOP TIP

Atchoo!

Occasionally clients start sneezing when you tweeze hairs at the bridge of the nose. If this happens, leave this area till last.

ALWAYS REMEMBER

New hair growth following treatment

Twenty per cent of hairs are not visible above the skin's surface at any one time. Explain this to the client so that they understand why stray hairs may appear shortly after treatment.

14   At regular intervals during shaping, brush the brows to check their shape. Apply antiseptic lotion or gel to a clean, dampened cotton wool pad, and wipe this gently over the eyebrow tissue to reduce sensitivity and to sanitize the area.

15   When the bulk of excess hair has been removed, manual tweezers may be used to take away any stray hairs and to define the line. Long hairs may be trimmed with scissors if necessary. Any discoloured, coarse, long, curly or wavy hairs may be removed, as long as this does not alter the line or leave a bald patch.

Brush the brows into shape and show the client the finished effect. The client may wish further hairs to be removed. Ask them to identify these. If you think this would be unsuitable explain why.

16   On completion of brow shaping, wipe the eyebrows with the antiseptic soothing lotion or gel, applied with clean, damp cotton wool. Apply a mild antiseptic cream to the area, using clean, dry cotton wool, to reduce the possibility of infection.

17   The hairs that have been removed should be disposed of hygienically.

18   Record details of the treatment on the client's record card.

STEP-BY-STEP: EYEBROW SHAPING

4 Protecting client's hair with headband – good hygiene working practice

5 Cleansing the eyebrow

6 Brushing the eyebrow

7 Measuring the eyebrow: the inner corner of the eye

7 continued. Measuring the eyebrow: the outer corner of the eye

7 continued. Measuring the eyebrow: the arch

10 Tweezing at the bridge of the nose using automatic tweezers

10 continued. Tweezing at the outer corner of the eyebrow using automatic tweezers

10 continued. Tweezing using manual tweezers to define the finished eyebrow shape

13 Applying antiseptic and soothing lotion

14 Brushing the eyebrow into shape

16 The complete eyebrows after shaping

Tinting the eyebrows and lashes

How to prepare the client

The client should be shown through to the cubicle after the record card has been completed.

1 Position the client comfortably, in a flat or slightly elevated position considering client preference. If they are wearing contact lenses, these must be removed.

2 Drape a towel across the client's chest and shoulders, and protect their hair with a clean headband.

3 Wash your hands, which assures the client that the treatment is beginning in a hygienic and professional manner.

4 Consult the client's record card, then check the area for any visible contra-indications or abnormalities before proceeding.

5 Cleanse the area to be treated with a cleansing milk to dissolve facial make-up (if worn). Then use a non-oily eye make-up remover to remove eye products: apply this with clean, damp cotton wool.

6 To ensure that the area is thoroughly clean and grease-free, apply a mild toning lotion, stroked over the lash or brow hair.

Knowledge Check

How can you ensure that the hairs are removed at their root?

Refer to page 295, procedure no 11 to help you.

CourseMate video: Eyebrow Tinting

7 Blot the eyelashes or eyebrows dry with a clean facial tissue. This ensures that the tint is not diluted, and also prevents the tint from being carried into the eye. Brush through the brows to separate the hair using a disposable brush. Note the fair root at the lash base.

8 Prepare the pre-shaped eye shields by applying petroleum jelly to the inner surface of each eye shield (the surface that comes into contact with the skin).

9 Ensure that the light is not shining directly into the client's eyes. If it were, the eyes might water, carrying the tint into the eye or down the face (causing skin or hair staining).

10 Finally, check that the client is comfortable before beginning the tint application.

11 Best practice is to wear disposable gloves to avoid contact with the tint that could lead to skin staining and possibly **contact dermatitis**. If worn, put on at this stage.

STEP-BY-STEP: PREPARING THE CLIENT

5 Cleansing the eye

6 Apply a mild toning lotion

7 Blotting the brow hair to remove moisture

Tinting the eyelashes

1 Remove some petroleum jelly from its container, using a new disposable spatula.

2 Working from behind the client, ask the client to open their eyes and to look upwards towards you. Using a disposable brush, apply petroleum jelly underneath the lower lashes of one eye, ensuring that it extends at the outer corner of the eye. (This is in case the client's eyes water slightly during service, which might otherwise lead to skin staining.) The petroleum jelly must not come into contact with the lash hair, where it would create a barrier to the tint.

3 Place the prepared eye shield on the skin under the lower lashes, ensuring that it adheres to the petroleum jelly and fits 'snugly' to the base of the lower lashes.

4 Repeat the above process for the other eye.

5 Ask the client to close their eyes gently. Instruct them not to open them again until you advise them to do so, in about 10 minutes' time.

6 Apply petroleum jelly to the upper eyelid, in a line on the skin at the base of the lashes.

7   Considering the length and density of the client's eyelashes, mix the required amount of tint with 10-volume (3%) hydrogen peroxide. As a guide, a 5mm length of tint from the tube, mixed with two or three drops of hydrogen peroxide, is usually sufficient. Mix the products to a smooth cream in the tinting bowl, using the disposable brush. Always recap bottles and tubes tightly after use, to avoid deterioration of materials.

8   Wipe excess tint off the brush onto the inside of the bowl. Apply the tint thinly to each hair. Work from the base of the lash to the tip, ensuring that each hair is evenly covered. Press down gently with the applicator to ensure that the lower lashes also are covered. The few inner and outer lashes should also be covered, down to the base. Remove any excess tint from the skin with a clean cotton bud.

9   Allow the tint to process, for approximately 5 to 10 minutes from the completion of application. Discard any unused mixture as soon as the tint has been applied.

10 On completion of processing, remove the eyelash tint by applying clean, damp cotton wool pads over each eye, wiping away most of the tint and removing the protective eye shield in one movement, an outward sweep. Using fresh dampened cotton wool pads, gently stroke down the lashes from roots to tips, until all excess tint has been removed. With a sweeping action on each eye and using one cotton wool pad, wipe from the side to the middle against the lash growth, while the other hand supports the eye tissue. ***All tint must be thoroughly removed before the client opens their eyes.***

11 Ask the client to open their eyes. If removal has been correctly carried out, the lashes and their bases will be free from tint. (While training, if any tint remains at the base of the lashes after the eyes have been opened, ask the client to close her eyes again and finish the removal process using clean, damp cotton wool.) Check that every lash has been tinted, especially the base of each lash and the inner and outer corner lashes. Show the client the result, ensuring the colour is dark enough and that they are satisfied with the final effect.

12 Once you are satisfied that all tint has been removed, place a cool, damp cotton wool pad over each eye for 2 to 3 minutes to soothe the eye tissue.

13 Record details of the treatment on the client's record card.

ALWAYS REMEMBER

Protection of work surfaces

Make sure that work surfaces are protected with disposable coverings, to prevent permanent staining following spillages.

TOP TIP

Client communication during eyelash tinting procedure

Speak to your client as you apply the eyelash tint. Check that they are comfortable and understand what you are doing. Remember: the eyes are very sensitive and will water readily.

CourseMate video: Eyelash Tinting

HEALTH & SAFETY

Using tints Always read the manufacturer's instructions carefully before using a permanent tint. Instructions on usage may vary between brands.

STEP-BY-STEP: TINTING THE EYELASHES

1 Use a disposable spatula for the petroleum jelly

2 Apply petroleum jelly to prevent skin staining

3 Placement of eye shield

6 Application of petroleum jelly to upper eyelid

7 Mix the tint and hydrogen peroxide according to manufacturer's instructions

8 Applying the tint to the eyelashes

8 continued. Removal of any excess tint with a cotton bud

9 Processing the tint

10 Removing the tint

12 The completed eyelash tint

TOP TIP

Thorough tint removal

Use a cotton bud to remove any excess tint from along the lash line on removal.

HEALTH & SAFETY

Client comfort The client should not be left during the lash-tinting service. You must be available both to offer reassurance and to take the necessary action if the eyes water.

If the eyes do water while the eyes are closed, hold a tissue at the corner of the eye to soak up the moisture. Take further action if watering persists and the eyes begin to sting.

Tinting the eyebrows

1 Remove some petroleum jelly from its container, using a new disposable spatula.

2 Brush the brow hair away from the skin, using a disposable brow brush (as shown in the picture).

3 Using a disposable brush, surround each eyebrow with petroleum jelly, as close as possible to the brow hair (to avoid skin staining).

4 Mix approximately 5 mm of the chosen tint colour with two or three drops of 10-volume (3%) hydrogen peroxide in a tinting bowl. Ensure that the tint is mixed thoroughly to a creamy consistency, according to the manufacturer's instructions.

5 Wipe excess tint off the brush onto the inside of the tinting bowl. Apply the tint neatly and economically to the brow hair of the first eyebrow; ensuring that the brow hairs, from the base to the tips, are evenly covered (as shown in the picture).

6 Apply the tint to the second eyebrow; following the same procedure.

7 Immediately after application of the tint to the second eyebrow, remove the tint from the first eyebrow. Use a clean dampened cotton wool pad. Place it on the eyebrow, then wipe it across the eyebrow in an outward sweep, removing the excess tint. Ensure that all traces of excess tint have been removed, to prevent skin staining.

Never leave tint on the eyebrows for longer than 2 minutes. Eyebrow hair colour develops much more quickly than lash hair.

8 Remove the tint from the second eyebrow in the same way.

Show the client the effect of the tinted eyebrows. If the brow hair is not dark enough, reapply the tint to the eyebrow hair, following the same application and removal procedure. Note this on the client's record card.

When you are both satisfied with the colour of the tinted eyebrows, complete the client's record card by recording details of the service.

9 The completed effect, showing both eyelash and eyebrow tint.

TOP TIP

Application of tint to brow hair

To ensure even coverage of brow hair, use a brush to lift the hair to enable application at the roots of the hair to mid-length of the hair shaft.

Knowledge Check

How should you select the tint colour when carrying out a permanent tinting service?

Refer to pages 287–288 to help you.

ALWAYS REMEMBER

The effect of tinting depends on the natural colour:

◆ *Blonde hair* develops colour rapidly – if the tint is left on the eyebrow too long, a harsh, unnatural appearance will be created.

◆ *Red/grey hair* is more resistant to the tint, and developing will take a little longer – allow 15 minutes' processing time when tinting lash hair.

◆ *Dark hair* requires tinting to increase the intensity of the natural eyebrow colour, giving a glossy, conditioned appearance.

HEALTH & SAFETY

Skin stains If skin staining accidentally occurs, use a professional skin stain remover designed for this purpose. Afterwards, use plenty of clean, dampened cotton wool pads to avoid skin irritation.

Skin stains

Skin stains

STEP-BY-STEP: TINTING THE EYEBROWS

2 Brush the brow hair away from the skin

3 Apply petroleum jelly to prevent skin staining

5 Apply the tint to the brow hair of the first brow

6 Apply the tint to the brow hair of the second brow

7 Remove the tint from the first eyebrow

8 Remove the tint from the second eyebrow

9 The completed eyebrow tint

Client suitability is checked at the start of treatment when the client's requirements are confirmed

Applying false lashes

How to prepare the client

Show the client through to the prepared work area after the record card has been completed. Consult the record card and check the area for any contra-indications to treatment.

1 Position the client comfortably on the treatment couch or beauty chair (which should be slightly elevated). If the client wears contact lenses, these must be removed before the treatment begins.

2   Drape a clean towel across the client's chest and shoulders. Protect their hair with a clean headband.

3   Wash your hands, which indicates to the client that treatment is beginning and in a hygienic and professional manner.

4   It is usual to carry out a full facial cleanse (rather than cleansing only the eye area), as make-up is usually applied to complement the false individual flare eyelashes. Use a cleansing milk to dissolve facial make-up, followed by a non-oily eye make-up remover to cleanse the eye area. Both products should be removed with clean, damp cotton wool.

5   To ensure that the eye tissue and eyelashes are thoroughly clean and grease-free, apply a mild oil-free toning lotion: stroke this over the skin using clean, damp cotton wool.

6   Blot the lashes dry, using a fresh facial tissue for each eye. (Any moisture left on the natural lashes will reduce the effectiveness of the eyelash adhesive.)

7   Apply make-up to complement the effect achieved. Brush the natural lashes to separate them before application.

Special occasion make-up is applied and the natural lashes are brushed before application of individual flare false lashes

How to apply false individual flare lashes

STEP-BY-STEP: FALSE INDIVIDUAL FLARE LASH APPLICATION

7 False individual flare lash positioned

8 Apply the false lashes one at a time

1   Check that everything you need is on the trolley.

2   Check that the back of the couch or beauty chair is slightly raised, at a height that is comfortable for you.

3   Discuss the service procedure with the client. Explain that they will be required to keep their eyes open during the service. Reassure them that they may blink during application. Very often clients feel that they shouldn't, and their eyes begin to water.

ALWAYS REMEMBER

False lash adhesive

Do not prepare the lash adhesive until you are ready to use it. It tends to dry on contact with air.

TOP TIP

Positioning

When applying the false individual flare lashes to the inner portion of the eyelid, hold the skin taut, stretching the skin slightly. This will enable you to position the false lash more easily.

TOP TIP

Keep a grip

Use a clean pair of tweezers to remove the false individual flare lashes from their container when required. Holding the tweezers firmly, grip each lash near its base (this avoids misshaping the outer lash hairs).

TOP TIP

Clean tweezer tips

To ensure efficient false lash application, don't get adhesive on the points of the tweezers.

TOP TIP

Practice makes perfect

Positioning the false individual flare lashes correctly requires experience. It is a good idea initially to practise application without adhesive.

Step **10** Finished look. Short false individual flare lashes applied to thicken the natural lashes

CourseMate video: False Individual Flare Lashes

Step **3** Individual lashes

4 Ask them to tilt their head downwards very slightly. This tends to lower the upper eyelids, making application easier.

5 Depending on the effect required, you may start application of the false individual flare lashes at different positions along the natural lash line. In general, apply shorter lashes to the inner corners of the eyelid, and longer lashes to the outer corners; this creates a realistic effect and ensures client comfort. If you are applying false individual flare lashes to the entire upper lid, it is practical to start application at the inner corner of the eyelid and work outwards: this follows the natural contour of the eye.

6 With the sterile tweezers, select a lash from the package, holding it near its centre. Brush the underside of the false individual flare lash, at the root, through the adhesive. The adhesive should extend slightly beyond the root. You need sufficient adhesive, but not too much – excess adhesive should be removed by wiping the lash against the inside of the adhesive container.

7 Working from behind and at the side of the client, hold the tweezers at the angle at which the false lashes will be applied to the natural lash line. Hold the brow tissue with your other hand to steady the eyelid.

Using a stroking movement, place the underside of the false lashes on top of the natural lash. Stroke the adhesive along the length of the natural eyelash. Guide the false lashes towards the base of the natural lash, so that the false lash rests along the length of the natural lash. Wait a few seconds to allow the adhesive to dry (to prevent the lashes from sticking together). Continue placing further false lashes side by side until the desired effect is achieved.

During application, keep checking your work. If a lash is out of line, remove it while the adhesive is still soft. If the adhesive has set, the lash will need to be removed using adhesive solvent.

8 Apply the false lashes one at a time, to each eye alternately. This avoids sensitizing the eye, and makes it easier for you to create a balanced effect.

9 If the client requires false lashes to be applied to the *lower* lid, the application technique is slightly different.

Work facing the client, with the client looking upwards, their eyes slightly open. Follow the same general procedure for applying the false eyelashes; here, however, the lashes curve downwards and the adhesive is applied to the upper surface of the lash.

Lashes applied to the lower eyelid are usually shorter than those chosen for the upper lid, and more adhesive is required for the lashes to be secure and have maximum durability.

10 When you have completed the lash application, ask the client to sit up, and show them the completed effect.

11 If the client is satisfied with the result, you can apply a water- or powder-based eye make-up at this stage if desired. Do not apply mascara, as this will reduce the adhesion to the natural lash. Mascara also clogs the lashes together; and is difficult to remove without affecting the **eyelash adhesive**. There are specially formulated mascaras available to be used with false lashes. On completion, the lashes can be gently brushed – using a disposable brush – to remove particles of eye shadow.

How to apply false strip lashes

Strip false eyelashes may be applied *before* carrying out the eye make-up – this avoids the eye make-up being spoilt if the eyes water slightly during application.

1 Check that everything required for the false eyelash application is available on your trolley.

2 Carefully apply moisturizer and foundation, taking care not to get any cosmetic products on the lashes. (If you do, gently wipe over the lashes with the non-oily eye make-up remover, and blot the eyelashes dry again with a clean facial tissue.)

3 Brush the lashes to separate them, using a clean disposable mascara brush. This makes application of false lashes easier, and removes any fine particles of loose powder.

4 Remove the false strip lashes from their container; and place them on a clean, disinfected palette. Each strip is designed to fit either the left or the right eye: remember which is which when placing them on the palette.

5 Check the length of the strip against the client's eyelid. The strip should never be applied directly from one corner of the eyelid to the other; but should start about 2 mm from the inner corner of the eye, and end 2 mm from the outer corner. This ensures a natural effect and maximizes the durability of the false lashes.

When you remove the false strip lash from the package you will find that there is adhesive on the backing strip, which fixes the lash in the container: this adhesive is sufficient to hold the lash onto the client's natural lash while you measure the length.

6 To trim the false strip lashes you require a sharp pair of scissors. First correct the length of the *strip* if necessary. Hold the lashes securely with one hand, and then trim the strip at the outer edge. Then trim the lashes themselves, if necessary. Never reduce the length of the lashes by cutting straight across them: the result would not look natural. Natural eyelashes are of varying lengths, due to the nature of the hair growth cycle; it is this effect that you must simulate. To shorten the lash, 'chip' into the lash. Use the *points* of the scissors to shorten the lash length. Cut the lashes so that the shorter lashes are at the inner corner of the eyelid, gradually increasing toward the outer corner.

7 The couch or beauty chair should be in a slightly raised position. During the treatment, you will be working from behind the client: the height must be comfortable for you.

8 Discuss the treatment procedure with the client. Explain to her that she will be required to keep her eyes open during the application. Ask her to tilt her head downwards very slightly – this lowers the upper eyelids, making application easier.

9 Using the sterile tweezers, remove one of the eyelash strips from the palette. Handle it very carefully, as it can easily become misshapen.

Remembering that the strip is designed to fit either the right or the left eye, place it against the appropriate eyelid and check the length (with the client's eyes closed).

10 Once satisfied that the length of the false strip lash is correct (see step 6 for reducing the length), remove the adhesive tape used to hold it in the container.

11 Place a small quantity of false strip lash adhesive on the disinfected palette. Alternatively the adhesive can be directly applied to the base of the false lash.

ALWAYS REMEMBER

Bottom lashes don't last as long

Tell the client that false lashes applied to the lower lashes tend to fall off after one week. (This is probably due to the natural watering of the eye affecting the adhesive.)

HEALTH & SAFETY

False strip lash length If the lashes were not shorter at the inner corner of the eyelid, they would irritate the client's eye.

TOP TIP

Dealing with downward growing lashes

If a client has straight eyelashes that grow downwards, curl them slightly using eyelash rods. If you don't, a gap will be visible between the real lashes and the false strip lash.

Step 6 Trimming the false strip lashes

Step **12** Adhesive applied to the false strip lash base

Step **12** Positioning the false strip lash

Step **18** Finished effect

12   Ask the client to look down slightly, with their eyes half open. With one hand lift their brow to steady the upper eyelid.

Holding the false strip lash with the sterile tweezers at its centre, drag it at its base through the adhesive. (The adhesive must be moist.) It is usually white, but when it dries it becomes colourless. Alternatively the adhesive may be applied to the false strip lash base as shown.

Position the base of the false strip lash as close as possible to the base of the natural eyelash, ensuring that it is about 2 mm in from the inner and outer corners of the eye. *Gently* press the false and natural eyelashes together with your fingertips, along the length of the lash and at the outer corners.

13   When you are sure that the first false strip lash is secure, apply the second in the same way.

14   If false strip lashes are to be applied to the bottom lashes also, apply these now, in the same way as the upper lashes. (False strip lashes for the lower lids are fine, with an extremely thin base. These lashes should be trimmed as before to ensure comfort and durability in wear.)

15   Allow 3 to 5 minutes for the adhesive to dry.

16   Gently brush the lashes from underneath the natural lash line, using a clean disposable mascara brush. This will blend the natural and false lashes together Check that both sets of lashes are correctly positioned, and that a balanced look has been achieved.

17   False lashes look more realistic if eyeliner is applied to the client's eyelid: this disguises the base of the false strip lash.

18   Show the client the finished effect.

19   When you are satisfied, record the details on the client record card.

TOP TIP

Heavy false strip lashes

Heavy false strip lashes are not suitable for fine short lashes. Extra glue may be required to ensure effective adhesion.

TOP TIP

Prevent lifting in the perm rod

Extra glue (although not excessive) may be applied to the ends of the lashes to prevent lifting while wearing them.

HEALTH & SAFETY

False individual flare lash application

Check the eyelash application as you work. Ensure that the lower and upper lashes are not stuck together, and that the eyelashes are accurately and evenly applied.

Eyelash Perming

How to prepare the client

The client should be shown through to the cubicle after the record card has been completed.

1   Position the client comfortably, in a flat or slightly elevated position. If they wear contact lenses, these must be removed.

2   Drape a towel across the client's chest and shoulders, and protect their hair with a clean headband.

3   Wash your hands. This assures the client that the treatment is beginning in a hygienic and professional manner.

4   Consult the client's record card, then check the area for any visible contra-indications or abnormalities before proceeding.

5   Cleanse the surrounding eye area with a suitable make-up cleanser (oil-free) to dissolve facial make-up. Then use a non-oily eye make-up remover to remove eye products: apply this with clean, damp cotton wool.

6   Blot the eyelashes dry with a clean facial tissue. This ensures that the perm lotion is not diluted, and also prevents the perm lotion being carried into the eye.

7   Explain the procedure to the client and tell them about the sensations they may experience during eyelash perming. Warn them that they will need to keep their eyes closed for a long period. Some clients may find this difficult, while others will enjoy this as a time of relaxation!

> **TOP TIP**
>
> **Continuing professional development**
>
> As part of your progression you may develop your skills further in the application of false lashes by learning the Level 3 Unit Single lash extensions.

> **TOP TIP**
>
> **Optimal results**
>
> If possible, after cleansing leave the eyelashes to dry for 10 minutes before perming, to ensure that the lashes are completely dry. Comb through the lashes to ensure they are evenly separated and dry. This will optimize the results.

Eyelash perming

1   Comb through the lashes to ensure they are evenly separated and dry. This will optimize the results.

2   Cleanse the eye area.

3   Ask the client to look upwards whilst you protect lower eyelashes with damp cotton wool or alternative suitable eye shield.

4   Select the correct size of rod for the client's lash length. Bend it so that it fits the contour of the eye. If the rod is too long it may be trimmed see image page 293.

5   Place the rod at the base of the upper lashes, near the inner tear duct.

6   Gently curl the natural lashes around the rod, using the disposable stick. Ensure that the lashes do not overlap each other and are straight or the ends will be 'crooked', spoiling the overall effect and appearance. A specialized adhesive may be applied to secure the lashes to the rod and keep them even and straight so that the upper and lower lashes do not come into contact.

7   When you are satisfied that the lashes are straight and that the client is comfortable, apply the perm lotion evenly to the upper lashes, using a brush, avoiding contact with the skin.

The lashes may be covered with a plastic film (clear wrap) or dry lint pads. This creates warmth which aids the perming process. Allow:

◆ 7–10 minutes for fine or previously tinted hair

◆ 10 minutes for coarse hair.

Follow manufacturer's guidance on timing as this may vary.

CourseMate video: False Strip Lash and Removal

> **TOP TIP**
>
> **Protect lower lashes**
>
> A protective damp cotton wool pad may be placed over the lower lashes to form a barrier to the perm lotion when it is being applied to the upper lashes.

> **Knowledge Check**
>
> What are the differences between the application of false strip lashes and the application of false individual flare lashes?
>
> Refer to pages 302–306 to help you.

8 Check for the desired curl before removal. Separate a couple of eyelashes from the rod, leave for 2–3 minutes longer if the curl required has not been achieved.

9 Remove the perm lotion using dry lint-free pads, gently blotting the lashes.

10 Apply the fixing/neutralizing lotion with a clean brush or applicator.

11 Cover the eyelashes with plastic film (clear wrap) or dry lint-free pads for 10 minutes, following the manufacturer's guidance.

12 Gently remove the fixing/neutralizing lotion from the eyelashes, using dry lint-free pads.

13 When all the fixing/neutralizing lotion has been removed, gently remove each rod, rolling downwards. A moisturizing agent may be applied with a cotton bud to the eyelashes to aid the removal of the rods. Wipe excess product from the lashes with damp, clean cotton wool. Brush gently though the eyelashes to define their shape and appearance.

14 Show the client the effect of their permed eyelashes in a mirror. When you are both satisfied with the result, finalize details on the client's record card. Take the client to reception to book their next appointment.

STEP-BY-STEP: EYELASH PERMING

2 Cleanse the eye area

3 Protect lower eyelashes with an eye shield

4 Select the correct size of rod for the client's lash length

6 Curl the natural lashes around the rod

6 continued Specialised adhesive application

10 Apply the fixing/neutralizing lotion

12 Remove the fixing/neutralizing lotion

13 Apply a moisturizing lotion

14 The completed permed eyelashes

Aftercare advice

Advise the client on skincare preparations to use at home to enhance the appearance of the eyebrows and lashes.

The following aftercare advice, specific to the eye treatment received, should be given to clients.

Eyebrow shape aftercare advice Advise the client to receive the treatment as follows:

◆ eyebrow maintenance every 1–2 weeks

◆ eyebrow reshaping every 3–4 weeks.

While a client receives an eyebrow shape it is an ideal opportunity to promote an eyebrow/eyelash tint.

An eyebrow pencil or powder matt cosmetic can be recommended to disguise bald patches, e.g. scars. Sparse eyebrows can be made to appear thicker. These products can also be used to simulate hairs, when the length needs to be increased. Colour should always complement hair colour. Darker colour creates a dramatic effect appropriate for evening make-up looks.

Wax sealer, a cosmetic for the brows, keeps the hair in place and can be applied over brow powder to define the brow. This is a good product to have available for retail.

Explain how to care for the area following the treatment to avoid an unwanted reaction – a contra-action. Advise the client not to wear eye make-up for at least 6 hours following the eyebrow-shaping treatment. The hair follicle has been damaged where the hair has been torn out: it will be susceptible to infection unless the area is cared for while it heals. It should not be necessary for the client to continue using antiseptic lotion at home, but they should be advised to carry out these instructions if discomfort or continued reddening occurs:

1 Explain to the client the action to take in the event of a contra-action.

2 Cleanse the eyebrow area using a mild antiseptic lotion or witch hazel, applied with a small piece of clean, dampened cotton wool.

3 Apply an antiseptic soothing lotion, cream or gel with clean, dry cotton wool.

4 Gently remove excess antiseptic lotion, cream or gel using a clean, soft facial tissue or clean damp cotton wool.

5 Repeat as necessary, approximately every 4 hours. *If the reddening does not subside in the next 24 hours, contact the salon*.

6 Eye make-up may be worn as soon as the redness has gone – usually after 8 hours.

Eyelash perming aftercare

◆ Recommend that the client receives the treatment every 2–3 months.

◆ A skin sensitivity test is required before each perming treatment.

HEALTH & SAFETY

Avoiding the possibility of secondary infection Remind the client to avoid touching the area immediately following an eyebrow shaping treatment. This is because the area is susceptible to infection and the fingers may transfer dirt, causing secondary infection.

If excess antiseptic lotion or cream is left on the area, this may attract small particles of dust, which could cause infection.

HEALTH & SAFETY

False eyelash adhesive solvents Although solvents are formulated to remove false lashes from the natural lash, great care must be taken to avoid skin/eye irritation.

TOP TIP

False eyelash solvent application

Disposable cotton buds are ideal for applying eyelash adhesive solvent.

HEALTH & SAFETY

Eye care when using false lash glue solvent Do not allow eyelash adhesive solvent to come into excessive contact with the eye tissue – it could cause irritation of the skin. Ensure that there is sufficient solvent only on the applicator: it should be moist but not dripping wet or the solvent might enter the eye.

Knowledge Check

What aftercare advice should be given to a client following an eyebrow shaping treatment?

Refer to page 309 to help you.

HEALTH & SAFETY

Client comfort Never attempt to remove the false individual flare eyelashes until they have begun to loosen – if you do, the client's natural eyelashes will also be removed, causing them discomfort.

HEALTH & SAFETY

Client comfort When removing the false strip lash, avoid pulling the natural lashes with the false lashes.

◆ Advise your client not to apply make-up for at least 24 hours to the lash area.

◆ Similarly, they should not receive any other eye treatments for at least 24 hours.

◆ Subsequently however, eyelash tinting will enhance the effect of the newly permed lashes so you can promote this treatment to the client.

Tint eyebrow and lash aftercare advice If an unwanted reaction occurs (a contra-action, e.g. irritation or redness), apply cool water or a damp cotton wool pad compress to the area.

If reddening continues after 24 hours contact the salon.

Advise the client to receive the treatment as follows:

◆ eyelash tinting every 4–6 weeks

◆ eyebrow tinting every 3–4 weeks.

False eyelash aftercare advice

◆ Provide advice on the action to take if an unwanted reaction, a contra-action, occurs.

◆ Avoid rubbing the eyes, or the lashes may become loosened.

◆ Do not use an oil-based eye make-up remover as its cosmetic constituents will dissolve the adhesive.

◆ Use only dry or water-based eye make-up (as these may readily be removed with a non-oily eye make-up remover).

◆ If the lashes are made of a synthetic material, heat will cause them to become frizzy. Advise the client to avoid extremes of temperature, such as a hot sauna.

◆ Do not touch the eyes for 1½ hours after application, while the adhesive dries thoroughly.

If the client has had false *individual* flare lashes applied, the following homecare advice should be given on caring for the lashes:

◆ use a non-oily eye make-up remover daily to cleanse the eyelids and eyelashes. Avoid contact with oil-based preparations in the eye area, such as moisturizers and cleansers – the oil content will dissolve the adhesive, and the lashes would become detached

◆ do not attempt to remove the false lashes – pulling at false lashes will also pull out the natural eyelashes

◆ after bathing or swimming, gently *pat* the eye area dry with a clean towel

◆ a disposable spiral applicator brush may be used to comb through the lashes to separate.

Clients with false individual flare eyelashes should have the false lashes maintained by regular visits to the salon. Lost false individual flare lashes can be replaced as necessary; this is often described as an eyelash *infill* treatment. Schedule this for every 10–14 days.

If the client wishes to have the individual false lashes removed, this should be done professionally.

How to remove false individual flare eyelashes

1   Position the client lying on the couch.

2   Wash your hands.

3   Remove make-up from the eye area, cleansing the skin with a suitable eye make-up remover.

4   While the client's eyes are open, place a pre-shaped eye shield underneath the lower lashes of each eye. (This will protect the eye tissue from the solvent.) Position the eye shields so that they fit snugly to the base of the lower lashes.

5   Ask the client to close their eyes gently, and not to open them again until you tell them to do so.

6   Prepare a new disposable orange stick by covering it at the pointed end with clean, dry cotton wool (or alternatively a cotton bud may be used).

7   Moisten the cotton wool with the false eyelash adhesive solvent.

8   Treating one eye at a time, gently stroke down the false eyelashes with the adhesive solvent until the adhesive dissolves and the false eyelash begins to loosen.

9   When you are satisfied that the eyelash adhesive has dissolved, gently attempt to remove the false eyelash. Support the upper eyelid with the fingers of one hand, using the other hand to remove the false lash with a sterile pair of manual tweezers. If the adhesive has been adequately dissolved, the eyelash will lift away easily from the natural eyelash. If there is any resistance, repeat the solvent application until the eyelash comes away readily.

10   As the false eyelashes are removed, collect them on a clean white facial tissue or a clean pad of cotton wool.

11   Having removed all of the false eyelashes from one eye, soothe the area by applying damp cotton wool pads soaked in cool water. (This will also remove any remaining solvent.) A damp cotton wool pad may be placed over the eye, while you remove the false lashes from the other eye.

How to remove false strip lashes

If a client wears strip false lashes, they will need instructions on how to remove and care for the false lashes themselves.

1   Use the fingertips of one hand to support the eyelid at the outer corner. With the other hand, lift the lash strip base at the outer corner of the eye. Gently peel the strip away from the natural lash, from the outer edge towards the centre of the eyelid.

2   Peel the adhesive from the backing strip, using a clean pair of manual tweezers. Take care to avoid stretching the false strip lash.

HEALTH & SAFETY

Eye care when using false lash glue solvent Do not allow eyelash adhesive solvent to come into excessive contact with the eye tissue – it could cause irritation of the skin. Ensure that there is sufficient solvent only on the applicator: it should be moist but not dripping wet or the solvent might enter the eye.

HEALTH & SAFETY

Client comfort When removing the strip false lash, avoid pulling the natural lashes with the false lashes.

HEALTH & SAFETY

Removing false individual flare lashes Never attempt to remove the artificial eyelashes until they have begun to loosen – if you do, the client's natural eyelashes will also be removed, causing them discomfort.

Removing false strip lashes from the outer corner of the eye

Support the eye as you peel the false strip lash inwards to wards the nose

HEALTH & SAFETY

False individual flare lashes The client should be advised to return to the salon for these lashes to be removed professionally due to the semi-permanent nature of the adhesive used.

Knowledge Check

What is the correct method for removing false strip lashes and false individual flare lashes?

Refer to pages 310–311 to help you.

3   Clean the false strip lash in the appropriate way.

◆ **Strips made from human hair** Clean with a commercial lash cleaner or 70% alcohol. This removes the remaining adhesive and the eye make-up.

◆ **Synthetic strips** Place in warm, soapy water for a few minutes, to clean the lashes and remove the remaining adhesive. Rinse in tepid water.

4   After cleaning, the false strip lashes should be recurled.

How to recurl false strip lashes

For reasons of hygiene and because of the time involved, this treatment will not be offered by the salon. The client, however, will need advice on how to recurl the lashes at home.

1   On removal from the water, place the lashes side by side, ensuring that the inner edges are together inside a clean facial tissue.

2   Wrap a tissue around an even, barrel-shaped object such as a felt-tip pen, and secure it with an elastic band.

3   The false lashes, inside the facial tissue, should then be rolled around this object. Keep the base of the lash straight, so that the whole lash length curls around the object.

Once recurled, the false strip lashes can be returned to their original container and stored for further use.

Recurling false strip lashes

ASSESSMENT OF KNOWLEDGE AND UNDERSTANDING

You have now learnt how to provide eyelash and brow treatments in the beauty therapy workplace. To test your level of knowledge, answer the following short questions. These will prepare you for your summative (final) assessment.

1. An allergic reaction to a skin sensitivity test is known as a:
   a. positive skin sensitivity test
   b. negative skin sensitivity test

2. The following is a contra-indication that restricts an eyebrow shaping treatment:
   a. client is undergoing chemotherapy treatment
   b. diabetes
   c. conjunctivitis
   d. severe psoriasis

3. A skin sensitivity test is carried out:
   a. 48 hours before each treatment
   b. 24–48 hours before each treatment
   c. the first time the client ever has the treatment
   d. if the client has a sensitive skin

4. If the client has a round face, an unsuitable eyebrow shape would be?
   a. round
   b. straight
   c. oblique
   d. arched

5. The method of sterilization for tweezers is:
   a. an UV cabinet
   b. a chemical disinfectant
   c. a glass bead sterilizer
   d. an autoclave

6. How often would you recommend that a client returns to the salon for an eyebrow trim?
   a. once a week
   b. every 2 weeks
   c. every 3 weeks
   d. every month

7. When applying false individual flare lashes, if the client has close-set eyes:
   a. place longer lashes at the outer third of the eyes
   b. apply medium-length lashes at the inner corner of the eye and the centre of the lash line
   c. apply longer lashes along the length of the lash line
   d. apply shorter lashes at the outer corner of the lash line and medium from the centre to the inner third of the eye

8. The small dye molecules used in permanent tinting swell and join together, trapped permanently in the:
   a. cuticle of the hair
   b. the medulla of the hair
   c. the cortex of the hair
   d. the papilla

9. How often would you recommend that a client has their eyelashes permed?
   a. every month
   b. every 2–3 months
   c. every 2 weeks
   d. every 4–6 months

10. Hair maintains its shape and strength by chemical cross bonds in the cortex (the thickest layer of the hair) called what?

9 Threading

LEARNING OBJECTIVES

There are two learning outcomes to achieve for this optional unit:

1 Be able to prepare for threading.

2 Be able to provide threading.

The assessment range applied requires you to:

◆ Use consultation techniques to identify the client's treatment objectives.

◆ Use suitable products, tools and equipment.

◆ Ensure the environmental conditions are appropriate.

◆ Identify contra-indications that may affect if and how the treatment can proceed.

◆ Communicate and behave in an appropriate and professional manner.

◆ Follow all relevant health and safety working practices.

◆ Use threading techniques to suit hair removal needs and their skin type/condition.

◆ Provide relevant aftercare and contra-action advice.

KEY TERMS

aftercare advice

client care

clinical waste

communication (verbal and
     non-verbal)

consultation

contra-action advice

contra-actions

contra-indication advice

cross-contamination

erythema

folliculitis

hand technique

health and safety

mouth technique

neck technique

threading

treatment objectives

treatment plan

Unit Topic

Provide threading treatments for hair removal

This VRQ unit is linked to the Beauty Therapy NOS Unit B34.

INTRODUCTION

This unit is about temporarily removing hair from areas of the face using threading techniques. Threading involves the use of a loop of twisted cotton thread which is passed across the skin to trap the hairs and so 'pluck' them from their follicles. There are three main methods of threading, the mouth technique, neck technique and hand technique which are discussed later in the chapter. Reference is made in the chapter to the technical skill eyebrow shaping in order that you are able to achieve different eyebrow shapes clients may require and to be able provide advice to the client on how to maintain the finished look. For further information on eyebrow shaping using tweezer hair removal technique, see Chapter 8.

Dealing with people in a polite, efficient manner and using good communication and questioning skills to find out exactly what they require from the threading treatment forms an important part of this technical treatment.

You must be able to show you have the necessary practical skills and underpinning knowledge to provide threading treatments for hair removal.

INDUSTRY ROLE MODEL

SHAVATA SINGH Founder of Shavata Brow Studios

" My career began as a beauty therapist at Michaeljohn Salon on Mayfair's Albemarle Street where I was the only threader on the team. Clients loved the results and kept coming back and this is how brows found me. Threading is a vital component of the treatments I offer in my brow studios. I maintain excellent service and the very best treatments as a central part of my business in all my studios. This philosophy reaps benefits for both clients and staff.

ANATOMY & PHYSIOLOGY
Essential anatomy and physiology knowledge requirements for this chapter are identified on the checklist chart on page 33

TOP TIP

Gentle on the skin

Threading creates less trauma on the skin than other hair removal treatments, e.g. waxing, which can cause irritation from heat, allergic reactions and possible skin removal.

HEALTH & SAFETY

Extra protection Some specialist threading thread has an anti-bacterial coating added to it during the manufacture process to give protection to the skin while performing the treatment and so reduce the risk of infection.

Introduction

History

Threading has been used for many centuries. Its origin is a little uncertain but it is believed that it was originally used in Arabia, Turkey and India.

Threading is an ancient manual method of temporary hair removal, similar to tweezing. A loop of twisted cotton thread is passed across the skin to trap the hairs and so 'pluck' them from their follicles.

Benefits of threading

Threading is simple, natural and inexpensive whilst being an efficient way of removing unwanted hair with minimal pain and skin irritation. Neat results are achieved, with hair regrowth usually seen between 2 to 6 weeks, dependent upon hair growth and type. An advantage of threading to other hair removal systems, such as waxing, is that very short hair can be removed with little irritation to the skin in the area, as the thread only removes the hair – not skin. This also makes it possible to go over the treatment area more than once. Hair can be removed individually or in 'lines', creating a precise, defined shape and can be removed from both above and below the eyebrow. This gives the threaded eyebrow its characteristic groomed appearance. Threading is also good for individuals that have undergone strong acne treatments, e.g. roaccutane, retin A, where the skin becomes very delicate, or those that have other contra-indications to waxing, i.e. due to allergies to ingredients contained such as resin.

What type of thread is used for threading?

A specialist 100 per cent cotton thread is used for threading. This thread allows strength but resilience during the treatment which is important in order to perform threading to a high standard.

Advantages	Disadvantages
◆ Only removes hair not skin	◆ Some clients may experience side-effects following the treatment; these include excessive skin reddening (erythema) and short-term puffiness of the skin tissue treated
◆ Good for removal of short hairs	◆ The area may be uncomfortable for a short while
◆ Can isolate one hair at a time	◆ Itching may occur following hair removal
◆ Can go over an area more than once without causing skin irritation	◆ Ingrowing hair may occur when the hair regrows or as a result of poor technique
◆ Sharp, defined shape can be achieved	◆ Infections may occur (e.g. folliculitis), if homecare advice is not followed as the follicle will remain open for up to 24 hours following the treatment
◆ Inexpensive to perform as minimal resources required	
◆ Fast results	
◆ Ideal for eyebrows and facial hair	
◆ Minimal skin irritation – good for delicate, sensitive skin types	

What areas can be threaded?

Threading is mainly performed on the face (eyebrows, upper lip, chin, sides of face, nose, ears, neck and forehead) but can be used all over the body if desired.

Like tweezing, threading can be combined with other eye treatments to enhance the treatment. A good example would be to tint the eyebrows (ensure skin sensitivity test has been completed 48 hours in advance of the treatment with a negative result obtained) before performing the threading treatment.

To further enhance the eye area, false eyelashes may be applied.

For male grooming an eyebrow threading treatment can combine with a barbering treatment. Hair can also be removed from the tops of the cheeks, nose and ears.

Knowledge Check

What are the three layers of terminal hair called?

Refer to page 64 to help you.

Specialist threading thread shown

Outcome 1: Be able to prepare for threading

Learn how to prepare for threading

PRACTICAL SKILLS	UNDERPINNING KNOWLEDGE
Prepare yourself, client and work area for threading	Describe workplace requirements for preparing yourself, the client and the work area
Use suitable consultation techniques to identify treatment objectives	State the environmental conditions suitable for threading
Provide clear recommendations to the client	Describe different consultation techniques used to identify treatment objectives
Select products, tools and equipment to suit client treatment needs	Describe how to select products, tools and equipment to suit client treatment needs
	Describe the contra-indications which prevent or restrict threading

Preparing the work area

Before beginning threading, check that you have the necessary products, tools and equipment to hand and that they meet the legal hygiene and industry requirements for threading treatment.

Products, tools and equipment

- ◆ **Couch or chair** With neck and foot support
- ◆ **Trolley** On which to place everything
- ◆ **Bright lighting and magnifying lamp** To optimize visibility

- ◆ **Disinfecting solution** For storing sterilized tweezers and scissors
- ◆ **Headband (or clips)** To hold the hair from the client's face
- ◆ **Specialist threading thread** To remove hair when performing threading techniques
- ◆ **Powder** Purified talc or other specialist powder supplied by the manufacturer for threading

Magnifying lamp

Specialist threading thread

Disinfecting solution

◆ **Scissors** Specialist stainless steel scissors for trimming long hairs

◆ **Disposable non-latex (nitrile or PVC) powder-free gloves** Worn to reduce the possibility of cross-contamination

◆ **Cotton wool** To cleanse the treatment area and apply the preferred soothing aftercare product

YOU WILL ALSO NEED:

◆ **Mirror** To show the client the finished result

◆ **Skin disinfectant** To cleanse and disinfect the client's skin

◆ **Antiseptic soothing lotion or gel** With healing and antiseptic properties, suitable for facial skin

◆ **Medium sized towels (1)** To protect the client's clothes

◆ **Client record card** To record confidential details of each client registered to the salon including personal details, products used and details of the treatment

◆ **Eyebrow brush** To brush the eyebrows into shape before and after treatment

◆ **Waste container** This should be a lined metal bin with a lid

◆ **Disposable tissue (such as bedroll)** To cover the work surface and couch or chair

Sterilization and disinfection for threading

Hygiene must be maintained in a number of ways:

◆ client hair and clothing is protected and any clothing and accessories are removed where necessary

◆ always wash hands before treatment. Wear disposable gloves to avoid cross-contamination and infection when possible; however, gloves can hinder technique

◆ ensure the skin is clean and grease free. Apply a mild ethanol skin disinfectant

◆ ensure that the client's hands do not come into contact with the treatment area whilst stretching the skin to avoid the possibility of infection

◆ select a new piece of thread for each treatment area

◆ if used, metal tools such as scissors and tweezers must be sterilized before use on each client

◆ maintain accepted industry hygiene and safety working practices throughout the treatment.

Reception

When a client makes an appointment for a threading treatment, the receptionist will need to check which area the client would like treated, to allow sufficient time.

As contact lenses should be removed when performing eyebrow threading, inform the client of this in order that they can store them safely on removal.

All staff, especially the staff communicating with clients at reception, should be familiar with the different pricing structures for the range of threading treatments and products available for retail.

Commercially, 10 minutes is allowed for threading to the upper lip or chin and 20 minutes for an eyebrow reshape.

HEALTH & SAFETY

Waste Contaminated waste must be disposed of in accordance with the Environmental Health Department of your local council.

TOP TIP

Powder

Cornflour is traditionally used as an alternative to talc, to dry the skin, absorbing any moisture and lift the hair before the treatment. Some threading specialists use the powder to ensure the smooth gliding of the thread on the skin's surface.

TOP TIP

Hygiene

Disposable mascara brushes can be used to brush the eyebrows as an alternative to a brow brush, which can then be hygienically disposed of immediately after use.

Disposable mascara wands

Consultation

As with all treatments, **consultation** is essential and should be carried out in a comfortable and quiet area where the client is able to ask any questions and clarify points if necessary. All details should be recorded and signatures obtained.

Consult with the client ensuring there is a clear understanding of the area to be treated and what is realistically achievable both short- and long-term. Explain to the client that they will be required to support the skin to assist hair removal as instructed. You may wish to demonstrate this to confirm understanding at consultation. Encourage clients to ask questions to clarify any points.

Check client suitability, certain contra-indications will prevent or restrict threading.

If the client is a minor under the age of 16, it is necessary to obtain parent/guardian permission for the threading treatment. The parent/guardian will also have to be present when the treatment is received.

Contra-indications

Although threading is considered to be more suitable for individuals with skin sensitivities resulting from conditions like psoriasis, eczema, dermatitis and diabetes, as with all hair removal techniques contra-indications will apply and will be the same as other hair removal techniques (e.g. waxing and tweezing, refer to Chapter 8 Eyelash and Brow Treatments and Chapter 15 Waxing Treatments).

There is also the possibility that **contra-actions** may arise. This can be avoided by ensuring a thorough consultation prior to the treatment to assess client's suitability for the treatment and giving clear aftercare instructions on completion of the treatment.

Contra-actions

Examples of possible contra-actions:

- **folliculitis**
- **erythema**
- ingrowing hairs
- bruising
- blood spots
- broken hair
- histamine (allergic reaction)
- severe swelling
- severe erythema.

The record card should be signed and dated following the consultation to confirm the suitability and consent with the agreed threading treatment. It is important that accurate records are kept and stored in compliance with the Data Protection Act for future reference. Any additional details are to be recorded on the reverse of the card. Existing clients will need to indicate whether there have been any changes since their last treatment, which must also be noted down on the record card.

Please refer to the sample client record card on pages 283–284.

Preparing the client

Preparation of the client for the treatment is as important as the preparation of the beauty therapist (see pages 114–116) and must be carried out thoroughly and professionally:

1 Escort the client to the treatment area and assist with removal of clothing/accessories in the area (e.g. jewellery, scarves, etc.) and help the client onto the couch where necessary. Ensure that they are comfortable and positioned at the correct height for you to work.

2 Confirm required hair removal discussed at consultation and advise further where necessary.

3 Disinfect your hands and if worn apply disposable gloves.

Knowledge Check

How should you prepare yourself hygienically for threading treatment to prevent cross-infection or contamination?

Working in a professional environment means arriving 10 minutes early to work, looking smart, working hard and learning from those around you and remembering at all times that you are representing a brand and yourself and this can affect your future.

Shavata Singh

Outcome 2: Be able to provide threading

Learn how to provide threading

PRACTICAL SKILLS

Communicate and behave in a professional manner

Follow health and safety working practices

Position themselves and client correctly throughout the treatment

Use products, tools and equipment and techniques to suit client's treatment needs

Complete the treatment to the satisfaction of the client

Record the results of the treatment

Provide suitable aftercare advice

UNDERPINNING KNOWLEDGE

State how to communicate and behave in a professional manner

Describe health and safety working practices

State the importance of positioning yourself and the client correctly throughout the treatment

State the importance of using product, tools, equipment and techniques to suit client's treatment needs, skin types and conditions

Describe how treatments can be adapted to suit client treatment needs

State the contra-actions that may occur during and following treatments and how to respond

State the importance of completing the treatment to the satisfaction of the client

State the importance of completing treatment records

State the aftercare advice that should be provided

Describe the structure and functions of the skin

Describe the structure and function of the hair

Eyebrow threading

1   First remove any facial creams or cosmetic products from the area to be treated by using clean cotton wool and cleanser, followed by a skin disinfecting product, e.g. a mild formulation of ethanol, and then blot dry with a clean tissue, disposing of both in a lined metal waste bin. Moisture left on the area will reduce the effectiveness of the thread gripping the hair.

2   For eyebrow shaping, brush the eyebrows in an upwards and then downwards direction to ensure the hairs are laying flat, and trim any long hairs that may spoil the finished result. Brush eyebrows back into place.

3   With a clean piece of cotton wool, apply a light dusting of powder (optional) to the area – this will enable the thread to glide over the skin and is particularly good when the skin is hot and moist.

4   Decide the method of threading to be used (examples are described on the following page) and prepare the cotton. Shorter lengths of thread are easier to handle whilst developing your skills or if you have smaller hands.

5   The client must now support the area to be treated – for eyebrows one hand should be over the eye and one over the top of the eyebrow (see step 5 image on page 323). The area should be supported firmly in order to avoid the skin being pinched or cut by the thread.

6   The hairs are removed against the direction of hair growth, with the thread firmly placed onto the skin ensuring even tension throughout the treatment. This will enable effective and accurate removal of the hair from the root, avoiding snapping while reducing any discomfort to the client.

7   Remove all hairs as necessary, using the thread to brush away any loose ones dropping onto the skin during the treatment. Keep checking the threaded area to ensure symmetry of both eyebrows. If completing a reshape show the client the eyebrow shape as the treatment progresses to ensure client satisfaction.

8   On completion of the treatment and when the treatment is to the satisfaction of the client, apply a soothing aftercare product to the area using clean cotton wool to remove loose hairs and soothe the area and then dispose of in a lined bin.

9   Brush the eyebrows into shape and show client the finished result.

10   Assist client from the treatment chair/couch and provide appropriate **aftercare advice**.

STEP-BY-STEP: EYEBROW THREADING

1 Cleanse the area to be treated

2 Trim long hairs if necessary

5 Get the client to support the area being treated

7 Thread against hair growth

8 Wipe over area to remove loose hair and apply aftercare antiseptic soothing product

9 Brush eyebrow and show client finished result

Threading techniques

There are three techniques that are commonly used:

1   **Mouth technique** – Hair removal using thread where one part of the thread is anchored in the mouth, held between the teeth and lips and the other part is looped in the hands. Using the index and middle fingers of the working hand, the loop is widened and drawn over the skin's surface. The thread is then opened by widening the fingers and thumb of one hand, this action removes the hair. This is the most commonly used technique, originating from the Far East and is also known as the Asian or single looped method.

2   **Neck technique** – A substitute for the mouth technique where one part of the thread is anchored around the neck and the other part is looped in the hands. This technique originates from the Middle East and is also known as the Arabian or single looped method.

> Work hard and talk! Some of my best opportunities have come about as a result of hard graft and conversation. I have got some incredible 'leads' as a result of chatting to clients and you never know where it could take you and your business, next.
>
> *Shavata Singh*

TOP TIP

Client satisfaction

To ensure client satisfaction, especially when reshaping a thick eyebrow shape, it is advisable to show the client the shape as it is developing.

TOP TIP

Retail opportunities

On completion of the treatment you could recommend a retail product or further eye treatment, e.g. demonstrate the use of a suitable aftercare cream to enhance the treatment.

1 The mouth technique

2 The neck technique

3 The hand technique (self-threading)

3 **Hand technique** – Hair removal using thread which is held between the index and middle finger of one hand and then the other hand twists the looped thread. The action of widening the thread with the index finger and thumb of one hand traps and removes the hairs as it is moved over the area. Commonly used by practitioners on themselves. This technique is also known as cat's cradle, doubled looped or self technique.

Aftercare advice

Aftercare advice is essential not only to avoid contra-actions but in order to maintain the treatment results. It is important to give general as well as specific advice.

For the next 12–24 hours it is important to avoid activities or actions that could lead to skin irritation/infection:

◆ swimming

◆ heat treatments, e.g. hot water, sauna, steam

◆ UV light exposure, natural or artificial

◆ perfumed products applied to the area treated

◆ facial treatments/exfoliation

◆ touching the area

◆ excessive sweating

◆ applying make-up to the area.

To avoid ingrowing hairs it is important to gently exfoliate the area after 3 days and twice weekly thereafter.

If needed, the area can be soothed with either a recommended product or a soothing and calming product, e.g. aloe vera gel.

Recommend the application of cosmetic colour to define the brows, especially if the brow hair is sparse or a different shape is to be achieved requiring additional hair growth. This may be a brow pencil or brow powder of a suitable colour.

Recommend other treatments which will further enhance the eye area such as permanent tinting to the eyebrow/eyelashes and artificial lashes.

If there is a contra-action following treatment, advise the client what appropriate action should be taken. Advise the client to receive the treatment in the specified time according to their hair growth cycle. Repeat bookings vary according to the natural hair regrowth and client requirements.

Ensure that the client's records are up-to-date, accurate and complete following the threading treatment. Provide written instructions in an aftercare leaflet.

ALWAYS REMEMBER

Appointments

To schedule the client's next appointment as part of the aftercare advice.

Knowledge Check

What are the three techniques of threading that you can use?

Refer to page 324 to help you.

Knowledge Check

Why is exfoliation to the area following threading treatment important as part of the aftercare advice?

ASSESSMENT OF KNOWLEDGE AND UNDERSTANDING

You have now learnt how to provide threading treatments in the beauty therapy workplace. To test your level of knowledge, answer the following short questions. These will prepare you for your summative (final) assessment.

1. The part of the skin where the hair is removed from when performing threading is the:

   a. papillary layer
   b. reticular layer
   c. subcutaneous layer
   d. cornified layer

2. The growing active stage of the hair growth cycle is known as:

   a. catagen
   b. telogen
   c. anagen

3. Hair that is coarse and usually pigmented is known as:

   a. terminal hair
   b. vellus hair
   c. lanugo hair

4. What are the three popular threading techniques for removal?

   a. mouth, neck and hand
   b. lip, chin and eyebrow

   c. mouth, neck and foot
   d. two-handed threading, hand and mouth threading

5. Good working practice will avoid RSI. What does this stand for?

6. What is a normal, expected skin reaction to hair removal threading?

7. To avoid hair breakage, coarse hair will require the thread tension to be:

   a. more
   b. less

8. Why is powder applied to the skin?

9. What is the best method of sterilization for threading scissors?

   a. a chemical disinfectant
   b. an autoclave
   c. an UV cabinet
   d. surgical spirit

10. As the thread moves along the skin it removes hair from the hair follicle:

    a. with hair growth
    b. against hair growth

10 Part 1: Make-up

LEARNING OBJECTIVES

There are two learning outcomes to achieve for this mandatory technical unit:

1 Be able to prepare for make-up.

2 Be able to apply make-up.

The assessment range applied requires you to:

◆ Use consultation techniques to identify treatment objectives.

◆ Use products, tools and equipment as appropriate.

◆ Treat all skin types and conditions.

◆ Apply make-up to meet the objectives for different occasions.

◆ Ensure the environmental conditions are suitable.

◆ Identify contra-indications that may affect if and how the treatment can proceed.

◆ Communicate and behave in an appropriate and professional manner.

◆ Follow all health and safety working practices.

◆ Apply corrective methods, taking into account age, facial shape, eye and lip shape and if the client wears glasses or contact lenses.

◆ Provide relevant aftercare and contra-action advice.

KEY TERMS

aftercare advice

age groups

blushers

bronzing products

client care

colour correctors

communication (verbal and
    non-verbal)

concealer

consultation

contra-action advice

contra-actions

contra-indication advice

contour cosmetics

corrective methods

eye shadow

eyebrow colour

eyeliner

face shape

facial features

foundation

health and safety

highlighters

lip balm

lip glosses

lip liner

lip stain

lipstick

make-up

make-up objectives

make-up products

mineral make-up

pigment

primers

powder

shaders

skin conditions

skin type

treatment plan

triangle

Unit Topic

Apply make-up

This VRQ unit is linked to the Beauty Therapy NOS Unit B8.

INTRODUCTION

This unit is about how to achieve professional make-up. Make-up may be applied for a variety of different occasions or events including day, evening and special occasions. The choice and application of make-up products and techniques will take into account your client's treatment needs and the look to be achieved. The choice and application of make-up products and techniques will differ according the type of light the make-up is to be seen be in. At the end of this chapter there is a practical assignment for you to complete. You must be able to show you have the necessary practical skills and underpinning knowledge to apply make-up.

Dealing with people in a polite, efficient manner and using good communication and questioning skills to find out exactly what they require from their make-up treatment forms an important part of this technical service.

INDUSTRY ROLE MODEL

CHARLOTTE GABRIELLA SAVOURY Key Artist for Illamasqua

" My Key Artist role allows me to cover many areas within Illamasqua. From designing looks inspired by specific briefs, working with and training the teams across the UK, holding events/master classes to help educate students and supporting research in the development of new products and collections.

My highlights at Illamasqua include being able to showcase my own art work and have full creative input into design projects.

I work alongside Illamasqua Creative Director Alex Box and created one of the visuals for the I'mperfection campaign. I was appointed Key Artist for the Sorapol Fashion Show, opening one of our stand-alone stores in Dubai and creating the make-up for external fashion campaigns, such as Tatty Devine's S/S13 range.

ANATOMY & PHYSIOLOGY
Essential anatomy and physiology knowledge requirements for this chapter are identified on the checklist chart on page 33

Purpose of make-up treatment

Make-up is used to disguise, enhance and accentuate the facial features to make us appear more attractive – which in turn makes us feel more confident. Balance in the face is created by the skilful application of different cosmetic products.

Each client is unique, so each requires an individual approach for their make-up. The overall effect should be attractive, complementing the client's personality, lifestyle and the context for which the make-up is to be worn. Make-up looks and colours change in trend to complement each season's fashions. It is therefore important to keep up-to-date and be aware of how to achieve these different looks. Retail products should be available for the client to purchase if they wish to achieve or maintain the look for themselves.

Make-up products can also improve the appearance and condition of the skin. Products should be selected to suit the client's skin type, colouring, condition and age.

Preparing the work area

The make-up work area should be decorated in light, neutral colours to avoid creating unnecessary shadows. The area where the make-up is to be applied should be well lit, ideally with the same kind of light as that in which the make-up will be seen.

If provided, background music should be at a sound level that allows effective communication with your client.

Place all the products, tools and equipment required on the trolley or work surface, in front of a make-up mirror. Make-up brushes may alternatively be placed in a make-up tool belt worn around the waist. If you are displaying the make-up on a trolley, place the cosmetic products on a lower shelf until required, when they can be moved to the top shelf. This avoids cluttering the working area.

Keeping the work area tidy promotes an organized and professional image, and prevents time being wasted as you try to find resources. The work area should always be in a condition to provide further make-up treatments.

TOP TIP

Keep up-to-date

Purchase professional magazines or subscribe to professional websites that can make you aware of make-up looks, make-up tools, equipment and products, future trends and related technical training.

Outcome 1: Be able to prepare for make-up

Learn how to prepare for make-up

PRACTICAL SKILLS

Prepare yourself, client and work area for make-up

Use suitable consultation techniques to identify treatment objectives

Carry out a skin analysis

Provide clear recommendations to the client

Select products, tools and equipment to suit client treatment needs, skin types and conditions

UNDERPINNING KNOWLEDGE

Describe workplace requirements for preparing yourself, the client and work area

State the environmental conditions suitable for make-up

Describe different consultation techniques used to identify treatment objectives

Describe the importance of carrying out a detailed skin analysis

Describe how to select products, tools and equipment to suit client treatment needs, skin types and conditions

Identify skin types, conditions and characteristics

Describe the contra-indications which prevent or restrict make-up application

Lighting You need to know the *type* of light in which the proposed make-up will be seen: this is important when deciding upon the correct choice of make-up colours, because the appearance of colours may change according to the type of light. Is the make-up to be seen in daylight, in a fluorescent-lit office or a softly-lit restaurant?

White light (natural daylight) contains all the colours of the rainbow. When white light falls on an object, it absorbs some colours and *reflects* others: it is the reflected colour that we see. Thus, an object that we see as red is an object that absorbs the colours in white light except red. A *white* object reflects most of the light that falls on it; a *black* object absorbs most of the light that falls on it.

Always be prepared
Often I have had people change their minds last minute. Whether it be a bride or on set, you will sometimes have to come up with a new look or change the existing one quickly, so it's essential that you carry your full kit with you and extras just in case.

Charlotte Savoury

Make-up work station

If the make-up is to be worn in natural light, choose subtle make-up products in neutral colours as daylight intensifies colours. Any imperfection will be clearly seen. Avoid heavy shading and contouring techniques which will appear exaggerated.

If the make-up is to be worn in the office, it will probably be seen under fluorescent light. This contains an excess of blue and green, which have a 'cool' effect on the make-up: the red in the face does not show up and the face can look drained of colour. Reds and yellows should be avoided, as these will not show up; blue-toned colours will. This light also sharpens colours. This light also sharpens colours. Don't apply dark colours, as fluorescent light intensifies these. Choose lighter textured products in natural and neutral colours.

In the workplace a warm fluorescent tube covered with a diffuser is preferable to simulate natural lighting and provide a truer representation of colour.

Evening make-up is usually seen in incandescent light – light produced by a filament lamp. This produces an excess of red and yellow light, which creates a warm, flattering effect. Almost all colours can be used in this light, except that browns and purples will appear darker. Choose a lighter foundation than normal to reflect the light, and use frosted highlighting products where possible for the same reason.

Because it is necessary to choose brighter colours and to emphasize facial features using contouring cosmetics, evening make-up will appear very obvious and dramatic in daylight. Explain to the client the reasons for the effect created, so that when she leaves the salon in daylight she won't feel that the make-up is inappropriate.

Before beginning the make-up application, check that you have the necessary products, tools and equipment to hand and that they meet the legal hygiene and industry requirements for make-up application.

You will need to have to hand a good range of make-up, suitable for clients with known skin allergies to cosmetics, for contact lens wearers, for different skin types, conditions, ages and skin colours including:

◆ concealing and contouring cosmetics (shaders, highlighters and blushers)

◆ foundations

◆ translucent powders

◆ eye shadows

◆ eyeliners

◆ brow liners

◆ mascara

◆ lipsticks

◆ lip glosses

◆ lip liners.

Products, tools and equipment

- **Couch or make-up chair** With sit-up and lie-down positions and an easy-to-clean surface
- **Trolley** Or other surface on which to place everything
- **Non-oily eye make-up remover** To remove eye make-up and prepare the skin for make-up application
- **Toning lotion** Suitable for different skin types. To remove excess cleanser and restore the skin's pH balance
- **Lightweight moisturizer or primer** Suitable for different skin types. To facilitate make-up application and create a barrier between the skin and make-up
- **Dry cotton wool** Stored in a covered jar, to apply loose face powder
- **Large white facial tissues** To blot the skin after facial toning, and to protect the skin during make-up application
- **Make-up (a range)** To suit different skin types, tones and age groups
- **Bright lighting and magnifying lamp** To inspect the skin after cleansing and check for areas requiring special attention, e.g. broken capillaries that require concealer
- **Make-up brushes (assorted – at least three sets)** To allow for disinfection after use
- **Applicators and brushes** Where possible use disposable, for example for mascara and the application of eye shadow and lipstick
- **Headband (clean) or hair clips** To protect the client's hair while cleansing the skin. Alternatively if the hair has been styled it will be necessary to secure the hair away from the face with hair clips
- **Cleansing lotion/make-up remover** Suitable for different skin types. To clean and prepare the skin for make-up application

- **Non-latex cosmetic sponges** For applying foundation and other facial cosmetic preparations
- **Make-up palette** For preparing and dispensing cosmetic products prior to application
- **Pencil sharpener** For cosmetic pencils
- **False eyelashes** To enhance the eyes as required
- **Small spatulas (several)** For removing make-up products from their containers
- **Brush cleanser** A proprietary brand cleaner to care for and maintain brushes hygienically
- **Eyelash curlers** Tool used to temporarily curl the eyelashes

YOU WILL ALSO NEED:

- **Disposable tissue (such as bedroll)** To cover the work surface and the couch or beauty chair
- **Towels (2)** Freshly laundered for each client – one to be placed over the head of the couch or chair, the other over the client's chest and shoulders to protect their clothing
- **Damp cotton wool** Prepared for each client and used during skin cleansing
- **Bowls** To hold the prepared cotton wool
- **Bowls and lined metal pedal bin** For waste materials
- **Hand mirror (clean)** To show client the make-up during and after application to ensure satisfaction
- **Client record card** To record confidential details of each client registered at the salon, including personal details, products used and details of the treatment.

> **Mark your kit/ brushes**
> It can get pretty hectic on jobs and things can often run late especially on photo shoots where everything needs to be packed away quickly. So to make sure nobody runs off with any of your brushes or make-up, mark them with a brightly coloured nail polish or small sticker so they can be clearly identified.
>
> *Charlotte Savoury*

Trolley setup

Range of make-up brushes

Name	Description
Large face powder dusting brush	To remove excess face powder or to apply specialized powders such as bronzing and shimmer powders
Foundation brush	To apply foundation to specific areas
Contouring blush brush	To apply facial contouring products to highlight and shade areas of the face. This is achieved as the bristles have a blunt cut or angled end
Blusher brush (large to medium)	To apply powder colour to the face and for blending
Small flat angle-edged eye shadow brush	To apply and blend powder eye make-up products in the socket area of the eye
Small rounded-edged eye shadow brush	To apply eye shadow, blend and shade
Medium firm eye shadow blending brush	To blend powder eye colours and soften harsh lines and colour
Small concealer brush	For exact placement of concealing product in areas such as around the nose and mouth. The brush has a flat surface with a round end; a smaller version of the foundation brush
Eyebrow brush	To remove excess make-up from the brow hair and to add colour, blend eyebrow pencil and groom the brow hair into shape
Eyeliner brush	A fine brush used to apply make-up eye liner colour to contour the eyes, creating a precise line. A line and define brush is shown
Mascara wand/comb	To apply mascara and remove excess mascara to separate the lashes
Lip brush	To apply lip products and ensure a definite, balanced outline to the lips. These are available in different shapes including angled for coverage, fine-tipped for applying a lip line, flat and diamond-tipped

Make-up brushes

Make-up brushes consist of a handle, a metal ferrule which attaches to the handle and holds the brush fibre bristles in place, and the actual bristles. They are available in a variety of shapes and designs and are made from different fibres which may be synthetic (from fabric and chemical sources) or naturally sourced from animals including camel, sable, squirrel, pony and goat, and contain blends of different animal hairs. Synthetic brushes are non-absorbent and are better for the application of cream or gel textured products as they control the application of the product more. Powder and blusher brushes are usually made from soft animal hair but for the purposes of contouring and blending you will need firmer brushes.

When buying make-up brushes make sure the fibres are securely attached to the handle. Test the comfort of the fibres on the skin by stroking the brush on the back of your hand.

You will need to have more than one set of brushes so one set can be used whilst the other is being disinfected. To avoid cross-contamination all brushes must be cleaned after each use.

Sterilization and disinfection

Hygiene must be maintained in a number of ways:

◆ ensure that tools and equipment are sterile before use

◆ disinfect work surfaces after every client

◆ always follow hygienic work practices

◆ maintain a high standard of personal hygiene.

TOP TIP

Fibre optic brushes

Fibre optic brushes are a mixture of animal hair at the base and synthetic hair at the ends. This combination is great for powder make-up product application as the animal hair holds the powder product and the synthetic end achieves a light final coverage of the make-up product.

Fibre optic brush

TOP TIP

Make-up case

If you intend to apply make-up at different locations, buy a large make-up case so that you can transport the make-up easily and hygienically.

Make-up case

Knowledge Check

Why is it important to match lighting with the occasion for which the make-up is to be worn?

Refer to pages 329–330 to help you.

TOP TIP

Positive promotion

Where possible, use make-up that you also sell in the salon, so that the client can buy the products for home use if they wish. Use attractive visual aids such as posters and displays to raise awareness and interest in the products.

Lipstick retail products

TOP TIP

Make-up instruction

If you provide make-up instruction to a client, do so in front of a large mirror so that the client can watch the various stages of make-up application.

Record the make-up used and the advice given on a separate record, for the client to take away with them.

HEALTH & SAFETY

Maintaining hygiene If you drop a make-up tool on the floor, discard it – don't use it again until it has been disinfected and sterilized.

Application of a professional brush cleaner. PPE is worn to protect the hands when using sterilizing products which could dry and irritate the skin leading to possible skin disorders such as dermatitis.

Hygienic removal of make-up product and placement onto a make-up palette

Where possible, use disposable applicators during make-up application, costing these into the treatment price. Disinfect non-disposable make-up brushes after each use: wash them in warm water and detergent, rinse them thoroughly in a disinfecting solution and then rinse in clean water, and allow them to dry naturally. Once dry, place the brushes in an UV light cabinet ready for use. An alcohol-based brush cleaner is recommended to clean as well as care for your brushes as they contain oils which condition the bristles. Use brush cleaner following the manufacturer's instructions.

All cosmetic products should be removed from their containers using a clean spatula and placed on the clean plastic make-up palette before application. (This avoids contamination of the make-up with bacteria from unclean make-up applicators.)

The make-up palette should be cleaned with warm water and detergent, then wiped with a disinfectant solution applied with a suitable disposable material i.e. clean cotton wool. It should be stored in the UV cabinet.

Mascara should be applied using a disposable brush applicator, fresh for each client. Sharpen cosmetic pencils with a pencil sharpener before each use.

Make-up consumables, which are disposed of after use

Make-up sponges should be disposed of after use, or washed in warm water and detergent, then placed in a disinfectant solution and rinsed. Allow them to dry, then place them in the UV cabinet, with each side being exposed for at least 20 minutes.

> **Perfect hygiene**
> Always ensure you have enough hygiene with you for the day especially disposable mascara wands as double dipping mascaras/lip glosses is a huge no-no. Beauty sprays are a great way of sanitizing products both before and after use to keep your customers happy and your kit clean.
> *Charlotte Savoury*

TOP TIP

Lighting

If working under artificial light, use warm white fluorescent light for day make-up, as this closely resembles natural light.

A diffuser may be used to cover the fluorescent tube. This softens the cool effect on the make-up and reduces the effects of shadows.

Reception

When a client makes an appointment for make-up, the receptionist will need to check the purpose of the make-up application.

Make-up application is offered for different purposes, called **make-up objectives**.

◆ *A make-up lesson* A chance for the client to learn from a professional how to apply make-up that suits them and to learn new techniques.

◆ *Special occasion make-up* Applied to suit the occasion for which it is to be worn, such as a wedding. If the make-up is for a bride, advise the client to visit the salon for a consultation and a practice session so that you can decide together on appropriate make-up. Ask the client if she can bring a swatch of the dress material with her, so that you can select colours to complement this and to co-ordinate with the accessories.

◆ *Evening make-up* Generally will be seen under artificial lighting. The effect this has on the appearance of the make-up will depend upon the light source, which must be considered when applying evening make-up. Generally, evening make-up is heavier in application and stronger colours may be applied. Placement of some brighter colour tones and finishes should be introduced. Include products to emphasize and highlight, such as frosted eye shadows and lip glosses.

◆ *Corrective make-up* May be applied for concealing purposes, using camouflage products to cover facial disfigurements or birth marks, and the client may be advised if qualified how to do this themselves.

◆ *Photographic make-up* Applied for many reasons including magazine shoots, portrait work and fashion shows. Make-up application must be skilful to achieve the right end result as the location may be a photographic studio or outdoors on location.

◆ *A professional look* Some clients simply wish to have their make-up professionally applied just as they would have their hair professionally styled.

All staff, especially the staff communicating with clients at reception, should be familiar with the different pricing structures for the range of make-up treatments and products available for retail. Be aware of market trends – a client may request they only have eye make-up application. If offered, this would have to be priced accordingly.

In the salon, advise the client that if they intend to have their hair washed and styled, this should be done before they have the make-up applied.

If a client requests a deep cleansing facial followed by make-up application, suggest that they have the facial at least 5 days prior to the make-up. The facial will stimulate the skin, increasing its normal physiological functioning such as localized blood circulation and increased sebaceous gland activity. This will affect how long the make-up lasts; it may even cause the colour of the foundation to change.

Do not reshape the eyebrows at the same treatment as make-up application – secondary infection could occur; also the skin in the area will become very red or darker, depending upon skin colour, altering the colour and thus the effect of eye shadow. This is because of an increase in blood circulation in the local area.

TOP TIP

Ensure suitable make-up application

When applying make-up it is important that you fully understand the effect to be achieved. Good communication is essential. Ensure you understand what the final result should look like.

It is also important that you check that the client does not have allergies to any products to avoid a possible contra-action.

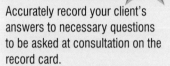

Knowledge Check

Give five examples of how the work area should be prepared for the next client following make-up application.

Refer to pages 333–334 to help you.

ALWAYS REMEMBER

Accurately record your client's answers to necessary questions to be asked at consultation on the record card.

◆ 'Do you normally wear make-up?'

◆ 'For what occasion is the make-up to be worn?'

◆ 'What colour are the clothing and accessories to be worn on this occasion?'

◆ 'Are there any colours that you particularly like or dislike?'

◆ 'What effect would you like the make-up to create?' (This question may be asked in many contexts – the client may wish to achieve a natural or a glamorous effect, or to emphasize or diminish certain facial features.)

◆ Are there any products that you are allergic to?

◆ Do you wear contact lenses?

ALWAYS REMEMBER

Treatment timings

Make-up lesson: allow 1 hour.

Special occasion or evening make-up: allow 45 minutes to 1 hour.

Day make-up: allow 45 minutes.

Knowledge Check

In order to select the correct skincare and make-up products to suit the client's skin, it is necessary to correctly identify the skin type. What are the facial skin characteristic conditions of the following skin types that you learnt about in Chapter 7 Facial Skincare:

◆ oily skin

◆ dry skin

◆ combination skin.

Refer to pages 204–206 to help you.

ACTIVITY

Recognizing contra-indications

What skin disorders can you think of that would contra-indicate, preventing make-up application?

> **Good communication**
>
> It is essential that you communicate and ask questions if you are unsure on specific briefs. You need to make sure you are fully prepared and can have a practice run of looks beforehand, ensuring you can tackle any problems with the look rather than encountering them on the day and trying to figure them out while on set. Time is limited so this will ensure everything runs smoothly and you know exactly what you're doing.
>
> *Charlotte Savoury*

The consultation

Complete a record card noting the client's personal details. This will be used to record details of the make-up applied. A sample record card for make-up is found on pages 337–338.

If the client is a minor under the age of 16, it is necessary to obtain parent/guardian permission for the make-up treatment. The parent/guardian will also have to be present when the treatment is received.

Discuss your make-up plan with the client to ensure that the make-up will meet their requirements or make-up treatment objectives. You may need to ask questions such as those listed in the Always remember box on page 335, but of course the questions depend on the purpose of the make-up application.

If the client wears glasses, check the function of the lens, as this can alter the effect of the make-up.

Provide the opportunity for your client to ask any questions relating to the make-up treatment.

The record card should be signed and dated following the consultation to confirm the suitability and consent with the agreed make-up treatment.

It is important that accurate records are kept and stored in compliance with the Data Protection Act for future reference.

Contra-indications

Certain contra-indications prevent make-up application. These include bacterial, fungal, parasitic and viral infections, which are described in more detail in **Chapter 2**, where contra-indications are illustrated and discussed. Check for these at the consultation, and if any of the following are present on inspection of the skin, do not proceed with make-up application.

ALWAYS REMEMBER

Each client make-up will be different. Examples of make-up application modification include:

◆ choice of make-up products and application techniques for corrective work

◆ choice of make-up to suit the client's skin type and condition

◆ disguising minor skin imperfections

◆ using hypo-allergenic products for a client with cosmetic sensitivity

◆ age of client, using light-reflecting make-up products for a mature skin or one showing signs of premature ageing.

A sample client record card

Date	Beauty therapist name	
Client name	Date of birth (identifying client age group)	
Home address	Postcode	
Email address	Landline phone number	Mobile phone number
Name of doctor	Doctor's address and phone number	
Related medical history (conditions that may restrict or prohibit treatment application)		
Are you taking any medication? (This may affect skin sensitivity)		

CONTRA-INDICATIONS REQUIRING MEDICAL REFERRAL
(Preventing the application of make-up.)

- ☐ bacterial infections (e.g. impetigo, conjunctivitis)
- ☐ viral infections (e.g. herpes simplex)
- ☐ fungal infections (e.g. tinea corporis)
- ☐ parasitic infestations (e.g. pediculosis and scabies)
- ☐ severe skin conditions e.g. eczema and psoriasis

CONTRA-INDICATIONS WHICH RESTRICT TREATMENT
(treatment may require adaptation)

- ☐ cuts and abrasions
- ☐ recent scar tissue
- ☐ skin allergies
- ☐ styes
- ☐ watery eyes
- ☐ bruising and swelling
- ☐ eczema
- ☐ vitiligo
- ☐ hyper keratosis
- ☐ epilepsy

MAKE-UP CONTEXT

- ☐ day
- ☐ evening
- ☐ special occasion

SKIN TYPE

- ☐ normal
- ☐ oily
- ☐ dry
- ☐ combination

SKIN CONDITION

- ☐ sensitive
- ☐ mature
- ☐ dehydrated

CONCEALER

- ☐ cream
- ☐ stick
- ☐ liquid

FOUNDATION

- ☐ liquid
- ☐ stick
- ☐ mineral
- ☐ compact
- ☐ cream
- ☐ tinted moisturizer

POWDER

- ☐ loose
- ☐ compact
- ☐ mineral

BRONZING PRODUCTS

- ☐ powder
- ☐ gel
- ☐ liquid

EYE PRODUCTS FOR EYE AREA

- ☐ cream eye shadow
- ☐ pencil eyeliner
- ☐ kohl eyeliner
- ☐ liquid eyeliner
- ☐ cake eyeliner
- ☐ powder eye shadow
- ☐ mineral and pigment
- ☐ eye shadows
- ☐ gel eye shadow
- ☐

EYE PRODUCTS FOR BROW AREA

- ☐ pencil
- ☐ shadow
- ☐ liquid
- ☐ eyebrow mascara

EYE PRODUCTS FOR EYELASHES

- ☐ waterproof mascara
- ☐ false lashes
- ☐ non-waterproof mascara
- ☐ lash curling

CHEEK PRODUCTS

- ☐ highlighter
- ☐ shader
- ☐ blusher

LIP PRODUCTS

- ☐ pencil lip liner
- ☐ lipstick
- ☐ lip gloss
- ☐ lip balm

Record of make-up products applied

Mascara
Eyeliner
Lip liner
Lip product
Foundation
Powder
Eyebrow colour
Browbone
Socket
Eyelid
Blusher
Contour

Beauty therapist signature (for reference)
Client signature (confirmation of details)

(Continued)

A sample client record card (continued)

TREATMENT ADVICE	TREATMENT PLAN
Make-up application, day make-up – allow 45 minutes Special occasion make-up – allow 45– 60 minutes Make-up lesson – allow 1 hour	Record relevant details of your treatment and advice provided for future reference. Ensure the client's records are up-to-date, accurate and fully completed following treatment. Non-compliance may invalidate insurance.

DURING

Find out:

◆ what products the client is currently using to cleanse and care for the skin of the face and neck.

Discuss:

◆ the importance of a good skincare routine in relation to make-up application

◆ current satisfaction with the client's make-up technique

◆ tips and explain each stage of the make-up application to enhance the client's understanding.

Note:

◆ any adverse reaction, if any occur.

AFTER

Record:

◆ any modification to make-up application that has occurred

◆ what products have been used in the make-up application

◆ the effectiveness of the make-up result

◆ any samples provided (review their success at the next appointment).

Advise on:

◆ how to reapply products to achieve/maintain the result

◆ correct make-up removal technique.

RETAIL OPPORTUNITIES

Advise on:

◆ products that would be suitable for the client to use at home to care for their skin

◆ the benefits of each make-up product clearly and logically during application

◆ recommendations for further make-up treatments

◆ further products or treatments that the client may or may not have received before.

Note:

◆ any purchase made by the client.

EVALUATION

Record:

◆ comments on the client's satisfaction with the treatment

◆ if poor results are achieved, the reasons why.

HEALTH AND SAFETY

Advise on:

◆ avoidance of activities or product application that may cause a contra-action

◆ appropriate necessary action to be taken in the event of an unwanted skin reaction.

Remember that not all contra-indications are visible – a current bone fracture, for example, would not be. The following disorders may contra-indicate or restrict make-up applications. If you suspect the client has any disorder from the list below, do not attempt a diagnosis but refer the client tactfully to their GP without causing concern:

◆ *pediculosis capitis (head lice)*

◆ *pediculosis corporis (body lice)*

◆ *acne vulgaris (active)*

◆ *herpes simplex (cold sore)*

◆ *impetigo*

◆ *styes or hordeola*

◆ *conjuncitivitis (pink eye)*

◆ *watery eye or epiphora*

◆ *blepharitis.*

The following conditions also contra-indicate make-up application:

◆ *skin disorders* including those not listed in the above list, such as bacterial infections (e.g. boils), viral infections (herpes zoster), and fungal infections (e.g. tinea corporis)

◆ *active psoriasis* and *eczema*

◆ *bruising* in the area

◆ *recent haemorrhage*

◆ *swelling and inflammation* in the area

◆ *recent scar tissue*

◆ *sensory nerve disorders*

◆ *cuts or abrasions* in the area

◆ *a recent operation* in the area

◆ *eye disorders* including those not listed in the chart

◆ *parasitic infestation* such as pediculosis capitis and corporis and scabies.

Ask the client whether they have any known allergies to cosmetic preparations. Note the answer on the record card. Care must be taken to avoid contact with an allergen.

Remember, never name a contra-indication, you may be wrong. Refer the client to their GP whose role it is to identify and advise.

In the case of the skin disorder herpes simplex, the make-up treatment may be received when the skin is healed and clear.

HEALTH & SAFETY

Make-up tool/product hygiene at home Advise clients to keep their own make-up clean. Dirty brushes spoil effective make-up application, and offer breeding grounds for bacteria.

Make-up generally has a shelf life of 2 years and is then past its best and becomes unhygienic. Some products require to be replaced more frequently. It is recommended that mascara be replaced every 6 months.

Contra-actions

Certain cosmetic ingredients are known to cause allergic reactions in some people. These ingredients are known as allergens. Allergens may cause irritation, severe erythema, inflammation and swelling, known as a contra-action. This may occur during or following treatment.

ACTIVITY

The record card

Why is it important to complete a record card? What information should be recorded on it?

Knowledge Check

Name three skin disorders and three eye disorders that would contra-indicate make-up application.

Refer to pages 336–337 to help you.

HEALTH & SAFETY

Allergies Where possible, before using a new cosmetic, a client with known allergies should first receive a skin sensitivity test, or be given a small sample of a product to try on a less sensitive area of the skin, to assess the skin's tolerance. If an allergic reaction occurs, medical attention must be sought immediately.

It is possible that clients may grow out of an allergy to a given product. It is also possible, however, suddenly to become allergic to a product that has not given problems before.

TOP TIP

Hair clips

If the client has had their hair styled it may be better to clip the hair out of the way rather than using a headband.

Known cosmetic allergens include the following:

◆ *Lanolin* This is similar to sebum, and is obtained from sheep's wool. It is added to many cosmetics as an emollient.

◆ *Mineral oils* Examples are oleic acid and butyl stearate.

◆ *Eosin (bromo-acid dye)* A staining **pigment**, used in some lip cosmetics and perfumes.

◆ *Paraben* An antiseptic ingredient, used as a preservative in facial cosmetics.

◆ *Certain colourants* One example is carmine.

◆ *Perfume* This is added to most cosmetics, and is a common sensitizer.

Products should be selected without the allergen where identified.

Other contra-actions include:

◆ *Watery eyes* The client's eyes water excessively. If the client has watery eyes, a tissue may be placed at the corners until the irritation has ceased. If the client's eyes continue to water, remove eye make-up and discontinue treatment.

◆ *Excessive perspiration* Some clients may perspire, which will affect adherence of the make-up and its finished result. Blot the skin with soft facial tissue and apply more loose face powder to absorb perspiration. If the client continues to perspire, discontinue treatment.

External contact with an allergen may cause urticaria, also known as hives, and eczema or dermatitis. If an allergy occurs, the product should be removed from the skin and a soothing substance applied. The client should be advised not to use the product again. Always record any allergies on the client's record card so that the offending product may be avoided in the future.

Preparing the client

Take the client through to the make-up work area. Make-up application may take place either at the make-up chair, in front of a mirror, or at the treatment couch/chair. Before you start the make-up, discuss and plan the make-up with the client, recording significant details on their record card.

Before preparing the client for the treatment, clean your hands using an approved hand cleansing technique in front of your client who will observe hygienic procedures being carried out. The client need remove only their upper outer clothing, to their underwear. Offer the client a gown, or drape a clean towel or make-up cape across their chest and shoulders. Place a headband or hairclips around the hairline, to protect the hair and keep it away from the face. Any jewellery in the treatment area should be removed. Refer to the record card to check for any known allergies to cosmetic products.

Ensure that the client is comfortable.

After preparing the client, and before touching the skin, clean your hands again.

Now cleanse and tone the skin, using products appropriate to their skin type. Just as skincare products vary in their formulation to suit the various skin types, so make-up products are designed for different skin types and conditions. Record all relevant details on the record card.

Perform a skin analysis by inspecting the skin; if necessary use a magnifying lamp. Identify any areas that require specific attention, i.e. broken capillaries, pustules, papules, dark circles, hyperpigmentation, hypopigmentation and scarring. Touch the skin to assess tone and levels of hydration.

Apply a light-textured moisturizer before make-up application. This has the following benefits:

◆ it prevents the natural secretions of the skin changing the colour of the foundation

◆ it seals the surface of the skin, and prevents absorption of the foundation into the skin

◆ it facilitates make-up application by providing a smooth base.

Remove excess moisturizer by blotting the skin with a soft facial tissue.

Special lotions may be applied to improve the skin texture and increase make-up durability. These include skin **primers** and oil control lotions.

Skin primers are silicone-based, creating a film on the skin's surface. They refine the skin's appearance, minimizing open pores and the appearance of fine lines. The formulations can vary to suit the client's skin type and may contain pigments to correct skin tone. The primer provides a base and acts as a barrier, preventing absorption of the make-up products into the skin. Primers are applied the same way as moisturizers, but less is required.

Oil control lotions contain **powder** ingredients which absorb the skin's natural oil, reducing shine and producing a matt finish. They are ideal to prepare an oily or combination skin before make-up application.

Blotting the skin

HEALTH & SAFETY

Contact lenses If the client wears contact lenses, ask them whether they wish to remove them before the skin is cleansed. (The need for this will depend on the sensitivity of the eyes.)

TOP TIP

Headbands

If a headband is used, it is a good idea to remove it directly after the facial cleanse so that it doesn't flatten and spoil the hair.

TOP TIP

Removing eyeliner

Existing cosmetic eyeliner is sometimes difficult to remove. Use a cotton bud soaked in eye make-up remover: gently stroke this along the base of the lower eyelashes, in towards the nose.

Removing eyeliner

ALWAYS REMEMBER

Erythema

Avoid excessive pressure and stimulation of the skin while cleansing and preparing the skin for make-up application.

The skin will become too warm, affecting durability and erythema of the skin will occur – skin reddening requires correction.

ALWAYS REMEMBER

Order of application

Make-up is applied in a specific sequence to ensure:

◆ a balanced look is achieved

◆ products are applied effectively, i.e. cream on cream, powder on powder, which allows products to be blended and set appropriately

◆ the client's understanding, e.g. when carrying out a make-up lesson or demonstrating how to achieve a certain look

◆ durability and the optimum look of the make-up is maintained.

Outcome 2: Be able to apply make-up

Learn how to apply make-up

PRACTICAL SKILLS

Communicate and behave in a professional manner

Follow health and safety working practices

Position yourself and client correctly throughout the treatment

Use products, tools, equipment and techniques to suit clients treatment needs, skin types and conditions

Complete the treatment to the satisfaction of the client to suit a range of occasions

Record the results of the treatment

Provide suitable aftercare advice

UNDERPINNING KNOWLEDGE

State how to communicate and behave in a professional manner

Describe health and safety working practices

State the importance of positioning yourself and the client correctly throughout the treatment

State the importance of using products, tools, equipment and techniques to suit client's treatment needs, skin type and conditions

Describe how to use corrective methods to suit client treatment needs, skin types and conditions

State the contra-actions that may occur during and following treatments and how to respond

State the importance of completing the treatment to the satisfaction of the client

State the importance of completing treatment records

State the aftercare advice that should be provided

Describe the structure and functions of the skin

Describe diseases and disorders of the skin

Explain how natural ageing, lifestyle and environmental factors affect the condition of the skin and muscle tone

State the position and action of the muscles of the head, neck and shoulders

State the names and position of the bones of the head, neck and shoulders

Describe the structure and function of the blood and lymphatic system for the head, neck and shoulders

Applying make-up products

The make-up sequence

The correct sequence for applying make-up is as follows.

1 Conceal any blemishes.

2 Apply foundation.

3 Contour the face (with cream liquid products).

4 Apply powder.

5 Contour the face (with powder products).

6 Apply blusher.

7 Apply eye shadow.

8 Make up the eyebrows.

9 Apply mascara.

10 Make up the lips.

11 Contour products, used to shade and highlight the face and features, can be applied in powder or cream formulation. Application sequence for contouring will depend upon product formulation chosen.

Age of the client

When applying make-up, consider how skin changes with age. This will influence the imperfections and skin conditions that may be present and require correction.

Appearance and age table

Age	Appearance
<15	Nearly perfect skin. Smooth texture, pores small
15–24	Acne key factor in surface texture. Fine lines start to appear, pore size increasing
25–45	More fine lines and appearance of first wrinkles (photodamage). Early signs of sagging near the eye. Some loss of elasticity. Adult acne
46–55	More wrinkles, rough texture. Sallow yellow colour begins to appear. Pores and age spots enlarge and define. Sagging near eye and cheek
56+	Wrinkles and fine lines in abundance. Uneven colour, pigmentation. Sagging worsens. Dark circles under eye

DR JOHN GRAY, THE WORLD OF SKINCARE

Knowledge Check

How should the skin be prepared before the make-up application?

Refer to pages 340–341 to help you.

ALWAYS REMEMBER

Manufacturer's instructions

Use all products following manufacturer's instructions to ensure the optimum make-up is achieved and unwanted reactions – contra-actions – are avoided.

Applying concealer before foundation application to minimize the appearance of a skin papule

Applying concealer after foundation application to minimize the appearance of dark circles under the eye

Various types of make-up concealer

Applying foundation

Concealer

Before you begin to apply make-up to the face, inspect the skin and identify any areas that require concealing, such as blemishes, uneven skin colour, dark circles under the eyes or shadows.

Foundation may be used to disguise minor skin imperfections, but where extra coverage is required it is necessary to apply a special concealer, a cosmetic designed to provide maximum skin coverage. Concealers may be applied directly to the skin after skin moisturizing, or following application of the foundation. They can also be used for contouring as highlighters and shaders.

Choose a concealer that is one to two shades lighter than the client's skin tone. In the case of pigmentation this may vary however, according to the colour difference between the area being concealed and the skin's natural colour.

Concealers designed for use around the eye area are light in texture, lighter in colour than the foundation with a yellow tone to minimize the appearance of dark circles. Concealers designed for covering blemishes are unsuitable for application around the eyes.

Concealer can contain pigment to help correct skin tone.

◆ *Green* helps to counteract high colouring, and to conceal dilated capillaries.
◆ *Lilac or pink* counteract a sallow skin colour.
◆ *Peach and pink* counteract dark circles around the eyes and are suitable for darker skin tones.
◆ *White or cream* help to correct unevenness in the skin pigmentation.
◆ *Yellow* helps to counteract the appearance of dark circles around the eyes.

Concealers come in a range of colours and consistencies including liquid, cream, stick and tube, to suit all skins and differences in skin texture. Mix different colours together to obtain the required colour.

Colour correctors target problem areas and contain pigments which balance skin tone. Select lighter shades, e.g. light pink for lighter skins, if the skin is darker select shades of peach. Peach is particularly effective to counteract bluish under-eye shadows. Green correctors counteract areas of redness. Yellow counteracts pink tones.

Correctors are applied like concealer and may be followed with concealer or foundation.

Applying concealer   Remove a small quantity of the concealer from its container, using a clean disposable spatula. If it has a brush applicator attached to the product, for reasons of hygiene this cannot be used.

ALWAYS REMEMBER

Common racial skin problems

◆ White skin – easily damaged by exposure to high temperatures and UV light, leading to broken veins and pigmentation disorders.
◆ Oriental skin – prone to uneven pigmentation on UV light exposure.
◆ Asian skin – often has uneven pigmentation skin tones; darker skin is often found around the eyes.
◆ Black skin – melanin is present in all layers of the epidermis; this can cause scarring following skin damage, possibly leading to uneven pigmentation, vitiligo and keloids.

TOP TIP

Blending concealer

Avoid rubbing the product while blending it, or it will wipe off. Any contact with the skin should be light.

Apply the concealer to the area to be disguised, using either a clean make-up sponge or a concealer make-up brush. Blend the concealer to achieve a realistic effect. Reapply concealer as necessary until correction is achieved.

Foundation

Foundation is applied to produce an even skin tone, to disguise minor skin blemishes, and as a contour cosmetic. Black skin in particular often has an uneven skin tone, requiring certain parts of the face to be lightened and others darkened to produce an even skin tone.

Foundation is available as cream, liquid, compact stick, gel, cake, mousse, powder, mineral-based and tinted moisturizer.

Foundations can contain 'anti-ageing' ingredients such as vitamins A, C and E. These are to neutralize free radicals, natural chemicals thought to be responsible for damaging the skin and producing the signs of ageing – the lines and wrinkles! Sunscreens and moisturizers are commonly included in foundations to protect the skin from the environment.

Silica beads can be included in the formulations, especially for combination/oily skin, to absorb the skin's natural sweat and oil.

Kinds of foundations

Each foundation differs in its formulation to suit a particular skin type. The correct choice will guarantee that the foundation lasts throughout the day.

Cream foundation Cream foundations are oil-based and blend easily on application. They provide a heavy coverage, and have these specific treatment uses:

- ◆ dry skin
- ◆ normal skin
- ◆ mature skin.

Liquid foundation Liquid foundations are oil- or water-based, providing light to medium coverage. Oil-based liquid foundations have these specific uses:

- ◆ dry skin
- ◆ normal skin
- ◆ mature skin
- ◆ combination skin (apply the foundation to the *dry* areas).

Water-based liquid foundations have the following uses:

- ◆ normal skin
- ◆ oily skin
- ◆ combination skin (apply the foundation to the *oily* areas).

Foundation products

Liquid foundations are composed of water, powder, oil, humectant (such as glycerol), pigments and additives.

Water-based foundations do not spread very easily because the water content rapidly evaporates, so these foundations must be applied quickly.

TOP TIP

Specialist foundations

Special ingredients may be included in a foundation for oily skin, selected to avoid clogging the pores and thereby causing congestion.

On a black skin, avoid powder-based foundations as these will make the skin look grey and dull. Use a transparent gel foundation instead.

Gel foundation Gel foundations provide sheer, oil-free non-greasy coverage and a matte finish. Light reflective properties are achieved through the addition of pigments. They have these specific uses:

◆ black, unblemished skin

◆ tanned skin

◆ skin on which a natural effect is required.

Compact skin or cake foundation Compact skin or cake foundations may have an oil, wax or powder base. They give a heavy coverage, and have these specific uses:

◆ dry skin

◆ normal skin

◆ badly blemished or scarred skin.

Mousse foundation Mousse foundations provide light to medium coverage depending on application technique. They have a mineral oil base. Their specific uses are:

◆ normal skin

◆ combination skin.

Care must be taken to apply the mousse foundation to an area of the skin and blend quickly or it may start to dry on the face, creating a chalky appearance.

Mineral-based foundation Mineral liquid foundation contains the natural light-reflecting properties of micro-minerals. It provides a low to medium coverage, with a skin enhancing, slightly luminous look:

◆ it helps make the skin appear healthy and fresh

◆ it is suitable for all skin types, especially normal to dry skin.

Mineral powder foundation contains micro-minerals in a solid powder with a binding ingredient such as algae. Again, suitable for all skin types providing a heavier coverage through layer application.

Compact foundation

Liquid mineral

Mineral make-up is created from finely ground minerals, a process called micronization. Pure mineral make-up allows the skin to breathe as it does not contain synthetic powders and oils.

The make-up may contain a selection of the following minerals which all contribute an effect to the finished look of the make-up:

◆ titanium oxide, a natural white mineral powder providing opacity – titanium is also an ingredient used in cosmetics for its sun protection factor (SPF) effect

◆ zinc oxide, a natural white mineral powder which enhances the appearance of the crystallized minerals; mica, a natural mineral which has light-reflecting properties showing a range of colours (It also affects the finished formulation, providing slip to facilitate make-up application.)

◆ bismuth oxychloride, a synthetic white mineral with a silvery metallic sheen providing coverage to the make-up; iron oxide, a synthetic mineral iron used to add colour.

Tinted foundation Tinted foundation provides a moist, light to medium coverage available in a range of shades. It offers protection from the environment with added sunscreen and skin moisturizers.

◆ It helps make the skin appear natural, healthy and fresh.

◆ It is suitable for all skin types in oil or oil-free formulation.

Foundation colour

The colour or shade of the foundation should match the client's natural skin colour. Test the foundation for compatibility on the client's jaw line or forehead. If an incorrect colour is selected, or if the foundation is insufficiently blended on application, there will be a noticeable demarcation line.

Skin tones may vary on the face with lighter and darker areas, especially on black skin. If the lighter tones are to be emphasized, a lighter coverage foundation product should be selected allowing the skin's natural tone to show. Multi-ethnic skin will require mixing products and shades to create a balanced look. Remember, products can be layered to increase coverage.

Applying the foundation

If the foundation is in a container with a lid, remove some using a clean disposable spatula, placing it on a clean make-up palette.

TOP TIP

Mineral make-up

Mineral make-up can be applied following a facial as the blend of minerals and pigments form microscopic flat crystals due to its formulation which allows the skin to breathe and function.

Mineral make-up products

Skin colour	Foundation colour
White	Ivory or light beige, with warm tones of pink or peach
Olive	Dark beige or bronze
Suntanned	Bronze (to suit skin colour)
Florid	Matt beige with a green tint
Sallow	Beige with a pink tint
Light brown	Light brown foundation with a warm tone
Medium brown	Light brown with a yellow/orange tone
Dark brown	Deep bronze foundation with a yellow/orange tone
Black	Dark golden bronze (usually a gel)

Foundation may be applied using either a large soft foundation brush, which is stroked over the surface of the skin, or a cosmetic sponge. It should be applied to one area of the face at a time, with an outward stroking movement.

Also use a cosmetic sponge to blend the foundation. Take care that you blend it at the hairline and at the jaw line. Avoid clogging the eyebrows with foundation. The cosmetic make-up wedge is designed to apply varying amounts of pressure to the different areas of the face, and to ensure even coverage of the foundation.

When applying foundation around the eye area, use a foundation brush or the angular edge of a cosmetic sponge. This will help you achieve accuracy in application.

The extent of coverage can be controlled by the method of application. If the cosmetic sponge is damp, coverage is light and sheer. To achieve a heavier coverage, use a dry latex-free make-up sponge.

Apply foundation to cover the entire face, including the lips and the eyelids. Do not extend the make-up past the jaw line unless the occasion requires this – for example, if a bride's dress exposes part of the upper chest – because the foundation will mark clothes at the neckline.

Some areas of pigmentation, such as dark circles under the eyes, may require concealing with a concealer product following foundation application.

Contouring

Contour cosmetics

Changing the shape of the face and the facial features can be achieved with the careful application of **contour cosmetics**. These products draw attention either towards or away from facial features, and can create the optical illusion of perfection.

Each face differs in shape and size, so each requires a different application technique.

Contour cosmetics include **highlighters**, **shaders** and **blushers**. They are available in powder, liquid and cream forms.

◆ **Highlighters** Draw attention towards – emphasize.
◆ **Shaders** Draw attention away – minimize.
◆ **Blushers** Add warmth to the face and emphasize the facial contours.

Some blushers appear very vibrant in the container, yet when they are applied to the skin they are subtle.

Before applying these products, decide on the effect you wish to achieve. Study the client's face from the front and side profiles, and determine what facial corrective work is necessary.

The colour should brighten the face. Hold different blusher shades next to the face to identify a suitable colour. Consider the age of the client: natural shades are preferable to bright fashion colours.

Blushers are available in powder, cream and liquid formulations.

Powder blushers Mineral powder blusher is formulated using pigments to add colour and warmth to the skin. Alternatively, synthetic or natural pigments are formulated with a face powder with a talc base to add bulk, and zinc stearate to bind the ingredients together with various skin conditioning agents. A softer look is achieved with powder blusher.

Blusher contour product

Cream blushers A cream or wax base holds the pigment colour. Silicone is added to cream blushers to facilitate application. Cream blushers are highly pigmented so consider this when applying.

Liquid blushers Pigment providing the tint shade is suspended in a liquid containing water, glycerine, silica and alcohol.

If liquid or cream cosmetics are used, these must be applied on top of a liquid or cream foundation before powder application. (If powder contour products are used, these should be applied after the application of the loose face powder. The rule of contour cosmetic application is: powder on powder; cream on cream.)

Shader/blusher contour product

Mineral powder blushes Minerals are refined to a lightweight, sheer application where colour is achieved by layering. Ideal to use for a mature skin.

How to apply powder blushers

Stroke the contour brush over the powder blusher. Tap the brush gently to dislodge excess blusher.

Apply the blusher to the cheek area, carefully placing the product according to the effect you wish to create. The direction of brush strokes should be upwards and outwards, towards the hairline. Keep the blusher away from the nose, and avoid applying blusher too near the outer eye. Ensure the edges of the blusher application are blended and softened.

Apply more blusher if necessary. The key to successful blusher application is to build up colour slowly until you have achieved the optimum effect.

If too much blusher is applied, tone down with the application of a loose face powder.

How to apply cream blushers

Remove the cream blusher hygienically from its container.

Apply the cream blusher after foundation application. Using the fingertips dot the cream blush colour sparingly onto the fullness of the cheek area and blend towards the hairline.

> ### TOP TIP
> **Blusher**
> Blusher can be applied to the cheeks and temples to add warmth to the face.

Blusher application

Cream blusher is suited to all skin types except oily. Place a loose translucent powder over the cream blusher to set if required. Alternatively it can be left unpowdered for a 'dewy' effect.

How to apply liquid blushers

Liquid blusher provides a sheer to strong, stained look, dependent upon product usage. It is best to apply to a normal skin as it is difficult to blend and would be generally unsuitable on a dry skin type.

Dot the liquid blush on the cheek area and blend well. Remember it must be worked with quickly, if left in an area too long it will stain.

To assess the client's **face shape**, take the hair away from the face – hairstyles often disguise the face shape. Study the size and shape of the facial bone structure. Consider the amount of excess fat and the muscle tone.

Oval *Bone structure* This is regarded as the perfect face shape.

Corrective make-up Corrective make-up application usually attempts to create the *appearance* of an oval face shape. Draw attention to the cheekbones by applying shader beneath the cheekbone, and highlighter above. Blusher should be drawn along the cheekbone and blended up towards the temples.

Round *Bone structure* Broad and short.

Corrective make-up Apply highlighter in a thin band down the central portion of the face to create the illusion of length. Shader may be applied over the angle of the jaw to the temples. Apply blusher in a triangular shape, with the base of the triangle running parallel to the ear.

Square *Bone structure* A broad forehead and a broad, angular jaw line.

Corrective make-up Shade the angles of the jawbone, up and towards the cheekbone. Apply blusher in a circular pattern on the cheekbones, taking it towards the temples.

Heart *Bone structure* A wide forehead, with the face tapering to a narrow, pointed chin, like an inverted triangle (heart shape is also known as an inverted **triangle** – a triangle on its point).

Corrective make-up Highlight the angles of the jawbone and shade the point of the chin, the temples and the sides of the forehead. Apply blusher under the cheekbones, in an upward and outward direction towards the temples.

Diamond *Bone structure* A narrow forehead, with wide cheekbones tapering to a narrow chin.

Corrective make-up Apply shader to the tip of the chin and the height of the forehead, to reduce length. Highlight the narrow sides of the temples and the lower jaw. Apply blusher to the fullness of the cheekbones to draw attention to the centre of the face.

Oblong *Bone structure* Long and narrow, tapering to a pointed chin.

Corrective make-up Apply shader to the hairline and the point of the chin to reduce the length of the face. Highlight the angle of the jawbone and the temples to create width. Blend blusher along the cheekbones, outwards towards the ears.

Face shapes

Oval face   Round face   Square face   Heart face

Diamond face   Oblong face   Pear face

Pear *Bone structure* A wide jaw line, tapering to a narrow forehead. Also known as triangular face shape.

Corrective make-up Highlight the forehead and shade the sides of the chin and the angle of the jaw. Apply blusher to the fullness of the cheeks, or blend it along the cheekbones, up towards the temples.

> ##### Practice Makes Perfect
> It's true when they say practice makes perfect. A lot of people rely on 'models' to practice on. The best practice I have is when I am working on counter; every person who sits in my chair is unique. No face is the same so the more people you see the more practice you get. This will prepare you for jobs when you are meeting models for the first time. You have to adapt quickly and practising on all different types of people is perfect for mastering your techniques.
>
> *Charlotte Savoury*

ACTIVITY

Correcting nose shapes

Think of the different nose shapes you may encounter, such as Roman, turned up, bulbous, or with a long tip. Which contour cosmetics would you select to correct each? Where would you apply them?

TOP TIP

Blusher

Keep blusher away from the centre of the face to avoid accentuating the breadth of the face.

ACTIVITY

Contouring

Study three different clients or colleagues. Identify their face shapes. Where would you apply the contouring cosmetics for each face shape, and why?

TOP TIP

Asian faces

An Asian face may appear as a flat plane: the skilful application of shading and highlighting products can create highs and lows.

Features

Noses

- **If the nose is too broad**: apply shader to the sides of the nose.
- **If the nose is too short**: apply highlighter down the length of the nose from the bridge to the tip.
- **If the nose is too long**: apply shader to the tip of the nose.
- **If there is a bump on the nose**: apply shader over the area.
- **If there is a hollow along the bridge of the nose**: apply highlighter to the hollow area.
- **If the nose is crooked**: apply shader over the crooked side.

Foreheads

- *If the forehead is prominent*: apply shader centrally over the prominent area, blending it outwards toward the temples.
- *If the forehead is shallow*: apply highlighter in a narrow band below the hairline.
- *If the forehead is deep*: apply shader in a narrow band below the hairline.

Chins

- *If the jaw is too wide*: apply shader from beneath the cheekbones and along the jaw line, blending it at the neck.
- *If the chin is double*: apply shader to the centre of the chin, blending it outwards along the jawbone and under the chin.
- *If the chin is prominent*: apply foundation to the tip of the chin.
- *If the chin is long*: apply shader over the prominent area.
- *If the chin recedes*: apply highlighter along the jaw line and at the centre of the chin.

Necks

- *If the neck is thin*: apply highlighter down each side of the neck.
- *If the neck is thick*: apply shader to both sides of the neck.

Face powder

Face powder is applied to set the foundation, disguising minor blemishes and making the skin appear smooth and oil-free. It protects the skin from the environment by acting as a barrier. It also allows the application and smooth blending of other powder products such as blusher and eye shadow.

Most powders are based on talc as the main ingredient, but talc particles are of uneven size, and substitutes such as mica are now becoming popular. These give a more natural, flattering appearance to the skin.

Powder adheres to the foundation through the addition of zinc, magnesium stearate or fatty esters. These chemicals set the make-up and remove tackiness. Further powder products can then be applied to the skin.

Face powder contains absorbent materials such as precipitated chalk, rice powder or nylon derivatives. These absorb sweat and sebum throughout the day, reducing shine and giving the foundation greater durability.

Light-reflecting ingredients such as mica and moisturizing ingredients are popular to reduce and soften the signs of ageing such as fine lines.

Shine-control ingredients or 'blot powder' is created for use in professional situations and for touch-ups. Blot powder contains crystallized minerals and silica to absorb excess oils and reduce shine on the skin's surface.

HEALTH & SAFETY

Avoiding contamination Before application, always remove sufficient loose powder from the container. This minimizes the chances of bacteria entering the powder.

Kinds of face powders

There are two basic products: loose powders and compact powders.

Loose powders Loose powders do not contain any oils or gums to bind the powder together. They are available in a range of shades, with different pastel pigments added to counteract skin imperfections. Colours include pink and lilac, which are flattering when viewed under artificial lights; yellow, which enhances a tanned skin; and green, which counteracts a red skin. Iridescent ingredients may be included to produce shimmering and highlighting effects. Translucent powder has no colour.

Many cosmetic products contain titanium dioxide, an opaque white pigment, to provide coverage. When applied to black skin, this can give the skin a chalky appearance. When selecting products for black skin, bear in mind not just the shade but also the ingredients.

Compact powders Compact powders contain a gum, mixed with the ingredients to bind them together. These powders provide a greater coverage, especially if they contain titanium dioxide. Pressed powders should be recommended mainly for a client's personal use, and then only to remove shine from the skin during the day, as required.

How to apply powder

Face powder is applied **after** the foundation, unless a water-based foundation or a combination powder foundation has been selected. Select a matt powder for a daytime make-up, and an iridescent shimmer powder for an evening make-up.

Don't apply face powder to excessively dry skin, as it would aggravate and emphasize the dry skin condition. Beware of applying powder if a client has superfluous facial hair, as it may emphasize this. If the skin appears too pale apply a facial bronzer to correct. Oily skin can make the powder darker. If this occurs apply a lighter powder to correct.

TOP TIP

Foreheads

Foreheads can be improved by a flattering hairstyle:

◆ *prominent forehead*: choose soft, flat, textured fringes

◆ *shallow forehead*: choose a shorter, soft fringe. Height will make the forehead appear longer

◆ *deep forehead*: choose a longer, soft fringe.

HEALTH & SAFETY

Home use If the client uses a pressed powder, advise them to wash and regularly replace the powder applicator to minimize the reproduction of bacteria.

TOP TIP

Mature skin

Some powders reflect light while appearing subtle and non-shiny. These are most flattering for mature skin, as wrinkles appear less obvious.

Light-reflecting mineral loose powder

Loose powder application

Removal of excess loose powder

Bronzing powder application

Loose face powder

1 Remove the loose powder from its container, using a clean spatula or, if the powder is in a shaker, by sprinkling it out. Place the powder on a clean facial tissue.

2 Ask the client to keep their eyes closed. Using a clean piece of cotton wool or velour sponge, press into the powder and then press the powder all over the face.

3 Remove excess powder using a large, disinfected facial powder brush. Direct the brush strokes first up the face, which dislodges the powder, then down the face, which flattens the facial hair and removes the final residue of excess powder.

Compact powder Apply powder with a brush or velour powder puff. Facial contouring using powder products may now be carried out.

Bronzing

Bronzing products are applied to create a healthy, natural or subtle tanned look. They are formulated to create a matt or shimmer effect and are also suitable as a highlighting contouring product.

Kinds of bronzing products

Bronzing products are available in powder, gel and liquid formulation. Powder bronzer, a tinted powder in different shades, gives skin natural colour effects and highlights. Ideal for enhancing a client's skin tone or tan and suitable for all skin types, although they can emphasize a dry or mature skin. Gel bronzer contains gel and glycerine in which the pigment is suspended. Gel bronzer is preferable for a dry, mature skin type and can be applied to the whole face or specific areas. Liquid bronzer is suitable for all skin types and contains a pearlized, light-reflective micro-fine powder with an oil-free formulation. Silicone enhances its application.

Apply bronzing products according to the effect you want to achieve after powder application or in the case of gel and liquid after foundation application. Remember you can use bronzers as a contour product also.

Powder Using a large powder brush apply the bronzer powder. Stroke the brush over the cheek area, followed by nose, chin and neck area.

Gel As for liquid blusher you need to blend the gel bronzer quickly over each area. Apply with the fingers or a damp sponge. Commence at the cheek area, forehead, nose and chin.

Liquid Apply as for gel bronzer.

Eye make-up

Make-up is applied to the eye area to complement the natural eye colour, to give definition to the eye area, and to enhance the natural shape of the eye.

Eye shadow

Eye shadow adds colour and definition to the eye area. The different types include matt, pearlized, metallic and pastel. They are available in cream, crayon or powder form. Eye shadows are composed of either oil-and-water emulsions or waxes containing inorganic pigments to give colour.

- ◆ *Powder eye shadows* have a talc base, mixed with oils to facilitate application. Lighter shades are produced by the addition of titanium dioxide – avoid these on dark skin as they contrast too harshly with the natural skin colour.

- ◆ *Cream eye shadows* contain wax, oil and silica.

- ◆ *Liquid eye shadows* contain water, mica, glycerine and butylene glycol to achieve the correct viscosity.

- ◆ *Crayon eye shadows* are composed of wax and oil, and are similar in appearance and application to an eye pencil.

Pearlized mineral eye shadows are created by the addition of bismuth oxychloride, a fine crystalline powder or mica, a light-reflecting mineral powder; a metallic effect is created by the addition of fine particles of gold leaf, aluminium or bronze.

TOP TIP

Bronzers for males

A bronzing powder especially for males is available which is matt and natural.

HEALTH & SAFETY

Eye cosmetics The eye tissue is particularly sensitive. Eye cosmetic products should be of the highest quality, and be permitted for use according to the Cosmetics Products (Safety) Regulations (2008).

ALWAYS REMEMBER

Too much powder

When applying powder colours, always tap the brush before application to remove excess eye shadow. If too much colour is deposited on the applicator, stroke it over a clean tissue to remove the excess.

Remember it is better to apply more product in stages until you create the look you want to achieve.

A selection of golden-hazel powder eye shadows

How to apply eye shadow

Eye shadow application will differ according to the eye shape of the client and the look to be achieved.

Powder eye shadow

1 Protect the skin beneath the eye with a clean tissue or loose powder to collect small particles of eye shadow that may fall during application.

2 Lift the skin at the brow slightly to keep the eye tissue taut, enabling you to reach the skin near to the base of the eyelashes.

3 Apply the selected eye shadow to the eyelid, using a sponge or an eye shadow brush applicator.

4 Highlight beneath the brow bone.

5 Using a brush, apply a darker eye shadow to the socket area, beginning at the outer corner of the eye. Blend the colour evenly, to avoid harsh lines.

6 Ask your client to open her eyes during application so that you can look at the effect created.

TOP TIP

Cream eye shadows

Cream eye shadows are less popular as they are more difficult to blend and quickly settle into creases. They are usually used by clients who have dry, mature skin.

ACTIVITY

Eye shadow application techniques

There are many different looks that can be created by the placement of eye shadow. Consider 'smoky' and 'winged'. Collect different images of techniques and practise their application.

3 Eye shadow application

4 Highlighter application beneath brow bone

5 Eye shadow application to contour the eye socket

5 continued. Blending eyeshadow to avoid harsh lines

Eyeliners

Cream eye shadow Apply over a base to hold the cream shadow in place. It may be applied with a brush and blended with the finger or brush.

Liquid eye shadow Apply the liquid shadow pearly colour with a brush stroking and blending over the eyelid where required.

Eyeliner

Eyeliner defines and emphasizes the eye area. It is available in pencil, liquid or powder form.

◆ *Eye pencil* Made of wax and oil, and contains different pigments which give it its colour.

◆ *Liquid and gel eyeliner* A gum solution, in which the pigment is suspended.

◆ *Powder eyeliner* A powder base with the addition of mineral oil.

Powder eyeliner is the most suitable choice for a client who is exposed to a warm environment, as it will not smudge. Sharpen the pencil if used to achieve a sharp point.

How to apply eyeliner If you are using a powder or liquid eyeliner, apply it with a clean eyeliner brush.

1 Lift the skin gently upwards at the eyebrows, to keep the firm and make application easier.

TOP TIP

Cotton buds

Have a clean cotton bud available so that you can remove the powder from any minor mistakes during application.

2   Draw a fine line along the base of the eyelashes (as close to the lashes as possible), as required. Start application at the outer corner of the eye and apply towards the inner corner of the eye. The length of the line applied and angle will differ depending on the look to be achieved.

3   If using an eye pencil or powder line, lightly smudge the eyeliner to soften the effect of the line. (This is not effective with liquid liner.) If required, a further application may be applied for a thicker line. Liquid liner is applied with a fine-tip brush. To help stability when applying, place the base of the hand on a tissue against the client's cheek.

4   Eyeliner may be applied to the inner eye, usually accompanying a 'smoky' eye shadow look. This technique is unsuitable on small eyes as it would make them appear smaller.

Eye pencil application to the upper eyelid

ALWAYS REMEMBER

Kohl eyeliner

Kohl was used by the Ancient Egyptians, a black cosmetic containing stibium. This is now banned. Iron oxide is a mineral ion commonly used today.

TOP TIP

Lasting eyeliner

Powder eye shadow may be applied over the eye pencil application to increase its durability, as heat and moisture can disturb the wax/oil content of a pencil.

Eyebrow colour

Eyebrow colour emphasizes the eyebrow, darkens the hair, alters its shape, disguises bald patches and can make sparse eyebrows look thicker. It is available in pencil, liquid or powder form.

◆ *Eyebrow pencil* Firmer than an eye pencil, and is composed of waxes that hold the inorganic pigments.

◆ *Powder brow colour* Composed of a talc base, mixed with mineral oil and pigments. This may be applied in conjunction with a specialized wax or gel.

◆ *Liquid eyebrow* A fluid, quick-drying eyebrow colour to define the brows.

◆ *Eyebrow mascara* Composed of mineral oil and waxes with pigment suspended in it. The mascara defines the brows and controls and shapes them.

Brow perfector

How to apply eyebrow colour

1   Select an appropriate colour of powder or eyebrow pencil. Brush the eyebrows with a clean brow brush to remove excess face powder and eye shadow. A specialized wax or gel can be applied which aids adherence of powder brow shadow and separates and defines the brow hair.

2   Simulate the appearance of brow hair by using fine strokes of colour, or disguise bald patches with a denser application. Use a pencil or liquid eyebrow to apply feathery strokes, or alternatively using a brush, apply powder to the prepared brow hair.

3   Brush the eyebrows into shape if necessary without disturbing product application.

Mascara

TOP TIP

Eyelash curling

The eyelashes may be temporarily curled with eyelash curlers before mascara application to open up the eye area.

ACTIVITY

Brow colour

What brow colour product would you select for the following and how would you apply it:

◆ blonde-haired client, day wear
◆ dark-haired client, evening make-up
◆ red-haired client, special occasion
◆ grey-haired client, sparse brow hair, day make-up.

HEALTH & SAFETY

Mascara Mascara when purchased is usually provided with a brush applicator. This applicator cannot be effectively cleaned and disinfected, however, so it should not be used. Instead use a disposable mascara brush for each client.

Mascara

Mascara enhances the natural eyelashes, making them appear longer, changed in colour and thicker. It is available in liquid, cream and block-cake forms. It is composed of waxes or an oil-and-water emulsion, and contains pigments which give it its colour. Other ingredients can be added to increase its durability, making it waterproof which will require a special eye make-up remover for waterproof mascara.

◆ *Liquid mascara* – a mixture of gum in water or alcohol; the pigment is suspended in this. It may also contain short textile filaments that adhere to the lashes and have a thickening, lengthening effect. Water-resistant mascara contains resin instead of gum, so that it will not run or smudge.

◆ *Cream mascara* – an emulsion of oil and water, with the pigment suspended in this.

◆ *Block mascara* – composed of mineral oil, lanolin and waxes, which are melted together to form a block on setting. It must be dampened with water before application.

HEALTH & SAFETY

Allergies If the client has hypersensitive eyes or skin, use hypoallergenic cosmetics that contain no known sensitizers.

Contact lenses If the client wears contact lenses, don't use either lash-building filament mascaras or loose-particled eye shadows, which have a tendency to flake and may enter the eye.

How to apply mascara Using a disposable mascara brush, apply mascara to the eyelashes:

1 Hold the brush horizontally to apply colour to the length of the lashes. Where the lashes are short and curly, or difficult to reach, hold the brush vertically and use the point of the brush.

2 Place a clean tissue underneath the base of the lower eyelashes, and stroke the brush down the length of the lashes from the base to the tips.

3 Lift the eyelid at the brow bone. Ask the client to look down slightly while keeping their eyes open. From above, stroke down the length of the lashes from the base to the tips.

TOP TIP

Clear mascara

Clear mascara makes the lashes appear thicker, while appearing very natural.

ALWAYS REMEMBER

Curly eyelashes

Curly lashes will require brushing, using a clean brush, both before mascara application and after each coat, to separate the lashes. A specialized gel may be applied before mascara application which, on drying, separates the lashes.

4 Using a zigzag motion, draw the brush upwards through the upper and lower surfaces of the lashes, from the base to the tips. Apply several coats to create a dramatic evening look.

5 Finally, separate the eyelashes with a clean brush or lash comb.

TOP TIP

Mascara accidents!

If you accidentally get mascara on the skin, remove with a cotton bud. If waterproof you may need a small amount of eye make-up remover on the bud. Apply any corrective make-up to follow and conceal.

Eye make-up for the client who wears glasses

If the client wears glasses, check the function of the lens, as this can alter the appearance and effect of the eye make-up.

◆ *If the client is short-sighted, the lens makes the eye appear smaller.* Draw attention to the eyes by selecting lighter colours. When applying eye shadow and eyeliner, use the corrective techniques for small eyes. Apply mascara to emphasize the eyelashes.

◆ *If the client is long-sighted, the lens will magnify the eye.* Make-up should therefore be subtle, avoiding frosted colours and lash-building mascaras. Careful blending is important, as any mistakes will be magnified!

How to apply corrective eye make-up

Dark circles

1 Minimize the circles by applying a concealing product.

Wide-set eyes

1 Apply a darker eye colour to the inner portion of the upper eyelid.

2 Apply lighter eye shadow to the outer portion of the eyelid.

3 Apply eyeliner in a darker colour to the inner half of the upper eyelid.

4 Eyebrow pencil may be applied to extend the inner browline.

Close-set eyes

1 Lighten the inner portion of the upper eyelid.

2 Use a darker colour at the outer eye.

3 Apply eyeliner to the outer corner of the upper eyelid.

4 Pluck brow hairs at the inner eyebrow – this helps to create the illusion of the eyes being further apart.

ALWAYS REMEMBER

Mascara wand

Never pump the mascara wand when loading it with mascara. This encourages air to enter and makes the mascara dry out.

Mascara application to the upper lashes

ACTIVITY

Choosing mascara

What colour mascara should be applied if the client has the following hair colouring: brown, red, black or grey?

Dark circles

Wide-set eyes

Close-set eyes

Round eyes

Round eyes

1   Apply a darker colour over the prominent central upper-lid area.

2   Elongate the eyes by applying eyeliner to the outer corners of the upper and lower eyelids.

Prominent eyes

Prominent eyes

1   Apply dark matt eye shadow over the prominent upper eyelid.

2   Apply a darker shade to the outer portion of the eyelid, and blend it upwards and outwards.

3   Highlight the brow bone, drawing attention to this area.

4   Eyeliner may be applied to the inner lower eyelid.

> **TOP TIP**
>
> **Prominent eyes**
>
> To make the eyes appear less prominent, select matt eye shadows – pearlized and frosted eye shadows will highlight and emphasize the eye.

Overhanging lids

Overhanging lids

1   Apply a pale highlighter to the middle of the eyelid.

2   Apply a darker eye shadow to contour the socket area, creating a higher crease (which disguises the hooded appearance).

Deep-set eyes

Deep-set eyes

1   Use light-coloured eye shadows.

2   Eye shadow may also be applied in a fine line to the inner half of the lower eyelid, beneath the lashes.

3   Apply eyeliner to the outer halves of the upper and lower eyelids, broadening the line as you extend outwards.

Downward-slanting eyes

Downward-slanting eyes

1   Create lift by applying the eye shadow upwards and outwards at the outer corners of the upper eyelid.

2   Apply eyeliner to the upper eyelid, applying it upwards at the outer corner.

3   Confine mascara to the outer lashes.

Small eyes

Small eyes

1   Choose a light colour for the upper eyelid.

2   Highlight under the brow, to open up the eye area.

3   Curl the lashes before applying mascara.

4   Apply a light-coloured eyeliner to the outer third of the lower eyelid.

5   A white eyeliner may be applied to the inner lid, to make the eye appear larger.

Narrow eyes

1   Apply a lighter colour in the centre of the eyelid, to open up the eye.

2   Apply a shader to the inner and outer portions of the eyelid.

Narrow eyes

Oriental eyes

1   Divide the upper eyelid in two vertically. Place a lighter colour over the inner half of the eyelid and a darker colour at the outer half.

2   Apply a highlighter under the eyebrow.

3   White eyeliner may be applied at the base of the lash line, on the lower inner eyelid.

Oriental eyes

TOP TIP

False eyelashes

False eyelashes should be available if you are applying an evening or special occasion make-up – you may wish to apply these to enhance the appearance of the eyes. Remember you will need to perform a skin sensitivity test in advance.

TOP TIP

Oriental clients

Eyelash curling is beneficial for Oriental clients who have short lashes that grow downwards.

The eyelashes

To emphasize the eyelashes, making them appear longer temporarily, curl them using eyelash curlers. If performing after mascara application it must be dry.

HEALTH & SAFETY

Eyelash curling Repeated eyelash curling can lead to breakage. The technique should therefore be used only for special occasions.

How to curl the eyelashes

1   Rest the upper lashes between the upper and lower portions of the eyelash curlers.

2   Bring the two portions gently together with a squeezing action.

3   Hold the lashes in the curlers for approximately 10 seconds, then release them.

4   If the lashes are not sufficiently curled, repeat the action.

The lips

Lip cosmetics add colour and draw attention to the lips. As the lips have no protective sebum, the use of lip cosmetics also helps to prevent them from drying and becoming chapped.

It is not uncommon for the lips to be out of proportion in some way. Using lip cosmetics and corrective techniques, symmetrical lips can be created. A careful choice of product and accurate application are required to achieve a professional effect.

Lip cosmetics

Lip cosmetics

The main lip cosmetics are lip liner, lipsticks, lip tints, lip balm and lip glosses. Sometimes the lips may be unevenly pigmented. The application of a lip toner or foundation over the lips corrects this.

Lip liner

Lip liner is used to define the lips, creating a perfectly symmetrical outline. This is coloured in with another lip cosmetic, either a lipstick or a lip gloss. The lip liner also helps to prevent the lipstick from 'bleeding' into lines around the lips.

Lip liner has a wax base which does not melt and can be applied easily. It contains pigments which give the pencil its colour.

When choosing a lip liner, select one that is the same colour as, or slightly darker than, the lipstick to be used with it.

Lipstick

Lipstick contains a blend of oils and waxes, which give it its firmness, and silicone, essential for easy application. It also contains pigment, to add colour, an emollient moisturizer to keep the lips soft and supple and perfume to improve its appeal. In addition it may include vitamins, to condition the lips, or sunscreens, to protect the lips from UV rays. Some lipsticks contain a relatively large proportion of water – these moisturize the lips and provide a natural look. The coverage provided by a lipstick depends on its formulation.

Lipsticks are available in the following forms: cream, matt, frosted and translucent. Frosted lipstick has good durability, as it is very dry. Some other lipsticks also offer extended durability, and are suitable for clients who are unable to renew their lipstick regularly.

When choosing the colour of lipstick, take into account the natural colour of the client's lips (it is best if it is the same colour tone), the skin and hair colours, and the colours selected for the rest of the make-up.

Lip gloss

Lip gloss provides a moist, shiny look to the lips. It may be worn alone, or applied on top of a lipstick. Its effect is short-lived. Lip gloss is made of mineral oils, with pigment suspended in the oil.

Note that mature clients often have creases on the lips that extend to the surrounding skin. If lip gloss is used it will often bleed into these lines.

Lip stain

Lip stain adds intense colour to the lips and is made of water, glycerine, skin-conditioning ingredients and mineral pigments. Prepare the lip with lip liner. Apply to lips quickly, using the fingertips or a make-up sponge. Build up the colour to achieve the result required.

Lip balm

Lip balm is a lip moisturizer containing oil and beeswax, vitamins C and E to help prevent dryness and improve skin texture, and pigment to add colour and sheen. Following the lip liner, apply to the lips with a brush. A gloss may then be applied to enhance the lips.

Dry lips Sometimes the lips become dry and chapped. Recommend that the client keeps them moisturized at all times, especially in extremes of heat, cold or wind. Some facial exfoliants can be professionally applied over the lips to remove dead skin.

If the client does not like to wear make-up during the day, or if the client is male, recommend that the lips be protected with a lip-care product.

How to apply corrective lip make-up

Thick lips Select natural colours and darker shades, avoiding bright, glossy colours.

1   Blend foundation over the lips to disguise the natural lip line.

2   Apply a darker lip liner inside the natural lip line to create a new line.

Thick lips

Thicker upper or lower lip

1   Use the technique described above to make the larger lip appear smaller.

2   Apply a slightly darker lipstick to the larger lip.

3   If the lips droop at the corners, raise the corners by applying lip liner to the corners of the upper lip, to turn them upwards.

Thick upper lip

Thick lower lips

Thin lips Select brighter, pearlized colours. Avoid darker lipsticks, which will make the mouth appear smaller.

1   Apply a neutral lip liner just outside the natural lip line.

Thin lips

Small mouth

1   Extend the line slightly at the corners of the mouth, with both the upper and the lower lips.

Small mouth

Uneven lips

1   Use a lip liner to draw in a new line.

2   Apply lipstick to the area.

Uneven lips

Lines around the mouth

1   Apply lip liner around the natural lip line.

2   Apply a matt cream lipstick to the lips. (Don't use gloss, which might bleed into the lines around the mouth.)

Lines around the mouth

How to apply lipstick

1   Select a lip pencil and lipstick to complement the client's colouring and the colour theme of the make-up.

2   Using a pencil sharpener, sharpen the lip pencil to expose a clean surface.

3   Ask the client to open her mouth slightly.

HEALTH & SAFETY

Lip brushes Disposable lip brushes are available to enable lip cosmetics to be applied hygienically.

Lip liner application

Lipstick application

CourseMate video: Day Make-up

The finished day make-up

4   Outline the lips, carrying out lip correction as necessary. Begin the lip line at the outer corner of the mouth, and continue it to the centre of the lips. Repeat the process on the other side of the lip, commencing at the outer corner of the mouth.

5   Remove sufficient lipstick using a clean spatula.

6   Using a disinfected lip brush, apply the lipstick to the lips.

7   Apply a clean facial tissue over the lip area, and gently press it onto the lips. This process, known as blotting, removes excess lipstick and fixes the colour on the lips.

8   The application of powder on the first application of lipstick will make the lipstick longer lasting.

9   A second light application of lipstick may then be applied.

10 If desired, lip gloss may be applied over the lipstick to add sheen, again using a disinfected lip brush.

Finished make-up

After applying the make-up, fix the client's hair and then discuss the finished result in front of the make-up mirror.

Wash your hands. Record details of the treatment on the client's record card.

Provide aftercare advice.

Finished results

Discussing the finished result - discuss how it can be maintained and how specific results have been achieved!

Aftercare advice

Following make-up application, recommend the correct skincare products to remove the products you have applied.

Eye cleansing advice

◆   Cleanse the eye area using a suitable eye make-up remover.

◆   Remove waterproof mascara, usually using an oily eye make-up remover.

◆   If false lashes have been applied, their removal must also be discussed (see pages 310–311).

Skincare advice

◆   Apply cleansing preparations to remove facial make-up with an appropriate cleanser in an upwards and outwards direction. Remove with damp cotton wool or clean facial sponges.

◆ Apply a suitable toner to suit skin type to remove excess cleanser.

◆ Apply day or night moisturizer in small dots to the neck, chin, cheeks, nose and forehead. Quickly and evenly spread a thin film over the face, using light upward, outward stroking movements.

◆ Blot the skin with a soft facial tissue to remove excess moisture.

Advise the client on application procedures to maintain the effect, e.g. removal of facial shine from the face with pressed powder, lip liner to stop 'bleeding', reapplication of blusher to add warmth.

Explain to the client that you can offer a make-up lesson in which you would discuss the reason for the selection of make-up products and colours, and the techniques for applying them. Recommend the correct skincare products to remove the products you have applied.

Have retail products available for the client to purchase. These include the products that you have used during the make-up application and skincare products for preparation and removal of make-up.

Share tips that will ensure that the client gets the best out of any products purchased. Explain how to use the product hygienically and when it should be replaced.

Explain what action to take in the event of a contra-action.

Finally, at the end of the make-up treatment ensure that the client's records are updated, accurate and signed by the client and beauty therapist.

Make-up objectives

Day make-up

The effect should be natural. Any corrective work carried out should be very subtle and kept to the minimum, as natural light makes any imperfections appear obvious.

Select a foundation the same colour as the skin – aim to even out the skin tone. Set the foundation with a translucent face powder.

Day make-up

Apply a subtle, warm blusher or bronzing product to add colour to the face. Avoid strong colours of cosmetics, especially on the eyes. The mascara colour should be chosen to complement the client's natural lash and skin colours. Mascara should be used to emphasize, but not exaggerate, the length and thickness of the eyelashes. Eyeliner may be used, but it should be carefully placed and blended.

Line the lips in a colour that will co-ordinate with the lipstick to be applied, which again should be quite natural. However, it may be bolder on occasions to follow a particular trend or to co-ordinate with an item of clothing or accessory.

Evening make-up

This should be applied bearing in mind the type of lighting in which the client will be seen. Artificial light dulls the effect, and changes the colour of the make-up: dark shades lose their brilliance, appearing 'muddy', so you need to use brighter colours. Emphasize the facial features with the careful placement of contouring cosmetics.

Evening make-up

Areas where shadows may be created, such as the eyes, should be emphasized using light, bright and highlighting cosmetic products. Add warmth to the face with an intense colour of blusher placed on the cheekbones. A highlighting or shimmer powder in a pearlized or metallic shade may be applied directly on top of or over the blusher. The client may like to try adventurous cosmetics such as metallics and frosted eye products.

Curl the eyelashes with eyelash curlers or apply false eyelashes to emphasize the eyes. Fashion shades of mascara may be selected, in purples, greens and blues, to complement the make-up and produce the effect required. Light shades of eyeliner may be used to frame the eyes and to 'open' them up.

Add a lip gloss to the lips, or apply a frosted lipstick to emphasize the mouth.

Colour the eyebrows, and carefully groom them to frame the eye area.

Special occasion make-up

A special occasion is usually an important event such as a wedding, day at the races, graduation ceremony or New Year's Eve party.

Whatever the occasion, whether daytime or evening, indoors or outdoors, you will need to consider the type of lighting the make-up will be viewed in – natural or artificial – and any other factors, such as how long it is to be worn for.

The selection of colours should co-ordinate with what the client will be wearing, and finally you need to know the effect they wish the make-up to create – should it be subtle or glamorous? Make-up products can then be selected and appropriately applied to suit the occasion.

Make-up to suit skin and hair colouring

White skin and blonde hair If the client has blonde hair and white skin, keep the skin colour natural. Apply a blusher in rose pink or beige.

Define the eyes with soft tones of browns and pinks. Apply a brown-black mascara.

Colour the lips with a rose-pink or peach lip colour. Generally, avoid lip colours lighter than the natural skin tone.

Oriental skin and black hair For creamy, sallow skin with dark hair, use blusher to add warmth and to brighten the skin, in either pink or brown.

The eyes are dark, with a prominent brow bone. Emphasize the socket of the eye with careful shading; extend this upwards and outwards. Place highlighter along the brow bone.

Pastel colours complement the eye colour. Select black mascara to emphasize the eyes. Deep pinks and orangey-reds suit the lips.

White skin and red hair Redheads usually have white skin with freckles (ephelides). The skin will flush and colour easily, probably requiring the application of a green-tinted moisturizer, concealer or face powder. Apply blusher in a warm rose or peach colour. Browns, rusts, greens and peach eye shadow colours suit this skin and complement the eyes. Brown mascara is preferable, to avoid making the eyes appear hard.

Special occasion make-up

White skin

Oriental skin and black hair

White skin and red hair

Black skin

Olive skin

For the lips, select a lipstick in peach, golden rust or pink.

Black skin and black hair A yellow-toned foundation is required: it may be necessary to blend foundations to obtain the correct colour. Avoid pink-toned foundations, which make the skin appear chalky.

Women with dark skin tend to have dark brown to brown-black eyes, and can use a wide range of heavily pigmented colours, especially browns and bronzes. Dark shades of blusher in red and plum may be chosen; eyeliner and mascara can be black, or any other dark shade.

Avoid lip colours lighter than the skin tone. A lip liner darker than the lip colour may be used.

Olive or white skin and dark hair Select a foundation to suit the basic skin tone. If the skin is fair, choose an ivory base; if it is sallow, select a foundation with a rusty, yellow tone. (With a sallow skin, avoid the use of pinks on the eyes – they make the eyes look sore.)

A beige blusher suits this skin colour, and is complemented by the selection of brown or green shades for the eyes. Black mascara should be used for the eyelashes.

For the lips, choose warm reds or beige.

Make-up for mature skin

As the skin ages it becomes sallow in colour and appears thinner. Small capillaries can be seen, commonly on the cheek area, and small veins may appear around the eyes. Pigment changes in the skin become obvious, and remain permanently.

At the make-up consultation, discuss your ideas with your client. Very often a mature client will have been using the same colours and the same cosmetics for many years, and they may not even be complementary. You will need to advise them tactfully on a fresh approach.

Select a foundation that matches the skin colour yet enhances the skin's appearance. An oil-based foundation is appropriate for use on mature skin: it keeps the skin supple and prevents the foundation from settling into the creases and emphasizing the lines and wrinkles.

A concealer may be applied to cover obvious capillaries and small veins, or a foundation may be selected which provides adequate coverage.

Knowledge Check

What aftercare advice should be given to a client following make-up application?

Refer to pages 364–365 to help you.

Knowledge Check

What are the differences in application between day, evening and special occasion make-up?

Refer to pages 365–366 to help you.

ALWAYS REMEMBER

Dark circles under eyes

Dark circles under the eyes can be minimized with concealer. Select a concealer lighter than the foundation to be applied.

The client's skin has been cleansed, toned, moisturized and blotted to remove excess moisturizer

A lighter foundation may be applied over wrinkled areas, to make them less obvious. These areas include:

◆ around the eyes (crow's feet)

◆ between the brows

◆ across the forehead

◆ between the nose and the mouth (nasolabial folds)

◆ around the mouth (the lip line).

With age, the contours of the face lose their firmness as the fat cells that plump the face reduce, and the facial muscles lose tone and sag. Poor muscle tone can be seen in the following areas:

◆ the cheek area

◆ loose skin along the jaw line

◆ loose skin under the brow and overhanging the lid

◆ loose skin on the neck.

The application of a shader, subtly blended, can improve the appearance of such areas.

Apply translucent powder. It may be preferable to avoid doing so in the eye area as it can emphasize lines around the eyes. To reduce the powdery effect, which may make the skin appear dry, you may direct a fine water spray from a suitable distance to set the make-up.

Apply a blusher with a warm tone – avoid harsh, bright shades. A cream blusher may be applied after the foundation. Place it high on the cheekbone and blend it upwards at the temples, drawing attention upwards rather than downwards.

The lip line becomes less obvious as one grows older, and lines often appear along it. Lip liner should be applied to redefine the lips and to prevent the lipstick from 'bleeding' into the lines. Select a lip liner that is the same colour as, or slightly lighter than, the lip colour. (A darker lip colour would create an unwanted shadow.) A special lip fixative may be recommended, and a durable cream lipstick applied. Avoid the use of a gloss lipstick, which emphasizes lines around the mouth.

The angle of the mouth may droop. Corrective techniques may be used to disguise this.

Powder matt eye shadows should be selected for use on the eyelid: these soften the appearance of any lines in the area. Choose natural, light shades. Dark colours can make the eyes appear small and tired.

Eyeliner should be used in neutral shades of brown and grey – avoid harsh, bright colours, which will give a hard appearance.

Eyebrows should be perfectly groomed, and arched to give lift to the eye. Bushy eyebrows give the eyes a hooded appearance. If eyebrow colour is required, select a colour that is slightly lighter than the brow colour, or a blend of two colours. If the client has grey hair, use grey and charcoal to provide a natural effect.

Eyelashes should be emphasized with a natural-looking shade of mascara, lightly applied. (If the eyelashes lose their colour, you can recommend that the client has their lashes professionally – and permanently – tinted. Individual flare false eyelashes may be recommended for corrective purposes.)

Mature client special occasion make-up application

Make-up is to be applied to a Caucasian client to achieve a glamorous appearance for a social evening. We allowed 45 minutes to achieve this look.

The client has dry skin as the sebaceous and sudoriferous glands have become less active as part of the ageing process. Noticeable facial skin characteristics include the following:

◆ dark circles appear around the eye area

◆ thin, delicate tissue is found around the eyes with small veins and capillaries showing through the skin

◆ habitual frown lines occur

◆ poor muscle tone has resulted in slack facial contours, e.g. double chin

◆ poor skin tone exists because the skin loses its elasticity, resulting in wrinkling and loss of firmness

◆ sallow skin colour is due to poor blood circulation.

The finished special occasion make-up

Client day make-up application

Corrective work completed is subtle, as natural daylight makes any imperfections seem more obvious.

The client's skin has been cleansed, toned, moisturized and blotted to remove excess moisturizer. Thirty minutes were allowed to achieve the look.

This is an oily skin type, where overactivity of the sebaceous glands in the skin is creating a shiny, sallow appearance. Darker skin underneath the eye area requires concealer correction.

STEP-BY-STEP: CLIENT DAY MAKE-UP APPLICATION

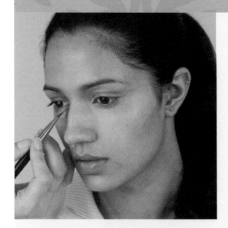

1 A concealer is applied with a brush underneath the eyes to disguise the darker skin tone.

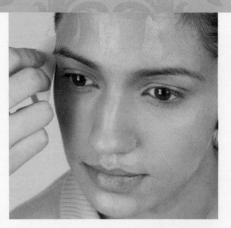

2 A liquid foundation matched to the client's skin tone is applied. Application is over the whole face, including the eyelids and lips, as this gives an even skin tone.

3 Following the application of loose powder, again matched to the client's skin tone, excess powder is removed using a large powder brush. Application is upwards and outwards.

4 Blusher colour is applied to accentuate the cheek area and add colour to the face.

5 Colour applied to the eye emphasizes the eye area. We used complementary colours in a purple range. A highlighting colour accentuates the brow bone.

6 The eyebrows are accentuated using a dark matt brown colour applied with a stiff eyebrow brush. This gives definition to the eyebrow, disguising sparse hair and gaps.

7 The lashes are lengthened using a lash-building mascara in black.

8 Lip liner colour is applied to define the desired lip contour. A co-ordinating lip colour is selected to match the lip liner and complement the eye make-up colour.

9 The lip colour is applied using a lip brush.

10 The final day make-up look.

Client evening make-up application

Make-up which will be seen under artificial lighting is applied. Stronger pigmented make-up colours have been selected, and the make-up effect emphasizes facial features through the choice and application of make-up products. Forty-five minutes were allowed to achieve the look.

The client's skin has been cleansed, toned, moisturized and blotted to remove excess moisturizer.

This is a combination skin type and the sebaceous glands are overactive in the T zone – forehead, nose and chin – and the pores appear larger in this area. The sebaceous glands are less active in the cheek, which results in dry skin with tight pores.

Other noticeable facial characteristics include the following:

◆ the skin tone of the face has uneven pigmentation

◆ the face shape requires balance, which can be achieved using shaded contour colour.

STEP-BY-STEP: CLIENT EVENING MAKE-UP APPLICATION

1 Foundation is selected to match the client's skin type and even the skin tone. A mousse foundation has been used to provide a medium coverage and has been blended quickly to avoid a chalky appearance.

2 A cream formulation shading product, in a darker shade than the foundation, is applied underneath the cheekbone and at the temples to accentuate the cheekbones and reduce the width of the face at the temples.

3 Loose powder matching the client's skin tone is applied to set the foundation and facilitate application of further powder products. Powder blusher is applied to the cheekbone.

4 Following application of a neutral eye shadow matt colour, a darker shading product is used to emphasize the eye socket.

5 The natural lash line is accentuated by eyeliner application. A steady hand is required!

6 The brows are defined.

7 Mascara application draws attention to the eyes.

8 Lip liner is applied to define the perfect lip line.

9 The lips are coloured in using a matt lipstick co-ordinated to suit the lip liner. Lip gloss achieves a final touch which will focus attention and add emphasis in darker lighting.

10 The final evening make-up look.

ASSESSMENT OF KNOWLEDGE AND UNDERSTANDING

You have now learnt the knowledge and skills required for applying make-up in the beauty therapy workplace. To test your level of knowledge, answer the following short questions. These will prepare you for your summative (final) assessment.

1. A facial feature to be diminished (made to appear less noticeable) would require the application of:

   a. highlighter contour product
   b. powder product
   c. shader contour product
   d. blusher contour product

2. If the client has large, full lips, such as the ones below, how can these be made to appear smaller?

3. The most suitable brush to apply eye shadow to cover the upper eyelid is:

   a. eyeliner brush
   b. medium firm eye shadow blending brush
   c. small rounded-edged eye shadow brush
   d. small flat-angle edged eye shadow brush

4. To test the colour of the foundation you should test it:

   a. on the client's forehead
   b. on the back of the client's hand
   c. on the client's jaw line
   d. on the client's cheekbone

5. If a cream blusher is to be applied, it should be applied:

   a. after the application of foundation
   b. after the application of powder

6. The following image shows dark circles under the eyes, these would be improved with the application of a _____ product.

7. The client below has a narrow jaw line. How can this be improved to look fuller?

8. A contra-action to make-up application may result in:

   a. an allergic reaction
   b. severe eczema
   c. a dry skin type
   d. erythema

9. The contour product blusher is applied to emphasize the following bones:

   a. parietal
   b. zygomatic
   c. maxilla
   d. tibia

10. The muscle that raises the eyebrows is the

   a. platysma
   b. orbicularis occuli
   c. corrugator
   d. frontalis

10 Part 2: Developing your make-up ideas

LEARNING OBJECTIVES

There are two learning outcomes to achieve for this optional unit:

◆ Be able to plan an image.

◆ Be able to create an image.

The assessment range applied requires you to:

◆ Develop a mood board based on a theme which clearly shows your ideas and influences and the research which guided you to create your final image to suit the requirements of the target audience.

◆ Explain the purpose of a mood board.

◆ Meet all preparation requirements for the implementation and presentation of the final theme based image.

◆ Communicate and behave in an appropriate and professional manner.

◆ Use technical skills to create a theme based image, for example hairstyling, make-up, nail art and nail enhancements.

◆ Follow all safe and hygienic working practices.

◆ Use different methods of evaluating feedback to assess the success of the treatment including observation, written, verbal, photographic and self-evaluation.

KEY TERMS

communication techniques

evaluative techniques

glitters

health and safety

hygiene requirements

marketing techniques

mood boards

team work

Unit Topic

Create an image based on a theme within the hair and beauty sector

INTRODUCTION

This unit is about developing your creative thoughts and ideas and consolidating these in order to present an image based on a theme. The image should be that which you feel best captures and represents the theme and your ideas. You may use this process for the purpose of advertising, and it is interesting to research the influences that led to the creation of different products in the beauty sector and how the final advertising image summarizes the concept. The ability to research, plan and create a range of images to a given brief, working together with others, is required in this unit. The ability to evaluate the results against the design plan is also required.

To carry out this unit you will need to maintain effective health, safety and hygiene practice throughout your work. You will also need to communicate the design concepts or ideas effectively with others involved in the project.

You must be able to show you have the necessary practical skills and underpinning knowledge to create an image based on a theme within the hair and beauty sector.

The unit will help you to plan and provide successful future promotional activities for the workplace. This will require the setting of clear objectives, realistic timescales to work to, attention to detail when planning and effective communication with all those involved with the activities implementation. Finally, engaging successfully with your audience to ensure that the promotion is a success and achieves its objectives.

Outcome 1: Be able to plan an image

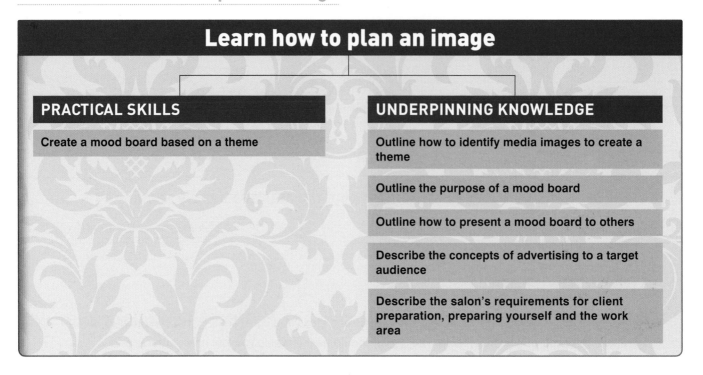

Learn how to plan an image

PRACTICAL SKILLS

Create a mood board based on a theme

UNDERPINNING KNOWLEDGE

Outline how to identify media images to create a theme

Outline the purpose of a mood board

Outline how to present a mood board to others

Describe the concepts of advertising to a target audience

Describe the salon's requirements for client preparation, preparing yourself and the work area

Knowledge Check

What are the health and safety requirements associated with make-up techniques?

Refer to pages 333–334 to help you.

The hair and beauty sector

The world of hair and beauty is an exciting and ever-changing one. It is essential that you keep up-to-date with current fashion and trends. What may be fashionable one season will change the next, and a look will quickly become outdated. This unit explains how images used in advertising campaigns can raise client awareness of a particular product or treatment you intend to gain interest in. This unit will enable you to creatively develop images which can best be used to advertise or represent a particular theme. To demonstrate this activity we are going to look at the concepts behind creating and presenting make-up looks.

Planning an image

In the workplace it is usual for you to work on activities and events with other people. You must therefore develop skills to work closely with other people. It is important for all to work towards, and aim for, the same agreed end result. Detailed and accurate planning is important so there are no misunderstandings and subsequent waste of resources including time and money.

You may choose to create a period-inspired make-up look or to use your imagination and artistic skills to create a fantasy or high-fashion effect. Photographic commercial make-up is created for advertising purposes and must not detract from the subject/medium being advertised. If it is the make-up being advertised, do not detract from the make-up with too many other fussy accessories. Always consider the design, scale and proportion of the image as a whole. Bridal or special occasion make-up must suit and please the individual wearing it, as well as looking great for photographic purposes. The stages for fashion and special occasion make-up activities will always be similar, although the techniques and

Bridal make-up

finished effects can be quite different. Your work in this area may include make-up looks for catwalk shows, music videos, commercials, bridal and special occasion make-ups.

Plan and design a make-up image based on a theme by:

1 Agreeing your ideas and image to be created with the relevant person(s) prior to commencing your design plan.

2 Clearly identifying the intended themed activity for which the make-up is required.

3 Using suitable sources of information to research ideas on themes for the make-up design.

4 Accurately sourcing and using suitable information to create your design.

5 Creating a design plan which:

◆ has clearly defined objectives which meet the requirements of the target audience

◆ uses **mood boards** suitable for the look(s) required

◆ identifies all resources required

◆ states how any risks to **health and safety** can be reduced

◆ takes into account any foreseeable problems and has noted ways of resolving them.

Preparation of products, tools and equipment

Make sure you are prepared, have everything you need, and that your tools, products and equipment are clean and well organized. Make sure the area is safe, comfortable and clean before you lay out your products, tools and equipment.

When you have completed your make-up, you may need to keep a few products on hand, such as powder and a powder puff, cotton buds, tissues and lip colour required to maintain the make-up look dependent upon the intended purpose of the make-up activity.

Mood boards

Having been told or decided upon the theme of the make-up you can then start to prepare and plan your ideas for the final look. This will require you to produce a mood board, which presents the ideas you have in mind and what you are trying to create/achieve for the overall image.

TOP TIP

Keep your client safe

◆ When planning your make-up, always ask the client if they have any known allergies to cosmetic products.

◆ Perform a skin sensitivity patch test if you have any doubts if using special effects make-up, or are using non-cosmetic products such as gold leaf.

◆ Become familiar with ingredients in skincare preparations and make-up products and their purpose.

◆ Use products intended for their purpose, e.g. don't use chunky glitter intended for use on paper near someone's eyes as it will be very abrasive. Only use cosmetic grade glitters.

ACTIVITY

Target audience groups

From your current experience of working in the beauty sector, what target groups could be encouraged to engage with your salon treatments/products? How could you promote this using a theme-based image?

HEALTH & SAFETY

Hazards

◆ Recognize potential hazards in the workplace and warn other colleagues and clients of them.

◆ Recognize steps that can be taken to minimize the risk of injury and cross-contamination at any practical activity.

A metallic themed mood board

An autumn themed mood board

Knowledge Check

Why should you research and plan thoroughly prior to the job and explain how you have created your make-up design plan?

Refer to pages 376–377 to help you.

TOP TIP

Effective communication

◆ Always be respectful and aware of differences in culture, age, disability and gender. Always strive where practicable to meet the needs of your clients.

◆ Listen carefully to others, communicate your own ideas, take on board feedback and be prepared to make changes.

Mood boards may be also referred to as concept boards or theme boards. They will help you to express your overall ideas. The result will be a collation, or collage, of images which have inspired your innovation and creativity. Items may include objects and items such as photographs, fabric swatches and make-up colour samples — anything that has progressed your ideas. The mood board is used to communicate and share ideas with your target audience, who can view it and decide whether they like the concepts represented by the board for the design theme.

Use additional media wherever possible to enhance the final image and complement it, such as painting nails to colour co-ordinate, along with clothing, accessories (props, headdresses, jewellery) and hairstyling. Carefully chosen accessories can really improve the look of the overall look. Record these ideas on your mood board.

Be creative (as long as you comply with health and safety); products can be adapted to suit effects required, for example, you may wish to dilute a creme foundation to make it into a tinted moisturizer, and lipstick could be used on eyelids etc.

You may need to research extensively for your target audience, using references such as magazines, books and the Internet. You must communicate your ideas effectively with the others before you agree to a final design plan and have your work checked over again at the end.

Developing images

Fantasy make-up

Fashion shoot creating the required image/look

Catwalk make-up

Fashion photoshoot make-up

Fantasy ice queen with use of additional media

Fantasy make-up with with use of additional media

Fantasy make-up with additional media

Themes

You may need to interpret a theme, e.g. an icy winter scene could imply using colours such as silvers, blues, greys and white. Or you may want a make-up created in brighter colours to 'warm up' a winter's day.

Consider the use of other components apart from the make-up, which will be visible and enhance the overall image. These items are referred to as 'additional media' and include:

◆ clothing

◆ hair

◆ nails

◆ accessories and props.

TOP TIP

Up your game!

If you are trained and proficient in hairstyling, fashion styling and/or nails, your chances of obtaining work will be increased, especially for smaller make-up assignments or where the budget is limited, as the client only has to pay one fee to one person. It pays to enhance your skills.

HEALTH & SAFETY

Hygiene Use hygienic practices – wash hands regularly, and use antibacterial hand cleanser or disposable tissue cloths when on location; use clean gowns, disposable gloves if working on someone with contra-indications; keep tools and equipment clean and sterile; never dip tools straight into make-up – remove with a spatula; wipe down working areas with anti-bacterial cleaner. Try to keep an aseptic working environment – a working environment which aims to eliminate bacteria.

HEALTH & SAFETY

Contra-indications Check your client for contra-indications. If they have the skin disorder herpes simplex for example, use disposables or their own brushes accompanied with hygienic practices, as you cannot cancel a shoot or wedding because of this!

Historical make-up looks

If creating an historical look, understanding the basic key make-up application points is important, such as:

◆ 1920s – pale skin, thin arched eyebrows, rounded eye shadow, blusher on the apples of the cheeks, red to dark red cupids bow style lips.

1920s make-up

1940s make-up

1950s make-up

1960s make-up

1970s make-up

1980s make-up

- 1940s – strong emphasis on the eyebrow shape and lips, typically lipstick was red.

- 1950s – strong angled eyebrows, thicker liner along the top eyelid, more eye shadow and lip colours available. Bright red glossy lips were popular.

- 1960s – pale skin, pale lipsticks, strong contouring in the eye socket in contrast with pale colour on the eyelid with the addition of heavy false eyelashes.

- 1970s – from disco glam, glitter and gloss, through to early punk at the other end of the scale.

- 1980s – strong make-up applied to the cheekbones, eyes and lips using multiple vibrant colours on the eyes. Mineral pigments were popular and used to create metallic colours for the lips and eyes.

Creating the final look

Invariably, you will work with other colleagues (like hair stylists) to create your final look, therefore good communication is important to ensure the overall look/effect is achieved. Distance and lighting need to be taken into consideration to please the relevant people viewing your work, for example, consider the differences between make-up competition judges who will scrutinize your work in close up, or audiences at a catwalk show who will view work from a distance – usually under stronger and coloured lighting effects.

Make sure you have acquired any relevant props, make-up and hair equipment in preparation. If you need any other additions to your kit, allow plenty of time to source them, contacting relevant suppliers. Make-up products and equipment can be sourced from professional make-up suppliers and department stores. Additional items such as lace, feathers, gems, etc. can be sourced from art, haberdashery and fabric stores.

If the client has not had their make-up done by another person before, explain the procedure to reassure the client and make them feel comfortable.

You may wish to practice in advance and take your own photographs to check the make-up and, if styled, the hair. Digital cameras enable you to see results instantly. You can print these out and place them on your mood board. Evaluate the look and its overall effectiveness, making any changes required. Make sure you have time and are able to adapt your design plan if any circumstances change.

As a result of assessment through self-evaluation, photographic evidence etc., you may see an opportunity to develop the initial image slightly. If you are working with a team, check with them before you go ahead and change anything as it is important that everybody is aware and in agreement with the change.

Retouching images

You should also be aware that today images are commonly 'retouched' or 'airbrushed', where the image taken is altered, often by the photographer or a graphic artist on a computer, generally using a 'Photoshop' program, after the shots have been taken.

Retouching has been common practice for many years and you will find that most images in glossy magazines have undergone this process. This procedure explains images of people with completely flawless skin, lack of under-eye shadows, wrinkles, slimline body, etc. Even the best make-up artist in the world cannot create that sort of magic!

You should, however, always aim for perfection using your make-up skills and never rely on your image being retouched afterwards.

HEALTH & SAFETY

Contra-actions If contra-actions occur (an unwanted reaction from the products), carefully remove make-up immediately and advise your client to seek medical advice if symptoms persist.

ACTIVITY

Research make-up trends from the Ancient Egyptians through to the present day. Include written information on how the make-up was applied, interesting ingredients used and colours worn in each era. Add as many images from each era as you can to build up your own photograph reference library.

> **Learn your craft**
>
> As an artist you never stop learning, the industry is constantly developing in terms of both products and techniques, so read blogs/books, watch videos and keep up-to-date with what's going on. With so many people becoming make-up artists it is essential that you continue to grow as an artist and knowledge is key.
>
> *Charlotte Savoury*

Evaluating the image

◆ Welcome feedback both positive and negative. Evaluate your make-up results. Ask for feedback from others as to the overall effectiveness and impact of your make-up, checking that it is conforming to the original design plan. If you are not 100 per cent sure of something, ask 'What do you think about this?'

◆ For your own self-development, check, evaluate and compare the development process and final result with the original themed image to identify opportunities for improvement in your design and application techniques. Is there anything you could have improved on? How? Have you used the products correctly to get the desired outcome?

◆ The final design should contribute to your professional profile.

Record the results of your evaluation for future reference. When you see the final image check everything carefully again.

Outcome 2: Be able to plan an image

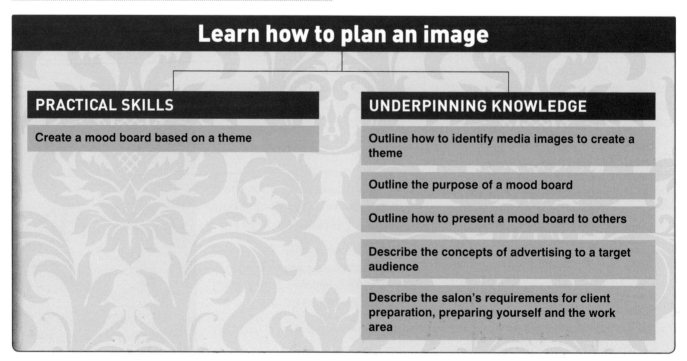

Learn how to plan an image

PRACTICAL SKILLS

Create a mood board based on a theme

UNDERPINNING KNOWLEDGE

Outline how to identify media images to create a theme

Outline the purpose of a mood board

Outline how to present a mood board to others

Describe the concepts of advertising to a target audience

Describe the salon's requirements for client preparation, preparing yourself and the work area

CASE STUDY: CREATE AN IMAGE BASED ON A THEME

Prepare and plan to create an image based on a theme. A make-up activity has been suggested but a choice could be made from any practical task within the hair and beauty sector.

◆ Develop a theme-based make-up of your choice. Suggestions for consideration include future catwalk trends; period make-up; special occasion make-up; make-up for a product advertisement; or make-up suitable for a competition brief (which you could enter!).

◆ Create a mood board to record your ideas and provide evidence of your research. Ensure this includes details of any additional media that you may be using.

◆ Do you have a budget to work to? If so, record what this is and itemize your expenditure.

◆ Provide a make-up work sheet that records the make-up products and application techniques you will use.

◆ Provide a brief description explaining and justifying how your make-up look promotes the chosen theme. Or, explain what the product stands for if it is to be used for an advertisement.

◆ Agree your final design plan with the relevant person(s) and record their comments for evaluative purposes. It may be necessary to make amendments. Note any changes made and the reasons for these changes.

Complete the make-up

◆ Complete the make-up, meeting all safety and hygiene requirements.

◆ Take pictures of the final result and evaluate its effectiveness.

◆ If necessary make any changes and update your worksheet. Inform the relevant person(s) of any changes made.

◆ Gather feedback from the relevant person(s); again you may want to make changes.

Summarize the success of the activity

◆ Were the objectives of the activity met?

◆ If working to a budget did you achieve this?

◆ Are you going to develop and use your image in the future?

◆ How could the idea be developed further?

◆ What have you learned or what experience have you gained?

◆ Did you encounter any issues and how were these dealt with?

Knowledge Check

How would you identify the effectiveness of your theme-based image and areas for improvement?

Refer to pages 381–382 to help you.

11 Manicure Treatments

LEARNING OBJECTIVES

There are two learning outcomes to achieve for this mandatory unit:

1 Be able to prepare for manicure treatments.

2 Be able to provide manicure treatments.

The assessment range applied requires you to:

◆ Use consultation techniques to identify the treatment objectives.

◆ Use products, tools and equipment as appropriate within the treatment.

◆ Treat all **skin types** and nail conditions.

◆ Ensure that the environmental conditions are suitable.

◆ Identify any contra-indications that may affect if and how the treatment can proceed.

◆ Communicate and behave in an appropriate and professional manner.

◆ Apply massage techniques.

◆ Follow all health and safety working practices.

◆ Provide relevant aftercare and **contra-action advice**.

KEY TERMS

aftercare advice	grit	nail shapes
base coat	hand and nail treatments	nail strengthener
bevelling	hand cream or oil	nail conditions
blue nail	hangnail	onycholysis
bruised nails	health and safety	onychophagy
buffer	hoof stick	onychorrhexis
consultation	joint manipulations	orange sticks
contra-action advice	leuconychia	paraffin wax
contra-actions	longitudinal ridges	psoriasis of the nail
cuticle knife	lifting	pterygium
cuticle nippers	manicure	ridge filler
cuticle cream or oil	massage	skin types
eggshell nail	muscles of the lower arm	top coat
emery board	and hand	transverse furrows
file	nail finish	treatment plan
frictions	nail polish	treatment objectives
foot creams/lotions	nail polish drier	verrucae or warts
gel	nail polish remover	warm-oil treatments

Unit Topic

Provide manicure treatments

This VRQ unit is linked to the Beauty Therapy NOS Unit N2.

INTRODUCTION

This unit is all about improving and maintaining your client's hands, nails and surrounding skin. A manicure includes filing the nails to shape, buffing the nail plate surface, using specialized nail products, cuticle products and treatments, massaging the lower arm and hand and providing an appropriate nail finish to suit the client.

Dealing with people in a polite, efficient manner and using good communication and questioning skills to find out exactly what they require from the manicure treatment service forms an important part of this technical service.

You must be able to show you have the necessary practical skills and underpinning knowledge to provide manicure treatments.

INDUSTRY ROLE MODEL

MARIAN NEWMAN Sessions Nail Technician, Industry Consultant, Author

"I have been in the professional nail industry for approximately 25 years. During that time I have been a salon owner, qualified FE teacher, written textbooks, been engaged in product development and am the Chair of the Nail Services Forum for Habia. In recent years I have worked mostly in the fashion/beauty media as a nail artist for advertising and editorial shoots, commercials and music videos. I am the lead nail artist for approximately 25 fashion shows each season in New York, London and Paris Fashion Weeks and am in my third year as a spokesperson for Chanel. I am also a judge for several national nail competitions each year.

Knowledge Check

What are the functions of blood?
Refer to page 93 to help you.

ANATOMY & PHYSIOLOGY
Essential anatomy and physiology knowledge requirements for this unit are identified on the checklist chart in Chapter 2, page 33.

Manicure products, tools and equipment

Manicure treatments

The word **manicure** is derived from the Latin words *manus*, meaning 'hand', and *cura*, meaning 'care'. A manicure therefore cares for the hands and nails and achieves the following effects:

◆ to improve the appearance of hands and nails

◆ to help to maintain and keep the nail plates healthy

◆ to keep the cuticles supple and healthy

◆ to keep the skin soft and smooth.

Preparing the work area

Ensure that all manicure tools, products and equipment are clean, sterilized and disinfected, as appropriate, and neatly organized on the work station which is suitably positioned.

Repetitive strain injury (RSI) is caused by repeated movements of a particular part of the body. This can result in injury to the skeleton and muscle of the upper body and limbs. A height adjustable chair with back support should be used ensuring that this is the correct height for the work station. Foot rests should be used for beauty therapists who cannot place their feet flat on the floor. All equipment, products and tools should be easily accessible between knee and shoulder height. Regular breaks should be taken to avoid fatigue.

TOP TIP

Benefits of manicure treatment

The beneficial effects of manicure treatment should be explained to a client at consultation and how regular manicure treatments will help to maintain healthy nails and skin.

Outcome 1: Be able to prepare for manicure treatments

Learn how to prepare for manicure treatments

PRACTICAL SKILLS

Prepare yourself, client and work area for manicure treatment

Use suitable consultation techniques to identify treatment objectives

Carry out a nail and skin analysis

Provide clear recommendations to the client

Select products, tools and equipment to suit client treatment needs, skin and nail conditions

UNDERPINNING KNOWLEDGE

Describe salon requirements for preparing yourself, the client and the work area

Describe the environmental conditions suitable for manicure treatments

Describe different consultation techniques used to identify treatment objectives

Explain the importance of carrying out a nail and skin analysis

Describe how to select products, tools and equipment to suit client treatment needs, skin and nail conditions

Identify nail and skin conditions

Describe the contra-indications which prevent or restrict manicure treatments

Keeping the working area tidy promotes an organized and professional image, and prevents time being wasted as you locate items you require. The work area should always be left in a condition suitable for further nail treatments.

A manicure treatment may be carried out at a purpose-built nail work station or over a treatment couch.

Prepare the area by placing a towel over the work surface, then fold another towel into a pad and place it in the middle of the work surface. The pad helps to support the client's forearm during treatment. Place the third towel over the pad, with more of the towel on the manicurist's side – this is used to dry the client's hands during treatment.

TOP TIP

Towels and disposable equipment

A tissue or disposable manicure mat may be placed on top of the towels, to catch any nail clippings or filings. This is thrown away later, for reasons of hygiene and to avoid irritation to the client from filings. All towels should be replaced with freshly laundered ones following each treatment.

Products, tools and equipment

Manicure trolley

◆ **Manicure table or trolley** On which to place everything

◆ **Emery boards** Used to shorten and shape the nail free edge

◆ **Hand cream or oil** Use hand cream or oil to massage the skin of the hand and arm

◆ **Base coat** To prevent nail staining, improve appearance and health of the nail and provide an even surface to improve nail polish application and adherence

◆ **Coloured nail polish (enamel)** A selection for the client to choose from in cream or and a varietly of finishes, e.g. shimmer, metallic, glitter

◆ **Top coat** To provide shine and strength to protect the nail polish. Reduces peeling and chipping and increases durability of the nail polish

◆ **Nail polish remover** To remove nail polish and excess oil or moisture remaining on the nail plate

◆ **Hoof stick** To gently tidy the softened cuticles

◆ **Cuticle nippers** To remove excess cuticle and torn skin surrounding the nail plate

◆ **Nail scissors** To shorten nail length

◆ **Orange sticks** (Orange sticks should be disposed of after each client, as they cannot be effectively sterilized.) Used to remove products from containers, and, when tipped at either end with cotton wool, to ease the cuticle back and clean under the free edge

◆ **Cuticle remover** Used to soften the skin cells and cuticle so excess epidermal skin can be easily removed

◆ **Cuticle oil or cream** Used to condition and rehydrate the skin of the cuticle; especially beneficial for dry nails and cuticles

◆ **Cotton wool** To remove nail polish and excess nail product preparations. Cotton wool may also be used to tip orange sticks for the purpose of nail product application and removal. Cotton wool filled gauze pads are also available which are more absorbent

◆ **Tissues** To protect client's clothing in the area, drying the treatment area and for drying tools after removal from the disinfectant solution etc.

YOU WILL ALSO NEED:

◆ **Medium-sized towels (3)** To dry the skin, nails, etc.

◆ **Small bowls (3)** Lined with tissues for storage and to dispense products into

◆ **A finger bowl** To place the fingers into a nail cleansing agent to soak, soften and cleanse the skin and nails

◆ **Cuticle knife** To remove excess cuticle from the surface of the nail plate

◆ **Buffers** Buffers are used to improve nail shine, stimulate blood circulation and superficial ridges when used with a buffing paste

◆ **Disinfecting solution** For all surfaces and mental implements

◆ **Skin sanitizer** To cleanse and disinfect the client's skin. Specialized sprays and gels are available for this purpose

◆ **Tow, three or four-sided buffer** To remove dead skin cells and impart shine improving the nail plate appearance

◆ **Client record card** To record confidential details of each client registered at the salon, including personal details, products used and details of the treatment provided.

◆ **Nail polish drier** An aerosol or oil preparation applied to speed up the drying process of nail polish

◆ **Waste container** This should be a lined metal bin with a lid to contain vapours from solvents

Additional equipment for further hand and nail treatments may include:

◆ Paraffin wax

◆ Hand masks

◆ Thermal mitts

◆ Exfoliators and warm oil

Products used in both manicure and pedicure treatments

Before beginning the manicure, check that you have the necessary products, tools and equipment and that they meet legal hygiene and industry requirements for nail treatments.

The following is a list of products that are used in both manicure and pedicure treatments and should be referred to when studying pedicure in Chapter 12.

Product	Ingredients	Uses
Nail polish remover	Acetone or ethyl acetate – solvent. Perfume – usually synthetic. Colour. Oil – emollient to reduce drying effect of solvent. Acetone-free **nail polish removers** are available made from soya- and corn-based agricultural chemical compounds called esters with the addition of an ingredient to reduce evaporation of the product such as the emollient glycerine	To remove nail polish. To remove grease from the nail plate prior to applying polish
Hand/foot lotion/oil	Vegetable oils (e.g. almond oil); synthetic chemical oils are also available. Perfume – synthetic or organic. Emulsifying agents (e.g. beeswax, gum tragacanth, glycerol stearate and cetyl alcohol). Emollients (e.g. glycerine, lanolin and shea butter). Preservatives	To soften the skin and cuticles. To provide slip during hand/foot massage
Nail bleach	Citric acid or hydrogen peroxide – bleaches the nail. Glycerine – emollient. Water	To whiten stained nails and the surrounding skin
Cuticle cream	Emollients (e.g. lanolin, beeswax or glycerine). Perfume. Colour	To soften and condition the nail cuticles and surrounding skin
Cuticle oil	Emollient oils such as lanolin and organic oils such as almond oil	To soften and condition the nail cuticles and surrounding skin

(Continued)

TOP TIP

Hand/foot lotion/oil

Therapeutic ingredients may be added to the basic formulation, such as lavender essential oil which can soothe dry sensitive skin on the hands. Peppermint oil and menthol are popular additions to foot lotion as they reduce redness and are refreshing, creating a cooling effect as it has vasoconstrictive effects on the localized blood capillaries in the area. These therapeutic ingredients should not be used on clients who are pregnant.

HEALTH & SAFETY

Preservatives

Ingredients are added to products to extend their shelf life such as isopropyl alcohol.

Always check how long the product will remain stable, in good condition and safe to use or retail.

ALWAYS REMEMBER

Pearlized polishes

Pearlized polishes are created by the addition of sparkling, reflective particles such as mica or a a synthetic product.

Pearlized polish

A range of cuticle knives

Product	Ingredients	Uses
Nail polish	Solvent (e.g. butyl alcohol) – creates a suitable consistency when applying, and to help polish dry at a controlled rate. Colour pigments – create nail polish colour. Resin – improves adhesion of polish to nail plate and flexibility	To colour nail plates. To provide some protection
	Toluene – solvent which dissolves ingredients in nail polish. Nitrocellulose – film-forming plastic which holds colour. Plasticizers – to provide flexibility after the polish has dried, reducing chipping. Pearlized particles – create a pearlized or crystalline effect	
Nail hardener	Formaldehyde – a plastic resin	To strengthen weak nails
Nail conditioners	Organic oils which are vitamin enriched and provide excellent emollient properties	Formulation designed to rehydrate, improving the appearance and health of the nail, encouraging nail growth
Cuticle remover	Potassium hydroxide – a caustic alkali. Glycerine – a humectant added to reduce the drying effect on the nail plate	To soften the cuticles
Nail polish drier	Mineral oil – assists drying Oleric acid or silicone – lubricant.	Increases the speed at which the polish hardens
Nail polish solvent	Ethyl acetate – thins nail polish consistency. Toluene – solvent which dissolves nail polish ingredients	Thins nail polish that has thickened, restoring consistency

Sterilization and disinfection

Hygiene must be maintained in a number of ways:

◆ ensure that tools and equipment are clean, disinfected and, where required according to legal requirements, sterile before use

◆ having sterilized or disinfected tools and equipment, store them in a chemical disinfectant, UV cabinet or closed container until ready for use. Remember, they will remain clean but will not be sterile after exposure to the air or once they have been touched.

◆ dispense products, e.g. creams and lotions, from containers with a clean, disposable spatula

◆ use disposable tools and equipment wherever possible.

Refer to Habia's Code of Practice for Nail Treatments for **health and safety** best practice guidance.

HEALTH & SAFETY

Disinfecting sprays

You can buy disinfecting sprays to disinfect the surface of the tools before further disinfection or sterilization. Any debris must first be removed using a detergent and hot water before the use of a disinfecting spray. Use in a well-ventilated area and avoid contact with flame and excessive heat.

TOP TIP

Nail treatments legal requirements

Habia provide a Code of Practice for Nail Treatments. You should refer to this to ensure that you are complying with relevant health and safety legislation.

ALWAYS REMEMBER

UV stabilizers

UV stabilizers are additives which prevent the polish changing colour on exposure to UV sunlight.

Metal tools when ready for use should be placed in a disinfecting solution. After the manicure treatment they must be washed with soap and water and disinfected.

Manicure and pedicure tools and equipment can be disposable or can be sterilized or disinfected if they have come into contact with bodily fluids by the following methods:

Tool/Equipment	Method	Term used
Cuticle knife	Autoclave	Sterilization
Cuticle nippers	Autoclave	Sterilization
Orange stick	Throw away after use	Disposable
Callus file	Autoclave	Sterilization
	Chemical (e.g. disinfectant)	Disinfection
Bowl	Chemical (e.g. disinfectant)	Disinfection
Emery board	Throw away after use	Disposable
Buffer	Wipe handle with chemical disinfectant	Disinfection
	Wash buffing cloth in hot (60°C) soapy water	Cleaned
Towel	Wash in hot soapy water (60°C)	Cleaned
Spatula	Throw away after use	Disposable
Nail clippers	Autoclave	Sterilization
Scissors	Autoclave	Sterilization
Hoof stick	Immerse in chemical (e.g. disinfectant)	Disinfection
Trolley	Wipe with chemical (e.g. disinfectant)	Disinfection

ACTIVITY

Stretching exercises to avoid RSI

Perform regular, daily stretching exercise to reduce tension and improve flexibility for the fingers, wrists, hands, arms, shoulder, neck and upper back.

Research simple stretching exercises for each of the above body areas.

Reception

When a client makes an appointment for a manicure treatment, the receptionist should ask a few simple questions that will help guide how long the treatment will take.

◆ Do they require nail polish? With drying time, this part of the treatment can last up to 20 minutes, so the client should be made aware of this.

◆ Are any nails damaged or in need of repair? Again extra time will need to be allowed for this work.

◆ Do they require any **hand and nail treatments** in addition to the manicure, such as exfoliation or paraffin wax? Allow extra time accordingly.

◆ Has the client had artificial nails applied previously which require removal? Allow approximately 20 minutes for this process.

◆ Commercial timing.

Allow 45 minutes for a manicure treatment.

Allow up to 1 hour for a specialist hand-nail treatment.

> " Education is the most important aspect of being a successful manicurist. As a beginner you will learn the basics. But this is just the start. You must continue learning by taking as many short courses as you can. Read the trade press and visit trade shows to keep up with latest products and developments. Have a basic understanding of all the most popular brands, products and technology even if you don't use them. Clients need to know that your knowledge is current and your advice comes from an educated viewpoint.
>
> *Marian Newman*

HEALTH & SAFETY

Metal in the autoclave
Any metal to be placed in the autoclave should be of a high-quality stainless steel, to prevent rusting. Always dry immediately to prevent damage.

All staff, especially the staff communicating with clients at reception, should be familiar with the different pricing structures for the range of manicure treatments and products available for retail.

The receptionist should also check the age of the client. If the client is a minor under the age of 16, it is necessary to obtain parent/guardian permission for treatment. The parent/guardian will also have to be present when the treatment is received.

Specialist hand and nail treatment: hand mask application

Assessing the nails and skin using a nail magnifier tool

Consultation

Before carrying out a manicure treatment, it is necessary to assess the condition of the client's skin, nails and cuticles. This is done in order that the most appropriate hand and nail treatments and products may be chosen. Also, by correctly assessing and analyzing the client's hand condition and writing this on their record card, you will be able to see over a period of time how the condition is improving and progressing.

Assess the condition of the following:

◆ **The cuticles** Are they dry, tight or cracked, or are they soft and pliable?

◆ **The nails** Are they strong or weak? Brittle, hard and non-flexible and shatter easily? Flaking? Are they dry, lacking moisture with visible ridges? Are they discoloured or stained? What shape are they – square, round, oval? Are they long or short? Are they bitten?

◆ **The skin** Is the skin dry, rough or chapped, or is it soft and smooth? Is the colour even?

While assessing the client's hands for treatment, you should also be looking for any *contra-indications* to manicure treatment.

Skin and nail disorders of the hands and nails

When a client attends for a manicure treatment, as part of the consultation and assessment of the client's needs, the beauty therapist should always look at the client's skin and nails to check that no infection or disease is present which might contra-indicate treatment. These include bacterial, fungal, viral and parasitic infections. These are described in more detail in Chapter 2, where contra-indications are illustrated and discussed.

If the client is wearing nail polish, this must be removed before inspecting the nail plate.

ALWAYS REMEMBER

Artificial nails

If the client has had several new sets of artificial nails applied this will damage the natural nail.

The nail plate may be thin, ridges may appear upon the nail plate and the removal technique, using acetone, will cause dehydration. All of these effects will need to be discussed with your client at consultation and an appropriate treatment plan discussed.

ACTIVITY

Making appointments

What questions could the receptionist ask when booking a client for manicure in order to make the appointments run more efficiently? Write down your answers.

ACTIVITY

Assessing the hands

Look closely at your own hands. Assess their condition and make notes about everything you see.

Then assess the hands of a colleague. How do they differ from your own?

Complete a record card and record the condition of the nails and surrounding skin. Design a suitable treatment plan for your client to meet their needs.

ANATOMY & PHYSIOLOGY
See The nails section on page 70

ACTIVITY

Communication skills

Communication is important. Give three examples of positive communication techniques used when performing a manicure consultation.

Contra-indications

The following disorders may contra-indicate or restrict manicure treatment. If you suspect the client has any disorder from the chart below, do not attempt a diagnosis, but refer the client tactfully to their GP without causing unnecessary concern.

Disorder	Description
 Broken bones	Injury resulting in a broken bone can often not be seen; confirm at consultation that there is no known injury in the treatment area
 Cuts or abrasions in the hands	Broken skin. Any cut or abrasion could lead to secondary infection and the area should not be treated until healed
 Diabetes	If a client has diabetic foot or hand condition, they are vulnerable to infection as they have slow skin healing. Care should be taken also with heat treatments due to impaired circulation. This could be problematic if the skin was accidentally broken during a pedicure treatment. Permission must be obtained from the client's GP before treatment can be received

Disorder	Description
 Paronychia	Infectious bacterial infection. Swelling, redness and pus appears in the cuticle area of the skin and surrounding the nail wall
 Scabies or itch mites	An infestation of the skin by an animal parasite. The animal parasite burrows beneath the skin and invades the hair follicles. Papules and wavy greyish lines appear, where dirt enters the burrows. Secondary bacterial infection may occur as a result of scratching the skin
 Severe eczema of the nail plate	Inflammation of the skin occurs. Differing changes to the nail may occur, including the appearance of ridges, pitting, onycholysis or nail thickening (hypertrophy)
 Severe eczema of the skin	Inflammation of the skin caused by contact internally or externally, with an irritant. Reddening of the skin occurs with swelling and blistering; the blisters leak tissue fluid, which later hardens and forms scabs
 Severe nail separation (onycholysis)	Lifting of the nail plate from the nail bed, may be caused by trauma or infection to the nail or surrounding area; where separation has occurred this appears as a greyish-white area on the nail as the pink undertone of the nail bed does not show
 Severe psoriasis of the nail	An inflammatory condition where there is an increased production of cells in the upper part of the skin. Pitting occurs on the surface of the nail plate. Nail plate separation from the nail bed (onycholysis) may also occur

(Continued)

Disorder	Description
Severe psoriasis of the skin	Red patches of skin appear covered in waxy, silvery scales. Bleeding will occur if the area is scratched and the scales are removed. The cause is unknown
Tinea corporis (body ringworm)	Fungal infection of the skin, which may occur on the limbs. Small scaly red patches, which spread outwards and then heal from the centre, leaving a ring
Tinea unguium	Fungal infection of the fingernails. The nail plate is yellowish-grey. Eventually the nail plate becomes brittle, crumbles and separates from the nail bed
Verrucae or warts	A viral infection. Small epidermal skin growths. Warts may be raised or flat depending upon their position. Warts vary in size, shape, texture and colour. Usually they have a rough surface and are raised. Plane wart – found on the surface of the hand

Knowledge Check

What is the cause of RSI and how can this be avoided when performing manicure treatments?

Refer to pages 113–114 to help you.

ALWAYS REMEMBER

Record keeping

Accurately record your client's answers to necessary questions to be asked at consultations on the record card. This is a legal requirement.

Below is a list of common disorders that may be seen on the hands. Not all of these contra-indicate treatment but they may restrict treatment.

Disorder	Cause	Appearance	Salon treatment	Home care advice
Blue nail	Poor blood circulation in the area. Heart disease	The nail bed does not appear a healthy pink colour but has a blue tinge	Permission to treat to be received from the client's GP. Regular manicure, including hand treatment to improve circulation	General manicure advice. Hand exercises and massage to improve circulation
Bruised nails	Trauma to the nail (e.g. trapping it in a door); severe damage can result in loss of the nail	Part of the nail plate may appear blue or black where bleeding has occurred on the new bed	Although this disorder does not contra-indicate treatment, it is advisable to postpone manicuring the nails until the condition is no longer painful. Nail polish may be used to disguise the damaged nail	Seek medical advice if swelling is present or if pain persists
Eggshell nail	Illness	Thin, fragile, white nail plate, curving under at the free edge	Permission for treatment to be received from the client's GP. Regular manicure	General manicure advice. Strengthening base coats
Hangnail	Biting the skin around the nails. Cracking of a dry skin or cuticle condition	Epidermis around the nail plate cracks and a small piece of skin protrudes between the nail plate and the nail wall, sometimes accompanied by redness and swelling: this condition can become extremely painful	Warm-oil treatments to soften the skin and cuticles. Remove the protrusion of dead skin with cuticle nippers: do not cut into live tissue	Regular use of a rich hand cream. Wear rubber gloves when cleaning and washing up. Wear warm gloves in cold weather. Ensure a balanced diet
Leuconychia	Trauma to the nail plate or matrix, due to pressure or hitting the nail with a hard object. Air pockets form between the nail plate and nail bed	White spots or marks on the nail plate: will grow out with the nail	General manicure treatment. Coloured nail polish application will disguise their appearance until the damaged area disappears as it grows towards the free edge	Be careful with the hands. Wear protective gloves when doing housework or gardening. Do not use the nails as tools!

(Continued)

Disorder	Cause	Appearance	Salon treatment	Home care advice
Longitudinal ridges in the nail plate (corrugated nails)	Illness. Damage to the matrix. Age, associated with the ageing process	Grooves in the nail plate running along the length of the nail from the cuticle to the free edge: may affect one or all nails	Abrasive buffing paste applied to smooth out the ridges. Use of a ridge-filling base coat prior to nail polish application	General manicure aftercare advice. Use of a ridge-filling base coat polish. Ensure a balanced diet
Minor nail separation (onycholysis)	Lifting of the nail plate from its bed. Can accompany a medical condition such as eczema or psoriasis or a fungal infection in the area	Where separation has occurred this appears as a greyish-white area as the pink undertone of the nail bed does not show through the nail plate	It is advisable to postpone manicuring for this nail until the condition is corrected. Refer the client to their GP to confirm cause	Be careful to avoid infection of the nail bed. Protect the nail with a protective dressing
Onychophagy	Excessive nail-biting	Very little nail plate; bulbous skin at the fingertip; nail walls often red and swollen, due to biting of the skin surrounding the nails	Regular weekly manicures. Cuticle treatment to maximize the visible nail-plate area. Nail conditioning treatments to prevent dry cuticles and hangnails	Bitter-tasting preparations painted onto the nail plate. Wear gloves to avoid biting in bed
Onychorrhexis	Using harsh detergents without wearing gloves. Poor diet. Not wearing gloves in cold weather	Split, flaking nails	Warm-oil manicures on a weekly basis	Regular use of a rich hand cream. Always wear rubber gloves when cleaning or washing up. Always wear warm gloves in cold weather. Ensure a balanced diet. Prescribe nail base coat to protect split, flaking nails
Pitting	Eczema. Psoriasis	Pitting resembling small irregular pin pricks appear on the nail plate	Refer the client to their GP for permission to treat if required. Regular manicure with gentle buffing	General manicure advice. Ridge-filling base coat polish

Disorder	Cause	Appearance	Salon treatment	Home care advice
Pterygium	Neglect of the nails	Overgrown thickened cuticles, often tightly adhered to the nail plate: if left untreated, this may lead to splitting of the cuticle and subsequent infection	Warm-oil or paraffin wax treatments weekly. Once softened, remove excess cuticle with cuticle nippers. If overgrown cuticle is excessive, refer client to their GP	Regular use of a rich cuticle cream. Wear rubber gloves when cleaning and washing up. Gently push back the cuticles with a soft towel when softened, e.g. after bathing
Transverse furrows in the nail plate (Beau's lines)	Temporary arrested development of the nail in the matrix, due to illness or trauma of the nail	Groove in the nail plate, often on all nails simultaneously, running from side to side: this will grow out with the nail	Regular manicure until normal cells replace the damaged cells	General manicure advice. Ensure a balanced diet

Contra-actions

Certain cosmetic ingredients are known to cause allergic reactions in some people. This is known as a contra-action and may occur during or following treatment.

The client – or the manicurist – may at some time develop an allergy to a manicure product that has been successfully used previously. This could be for a number of reasons, including new medication being taken or illness.

The symptoms of an allergic reaction could be:

◆ excessive redness of the skin (erythema)   ◆ skin irritation i.e. itching

◆ swelling   ◆ raised blisters.

The symptoms do not necessarily appear on the hands. In the case of nail polish allergy, the symptoms often show up on the face, which the hands are continually touching.

In the case of an allergic reaction:

◆ remove the offending product immediately, using water or, in the case of polish, nail polish solvent

◆ apply a cool compress and soothing agent to the skin to reduce redness and irritation

◆ if symptoms persist, seek medical advice. If the client receives medical advice, ask them to inform you of the advice and/or treatment received so you can include this in your records.

Always record any allergies on the client's record card, so that the offending product may be avoided in future.

Further **contra-actions** may occur as a result of poor manicure techniques, e.g. failing to check the temperature of **paraffin wax** before application, which if too hot could cause

Client with an allergic reaction that has affected the eyes causing redness and swelling

HEALTH & SAFETY

Diagnosis
You are not qualified to diagnose, this is the job of the GP.

Therefore if you are unsure about any nail or skin condition present refer the client to their GP.

Knowledge Check

What is the name of the infectious bacterial infection that may occur if the skin is broken as a result of the manicure treatment?

Refer to page 395 to help you.

HEALTH & SAFETY

Contaminated waste
If there is any tissue damage during the manicure procedure resulting in bleeding, this is *contaminated waste* and must be disposed of in accordance with disposal of contaminated waste regulations.

skin sensitivity, even burning! Tissue damage could result in blood loss, e.g. incorrect nipping removal technique when using cuticle nippers may result in pulling and tearing the skin. Incorrect positioning and use of the cuticle knife may lead to piercing the cuticle with the knife blade.

Avoid cutting the nails too short as again this can result in possible damage to the hyponychium the part of the epidermis under the free edge of the nail. This may affect its protective function leading to possible infection.

Treatment plan

After analyzing the client's nails and adjacent skin, a **treatment plan** should be considered and agreed with the client. In order to correct skin and nail problems, the client should attend the salon weekly. They should also be advised of the appropriate treatment preparations to use at home, so as to support the salon treatment. Specialist nail treatments to use will depend upon the nail and skin condition; they include:

◆ *Nail strengthener* This is used on brittle, damaged nails to strengthen, condition and protect them against breaking, splitting or peeling.

◆ *Ridge filler* This is used on nails with ridges to provide a more even surface, creating a bond between the **base coat** and polish, allowing a smoother application of polish.

◆ *Nail oil* This contains ingredients to rehydrate the nail and soften the cuticle.

◆ *Cuticle creams* These nourish the skin and restore the condition of the cuticle.

◆ *Hand and foot creams/lotions* Used to protect the skin, maintaining skin hydration and reducing the negative signs of dryness and neglect. In the foot area dry, cracked skin and on the hands rough, dry skin.

HEALTH & SAFETY

Contact dermatitis
Contact dermatitis is a skin problem caused by intolerance of the skin to a particular substance or a group of substances. On exposure to the substance the skin quickly becomes irritated and an allergic reaction occurs. This may occur when a manicurist's skin is exposed to dust and chemicals on a regular basis. Follow all HSE guidelines to reduce the risk of developing this skin disorder which could result in the need for a career change!

Always follow manufacturer's guidelines on the use of products.

A sample client record card

Date	Beauty therapist name	
Client name	Date of birth (identifying client age group)	
Home address	Postcode	
Email address	Landline phone number	Mobile phone number
Name of doctor	Doctor's address and phone number	
Related medical history (conditions that may restrict or prohibit treatment application)		
Are you taking any medication? (this may affect the sensitivity of the skin to the treatment)		

CONTRA-INDICATIONS REQUIRING MEDICAL REFERRAL
(preventing manicure treatment application)

☐ bacterial infections (e.g. paronychia)
☐ viral infections (e.g. plane warts)
☐ fungal infections (e.g. tinea unguium)
☐ parasitic infections, (e.g. scabies)
☐ severe nail separation
☐ severe eczema and psoriasis
☐ severe bruising
☐ severe skin conditions

CONTRA-INDICATIONS WHICH RESTRICT TREATMENT
(treatment may require adaptation)

☐ minor nail separation
☐ product allergies
☐ recent scar tissue
☐ severely damaged nails
☐ broken bones
☐ recent fractures and sprains
☐ undiagnosed lumps or swellings
☐ minor eczema and psoriasis
☐ severely bitten nails
☐ minor bruising or swelling
☐ minor cuts or abrasions

PRODUCTS, TOOLS AND EQUIPMENT

☐ nail and skin treatment tools
☐ abrasives (e.g. buffing cream)
☐ cuticle softeners
☐ nail and skin products
☐ nail conditioners (e.g. cuticle cream/oils)
☐ skin conditioners (e.g. hand cream)
☐ nail, skin and cuticle corrective treatments (e.g. paraffin wax)
☐ consumables

HAND AND NAIL TREATMENTS

☐ warm oil hand mask
☐ paraffin wax
☐ thermal mitts
☐ exfoliators

NAIL FINISH

☐ light colour
☐ dark colour
☐ French manicure
☐ buffing

COURSE OF TREATMENT

	Date	Date	Date
☐ improvement of skin	___	___	___
☐ condition products	___	___	___
☐ improvement of nail condition products	___	___	___

NAIL, CUTICLE AND SKIN CONDITION
Nails

☐ healthy
☐ dry
☐ ridged (horizontal or longitudinal)
☐ brittle
☐ weak
☐ split
☐ bitten (onychopag)y)

Nail shape

☐ oval
☐ tapered
☐ square
☐ squoval
☐ claw
☐ fan
☐ pointed

Cuticle

☐ healthy
☐ dry
☐ split
☐ hangnails
☐ overgrown (pterygium)

Skin

☐ healthy
☐ dry
☐ hard

MASSAGE MEDIUMS

☐ creams
☐ oils
☐ lotions

Beauty therapist signature (for reference)
Client signature (confirmation of details)

A sample client record card (continued)

TREATMENT ADVICE
Manicure – *allow 45 minutes*
Specialized hand/nail treatment – *allow up to 60 minutes*

TREATMENT PLAN
Record relevant details of your treatment and advice provided for future reference.
Ensure the client's records are up-to-date, accurate and fully completed following treatment. Non-compliance may invalidate insurance.

DURING
Discuss:

◆ details that may influence the client's nail condition, such as their occupation
◆ the products the client is currently using to care for the skin of the hands and nails, and the regularity of their use
◆ the client's satisfaction with these products
◆ relevant manicure procedures (e.g. how to file the nails correctly).

Note:

◆ any adverse (unwanted) reaction, if any occur during or after the manicure treatment.

AFTER
Record:

◆ results of treatment
◆ any modification to treatment application that has occurred
◆ what products have been used in the manicure treatment
◆ what hand and nail treatments have been used
◆ the effectiveness of treatment
◆ any samples provided (review their success at the next appointment).

Advise on:

◆ product application in order to gain maximum benefit from product use
◆ specialized products following manicure treatment for home care use
◆ general hand/nail care and maintenance
◆ the recommended time intervals between treatments
◆ the importance of a course of treatment to improve nail/skin conditions.

RETAIL OPPORTUNITIES
Advise on:

◆ progression of the treatment plan for future appointments
◆ products that would be suitable for the client to use at home to care for the skin of the hands and nails
◆ recommendations for further treatments
◆ further products or treatments that the client may or may not have received before.

Note:

◆ any purchase made by the client.

EVALUATION
Record:

◆ comments on the client's satisfaction with the treatment
◆ if poor results are achieved, the reasons why
◆ how you may alter the treatment plan to achieve the required treatment results in the future, if applicable.

HEALTH AND SAFETY
Advise on:

◆ appropriate necessary action to be taken in the event of an unwanted skin or nail reaction.

> Developing a good style of communicating with your clients is essential. This will develop with practice and experience but needs to start at the beginning of your education. Your clients should be confident in your professional skills and you need to be able to correctly identify their skin and nail conditions (without diagnosing medical-based conditions).Treat every client as an individual and not a series of 'step by steps'. Lead them through your consultation to make sure you understand what they actually want and balance that with what you believe they need.
>
> *Marian Newman*

Some hand creams contain UV filters to protect against UV damage and premature ageing.

◆ *Specialist hand and nail treatments* These may also be recommended within the manicure treatment to improve the appearance of the skin texture, nail and cuticle condition and provide a number of physiological benefits. These may be offered each time the client has a manicure treatment to maintain the condition of the nails and hands. Their use may be recommended as part of their home care routine e.g. a hand /foot exfoliant and mask.

Provide the opportunity for your client to ask any questions relating to the manicure treatment plan.

The record card should be signed and dated by the manicurist following the consultation to confirm the suitability and consent with the agreed manicure treatment.

It is important that accurate records are kept and stored in compliance with the Data Protection Act for future reference.

Cleaning the hands, beauty therapist

Cleaning the hands, client

Carrying out manicure treatments

Preparing the client

Ensure that the client is warm and comfortable when preparing them for a manicure.

Lighting must be good to avoid eyestrain and to allow the treatment to be performed competently. Avoid positioning the work station in direct sunlight however to prevent discomfort to client and manicurist. Heat can also spoil many manicure products. Always

TOP TIP

Modifying your treatment to meet your client's needs

Following your consultation, you may need to adjust your manicure to meet your client's needs by modifying:

◆ the depth of massage pressure when applying hand and arm massage and choice of massage movements applied, e.g. an elderly client's skin is thinner and has less elasticity and they may have reduced joint mobility
◆ the choice of massage medium, e.g. when client has excessively hairy arms
◆ the choice of nail polish product including base, colour and top coat to improve the nail condition and appearance.

store and handle products in the recommended way following manufacturer's guidelines and workplace policy.

Background music, if provided, should be at a sound level that allows effective communication with your client.

Consider the client's comfort with the location of the manicure treatment area. Some clients may require a more private area than a busy area with lots of traffic (people walking past). Check suitability of location with your client.

A lightweight gown may be offered to the client to cover their clothing. This will prevent damage to their clothes from accidental spillage of products during treatment. Ask them to remove any jewellery from the area to be treated, to prevent the jewellery being soiled or damaged by manicure products and to avoid obstructing **massage** movements. Place the jewellery where the client can see it. Alternatively, ask the client to take possession of it for safe-keeping – follow your workplace security policy. Ensure that the client is seated at the correct height, and close enough to avoid having to lean forward.

When the client is comfortably seated, clean your hands using an approved hand cleaning technique – preferably in view of the client, who will then observe hygienic procedures being carried out. This will assure them that they are receiving a professional service. The client should also wash their hands before the treatment commences. The client's skin can also be cleaned with a disinfectant gel or spray.

Consult the client's record card, and begin the treatment.

TOP TIP

Removal of artificial nails or UV cured gel polish prior to a manicure treatment

These are removed using a solvent containing acetone that softens the product, allowing removal from the natural nail. However, it is particularly drying to the natural nail which will later require rehydrating.

Procedure

◆ Remove any nail polish from artificial nails, and trim any excess length using clippers.

◆ Soak the nails in the recommended removal product. For artificial nails this is usually acetone for approximately 20 minutes, until the product has thoroughly softened.

◆ Remove the softened product with an orange stick.

◆ Wash the hands and nails thoroughly to remove acetone.

◆ The surface of the nail may require to be buffed lightly with a gentle abrasive file to remove excess product and provide a smooth nail surface.

◆ Continue with manicure treatment selecting products and treatments to restore nail condition.

Outcome 2: Be able to provide manicure treatments

Learn how to provide manicure treatments

PRACTICAL SKILLS

Communicate and behave in a professional manner

Follow health and safety working practices

Position yourself and client correctly throughout the treatment

Use products, tools, equipment and techniques to suit clients' treatment needs, skin and nail conditions

Complete the treatment to the satisfaction of the client

Record the results of the treatment

Provide suitable aftercare advice

UNDERPINNING KNOWLEDGE

State how to communicate and behave in a professional manner

Describe health and safety working practices

Explain the importance of positioning yourself and the client correctly throughout the treatment

Explain the importance of using products, tools, equipment and techniques to suit clients' treatment needs, skin and nail conditions

Describe how treatments can be adapted to suit client treatment needs, skin and nail conditions

Describe the different massage techniques and their benefits

State the contra-actions that may occur during and following treatments and how to respond

State the importance of completing the treatment to the satisfaction of the client

State the importance of completing treatment records

State the aftercare advice that should be provided

Describe diseases and disorders of the nail and skin

Describe the structure and function of the bones of the lower arm and hand

Describe the structure and functions of the nail and skin

STEP-BY-STEP: MANICURE PROCEDURE

This procedure briefly shows the stages in the manicure. Each step is discussed in detail later in the chapter. The procedure may start with the right or left hand.

1 Remove any existing nail polish with nail polish remover, using fresh cotton wool for each hand. Replace cotton wool as required to maintain its effectiveness.

2 Use a cotton wool-tipped orange stick to apply nail polish remover around the cuticle area if necessary to remove any excess nail polish. Avoid unnecessary contact with the skin to avoid drying out.

3 File the nails of the right hand to the desired length and shape.
Ensure the free edge is smooth by performing upward strokes with the file often referred to as bevelling.

4 Buff the nail plate of the right hand.

5 Apply cuticle cream or oil to the cuticle area.

6 Place a small amount of liquid soap formulated for use in manicures in the manicure bowl and add warm water when ready to use.

7 Place the right hand in the manicure bowl containing warm water and liquid soap. Repeat steps 3, 4, 5 and 7 for the left hand.

8 Remove the right hand from the manicure bowl and dry with a towel. Place the left hand into the manicure bowl.

9 Apply cuticle remover to the right hand. Avoid unnecessary contact with the product and the skin of the finger.

10 Push back the cuticle with a cotton wool-tipped orange stick or **hoof stick**.

11 Remove excess cuticle with nippers. Do not cut the living skin of the hyponychium.

12 Remove excess softened cuticle with a cuticle knife. The blade should be kept slightly wet to avoid scratching the nail plate.

13 Collect excess cuticle and skin tissue on a clean piece of cotton wool and dispose of it hygienically immediately following completion of this stage of the treatment. Wipe the nails with damp cotton wool to remove excess cuticle remover. This product could cause skin dryness and irritation.

14 Apply cuticle oil and massage it in with your thumbs. Repeat steps **9–13** for the left hand. Apply massage routine to both hands and forearms.
For more information on a hand and forearm massage routine see page 418.

15 Remove grease and excess nail products from the nail plate with a cotton wool pad soaked in nail polish remover.

16 Refile the nails as necessary to ensure they are smooth and even.

17 The client may find it convenient to pay for her treatment at this stage, to avoid smudging her polish later. Also, if jewellery has been removed ask her to replace it to avoid damage to the polish after application.

18 Confirm and apply the **nail finish**. If applying polish, apply: base coat (once); polish (twice); and top coat (once). If a pearlized polish is used, a top coat is not required and a third coat of polish may be applied. If the client doesn't want polish, buff to a shine with buffing paste or use a four-sided buffer.

19 Base coat may be applied under the edge of the nail to create a protective seal.

20a French manicure polish finish shown: neutral-coloured nail polish is applied in soft beige to evenly cover the nail plate surface. Apply one or two coats.

20b The free edge is painted white ensuring that the line is even. Apply one coat. If the nails are particularly stained the reverse of the free edge may be painted also.

20c Apply a top coat to seal and protect the nail polish.

21 The completed French manicure.

Gel polish application

UV cured gel application is increasingly a popular nail finish to traditional nail polish. A step by step procedure follows:

1   After preparing the nail by removing all cuticle on the nail plate and cleaning with a nail cleanser, you are ready to apply the UV **gel** base coat. Apply a VERY thin layer of base coat, making sure to go to the edges of the nail and capping the free edge.

2   Cure the first hand for the required time using the recommended UV lamp while you are applying the base coat to the nails on the other hand. Some lamps only cure four fingers at a time so place the thumbs under the lamp separately.

3   Apply a thin layer of the chosen colour to each nail on the first hand while the base coat on the second hand is curing under the lamp. Make sure to get close to the edges and cap the free edge. Don't worry if the colour is patchy as a thin layer is essential. Remove any colour from the skin using an orange stick. Cure for the required time while applying the colour to the second hand. Apply the second layer of colour to both hands and cure as before.

4   Apply the UV gel top coat to the first hand making sure all the colour layer has been covered and the free edge capped. Cure for required time and repeat for the second hand.

5   When the top coat is cured, saturate a cotton pad with gel cleanser and remove the sticky residue (inhibition layer) from each finger. Start with the little finger and wipe from the base of the nail to the tip to avoid getting any gel on the skin. Use a clean section of the pad or a new pad for the forefinger and thumb. Apply oil to the skin of each finger and massage in.

STEP-BY-STEP: GEL POLISH APPLICATION

2 Cure for the required time using the recommended UV lamp

3 Apply a thin layer of chosen colour

5 Remove the sticky residue

Gel polish removal

1   Collect together what you will need for the removal process

2   Saturate a cotton wool pad with gel polish remover (or pure acetone) and place on the nail. Wrap with foil, folding the end over the end of the finger.

3   The removal will take from 8-15 minutes depending on the brand and thickness of application. (If the client's hands are cold, wrap with a towel or place on a heated pad to speed up the process.)

4   After approximately 10 minutes, squeeze the cotton pad in the foil and rub from side to side to dislodge the gel polish. Remove the wrap. Most of the gel polish should have flaked away from the nail. If there are any flakes left, carefully lift from the nail using an orange stick. Take great care NOT to scrape the nail surface as it is very delicate at this stage and you will cause surface damage.

5   There will probably be some base coat and spots of colour left adhering to the nail plate.

6   To remove these, saturate a cotton wool pad with gel polish remover (or acetone) and firmly rub the nail plate to remove all traces of them.

7   Following removal massage nail oil into the nail plate and surrounding skin. There should be no surface damage or white spots on the nail.

HEALTH & SAFETY

PPE
When cutting the nail length, you may wish to wear safety glasses which protect the eyes from flying debris reducing potential injury.

TOP TIP

Client's jewellery

Keep the client's jewellery in full view throughout the treatment so they don't forget it when they leave.

Filing

The part of the nail that is filed is called the free edge. This should be filed to complement the nail and hand shape and the nail condition. When filing the natural nail, use a fine **grit emery board**. Very often emery boards have different degrees of coarseness on either side, indicated by different colours. Use the darker, rougher side to remove excess length, and the lighter, smoother side for shaping and removing rough edges. A flexible emery board is preferable to a stiff one as it generates less friction.

Filing the nails

> Practice and practice! Don't shy away from the French manicure because it's a bit tricky! Don't spend valuable practice time playing with nail art until you have honed your polishing skills. Beautifully polished nails will bring your clients back again and again.
>
> *Marian Newman*

Emery board

When shaping the nail always file the nails from the side to the centre, with the emery board sloping slightly under the free edge. If a square shape is required, file straight across the free edge in one direction to create a uniform square shape and then smooth the outside edges to remove roughness which may lead to accidental damage and breakage. Use swift, rhythmical strokes. Avoid a sawing action – this would generate friction and might cause the free edge to split.

Never file completely down the sides of the nail, as strength is required here to balance the free edge. Always allow about 4mm of nail growth to remain at the sides of the nail.

Knowledge Check

What shape are the nails shown in Step 21?

Refer to page 408 to help you.

TOP TIP

Emery boards

Cost the emery board into the manicure treatment, it is a consumable and cannot be used again. The client can keep the emery board for personal use. Instruct the client on how the nails should be filed to avoid nail damage.

TOP TIP

Nail filing

Some nail product suppliers consider the nails best filed after specialized oil application. It is considered less damaging than when filing the natural nail when dry.

ALWAYS REMEMBER

Nail shapes

When filing the nails ensure that the finished appearance complements the client's nail/hand.

If the fingers are long and thin, select a rounded/square shape and keep the nail length short.

If the fingers are short and fat, the nails should be filed into an oval shape and the nail length should be longer to elongate the fingers.

Oval shape

Square shape

Pointed shape

Squoval shape

Round shape

Fan shape

Cutting the nails

Where it is necessary to reduce nail length, it is more efficient to do so by cutting the nail free edge. This is performed using nail scissors or sometimes nail clippers. Support the nail wall with one hand on the free edge being cut. This minimizes client discomfort. Dispose of the trimmed nail plate hygienically in the metal lined waste bin. Make several small cuts across the free edge to avoid trauma to the nail and always file with a gentle emery board to smooth and seal the edges.

Nail shape The nail shape should complement the client's fingers and hand length and size. The shape of the free edge that will most compliment a client's nails is one that is similar to the shape of the nail at the base of the nail plate.

> **Oval** The ideal nail shape is oval. This is the shape that offers the most strength to the free edge.
>
> **Square** A fashionable shape chosen by many clients. The client should be informed, however, that if they have severe corners on the nails they will be more likely to catch and break them.
>
> **Pointed** One nail shape that should never be recommended is the pointed nail. This leaves the nail tip very weak and likely to break.
>
> **Squoval** A combination of oval and square nail shape. The nail is filed to a square finish at the free edge and is then gently curved or rounded at the corners.
>
> **Round** The free edge is rounded and is an ideal shape for short nails. This style is popular with male clients.

Tapered shape

Correcting natural nail shapes Sometimes the natural nail shape will require filing into a suitable shape to maintain nail strength, improve the look of the nail and create overall balance.

> **Fan** The nail becomes broader as it grows towards the free edge, appearing as a fan shape. The wider sides of the nail at the free edge should be shaped to achieve an oval shape.
>
> **Tapered nail** The free edge part of the nail plate is slimmer than that at the cuticle area which makes it weaker in strength. The free edge should be filed to a squoval shape to maintain strength.
>
> **Claw nail** Also referred to as hook or convex nail. The nail is excessively curved at the free edge. The nail should be kept short and filed to a round shape. Often this nail's shape can occur as a result of nail injury.
>
> **Spoon shape** Also referred to as ski jump or concave. The nail plate curves upwards as it grows from the free edge. File into an oval or squoval nail shape.

Claw shape

Spoon shape

Buffing using a traditional chamois leather covered buffer

Buffing

In manicure, buffing is used for these reasons:

◆ to give the nail plate a sheen

◆ to stimulate the blood supply in the nail bed, increasing nourishment and encouraging strong, healthy nail growth

◆ to smooth any surface irregularities.

Buffing manicure tools vary. A traditional chamois leather **buffer** may have a handle made of plastic and a replaceable convex pad covered with chamois or soft leather. Buffing paste is the cream used to help smooth out surface irregularities, and thereby give the nail a shine. It contains abrasive particles such as pumice, talc or kaolin.

The two, three or four-sided buffer: this is shaped like a thick emery board and has four types of surface, ranging from slightly abrasive to very smooth. It can be used to bring the nail to a shine without the need for buffing paste. It can be washed and sprayed with disinfectant after use.

Buffing is carried out after filing to stimulate healthy nail growth and before the nails are soaked in the finger bowl. It can also be used instead of polish at the end of the manicure, or as a **nail finish**. It is popular when performing a male manicure treatment as an alternative finish to nail polish application.

If it is being used, buffing paste is applied by taking a small amount out of the pot with a clean orange stick and applying this to each nail plate. With the fingertip, use downward strokes from the cuticle to the free edge to spread the paste without getting it under the cuticle (which would cause irritation). With the buffer held loosely in the hand, buff in one direction only from the base of the nail to the free edge, using smooth, firm, regular strokes. Use approximately six strokes per nail. Avoid excessive strokes which would cause friction and heat to the nail plate causing drying.

Knowledge Check

What is the nail condition known as where the cuticle becomes overgrown and thickened on the nail plate?

Refer to page 399 to help you.

HEALTH & SAFETY

Clinical waste
If you accidentally cut the skin causing bleeding at the cuticle area, protect your hands with disposable gloves and wipe the skin with a disinfectant wipe. Any waste is classed as clinical contaminated waste and should be disposed of in a yellow medical sealed bag in accordance with the **Environment Act 1990**.

See the *Habia Hygiene in Beauty Therapy* booklet for further guidance.

HEALTH & SAFETY

Hygiene
Use a fresh orange stick for each stage of the manicure treatment, and when working on different hands, to prevent contamination and cross-infection. The orange stick is disposed of after use.

Cuticle work

Cuticle work is carried out to keep the cuticle area attractive, healthy and also to prevent cuticles becoming overgrown and adhering to the nail plate, which could lead to splitting of the cuticle as the nail grows forward, and subsequently to infection of the area.

The work is carried out after soaking the nails in warm soapy water. This step loosens dirty particles from the free edge and softens the skin in the cuticle area.

How to carry out cuticle work

1   Take the fingers from the soapy water and pat them dry with a soft towel.

2   Apply cuticle remover to the cuticle and nail walls, using the applicator brush. (Cuticle remover is a slightly caustic solution that helps soften and loosen the cuticles and the eponychium from the nail plate.)

3   Gently loosen the cuticle from the nail plate with a cotton wool-tipped orange stick or hoof stick. (The cotton wool is to avoid splinters from the wood, and also may be easily replaced if necessary.) Use a gentle, circular motion to loosen the cuticle, holding the orange stick like a pen.

4   Hold the cuticle knife at 45° to the nail plate and stroke it in one direction only, gently loosening any eponychium and perionychium that has adhered to the nail plate: do not scratch it backwards and forwards. The **cuticle knife** should have a fine-ground flat blade which can be re-sharpened when necessary. Dampen it regularly in the manicure bowl to prevent scratches occurring on the nail plate.

5   Hold the nippers comfortably in the palm of the hand, with the thumb resting just above the blades – this gives firm control over what can be a dangerous instrument. Use the cuticle nippers to remove any loose cuticle, and to trim excess dead cuticle. Do not cut the living eponychium. If you do it may bleed and will also grow back thicker. Not every client will require the use of **cuticle nippers** – use them only when needed. Avoid trimming the eponychium, which can lead to overgrown, thickened skin.

TOP TIP

Diabetic clients

Avoid cutting the cuticles of a diabetic client unless you have experience. Their skin can be quite thin so if you nip them it can cause unexpected bleeding.

Using cuticle clippers

Pushing back cuticles using a cotton wool tipped orange stick

Using a cuticle knife

Pushing back cuticles using a hoof stick

TOP TIP

Choosing cuticle nippers

Cuticle nippers should have finely ground cutting blades to give a clean cut and to avoid tearing the cuticle. Check the quality of your nippers before you purchase, they should be of good quality and durable.

Knowledge Check

Which manicure tools are used to improve the condition and appearance of the cuticles?

Refer to page 413 to help you.

An oil/wax heater

Hand and nail treatments

In addition to a manicure, further hand and nail treatments may be included as appropriate to achieve the treatment plan aims.

Hand and nail treatments include:

◆ Warm-oil treatment involves gently heating a small amount of organic oil (such as almond oil) and soaking the cuticles in it for 10 minutes. This nourishes the nail plate, softens the cuticles and the surrounding skin, and is an excellent treatment for clients with dry, cracked cuticles.

◆ Warm oil may also be applied to the skin of the hand and forearm to improve skin texture, colour and blood circulation in the area.

Exfoliating treatment

An exfoliating treatment

Exfoliating treatment is carried out as part of the massage routine. The massage is performed as usual, using an exfoliant, a mildly abrasive cosmetic product. It may be applied prior to hand and arm massage also to expose new cells and aid the absorption of the massage oil/cream. This treatment offers the following benefits:

◆ the removal of dead skin cells

◆ improvement of the skin texture

◆ improvement of the skin colour

◆ increased blood circulation

◆ increased lymph circulation.

> " Cuticle work and preparation of the nail is very important. Sometimes this needs to take up the main part of the treatment. Good cuticle work is something that clients can rarely do for themselves. It is about thorough removal of the non-living cuticle from the nail plate and NOT about cutting the living skin at the base of the nail (nail fold). A good manicurist will prepare the nail perfectly and in such a way that is suitable for the specific nail condition. Don't take any short cuts on this part of the treatment. Anything you do after this stage, e.g. painting, will totally rely on your preparation
>
> *Marian Newman*

The abrasive particles must be thoroughly removed with hot, damp towels before continuing with the rest of the manicure.

Hand treatment mask

A hand treatment mask

An appropriate treatment mask may be applied, according to the client's treatment requirements. This may be either stimulating and rejuvenating, or moisturizing. The hands may be placed inside thermal mitts or hand gloves for 10 minutes to enable the mask to penetrate the epidermis. Several layers are applied. The mask is then removed, and followed with treatment massage cream. Some products may also be used as the massage medium.

Paraffin wax treatment

The paraffin wax is heated in a special bath to a temperature of 50–55°C. It is then applied to the hands and usually over the wrists too with a brush. It is then, covered with a plastic protective covering and left to set for 10–15 minutes before removal. Several layers are applied. This offers the following benefits:

Paraffin wax resources

◆ the heating effect stimulates the blood and lymph circulation

◆ eases discomfort of arthritic and rheumatic conditions

◆ softens the skin; improving the appearance and condition of the nails and dry skin

◆ soothes sensory nerve endings.

After use the wax is disposed of.

Thermal mitts

These are electrically heated gloves in which the hands are placed for approximately 10–15 minutes.

Thermal mitts

They are generally used following the application of a treatment within the manicure routine, e.g. a hand treatment mask. The hands are prepared by wrapping them in a plastic protective covering before placement in the mitts.

The treatment has the following benefits:

◆ decreases joint stiffness in the case of a client suffering from arthritis

◆ improves the condition of dry skin of the cuticles and hands by increasing the absorption of moisturizing products

◆ improves skin colour and blood and lymph circulation.

Always follow manufacturer's guidelines in the application procedure for hand and nail treatments.

Knowledge Check

Why would you choose to include exfoliation in your manicure treatment?

Refer to page 414 to help you.

CourseMate video: Specialist Hand and Nail Treatment

> A manicure is not just about sending a client away with lovely polished nails. It is also about improving the condition and appearance of the nails and surrounding skin. This usually takes some daily help. If you explain to your client what their own challenges are in an informative and interesting way you will automatically be retailing useful products without any hard sell techniques. They will also be impressed with your expert knowledge and care of them as your valued client.
>
> *Marian Newman*

Specialist hand treatments

Specialist treatments should be offered to your client when there is a specific treatment need or if they feel they would like to benefit from such a treatment.

Specialist training in these advanced techniques is usually offered by major product companies.

The model for this specialist hand and arm treatment is a mature client who suffers from the medical condition rheumatoid arthritis where the joints become inflamed and painful.

The following hand and arm treatment will:

◆ stimulate the blood and lymph circulation

◆ have a skin cleansing action

◆ remove dead skin cells (desquamation)

◆ improve the moisture content of the skin

◆ minimize discomfort caused by an arthritic, rheumatic condition.

Your treatments should be adapted to meet the treatment objectives for the client.

Allow 30 minutes for this specialist hand and arm treatment.

STEP-BY-STEP: SPECIALIST HAND AND ARM TREATMENT

1 The hands and arms are cleansed using warm towelling mitts infused with lime oil for its therapeutic, refreshing and energizing properties.

2 The hands are exfoliated to remove all dead skin cells and brighten the skin. A salt-based preparation with emollient, skin-softening ingredients is applied to the skin of each hand and is massaged gently over the skin's surface.

3 Towelling mitts are used to remove the exfoliating treatment. These have been steamed and are warm when used.

4 A skin-nourishing lotion is applied to each hand and arm. The lotion is particularly beneficial for dry, sensitive skin.

5 Massage movements are applied using effleurage and petrissage massage manipulations.

6 A further skin treatment product, hand mask, is applied. The hands are then placed in plastic bags to aid the absorption of the product.

7 The hands are then placed in electrically heated thermal mitts for 10–15 minutes. Remove the thermal mitts and plastic bags disposing of these and remove the product. Continue with a nail finish if required.

Hand and forearm massage

Hand massage is generally carried out near the end of the manicure treatment, just prior to nail polish application. It can also be carried out on its own if the client wants the effects of the massage but does not need or want treatment to their nails.

The massage incorporates classic massage movements, each with different effects:

◆ **Effleurage** – a stroking movement, used to begin the massage as a link manipulation, and to complete the massage sequence.

◆ **Petrissage** – movements including kneading where the tissues are lifted away from the underlying structures and compressed. Pressure is intermittent, and should be light yet firm.

◆ **Tapotement** – also referred to as percussion. Performed in a brisk, light and stimulating manner. Rhythm is important as the hands break contact with the skin. Movements include tapping used to increase blood supply and muscle/skin in the area.

◆ **Joint manipulations** – the joints of the wrists and hands are manipulated through their range of movement dependent upon the type of joint. This helps to maintain good mobility within the range of movement but must be avoided if the client has any joint disorders.

> "Client education is an important part of your nail service. You will find it amazing how much clients don't know about their nails and how to care for them! Without being a bore on the subject or too bossy, explain what you are doing and why and how they can, with a bit of easy home care, help to maintain the work you have done.
>
> *Marian Newman*

Knowledge Check

In Image 2, what is the name of the lymph node the beauty therapist is massaging located in the elbow area?

Refer to page 98 to help you.

TOP TIP

Link selling

Hand massage can be included during a facial while the mask is applied, maximizing treatment benefits and client relaxation. It also gives you the opportunity to promote another product or service to the client.

◆ **Frictions** – small circular movements using the pads of the fingers or thumbs. The skin and muscle below is massaged against the underlying bone. This can be used to loosen any adhesions in the tissues.

The beauty therapist can adapt the massage application according to the needs of the client. Either the speed of application, depth of pressure or choice of massage manipulation can be altered.

The reasons for offering massage during a manicure are as follows:

◆ to moisturize the skin with massage medium, improving skin hydration

◆ to increase blood circulation, transporting oxygen and nutrients to the lower arm and hand

◆ to increase lymph circulation, transporting waste products in the lymph from the lower arm and hand

◆ to help maintain joint mobility

◆ to ease discomfort from arthritis or rheumatism

◆ to relax the client

◆ to help remove dead skin cells (desquamation), exposing new cells.

STEP-BY-STEP: HAND AND FOREARM MASSAGE

1 Dispense the chosen massage medium into the hands, warm the product over the palms and apply to the client's skin using effleurage technique.

2 **Effleurage to the whole hand and forearm** Use long sweeping strokes from the hand to the elbow, moving on both the outer and the inner sides of the forearm.

Repeat step 2 a further five times.

3 Using a petrissage movement pick up the flexor and extensor muscles of the lower arm.

4 **Thumb kneading to the back of the hand and the forearm** Use the thumbs, one in front of the other, and rotate each thumb: one in a clockwise direction, the other anti-clockwise. Use a gently kneading action between each metacarpal bone. Move from the hand towards the elbow, massaging over the interosseus membrane located between the radius and ulna bone, then slide the thumbs back down to the hands.

Repeat step 4 a further two times.

5 Perform a scissoring, friction movement using both thumbs between each metacarpal bone in the hands.

6 Perform a 'knuckling' petrissage movement rotating the fingers in a small fist shape against the muscles in the palms of the hand.

7 Perform joint manipulations (Steps 7–9). Move the phalange bones of each finger, bending the finger at each joint and then straightening in a resistance movement.

8 Finger circulations, supporting the joints
Supporting the knuckles with one hand, hold the fingers individually and gently take each through its full range of movements, first clockwise and then anticlockwise. Move from the little finger to the thumb.

Repeat step 8 a further two times.

9 Wrist circulations, supporting the joints
Support the wrist with one hand and put your fingers between the client's, gently grasping their hand. Move the wrist through its full range of movement, first clockwise and then anticlockwise.

Repeat step 9 a further two times.

10 Effleurage to the whole hand and forearm Use the same movement as in step 2.

Repeat step 10 a further five times.

Nail polish application

Nail polish is used to coat the nail plate for a number of reasons:

◆ to decorate the nail

◆ to disguise stained nails

◆ to add temporary strength to weak nails

◆ to improve the condition or appearance of the natural nail

◆ to co-ordinate with clothes or make-up

◆ to create designs and effects, called 'nail art'.

Before nail polish is applied, the client's hand jewellery may be replaced, to avoid smudging afterwards.

Styles of polish application

◆ **Traditional application** This style is the one most commonly requested by clients: the entire nail plate is covered with polish in a block colour.

◆ **French manicure application** This style involves painting the nail plate of the nail bed pink or pale beige, and the free edge white. This can be adapted by painting a narrow block of colour along the free edge which is more complimentary for a shorter nail. This technique can also provide product strength to a weaker nail.

◆ **Moon application** This style involves applying polish over the whole nail plate except the area of the lunula.

◆ **Painted moon application** This style involves painting the lunula a contrasting colour.

◆ **Application to give the appearance of longer nails** This style creates an optical illusion that the nails are longer than they really are. The whole nail plate is painted, leaving a slightly larger gap than usual (usually 1.5mm) along the nail walls.

Tips for nail painting

◆ Ensure the surface of the nail is grease-free. If grease is present this will result in nail polish peeling or chipping.

◆ Select colours that suit the client's nail length, condition and skin colour.

◆ Dark colours will draw attention to the nails, and will make small/short nails appear smaller/shorter.

◆ If the nails are very broad leave a margin at the sides of the nail's wall free of polish, this will help them to appear slimmer.

◆ Avoid pearlized polish if the client's nail surface is uneven or ridged. The polish will emphasize the imperfection.

◆ Always apply a good quality base coat suited to the client's nail condition. This helps to prevent staining from pigment in the polish, and may strengthen the nail or smooth ridges depending on its formulation.

HEALTH & SAFETY

Joint mobility

If the client has any joint mobility restrictions, e.g. arthritis, you will need to modify your massage technique avoiding joint manipulation movements.

Knowledge Check

What are the terms used for the different types of massage used in manicure?

Refer to pages 416–418 to help you.

Manicured nails with a French application

TOP TIP

Fast-drying products

A nail 'fast-drying' product may be applied to reduce the time taken for the polish to dry.

TOP TIP

Choosing nail polish colours

For short nails, select a pale, neutral colour. Darker, more dramatic colours suit healthy, long nails, especially on clients with darker skin tones. Remember, it is always the client's choice, but you will often be asked to recommend.

◆ When applying nail polish colour, apply two coats, allowing the nails to dry between each coat to prevent the appearance of brush marks.

◆ Ensure good colour coverage.

◆ Ensure your polish is a good quality. If it has become thickened use a specialized solvent to restore to the correct consistency. This should be done 20 minutes prior to use to ensure an even consistency.

ALWAYS REMEMBER

Essential nail polish qualities

Nail polish should:

◆ adhere to the nail plate and be flexible to resist peeling and chipping

◆ have good durability on exposure to water, detergents and other chemicals it may come into contact with

◆ not stain the nail plate

◆ flow freely onto the nail plate and be easy to apply.

Reasons for peeling and chipping nail polish

Chipping may be explained by any of the following:

◆ the nail polish was not thick enough because of over-thinning with solvent

◆ no base coat was used

◆ grease was left on the nail plate prior to painting

◆ the nail plate is flaking

◆ the polish was dried too quickly by artificial means.

◆ The nail polish or the layers were too thick.

Peeling polish may have the following explanations:

◆ no top coat was used

◆ no base coat was used

◆ the nail polish was too thick, due to evaporation of the solvent

◆ grease was left on the nail plate prior to painting.

Nail polish storage

Nail polish should be stored in a cool, dark place, to avoid thickening, separation and fading. The caps and the rims of bottles must be kept clean, not only for appearance but also to ensure that the bottle is airtight. Always use stock rotation to ensure that the oldest product is used first, remember FILO – first in, last out.

If polish does thicken, solvent may be added to restore the correct consistency.

Knowledge Check

Identify the nail painting techniques shown:

Refer to page 421 to help you.

Cream and pearlized nail polish

Types of polish

The following types of polish may be used:

◆ **Cream** This has a matt finish, and requires a top coat application to give a sheen.

◆ **Pearlized, also known as crystalline** This has a frosted, shimmery appearance due to the addition of natural fish scales or synthetic ingredients such as bismuth oxychloride.

◆ **Base coat** This protects the nail from staining by a strong-coloured nail polish; it also gives a good grip to polish, and smooths out minor surface irregularities. Many base coats are formulated using ingredients to treat different nail problems such as weak, brittle, peeling or ridged nails.

◆ **Top coat** This gives a sheen to cream polish, and adds longer wear as it helps to prevent chipping.

Base coat

Contra-indications to nail polish

Do not apply polish in these circumstances:

◆ if there are diseases and disorders of the nail plate and surrounding skin

◆ if the client is allergic to nail polish.

In addition, pearlized nail polish should not be applied to excessively ridged nails as it may appear to exaggerate the problem. Short or bitten nails should be painted only with pale polishes, to avoid attracting attention.

Top coat

Painting the nail is a skill in its own right. It takes practice! Polishes differ and colours within the same range can differ. Even the temperature will make a difference. The longevity of polish will depend on the condition of the nail, e.g. a peeling nail will not hold polish as well as a smooth nail.

Marian Newman

TOP TIP

Cleaning the nail plate before polish application

Use a lint-free pad as cotton wool may leave fibres, which may spoil the application of nail polish.

STEP-BY-STEP: DARK POLISH APPLICATION

Confirm the client's choice of nail colour. A cream formulation has been demonstrated.

Ensure the free edge is smooth and the cuticles are neat and smooth.

1 Ensure that the nail plate is free from grease. Starting with the thumb, apply three brush strokes down the length of the nail from the cuticle to the free edge, beginning in the centre, then down either side close to the nail wall.

Take care to avoid touching the cuticle or the nail wall. If flooding occurs, remove the polish immediately with an orange stick and polish remover.

Apply one coat of base coat.

2 Apply the coloured polish, two coats are applied, followed by one coat of top coat.

3 The complete dark polish application.

Confirm with the client that the finished result is to their satisfaction.

Complete details on the client's record card.

CourseMate video: Dark Polish Application

Manicure for a male client

A man's hands differ slightly from a woman's usually in size, being larger, and there may be coarse terminal hair on the fingers. Males tend to wear their nails shorter too. Consider the following in your treatment plan:

◆ file the nails to a shorter length

◆ usually coloured nail polish is omitted. A nail treatment base coat may be included if advised or requested

◆ shape the nails square rather than oval

◆ buff the nails with paste, if a shine is required

◆ use unperfumed lotion for massage

◆ use a lotion or an oil rather than cream for massage, to avoid dragging body hair

◆ use deeper movements during hand and arm massage as the arms are more muscular.

HEALTH & SAFETY

Environment
Ensure the area is well ventilated to avoid inhalation of excessive fumes. Lighting should be good to enable you to avoid eyestrain. It is a good idea to use a table lamp when painting the nails.

ACTIVITY

Comparing hands

Write down as many differences as you can between the appearance of a male and female client's nails, hands and lower arms.

From your observations, can you think of any further adaptations or recommendations that may be necessary when manicuring a man's hands?

STEP-BY-STEP: MALE MANICURE

1 File the nails to a shorter length. The nails are usually filed to a square shape rather than oval.

2 Improve the appearance of the cuticles. Push back the cuticles gently after softening.

3 A cuticle knife is used to remove the excess eponychium from the cuticle area with cuticle remover if required. Remember to keep the blade dampened to avoid scratches to the nail plate.

4 Remove excess cuticle using cuticle nippers.

5 Buff the nails to improve blood circulation to the nail bed, giving a healthy appearance to the nail. Buff the nails with a buffing paste if a shine is required. This may be included at this stage or at the end of the manicure as a nail plate finish.

6 Specialist hand and arm treatments may be included if required. A hand massage is shown in the step-by-step that follows, but you may wish to include massage to the lower arm also.

After massage, the nail plate is cleaned with acetone if buffing is required as a finish, or a specialist nail polish finish is applied.

CourseMate video:
Male Manicure

STEP-BY-STEP: HAND AND FOREARM MASSAGE

1 Effleurage to the hand and forearm. This movement starts and concludes the hand and arm massage. Use long, sweeping strokes from the hand to the elbow, moving on both the outer and inner sides of the forearm.

2 Petrissage to the lower arm, picking up the flexor and extensor muscles.

3 Perform frictions over the back of the hand working between each metacarpal bone.

4 Perform small friction movements down the length of each finger (phalange).

5 Thumbs kneading movement to the palm of the hand.

6 Perform deep localized stroking to the palm of the hands using the thumbs. Repeat Step 1 effleurage to conclude the massage.

Aftercare advice

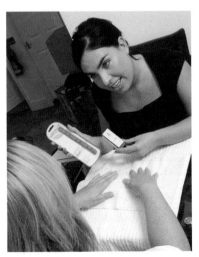

Recommending aftercare products to meet the client's needs

It is important when carrying out a manicure that the client knows how to care for their nails and hands at home. It is your duty as a beauty therapist to ensure that the correct aftercare advice is given. If it isn't, the client may unwittingly undo all the good work you have done during the treatment.

When giving aftercare advice you have a good opportunity to recommend retail products, such as nail treatment, polish or hand cream, thereby enhancing retail sales and the business's profit.

Aftercare advice will differ slightly for each client, according to individual needs, but generally it will be as follows:

◆ wear rubber gloves when washing up to avoid contact with harsh detergents, which may dehydrate the nails and skin

◆ wear protective gloves when gardening or doing domestic chores to avoid accidental damage

For each of the clients below, suggest a treatment routine. Detail the treatment plan to include: cause of the condition, aims of the treatment, products used, treatments recommended, relevant retail sales and aftercare advice.

◆ A hairdresser with very soft, weak, stained nails.

◆ An engineer with a bruised nail, overgrown cuticles and cracked skin on the fingers.

◆ A teenager with badly bitten nails.

◆ An elderly client with strong, ridged nails and dry skin on the hands.

A range of nail polishes for retail

> Few clients can paint their own nails beautifully. The polished nails are what your client will take away with them and see every day. They will forget the relaxing hand massage but will remember how beautiful their nails looked and how much longer the polish lasted as compared to when they do it.
>
> *Marian Newman*

◆ always wear gloves in cold weather: this will help maintain healthy blood circulation in the area

◆ dry the hands thoroughly after washing, and apply hand cream. Some hand creams contain UV filters which reduce hyperpigmentation (seen as darker areas of skin) occurring to the backs of the hands

◆ avoid harsh soaps when washing hands

◆ advise the client on how to file their nails

◆ do not use the fingernails as tools (for instance, to prise lids off tins)

◆ advise on appropriate nail/skincare products to remedy the problems present, e.g. dry skin, weak nails

◆ advise the client on what other professional treatments you could recommend

◆ advise the client on a treatment plan to improve the nail/skin condition and the time intervals recommended between each treatment.

It is also necessary to tell the client what to do in the event of a contra-action (see pages 399–400).

Have retail products available for the client to purchase. These include emery boards, coloured nail polishes, **nail polish remover** and nail/skin treatment products.

It is a good idea to have available the nail polish colours that you have used. The client can then touch up any accidental chips themselves.

Recommend the use of top coat applied every 3 to 4 days to protect the nail polish, increase its durability and impart shine.

Finally, at the end of the manicure treatment make sure the client's records are updated, accurate and signed by the client and manicurist. Ensure that the finished result is to the client's satisfaction and meets the agreed treatment plan.

Designing an aftercare leaflet

Devise an aftercare leaflet for clients, advising a suitable home care routine. It is good practice to provide the client with an aftercare leaflet outlining all recommendations following treatment.

Exercises for the hands

Hand exercises play an important role in the home care advice given to clients, for the following reasons:

◆ they keep the joints supple, allowing greater movement

◆ blood circulation is increased, encouraging healthy nail and skin growth

◆ good blood circulation helps to prevent cold hands

◆ exercises keep the client interested in their hands, and so more likely to keep regular salon appointments.

TOP TIP

Hand exercises

Remember, hand exercises should be performed by the manicurist also to keep the hands supple, reducing the possibility of the effects of RSI in the hands.

Hand exercises

Exercise routine

1 Rub the palms together, back and forth, until warm.

2 Make a tight fist with each hand, then slowly stretch out all the fingers as far as possible.

Repeat step 2 a further three times.

3 With the fingers extended, rotate the wrists slowly in large clockwise circles.

Repeat step 3 a further three times.

4 With the fingers extended, rotate the wrists slowly in large anticlockwise circles.

Repeat step 4 a further three times.

5 Play an imaginary piano vigorously with the fingers for 10 seconds.

6 With the hands together as if praying, gently widen the fingers as far as possible, then relax.

Repeat step 6 a further three times.

> Do not go straight from college into working on your own. Instead get a job in a salon for at least a year. This experience will be invaluable for you! You will learn how to deal with all sorts of clients, good and bad. You will learn other techniques from colleagues. You'll have a greater understanding of the business side and how to efficiently keep appointments running smoothly. Plus so much more!
>
> *Marian Newman*

ASSESSMENT OF KNOWLEDGE AND UNDERSTANDING

You have now learnt about the knowledge and skills for providing manicure treatment for the beauty therapy workplace. To test your level of knowledge, answer the following short questions. These will prepare you for your summative (final) assessment.

1. The nail condition shown below is called:

   a. onychia   b. onycholysis
   c. onychopagy   d. onychorrhexis

2. A hangnail is best removed with:

   a. cuticle nippers   b. nail scissors
   c. cuticle knife   d. an exfoliation product

3. Name the arteries shown on the diagram below.

4. The part of the epidermis found under the free edge of the nails is called:

   a. perionychium   b. cuticle
   c. hyponychium   d. eponychium

5. The image below shows a nail polish finish using:

   a. cream polish
   b. pearlized (crystalline) polish

6. Match the following tools with their use in manicure:

1) orange stick	a) used to trim away dead skin tissue
2) hoof stick	b) used to gently push back softened cuticle
3) cuticle nipper	c) used to add shine to the nail plate and smooth out ridges
4) chamois leather buffer	d) used to apply product, treating cuticle tissue or to clean under the free edge
5) scissors	e) used to shorten the free edge
6) cuticle knife	f) used to remove excess eponychium and perionychium from the nail plate

7. The nail product designed to loosen dead tissue from the nail plate so that it can be more easily removed from the nail plate is:

   a. acetone   b. cuticle oil
   c. cuticle remover   d. cuticle cream

8. The massage manipulation that is used when starting and ending the hand and arm massage is called:

   a. vibrations   b. frictions
   c. petrissage   d. effleurage

9. The nail is made of a hard protein called what?

10. To ease the discomfort of joint stiffness, which specialist hand and arm services would be best to use?

   a. paraffin wax   b. exfoliating treatment
   c. thermal mitts   d. hand mask

12 Pedicure Treatments

LEARNING OBJECTIVES

There are two learning outcomes to achieve for this mandatory unit:

1 Be able to prepare for pedicure treatments.

2 Be able to provide pedicure treatments.

The assessment range applied requires you to:

◆ Use all consultation techniques to identify the treatment objectives.

◆ Use all listed products, tools and equipment as appropriate within the treatment.

◆ Ensure that the environmental conditions are suitable.

◆ Identify and treat skin and nail conditions.

◆ Complete a consultation and skin inspection to identify any contra-indications that may affect if and how the treatment can proceed.

◆ Communicate and behave in a professional manner.

◆ Use a variety of massage techniques.

◆ Follow all health and safety practices.

◆ Provide relevant aftercare and contra-action advice.

KEY TERMS

aftercare advice

bunions

calluses

chiropodist

consultation

contra-action advice

contra-actions

Controlled Waste
  Regulations (1992)

corns

cuticle remover

diabetes

foot rasp

foot spas

eczema of the nail

foot and nail treatments

health and safety

ingrowing toenails

massage

nail conditions

nail finish

nail polish

nail polish remover

paronychia

pedicure

phlebitis

skin conditions

thermal booties

thrombophlebitis

tinea corporis (body ringworm)

tinea pedis (athlete's foot)

tinea unguium

treatment objectives

treatment plan

Unit Topic

Provide pedicure treatments

This VRQ unit is linked to the Beauty Therapy NOS Unit N3.

INTRODUCTION

This unit is all about improving and maintaining your client's feet, nails and surrounding skin condition. A pedicure includes filing the nails to shape, reducing nail length, using specialized nail, cuticle products and foot treatments, massaging the lower leg and foot and providing a complementary nail finish to suit the client's treatment objectives.

Dealing with people in a polite, efficient manner and using good communication and questioning skills to find out exactly what they require from the pedicure treatment forms an important part of this technical service.

You must be able to show you have the necessary practical skills and underpinning knowledge to provide pedicure treatments.

INDUSTRY ROLE MODEL

MARGARET DABBS Company founder and Chief Executive of Margaret Dabbs (Foot Care) London

" I am a fully trained Podiatrist, and recognized as a Global Leader in Foot Care. As company founder and Chief Executive of Margaret Dabbs London, my foot clinics are based in prestigious locations in London – and more recently Dubai – and have a reputation for excellence. In 1994 I created a range of results-driven luxury foot care products, which fuse both the health and beauty of the feet, and are used at some of the most prestigious destinations in the world.

ANATOMY & PHYSIOLOGY
Essential anatomy and physiology knowledge requirements for this unit are identified on the checklist chart on page 33

Pedicure treatment to improve skin condition of the feet

Pedicure tools and equipment

The purpose of a pedicure

The word **pedicure** is derived from the Latin word *pedis*, meaning 'foot' and *cura*, meaning 'care'. The treatment is very similar to manicure except that it is carried out on the feet instead of the hands. A pedicure therefore cares for the feet and nails and achieves the following effects:

◆ to improve the appearance of the foot and nails

◆ to keep the skin and cuticles soft and supple

◆ to reduce the amount of hard skin and prevent it from building in localized areas

◆ to relax tired, aching feet

◆ to keep the nails smooth and healthy.

Preparing the working area

All metal tools should be disinfected in a suitable solution prior to use. Prepare the products, tools and equipment neatly on the work station so that everything you need is to hand and the client need not be disturbed during treatment.

The work area should remain in a condition suitable for further nail treatments during the working day.

Place a towel on the floor between you and the client. The foot bowl or foot spa containing warm, soapy water should be placed on this towel. Exactly how you arrange the work area will depend upon how your work area is equipped to deliver the treatment resources.

Towels should be placed on your lap: one is for protection, the other is for drying the client's feet. Keep the other towels close by for wrapping the client's feet. Alternatively, the pedicure may be performed on a beauty couch or at a pedicure station. In this case towels are only required for drying and wrapping up feet.

When cutting the client's nails and removing hard skin, disposable tissue should be placed on your lap and then removed before continuing treatment.

PPE, e.g. safety glasses and synthetic powder-free gloves, may be worn for protection from skin and nail debris at this stage.

Outcome 1: Be able to prepare for pedicure treatments

Learn how to prepare for pedicure treatments

PRACTICAL SKILLS

Prepare yourself, the client and work area for pedicure treatment

Use suitable consultation techniques to identify treatment objectives

Carry out a nail and skin analysis

Provide clear recommendations to the client

Select products, tools and equipment to suit client treatment needs, skin and nail conditions

UNDERPINNING KNOWLEDGE

Describe salon requirements for preparing yourself, the client and the work area

Describe the environmental conditions suitable for pedicure treatments

Describe different consultation techniques used to identify treatment objectives

Explain the importance of carrying out a nail and skin analysis

Describe how to select products, tools and equipment to suit client treatment needs, skin and nail conditions

Identify nail and skin conditions

Describe the contra-indications which prevent or restrict pedicure treatments

When the client is comfortably seated, clean your hands using an approved hand cleaning technique, preferably in view of the client, who will observe hygienic procedures being carried out. This will assure them that they are receiving a professional treatment.

Before beginning the pedicure, check that you have the necessary tools, products and equipment to hand and that they meet the legal hygiene and industry requirements for nail treatments.

Tools and equipment

TOP TIP

Foot spa

Foot spas help to relax the feet by a combination of massage provided by an integral vibration feature, aeration of the water, creating a bubbling effect, and heating of the water. Some equipment can also alter the temperature of the water.

Footsie bath

Products, tools and equipment

◆ **Cotton wool** To remove nail polish and excess nail product preparations. Cotton wool may also be used to tip orange sticks for the purpose of nail product application and removal. Cotton wool filled gauze pads are also available and are more absorbent

◆ **Nail polish remover** To remove nail polish and excess nail care and skincare preparations from the nail plate

◆ **Scissors and toenail clippers** To shorten nail length

◆ **Emery boards** To shorten and shape the nail free edge

◆ **Cuticle oil or cream** Used to condition and rehydrate the skin of the cuticle; especially beneficial for dry nails and cuticles

◆ **Cuticle remover** Used to soften the skin cells and the cuticle so excess epidermal skin can be easily removed

◆ **Cuticle nippers** To remove excess cuticle and dead, torn skin surrounding the nail plate

◆ **Hoof stick or cuticle pusher** To gently push back the softened cuticles

◆ **Foot rasp or callous file** To remove excess dead skin from the foot

◆ **Foot massage lotion or oil** To massage the skin of the foot and lower leg

YOU WILL ALSO NEED:

◆ **Pedicure bowl or foot spa** To soak and cleanse the foot. The foot spa also revitalizes and refreshes the skin by stimulating the sensory nerve endings, and encouraging blood and lymph circulation

◆ **Small towels (5)** Used for protection and to dry the client's skin

◆ **Small bowls (3)** For storage etc.

◆ **Liquid soap** Specialized foot cleaning products to cleanse, soften and deodorize the feet

◆ **Skin disinfectant** To cleanse and disinfect the client's skin. Specialized sprays and gels are available for this purpose

◆ **Cuticle knife** To remove cuticle from the nail plate

◆ **Client's record card** To record confidential details of each client registered at the salon, including personal details, products used and details of the treatment provided

◆ **Base coat** Provides an even surface to improve nail polish application and adherence and prevent nail staining. Depending upon its formulation, it can also improve the appearance and health of the nail

◆ **Coloured nail polish (enamel)** A selection for the client to choose from in cream or pearlized (also termed crystalline) formulations

◆ **Top coat** To provide shine and strength to protect the nail polish, reduces peeling and chipping and increases durability of the polish

◆ **Tissues** To protect client's clothing in the treatment area and for drying tools after immersion in disinfectant solution

◆ **Disposable bedroll tissue** To collect waste and be replaced as necessary during the treatment

◆ **Orange sticks** Used to remove products from containers and, when tipped at either end with cotton wool, to ease the cuticle back and to clean under the free edge. Orange sticks should be disposed of after each client as they cannot be effectively sterilized

◆ **Disinfectant solution** To store small plastic and stainless steel sterilized tools

◆ **Nail polish drier** An aerosol or oil preparation applied to speed the drying process of nail polish

◆ **Disposable toe separators** Used to keep the toes separated during nail polish application. Alternatively, disposable items such as cotton wool or tissues may be used for this purpose

◆ **Disposable footwear (optional)** Enabling the client to move without smudging the nail polish application

◆ **Disinfecting solution** For all surfaces

◆ **Foot and nail treatment equipment** Including paraffin wax, foot masks, thermal boots and exfoliators

◆ **Waste container** This should be a lined metal bin with a lid to contain vapours from solvents

Products used in pedicure treatments

For full details of products used for both manicures and pedicures, their ingredients and uses, see the table on pages 389–390. In addition to these, an exfoliating pedicure scrub may also be used for the feet (see page 435).

Product	Ingredients	Use
Exfoliating pedicure scrub	Abrasive ingredients such as pumice, sea salt, detergent, water and water-soluble ingredients, added moisturizers, refreshing agents, e.g. peppermint oil	To remove dead skin cells, cleanse the skin, condition, soften and refresh the skin, improving blood circulation in the area

See the table on pages 389–390.

Disinfection

Hygiene must be maintained in a number of ways:

◆ ensure that tools and equipment are clean, disinfected and, where required, according to legal requirements sterile before use

◆ having sterilized or disinfected tools and equipment stored in a chemical disinfectant, UV cabinet or closed container until ready for use. Remember, they will remain clean but will not be sterile after after exposure to the air or once they have been touched

◆ dispense products from containers, e.g. creams and lotions, with a clean, disposable spatula

◆ use disposable tools, products and equipment wherever possible.

Refer to the Habia Code of Practice for Nail Services for **health and safety** best practice guidance.

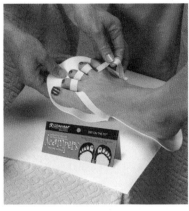
Disposable toe separators

ALWAYS REMEMBER

Disposable toe separators

Disposable toe separators are useful to prevent accidental damage following nail polish application and also to allow the client to move around the salon without walking on the flooring which would be unhygienic.

ACTIVITY

Why is personal presentation and best hygiene practice important to create a good impression?

Refer to the Habia *Code of Practice for Nail Services* to research recognized examples of good personal presentation and hygiene at www.habia.org

Reception

When a client makes an appointment for a pedicure treatment, the receptionist should advise the client how long the treatment will take. This will include sufficient time for the **nail polish** to dry before replacing footwear.

To allocate the appropriate length of time ask if they require a specialist foot treatment with their pedicure.

Ask the client whether they are currently receiving treatment from a chiropodist for conditions such as verrucas, athlete's foot or any fungal infections. These would contra-indicate treatment: the receptionist should advise the client to wait until the condition has cleared.

If the client is a minor under 16 years of age, it is necessary to obtain parent/guardian permission for treatment. The parent/guardian will also have to be present when the treatment is received.

Commercial timing:

◆ *allow 45 minutes for a pedicure treatment*

◆ *allow up to 1hour for a specialist foot treatment.*

Pedicure tools and equipment can be disposable or can be disinfected by the methods shown on page 390–391.

ALWAYS REMEMBER

GP referral

A client referred from their GP will usually have a letter. This would be the case when confirmation regarding suitability for treatment has been requested. This should be retained with the client's record card.

A sample client record card

Date	Beauty therapist name	
Client name		Date of birth (identifying client age group)
Home address		Postcode
Email address	Landline phone number	Mobile phone number
Name of doctor	Doctor's address and phone number	
Related medical history (conditions that may restrict or prohibit treatment application)		
Are you taking any medication? (this may affect the sensitivity of the skin to the treatment)		

CONTRA-INDICATIONS REQUIRING MEDICAL REFERRAL
(preventing pedicure treatment application)

☐ bacterial infections (e.g. paronychia)

☐ viral infections (e.g. plantar warts)

☐ fungal infections (e.g. tinea unguium, tinea pedis)

☐ parasitic infestations (e.g. scabies)

☐ severe skin conditions

☐ severe toenail separation

☐ severe skin disorders such as severe eczema or hyperkeratosis conditions such as psoriasis

☐ severe bruising

☐ diabetes

CONTRA-INDICATIONS WHICH RESTRICT TREATMENT
(treatment may require adaptation)

☐ minor toenail separation   ☐ broken capillaries

☐ minor eczema and psoriasis   ☐ moles

☐ recent scar tissue   ☐ product allergies

☐ broken bones   ☐ varicose veins

☐ recent fractures and sprains   ☐ cuts and abrasions

☐ minor cuts or abrasions   ☐ circulatory conditions

☐ minor bruising or swelling   such as phlebitis or

☐ undiagnosed lumps and   thrombophlebitis
    swellings

PRODUCTS, TOOLS AND EQUIPMENT

☐ toenail and skin treatment tools (scissors/clippers, foot file/ rasps, cuticle knife, cuticle nippers and hoof sticks)

☐ abrasives (e.g. buffing paste)

☐ cuticle softeners

☐ toenail conditioners (e.g. cuticle cream/oils)

☐ skin conditioners (e.g. foot cream)

☐ toenail, skin and cuticle corrective treatments (e.g. paraffin wax)

☐ consumables

FEET AND TOENAIL TREATMENTS

☐ paraffin wax   ☐ foot masks

☐ thermal booties   ☐ exfoliators

TOENAIL FINISH

☐ light colour   ☐ dark colour   ☐ French manicure

COURSE OF TREATMENT

	Date	Date	Date
☐ improvement of skin condition products used	_____	_____	_____
☐ improvement of toenail condition products used	_____	_____	_____

TOENAIL, CUTICLE AND SKIN CONDITION

Toenails

☐ normal   ☐ brittle   ☐ dry   ☐ weak   ☐ ridged

Cuticle

☐ normal   ☐ dry   ☐ split   ☐ overgrown
☐ hangnails

Skin

☐ normal   ☐ dry   ☐ hard

MASSAGE MEDIUMS

☐ creams   ☐ oils   ☐ oils

Beauty therapist signature (for reference)

Client signature (confirmation of details)

A sample client record card (continued)

TREATMENT ADVICE

Pedicure – *allow 45 minutes*

Specialized foot/nail treatment – *allow up to 60 minutes*

TREATMENT PLAN

Record relevant details of your treatment and advice provided for future reference.

Ensure the client's records are up-to-date, accurate and fully completed following treatment. Non-compliance may invalidate insurance.

DURING

Discuss:

- ◆ details that may influence the client's toenail condition, such as the client's level of exercise as this will affect the length of toenails
- ◆ the products the client is currently using to care for the skin of the feet and toenails
- ◆ the client's satisfaction with these products
- ◆ relevant pedicure procedures (e.g., how to file the toenails correctly).

Note:

- ◆ any adverse (unwanted) reaction, if any occur during or after the pedicure treatment.

AFTER

Record:

- ◆ results of treatment
- ◆ any modification to treatment application that has occurred
- ◆ what products have been used in the pedicure treatment
- ◆ what foot treatments have been used
- ◆ the effectiveness of treatment
- ◆ any samples provided (review their success at the next appointment).

Advise on:

- ◆ product application in order to gain maximum benefit from product use
- ◆ specialized products following pedicure treatment for homecare use
- ◆ general foot/toenail care and maintenance
- ◆ the recommended time intervals between treatments
- ◆ the importance of a course of treatments to improve toenail/skin conditions.

RETAIL OPPORTUNITIES

Advise on:

- ◆ progression of the treatment plan for future appointments
- ◆ products that would be suitable for the client to use at home to care for the skin of the feet and toenails
- ◆ recommendations for further treatments
- ◆ further products or treatments that the client may or may not have received before.

Note:

- ◆ any purchase made by the client.

EVALUATION

Record:

- ◆ comments on the client's satisfaction with the treatment
- ◆ if poor results are achieved, the reasons why
- ◆ how you may alter the treatment plan to achieve the required treatment results in the future, if applicable.

HEALTH AND SAFETY

Advise on:

- ◆ appropriate necessary action to be taken in the event of an unwanted skin or nail reaction.

HEALTH & SAFETY

Preventing injury and avoiding RSI Remember to consider your posture and prevent any awkward movements during delivery of the pedicure treatment. Ensure the work station is at the correct height to avoid stretching and straining your upper body and limbs. Adjust the client's seat to ensure you are comfortable when working and to avoid strain.

TOP TIP

Pedicure spa chair

Pedicure spa chairs provide comfort and luxury for the client. The client immerses their feet in a tray equipped with hydrotherapy jets to massage the feet, while the chair also features a vibrating massage system.

Knowledge Check

How many bones are there in the foot? How many can you name?

Refer to page 91 to help you.

All staff, especially the staff communicating with clients at reception, should be familiar with the different pricing structures for the range of pedicure treatments and products available for retail.

It is important that accurate records are kept and stored in compliance with the Data Protection Act for future reference.

Preparing the client

Ensure that the client is seated at the correct height, so that you can work comfortably and healthily and the client can enjoy the treatment without strain to the muscles and joints of the leg.

Make sure that the client is warm and comfortable when preparing for the pedicure. Client privacy and modesty should also be considered. Not all clients would be happy to be on view while receiving the treatment. Ensure that lighting is good to avoid eye strain and to enable the treatment to be performed competently. Avoid positioning the work station in direct sunlight however, to prevent discomfort to the client and pedicurist.

Before treatment begins, ask the client to remove their tights or socks, and any clothing that might restrict their lower leg movement, such as jeans or trousers. Cover their upper legs with a clean towel or provide a gown. This will help them to be more comfortable and allow you to work without restriction.

Ask them to remove any jewellery from the area to be treated, to prevent it being damaged by creams and to avoid obstructing **massage** movements. Place the jewellery where the client can see it. Alternatively, ask the client to take possession of it for safe keeping – following your salon security policy.

When the client is comfortably seated, clean your hands using an approved hand cleaning technique – preferably in view of the client, who will observe hygienic procedures being carried out. This will assure them that they are receiving a professional treatment.

Consultation

Before carrying out a pedicure treatment, it is necessary to assess the condition of the client's skin, nails and cuticles. This is done in order that the most appropriate **foot and nail treatments** and products may be chosen. Also, by correctly assessing and analyzing the client's foot condition and writing this on their record card, you will be able to see over a period of time how the condition is progressing.

Client Communication

The key to customer loyalty is all reliant on communication with your client. It is important that you introduce yourself – but not talk too much about yourself – that you explain what it is you are doing and why you are doing this. Promote the use of both your own skill and the products you are using, and show an interest in your client. Pride and compassion in what you are doing is what will shine through every time.

Margaret Dabbs

Assess the condition of the following:

◆ *The cuticles* Are they dry, tight, cracked or overgrown, or are they soft and pliable?

◆ *The nail* Are they strong or weak, thickened, discoloured or stained? Sometimes this may indicate a nail disorder. The nails of the foot should be filed straight across into a square shape. Shaping the nails at the corners can cause **ingrowing toenails**.

◆ *The skin* Is the skin dry, rough or cracked, or is it soft and smooth? Is the colour even? Also check the skin between the toes.

While assessing the client's feet, you should also be looking for any contra-indications to the treatment.

Skin and nail disorders of the feet

When a client attends for a pedicure treatment, as part of the consultation and assessment of the client's needs, the beauty therapist should always look at the client's skin and nails to check that no infection or disease is present which might contra-indicate treatment.

TOP TIP

Recommended footwear when receiving a pedicure treatment

Advise the client to wear open-toed shoes or sandals on the day of the pedicure to allow time for polish to dry completely before putting on shoes.

Ensure client is sitting at the correct height so they can enjoy the treatment without strain to the leg

Disorder	Description
Broken bones Cuts or abrasions on the feet Diabetes Paronychia Scabies or itch mites Severe eczema of the nail Severe eczema of the skin	*For full details, see pages 394–396.*
Severe nail separation (onycholysis) Severe psoriasis of the nail Severe psoriasis of the skin Tinea corporis (body ringworm) Tinea unguium	*For full details, see pages 394–398.*
Phlebitis	Recognized by swelling and pain in the leg caused by inflammation of the vein wall (veins transport blood from the tissues back towards the heart). If a vein becomes inflamed a blood clot commonly forms inside the inflamed area (termed **thrombophlebitis**). Venous problems can also lead to skin ulceration. Massage to the lower leg may cause a blood clot to move through the bloodstream, causing a blockage elsewhere which could prove fatal!

These include bacterial, fungal, parasitic and viral infections, which are described in more detail in **Chapter 2**, where contra-indications are illustrated and discussed.

If the client is wearing nail polish, this must be removed before checking.

Contra-indications The following disorders contra-indicate pedicure treatments. If you suspect the client has any disorder from the chart on page 440, do not attempt a diagnosis, but refer the client tactfully to their GP or a **chiropodist** without causing unnecessary concern.

Knowledge Check

What information should be recorded on the record card following a pedicure treatment?

Refer to page 437 to help you.

Knowledge Check

Why is diabetes considered a contra-indication to pedicure treatments?

Refer to page 394 to help you.

See also bruised nails, on page 397.

Disorder	Description
Ingrowing toenail	The sides of the nail penetrate the nail wall: redness, inflammation and pus may be present, depending on the severity of the condition. The client should be referred to a chiropodist for appropriate treatment. To prevent ingrowing toenails clients should be advised to cut the toenails straight across, and not too short
Tinea pedis (athlete's foot)	Fungal infection of the foot occurring in the webs of the skin between the toes. Small blisters form, which later burst. The skin in the area can become dry, with a scaly appearance
Verrucae or plantar warts on the feet	A viral infection Small epidermal skin growths. Warts occurring on the sole of the foot grow inwards, due to the pressure of body weight. Warts vary in size, shape, texture and colour. Usually they have a rough surface and are raised. Plantar wart – found on the sole of the foot

Below is a list of common disorders that may be seen on the feet. Not all of these contra-indicate treatment.

Disorder	Cause	Appearance	Salon treatment	Home care advice
Blue nail (shown on the fingernail)	Poor blood circulation in the area. Heart disease	The nail bed does not appear a healthy pink colour but has a blue tinge	Permission to treat to be received from the client's GP. Regular pedicure including foot treatment to improve circulation	General pedicure advice. Foot exercises and massage to improve circulation
Bunions	Long-term wear of ill-fitting shoes, especially those with high heels or pointed toe areas. A weakness in the arches of the feet. They can also be hereditary	The large joint at the base of the big toe protrudes, forcing the big toe inwards towards the other toes	None – refer the client to a chiropodist if the bunion is painful; gentle massage may help to ease any pain or discomfort	Try to keep pressure off the affected area

Disorder	Cause	Appearance	Salon treatment	Home care advice
Calluses	Incorrect footwear or client has not regularly removed build-up of hard skin	Thick, yellowish, hardened patches of skin, usually found on prominent areas of the foot such as the heel and the ball of toe; may be painful	Use a rasp or pumice stone gently to remove any build-up of hard skin: painful calluses should be treated by a chiropodist	Ensure that shoes fit correctly. Avoid standing for long periods. Alternate style of footwear regularly. Keep the skin of the foot moisturized with a specialized skin conditioner for the feet. Use a pumice stone regularly after bathing or showering to remove excess skin
Chilblains	Poor blood supply to the hands and feet, aggravated by cold weather	Fingers and toes may be red, blue or purple in colour; the client may complain of painful or itchy area	Regular pedicures, with special attention paid to massage which will help to improve the circulation	Keep affected areas warm and dry. Avoid tight footwear, which might restrict the circulation. If the condition is severe, seek medical advice
Corns	Incorrect footwear (corns are often found on toes which have been squeezed together by tight shoes)	Similar to calluses except that the affected area is smaller and more compact; corns often look white, and may be extremely painful	Small corns may be treated in the same way as a callus, but if the client has large or painful corns they should be treated by a chiropodist	Ensure that shoes fit correctly. Avoid standing for long periods. Alternate style of footwear regularly
Pitting (shown on the fingernail)	Eczema and/or psoriasis	Pitting, resembling small, irregular pin pricks, appear on the nail plate	Refer the client to their GP for permission to treat if required. Regular pedicure with gentle buffing	General pedicure advice. Ridge-filling base coat polish

Contra-actions

Certain cosmetic ingredients are known to cause allergic reactions in some people.

The client – or the pedicurist – may at some time develop an allergy to a pedicure product that has been successfully used previously. This could be for a number of reasons, including new medication being taken or illness. This is known as a contra-action. This may occur during or following a pedicure treatment.

The symptoms of an allergic reaction could be:

- excessive redness of the skin (erythema)
- skin irritation, e.g. itching
- swelling
- raised blisters.

The symptoms do not necessarily appear on the feet. In the case of nail polish allergy, the symptoms often show up on the face.

In the case of an allergic reaction:

- remove the offending product immediately, using water or, in the case of polish, nail polish solvent
- apply a cool compress and soothing agent to the skin to reduce redness and irritation
- if symptoms persist, seek medical advice. If the client receives medical advice, ask them to inform you of the advice and/or treatment received so you can include this in your records.

Always record any allergies on the client's record card, so that the offending product may be avoided in future.

Further **contra-actions** could occur as a result of incorrect use of pedicure tools, e.g. sore, sensitized skin following hard skin removal or sore, reddened skin in the cuticle area due to excessive trimming of the cuticle. Tissue damage could result in blood loss, e.g. incorrect nipping removal technique when using cuticle nippers may result in pulling and tearing the skin. Incorrect positioning and use of the cuticle knife may lead to piercing the nail fold with the knife blade.

Avoid cutting the nails too short as again this can result in possible damage to the hyponychium, the part of the epidermis under the free edge of the nail. This may affect its protective function, leading to possible infection.

Carrying out pedicure treatments

Treatment plan

Adding revitalizing spa agent to the foot spa water

After analyzing the client's nails and adjacent skin, a **treatment plan** should be considered and agreed with the client. In order to correct any skin and nail problems the client should attend the salon weekly. They should also be advised of the appropriate treatment preparations to use at home, so as to support the salon treatment. Specialist foot treatments to use will depend upon the skin and nail condition; they include:

- *Revitalizing foot spa agents* These may be in tablet form or as a foaming soak. They are dissolved in warm water, in which the feet are then immersed.
- *Exfoliator* This is used following immersion of the feet in the foot spa. It removes surface dead skin cells, preventing the formation of callus (excess dead tissue) tissue.
- *Massage lotion or cream* This is a massage preparation which includes refreshing essential oils such as peppermint. It is recommended for the relief of tired, aching feet.

◆ *Foot mask* A **mask** may be applied to cool and refresh the feet. Booties may be worn while the mask penetrates the epidermis.

◆ *Foot gel or spray* This may be applied to create an immediate cooling, refreshing effect.

Provide the opportunity for your client to ask any questions relating to the pedicure treatment plan.

The record card should be signed and dated by the client and pedicurist following the consultation to confirm the suitability and consent with the agreed pedicure treatment.

Knowledge Check

What advice would you give to a client who developed an allergic reaction to a product following a pedicure treatment?

Refer to pages 441–442 to help you.

Outcome 2: Be able to provide pedicure treatments

Learn how to provide pedicure treatments

PRACTICAL SKILLS	UNDERPINNING KNOWLEDGE
Communicate and behave in a professional manner	State how to communicate and behave in a professional manner.
Follow health and safety working practices	Describe health and safety working practices
Position yourself and client correctly throughout the treatment	Explain the importance of positioning yourself and the client correctly throughout the treatment
Use products, tools, equipment and techniques to suit client's treatment needs, nail and skin conditions	Explain the importance of using products, tools, equipment and techniques to suit client's treatment needs, nail and skin conditions
Complete the treatment to the satisfaction of the client	Describe the different massage techniques and their benefits
Record the results of the treatment	State the contra-actions that may occur during and following treatments and how to respond
Provide suitable aftercare advice	State the importance of completing the treatment to the satisfaction of the client
	Describe diseases and disorders of the nail and skin
	Describe the structure and functions of the nail and skin
	Describe the structure and function of the lymphatic vessels of the lower leg and foot
	Describe the structure and function of the arteries and veins of the lower leg and foot

HEALTH & SAFETY

Contamination Always remove products hygienically from containers to avoid contamination and cross-infection.

> Always think about first impressions. Dress properly for an interview and arrive on time. Make sure you research the company who are giving their time to interview you, and direct your questions carefully. It is important that you understand the position you are applying for and everything it will entail. Think about why you would like that job and why you think you are right for it. If you are loyal, hardworking, sincere and passionate about beauty, let them know!
>
> *Margaret Dabbs*

STEP-BY-STEP: PEDICURE PROCEDURE

This process briefly shows the stages in the pedicure. Each step is discussed in detail later in the chapter. The procedure may start with either the right or left foot.

1 Nails before pedicure procedure.

2 Clean your hands using an approved hand cleaning technique.

3 Wipe both feet (including between the toes) with cotton wool soaked in skin disinfectant (product example shown here) or a specialized hygiene spray for the feet. Use separate pieces of cotton wool for each foot.

4 Soak both feet in warm water to which a liquid soap or a similar appropriate product has been added. Take out left foot and towel dry it.

5 Remove any existing nail polish, and check again for contra-indications below the nail plate. (If a nail contra-indication is present treatment must not continue. Tactfully explain why and give appropriate referral advice.)

6 Cut the toenails straight across, using toenail clippers or scissors.

7 File the nails smooth with the emery board. Again do not shape the nails at the sides to avoid ingrowing nails.

8 Apply cuticle massage cream or oil.

9 Place the foot back in the water.

10 Remove the right foot and repeat steps 5–10.

11 Dry the left foot and apply **cuticle remover.** To avoid excessive application and contaminating the applicator apply to a cotton wool-tipped orange stick.

12 Push back the nail fold with a cotton wool-tipped orange stick or hoof stick.

13 Clean under the free edge with a separate cotton wool-tipped orange stick.

14 Use the cuticle knife where indicated to remove excess cuticle. Collect excess skin in a tissue or a clean piece of cotton wool and dispose of immediately.

15 Use cuticle nippers where necessary to remove excess cuticle.

16 Wipe off any remaining cuticle remover with damp cotton wool, and file the nails again if necessary. Apply cuticle oil.

17 Remove any hard skin. This may be done with exfoliating cream, pedicure callous file or a rasp, depending on the severity of the excess dry skin condition.

18 Wrap the foot in a dry towel to keep it warm.

19 Repeat steps 12–19 for the other foot.

20 Remove the foot bowl from the working area.

21 Perform a foot and lower leg massage. (See pages 450–451.)

22 Remove any grease from the nail plates with a cotton wool pad soaked in nail polish remover. Refile the nails as necessary to ensure they are smooth and even.

23 Place disposable toe separators or other hygienic equivalent to separate them and facilitate polish application.

23 Continued

23 Continued

24 Apply the polish: base coat (once), cream polish (twice) and top coat (once) where indicated. If a pearlized polish is used a top coat is not required and a third coat of polish may be applied.

24a Application of base coat.

24b Application of first coat of coloured cream polish.

24c Application of second coat of coloured cream polish. A cotton wool-tipped orange stick may be used to apply nail polish remover to remove any excess polish from the surrounding skin.

24d Application of top coat as the product is a cream polish, requiring a top coat.

25 The complete dark polish pedicure.

Complete nail treatment.

Knowledge Check

If you accidentally caused tissue damage resulting in bleeding, which legislation must you comply with in the disposable of any contaminated waste?

Refer to page 125 to help you.

HEALTH & SAFETY

Disposing of waste All waste should be disposed of as instructed by your local authority environmental agency requirements and the Industry Code of Practice for Nail Services.

Cutting and filing toenails

Toenails should be cut straight across, using nail clippers or strong sharp scissors, then filed smooth using the coarse side of the emery board. Do not cut nails in one go. Use several small cuts to avoid pressure on the side of the nails This helps to prevent ingrowing toenails. Do not cut too short to ensure there is adequate protection at the free edge to avoid discomfort and infection. Clients who wear trainers for exercise will need to have their nails, especially the big toenail, shorter than usual to prevent the pressure on the edge of the nail from tight fitting trainers which can cause the nail to lift from the nail bed

HEALTH & SAFETY

Cutting toenails Never cut toenails down at the sides. This increases the chance of ingrowing toenails, and may lead to infection.

HEALTH & SAFETY

If you accidentally cut the skin, causing bleeding at the cuticle area, protect your hands with disposable gloves and wipe the skin with an antiseptic wipe. Any waste is classed as clinical waste or contaminated waste and should be disposed of in a yellow medical bin liner in accordance with the Environmental Act (1990) and **Controlled Waste Regulations (1992)**.

See Habia *Hygiene in the Beauty Therapy* booklet for further guidance.

Cuticle work Cuticle work is carried out to keep the cuticle area attractive, healthy and also to prevent cuticles from becoming overgrown.

The work is carried out after soaking the feet in warm soapy water. This step loosens dirty particles from the free edge and softens the skin in the cuticle area.

Cutting toenails

Pushing back the cuticles

Using a cuticle knife

Using cuticle nippers

How to carry out cuticle work Cuticle work on the feet follows the same principles and cuticle work on the hands. For a detailed description, see page 413.

Removing hard skin

Hard skin develops on the feet as a form of protection, either from friction from footwear or from standing for long periods of time.

It is therefore not advisable to remove *all* the hard skin from an area, as this would remove the protective pad. Hard skin should be removed only to improve the appearance of the feet. Hard skin build-up that causes pain or discomfort should be referred to a chiropodist for treatment.

Excess hard skin may be removed from the feet in a number of ways, including exfoliators, pumice stones, callus files, chiropody sponges and corn planes. Exfoliators should be used with a deep circular massage movement: they are ideal when only a very small build-up of hard skin is present. Files, pumice stones and the rest should be used with a swift stroking movement in one direction only (similar to buffing). Sawing back and forth would lead to friction, and discomfort for the client.

Removing hard skin with a pumice file

Always finish off a hard skin removal procedure with the application of a specialized foot moisturizer or lotion, to soften the newly exposed skin.

Removing hard skin with a rasp

> Always arrive at work with plenty of time to ensure you are prepared for the day. Your managers will see from this that you are serious about your position and professional in your approach. Take an interest in your client list and always look at ways to maximize the treatment experience. It is important to follow a routine when performing a treatment so that you don't forget anything, and offer consistency to the results.

Margaret Dabbs

Foot and nail treatments

In addition to the pedicure, further treatments may be added as appropriate. Here are some examples:

◆ *Exfoliating treatment* is carried out prior to massage or as part of the massage routine. An abrasive massage product is massaged over the skin of the foot in circular movements, concentrating over the ball and heel of the foot. Exfoliation removes dead skin, increases blood and lymph circulation and improves the condition and appearance of the skin and the absorption of further treatment products.

Exfoliating treatment

◆ *Foot treatment mask* is applied according to the client's treatment requirements. The mask is applied to the skin, then covered with a plastic protective cover and the feet can then be wrapped in warm **thermal booties** to aid the absorption of the mask. The mask removes dead skin cells, improves blood circulation and improves the condition of the skin of the feet.

Foot treatment mask

◆ *Paraffin wax treatment* – this wax is heated in a special bath to a temperature of 50–55°C. The heating effect stimulates the blood and lymph circulation, eases the discomfort of arthritic and rheumatic conditions, soothes sensory nerve endings and softens the skin, improving the appearance and condition of dry skin.

After checking the client's tolerance to the wax temperature, the client's whole foot and ankle is covered with paraffin wax. The liquid wax is usually applied with a brush. The initial wax application quickly sets, becoming solid and then further layers of paraffin wax are applied to provide a waterproof covering. Once applied the feet should then be placed in a plastic protective covering and covered with towelling booties. The wax may be removed after 10–15 minutes. It is a good idea to remove the wax with the plastic covering, which is usually in one action. After use the wax is disposed of.

Paraffin wax tools and equipment

◆ *Thermal booties* are electrically heated booties. They are used to stimulate, rejuvenate and moisturize the skin of the feet. The feet are prepared with the application of a foot treatment mask, protected in a plastic covering and placed inside warm booties for 10 to 15 minutes to enable the mask to penetrate the skin of the epidermis.

Always follow manufacturer's guidelines in the application procedure for feet and nail treatments.

Pedicure products

Thermal booties

TOP TIP

Paraffin wax

Heat the wax at least half an hour before the client arrives to ensure it has melted properly. Paraffin wax may have essential oils added to enhance the therapeutic effects.

Specialist foot and leg treatment

Specialist treatments should be offered to your client when there is a specific need or if they feel they would like to benefit from such a treatment. Specialist treatment training in these advanced techniques is usually offered by major product companies.

The model for this specialist foot and leg treatment is a client who regularly visits the gym and wishes to benefit from a spa therapy revitalizing foot and lower leg treatment following a workout.

The following foot and leg treatment will:

◆ stimulate the blood circulation

◆ aid with the removal of toxins and waste products

◆ have a skin-cleansing action

◆ remove dead skin cells (desquamation)

◆ improve the moisture content of the skin

◆ relax tense/stiff muscles in the foot and leg.

Your treatments should be adapted to meet the **treatment objectives** of the client. Allow 30 minutes for the specialist foot and leg treatment below.

STEP-BY-STEP: SPECIALIST FOOT AND LEG TREATMENT

1 The skin of the feet and legs is cleansed using warm towelling mitts infused with lime oil for its therapeutic refreshing and energizing properties.

2 The feet and legs are exfoliated to remove all dead skin cells and brighten the skin. A sea salt-based preparation with emollient, skin softening ingredients is applied to each foot and leg.

3 Towelling mitts are used to remove the exfoliating treatment. These have been steamed and are warm when used.

4 A skin-nourishing milk lotion is applied to each foot and leg. The lotion is particularly beneficial for dry skin.

5 Massage movements are applied using effleurage and petrissage manipulations to introduce the massage medium into the skin.

6 A skin treatment mask product is applied and massaged into the skin. This will soften and condition the skin.

7 The feet are then placed in plastic bags before being placed in thermally heated booties for 10–15 minutes. The heat will help the skin to absorb the therapeutic ingredients of the mask.

Foot and lower leg massage

As with a manicure massage, the pedicure massage is carried out near the end of the treatment, prior to nail polishing. The pedicure massage includes the foot and the lower leg, and offers the following benefits to the client as follows:

◆ moisturizes the skin with the massage medium, cream, lotion or oil, improving skin hydration

◆ increases blood circulation transporting oxygen and nutrients to the lower leg and foot

◆ increases lymph circulation, transporting waste products in the lymph away from the lower leg and foot

◆ helps maintain joint mobility

◆ eases discomfort from arthritis or rheumatism

◆ relaxes the client

◆ muscle tone is improved as the muscles receive an improved supply of oxygenated blood, essential for cell growth

◆ helps remove any dead skin cells (desquamation) exposing new cells.

The massage incorporates classic massage movements, each with different effects:

◆ **Effleurage** – a stroking movement, used to begin the massage as a link manipulation, and to complete the massage sequence.

◆ **Petrissage** – movements, including kneading, where the tissues are lifted away from the underlying structures and compressed. Pressure is intermittent, and should be light yet firm.

◆ **Tapotement**, also known as percussion, may be included – tapotement movements are performed in a brisk, stimulating manner to increase blood supply and improve tone of the skin and muscles. Movements include cupping and tapping.

◆ **Joint manipulations** – ankle joints and toes are manipulated through their range of movement, dependent upon the type of joint. This helps to maintain good mobility within the range of movement but must be avoided if the client has any joint disorders.

◆ **Frictions** – small circular movements using the pads of the fingers or thumbs. The skin and muscle below is massaged against the underlying bone. This can be used to loosen any adhesions in the tissues.

The beauty therapist can adapt the massage application according to the needs of the client. Either the *speed of application* or *depth of pressure* can be altered.

STEP-BY-STEP: FOOT AND LOWER LEG MASSAGE

1 Dispense the massage medium into the hands, warm the product over the palms and apply to the client's skin using effleurage technique.

2 **Effleurage from the foot to the knee** Use long sweeping strokes from the toes to the knee, moving on both the back and the front of the leg. *Repeat step 2 a further five times.*

3 Flex the client's knee and using a petrissage movement in an upwards direction, pick up and gently squeeze the gastrocnemius muscle.

4 Slide the palm down to the ankle and using the thumbs knead gently upwards along the tibialis anterior muscles on the outer shin.

Knowledge Check

Which specialized foot treatment(s) would be best for an elderly male client who has little movement in his ankle joints and slightly distorted joints in his toes?

5 Using the pads of the fingers perform small circular kneading movements around the malleolus (ankle) bone. Massage both sides of the ankle bone at the same time.

6 **Thumb frictions to the dorsal aspect of the foot** Use the thumbs, one in front of the other, and move backwards and forwards in a gentle sawing action between each metatarsal bone. Move from the toes to the ankle, then slide back down to the toes.
Repeat step 6 a further two times.

7 **Thumb frictions to the plantar aspect of the foot** Use the same movement as in step 6, but on the sole of the foot, moving from the toes to the heel.
Repeat step 7 a further two times.

8 **Palm kneading to the plantar surface of the foot** Place the heel of the hand into the arch of the foot and massage with deep circular movements.
Repeat step 8 a further five times.

9 Support the foot with one hand and perform joint manipulations. Using the palm, cup the heel and perform a circular kneading movement.

10 Perform joint manipulations to the toes. Place the hand either side of the toes; gently press together and rotate all the toes three times clockwise and three times anticlockwise.

11 Effleurage from the foot to the knee. Use the same movements as in step 2.
Repeat step 11 a further five times.

Nail polishes

Nail polish application

Different types of nail polish are discussed on pages 421–424. Nail polish is applied to coat the nail plate for a number of reasons:

◆ to adorn the nail

◆ to disguise stained toenails

◆ to improve the condition and appearance of the nail

◆ to co-ordinate with clothes

◆ to create designs and effects called 'nail art'.

HEALTH & SAFETY

Lighting and ventilation Ensure the area is well ventilated to avoid inhalation of excessive fumes. Lighting should be good to enable you to avoid eyestrain. It is a good idea to use a table lamp, especially when painting the nails.

Styles of polish application

◆ *Traditional application* – This style is one of the most commonly requested by clients: the entire plate is covered with polish.

◆ *French application* – This style involves painting the nail plate of the nail pink or pale beige, and the free edge white.

See pages 421–422 for further information about nail polish application, including tips why it may chip or peel, and how to store.

Contra-indication to nail polish Do not apply polish in these circumstances:

◆ if there are diseases and disorders of the nail plate and surrounding skin

◆ if the client is allergic to nail polish.

STEP-BY-STEP: DARK NAIL POLISH APPLICATION

Confirm the client's choice of nail polish colour. A dark cream formulation has been demonstrated. Ensure the free edge is smooth and the cuticles are neat and smooth. Before nail polish is applied, any jewellery worn in the area should be replaced to avoid smudging the polish afterwards.

1 Place disposable toe separators or other hygienic equivalent to separate them and facilitate polish application.

2 After ensuring that the nail plate is free from oil apply a base coat to protect the nail plate from staining. You can then begin applying the dark polish, starting application with the big toe. Apply three to four brush strokes down the length of the nail from the cuticle to the free edge, beginning in the centre, then down either side close to the nail wall.

Take care to avoid touching the cuticle or nail wall. If flooding occurs, remove the polish immediately with an orange stick and nail polish remover.

2 Continued

3 Apply one base coat, two coats of coloured polish and one top coat. Top coat is required only after using cream polish; pearl polish does not need a top coat but a third coat of polish may be applied.

STEP-BY-STEP: FRENCH NAIL POLISH APPLICATION

1 After ensuring the nail plate is free from oil apply a base coat and, start application with the big toe. Apply three to four brush strokes down the length of the nail using a pink colour, cream formulation polish from the cuticle to the free edge, beginning in the centre, then down either side close to the nail wall.

2 Using a white polish, take the polish horizontally across the free edge, creating the appearance of a white free edge.

3 Continue application of white polish across the free edges of each nail. This becomes technically more difficult on the smaller nail of the little toe.

4 When all nails have been painted, apply a top coat to add gloss and durability to the finished nails.

Aftercare advice

Offering aftercare advice at the end of a pedicure treatment will help the client to look after their feet between salon visits, and is also an ideal opportunity to recommend retail products.

Aftercare advice will differ slightly for each client according to individual needs, but generally it will be as follows:

Knowledge Check

Can you list three retail products that you could recommend for a client to use at home?

◆ change socks or tights daily

◆ gently scrubbing the feet daily is recommended to avoid **skin conditions** such as athlete's foot. Apply moisturizing lotion daily to the feet, preferably after bathing when the skin is softened

◆ ensure that the feet are thoroughly dry after washing, especially between the toes

◆ apply talcum powder or a special foot powder between the toes to help absorb moisture

◆ foot sprays containing peppermint or citrus oil to cleanse and refresh are useful to refresh the feet during the day

◆ go barefoot wherever it is safe and practical to do so

◆ ensure that footwear fits properly. Foot problems such as bunions can be aggravated by incorrect footwear

◆ avoid wearing high heels for long periods of time. They can cause postural problems and increase hard skin callus formation

◆ advise on appropriate nail/skincare products to remedy the problems present, e.g. dry skin, nails, stained nails

◆ advise the client of any other professional treatments you could recommend

◆ advise the client on a treatment plan to improve the nail/skin condition and the time intervals recommended between each treatment

◆ when filing the nails, always file straight across in one direction

◆ if any pain is felt in the feet visit a chiropodist

◆ it is also necessary to advise the client what to do in the event of a contra-action (see pages 441–442).

Have retail products available for the client to purchase. These include emery boards, coloured nail polishes, **nail polish remover** and nail/skin treatment products.

It is a good idea to have the nail polish colours that you have used available for purchase. The client can then buy the matching colour to touch up any accidental chips themselves.

Recommend the use of a top coat applied every 3 to 4 days to protect the nail polish, increase its durability and impart shine.

Finally, at the end of the pedicure treatment ensure the client's records are updated, accurate and signed by the client and beauty therapist. Ensure the finished result is to the client's satisfaction and meets the agreed treatment plan.

Exercises for the feet and ankles
As part of the home care advice given to a pedicure client foot exercises should be mentioned – these can play a very important role in keeping the client's feet healthy. They help:

◆ to stimulate blood and lymph circulation

◆ to keep joints mobilized, allowing a greater range of movement in the toes and ankles

◆ to keep muscles strong, reducing the chance of fallen arches (flat feet).

Here are some examples of exercises:

1 Sitting on a chair with the feet flat on the floor raise the toes upwards and then relax.

2 Stand on tiptoes, and relax down again.

3 Sitting on a chair with the feet flat on the floor, lift one leg slightly and draw a circle with the toes so that the ankle moves through its full range of movement.

4 **Dorsiflexion:** bending the foot backwards towards the body.

5 **Plantar flexion:** pointing the foot down towards the ground.

6 **Inversion:** moving the foot inwards towards the middle of the body.

7 **Eversion:** moving the foot out towards the side of the body.

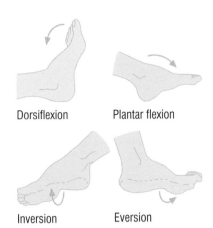

Dorsiflexion   Plantar flexion

Inversion   Eversion

Career Progression Tips

If you are passionate about what you do and work hard, you will inevitably do well. Learn from your superiors and always go the extra mile. When you are ready, take on more responsibility. If you have an avid interest in one area, develop your skills further with training courses. As you progress share your expertise with others, and think about where you would like to be in the future.

Margaret Dabbs

ASSESSMENT OF KNOWLEDGE AND UNDERSTANDING

You have now learnt the knowledge and skills for providing pedicure treatments in the beauty therapy workplace. To test your level of knowledge, answer the following short questions. These will prepare you for your summative (final) assessment.

1. The image below shows the nail being shortened with nail clippers. Nails are cut straight across to avoid causing _____ nails.

2. A cuticle pusher is shown performing cuticle work. The image shows the removal of cuticle at the sides of the nails, this is known as:

a. cuticle
b. hyponychium
c. perionychium
d. eponychium

3. One of the functions of a top coat is to make the nail polish:

   a. dry more quickly
   b. adhere to nail plate
   c. resistant to chipping
   d. appear smooth if uneven

4. A condition in which a blood clot forms under the nail plate, forming a dark purplish mark, usually due to injury, is called:

   a. eggshell nail
   b. bruised nail
   c. onycholysis
   d. pterygium

5. Thickened skin between the fingertip and free edge of the nail plate is the:

   a. hyponychium
   b. eponyichium
   c. nail mantle
   d. nail grooves

6. Thick-walled, large elastic tubes that carry oxygenated blood away from the heart are called the:

   a. capillaries
   b. arteries
   c. veins
   d. vessels

7. The image shown is called tinea unguium, this is a:

   a. bacterial nail condition
   b. viral nail condition
   c. fungal nail condition
   d. sebaceous gland disorder

8. The massage manipulation also known as percussion, performed in a brisk, stimulating manner to increase blood supply and improve tone of the skin and muscles is called:

   a. effleurage
   b. vibrations
   c. frictions
   d. tapotement

9. What are the names of the two bones of the lower leg labelled below?

10. Rearrange the following steps to place them in the correct order of sequence that they would be performed in the pedicure treatment:

   ◆ cut the toenails
   ◆ massage the foot
   ◆ remove excess cuticle with cuticle nippers
   ◆ exfoliate the skin of the foot

13 Provide and Maintain Nail Enhancement

LEARNING OBJECTIVES

There are two learning outcomes for this unit, which you must achieve through practical tasks and knowledge and understanding tasks to assess your capability and knowledge:

1 Be able to prepare for nail enhancement services.

2 Be able to provide nail enhancement services.

From the range statement, you must show that you have:

◆ Made sure that the environmental conditions are suitable.

◆ Used all consultation techniques to identify the treatment objectives.

◆ Met all requirements in client preparation for treatment.

◆ Completed a consultation and skin inspection to identify any contra-indications that may affect if and how the treatment can proceed.

◆ Shown how to communicate and behave in a professional manner.

◆ Followed all health and safety working practices.

◆ Used all listed products, tools and equipment.

◆ Adapted treatments to suit different objectives and nail conditions and nail shapes.

◆ Provided all types of relevant aftercare and contra-action advice.

KEY TERMS

acetone	infill	resin
aftercare advice	irritants	resin activator
'C' curve	liquid and powder	sensitization
catalyst	Lower arch	smile line
consultation	monomer	stop point
contra-action advice	nail bed	system
contra-actions	nail conditions	treatment objectives
corrosive	nail shapes	treatment plan
curing	nail wrap	UV gels
dehydrate	overlay	UV light cured
dermatitis	photoinitiator	vapours
fibre	polymer	white-tip powder
fibre mesh	Polymerization	wrap fabrics
health and safety	rebalance	zones

Unit Topic

Provide and maintain nail enhancement

This VRQ unit is linked to the Nail Services NOS Units N5, N6, N7 and N8.

INTRODUCTION

This unit is all about how to provide and maintain nail enhancements. Nail enhancements are a significant part of the beauty sector industry. The nail technician specializing in nail treatments are usually referred to as nail technicians. You will learn about a variety of technique procedures for application, removal and maintenance of nail enhancement systems including nail tips, wraps, acrylic and UV gel. The systems should be selected according to the nail condition and objective of the nail enhancement treatment.

Dealing with people in a polite, efficient manner and using good communication and questioning skills to find out exactly what they require from the nail enhancement treatment forms an important part of this technical service.

You must be able to show that you have the necessary practical skills and underpinning knowledge to provide and maintain nail enhancement.

INDUSTRY ROLE MODEL

LIZA SMITH Owner – Bodylines Salon
Owner and Head Educator – CND (Creative Nail Designs) Kent Academy
Director – Liza Smith Ltd

" I am one of the country's most respected Nail Artists. With over 25 years' experience of owning a salon and working as an educator for CND, I have a session work portfolio of high end fashion shows, shoots and celebrity clients, such as Victoria Beckham, Kate Moss and Naomi Campbell.

I hold 12 national trophies from competing with all systems of nail enhancements and have been ranked as fifth in the world in international competitions such as The Nailympics.

In 2010 I won 'Nail Professional of the Year', and my salon, Bodylines, was twice voted the 'British Nail Salon of the year' in 2012/2013.

ANATOMY & PHYSIOLOGY
Essential anatomy and physiology knowledge requirements for this unit are identified on the checklist chart on page 33.

TOP TIP

Minimum dimensions for the work area

The minimum worktop space needed is approximately 75 cm wide and 35 cm deep. The width should be not so wide that you need to stretch to reach the client's hands if the client is sitting back in their chair, nor should it be so narrow that it causes you to bend your neck down too far.

The purpose of nail enhancement

Nail enhancement treatments can provide the following benefits to the client:

◆ improve the appearance of the natural nail shape

◆ strengthen the natural nail

◆ improve the appearance of the fingers (e.g. short stubby fingers, by lengthening the free edge)

◆ motivate a nail-biter to break the habit – an acrylic/gel overlay or nail wrap will strengthen the nail and improve its appearance

◆ provide temporary length to the nails for a special occasion

◆ repair, in the case of flaking nails, free edge or flesh line break or severed free edge – the client can have the nail appearance balanced using the most appropriate nail **system**

◆ disguise a disfigured nail (that is not contra-indicated to treat) – a nail system can be applied for camouflage purposes

◆ an overlay placed over nail polish extends its durability.

Preparing for nail enhancement treatments

Whether the nail technician is working in a nail salon, a client's home, a beauty salon or a hair salon, a minimum amount of space is needed. Assess the space available before purchasing equipment. All equipment must be durable and easy to clean.

Outcome 1: Prepare for nail enhancement services

Learn how to prepare for nail enhancement treatment

PRACTICAL SKILLS

Prepare yourself, client and work area for nail enhancement services

Use suitable consultation techniques to identify service objectives

Carry out a nail and skin analysis

Provide clear recommendations to the client

Select products, tools and equipment to suit client treatment needs and nail conditions

UNDERPINNING KNOWLEDGE

Describe salon requirements for preparing yourself, the client and the work area

Describe the environmental conditions suitable for nail enhancement services

Describe different consultation techniques used to identify service objectives

Explain the importance of carrying out a detailed nail and skin analysis

Describe how to select products, tools and equipment to suit client treatment needs and nail conditions

Identify nail conditions

Describe the contra-indications which prevent or restrict nail enhancement services

The nail enhancement work station

When thinking about the space required for a nail technician in a salon, the work station is the first consideration. Ideally, the work station should have a couple of drawers for storage, and be very stable in construction.

Dust is one of the most important issues in **health and safety** for nail technicians. It is potentially more hazardous than any of the volatile products that are used. Dealing with the control of dust at the source, i.e. extraction of the dust at the work station, is the best method. Many nail work stations are available with built-in dust extraction systems. Whether built-in or independent to the work station, the dust extraction system should be on during treatment while any dust is being created, so a good flow of air is generated.

A nail work station

HEALTH & SAFETY

Cleaning the dust extractor Ensure that the filter is cleaned (according to manufacturer's instructions) very frequently. If it is an efficient extractor the filter will be full at the end of each day. The best system is made up of a fan that removes the dust that drops down into it, combined with a fan that takes the finer airborne dust (that is the most hazardous) from above the working area.

Work station with built-in dust and vapour extractor

Good working practices will minimize vapours generated from working with nail products. However, it is always worth investing in a system that helps remove these vapours from the atmosphere, again at the source.

Nail technician's chair

Seating

A comfortable seat is very important for both technician and client as you will be sitting for long periods of time. There are several exercises that a technician can do at various times throughout the day to help prevent strain, but, more than anything, sitting in the correct position and staying relaxed at all times is essential.

The chair for the client is as important as the one for the technician. The client must feel comfortable, as they could spend up to 2 hours in the same chair, but must also be in the right position for the technician. The height of the seat should be such that the client can rest their arms on the desk easily while keeping them and their shoulders in a relaxed position. They should also be able to get close enough to the desk so that their arm is still supported if they lean back into the chair. Make sure the client is sitting straight in front of the desk. This is important for the treatment because if the client is sitting at an angle, their hand will not be held straight in front of the technician. This could result in nail enhancements being applied unevenly.

HEALTH & SAFETY

Work position Always sit square to the desk without crossing your legs or leaning on one arm.

HEALTH & SAFETY

Electrical equipment Make sure all electrical equipment is subject to regular certified checks and PAT tests.

TOP TIP

Choice of chair

A chair must have the correct support for the user. The seat should be padded and of a depth that supports the legs. The tilt of the seat also affects how we sit. The backrest should give support to the back and the combination of the back and seat should encourage the user to sit upright with a slight hollow in the lower back. There are also 'posture' chairs available, on wheels and incorporating a rocking motion, that are designed to help those working at a desk.

ACTIVITY

There are several exercises that a technician can do at various times throughout the day, example shown below.

Research some further simple postural exercises that you could learn.

Lighting

It is essential to have excellent light, without glare, when providing any nail treatment to avoid eye strain and to be able to examine artificial nails for imperfections. This should be provided by a desk lamp, preferably one specifically designed for nail work. It is best to use halogen or low energy bulbs which do not get too hot when working with volatile products.

Ensure that all tools and equipment are clean, disinfected and hygienic using the methods described in the manicure chapter on pages 390–391, and that all necessary products, tools and equipment are neatly organized and easily accessible.

TOP TIP

Retail opportunity

Make sure there is plenty for the client to look at while they are sitting at your desk, especially retail lines. It will be something interesting for them and should encourage questions that could lead to sales.

HEALTH & SAFETY

Trip hazards Trailing wires in a workplace are a safety hazard, leading to trips and falls and should be avoided. Many work stations have a plug socket attached to them for electrical equipment. Always cover floor wires with a rubber conduit.

Product safety

Irritants and corrosive materials

The majority of nail products come under the category of hazardous chemicals and many of them are classed as **irritants**. Care must be taken when using these types of products. There are some irritants that are also classified as **corrosive** and these will cause a bad reaction with everyone.

◆ A common example of this type of chemical in the nail industry is an acid-based primer. This product, as the name suggests, is an acid that will sting and itch on contact with skin. Washing in running water will remove the chemical, but it is likely that the skin will be temporarily damaged. However, most modern products do not require the use of a primer.

◆ Many other commonly used products are irritants – for example, nail adhesive is an irritant, and every bottle and tube should carry a warning. The adhesive will bond to skin very easily and can cause injury to the skin if it is not removed carefully – acetone will debond the skin safely. If adhesive is spilt onto clothing and penetrates through to the skin, very severe burns can be caused. The chemicals in the adhesive react with fibres in clothing, and burns requiring cosmetic surgery have been known as a result of this accident.

Before beginning the nail enhancement treatment make sure you have the necessary products, tools and equipment to hand and that they meet the legal, hygiene and industry requirements.

TOP TIP

Files and buffers

Medium files (180 grit) are used for shaping or removing overlays and shortening artificial nails. Fine files (240–360 grit) are used for shaping natural nails. Buffers (400+ grit) are used to refine the shape and smooth the surface of the artificial nail.

HEALTH & SAFETY

Secure lids Make sure nail adhesive container lids are on securely and that there are no air pockets in the application nozzle that could cause the adhesive to spurt out. Clean the nozzle with remover before replacing the lid.

Products, tools and equipment

◆ Nail work station
◆ Files and buffers
◆ Cuticle knife
◆ Cuticle nippers
◆ Hoof stick
◆ Orange sticks
◆ Scissors
◆ Cuticle remover
◆ Cuticle oil or cream

◆ Cotton wool
◆ Tissues or disposal towels
◆ Disinfectant solution

YOU WILL ALSO NEED:
◆ Medium sized towels (3)
◆ Skin disinfectant
◆ Waste container
◆ Small bowls (3)
◆ Client record card

See the Products, tools and equipment list in CHAPTER 11 Manicure Treatments, for more details on each item of equipment.

Ensure that you have a MSDS for all chemicals in the salon

◆ It is a legal requirement for there to be warnings on many labels, but the absence of a warning does not necessarily mean a product is safe. All products should be treated with respect and all potentially hazardous products should have a MSDS available from the supplier (see Chapter 3 Health and Safety).

◆ As many nail products are classed as irritants, it is possible for individuals to develop a sensitivity (also known as a contra-action) to them at some time. As no one can tell how long this will take or how much of a specific product needs to come into contact with a person, it is important to take measures to avoid the possibility of a sensitivity occurring. It is also just as important to be able to recognize the signs – itchy skin, rash, headaches, etc. This happens when an individual has been exposed to too much of the product. Nail technicians can avoid developing a sensitivity by following good working practices. However, once a sensitivity has started, gloves must be worn when handling the relevant products. If a client develops a sensitivity, all the products must be removed immediately. Once the product has been removed, the condition may disappear. If the condition does not disappear within a few days or if it seems to get worse after the removal of all products, the technician or client affected should seek medical advice. Always note down the details of the allergic reaction and the action taken on the client's record card. If the client is willing, a different system could be tried which may be successful. If the initial reaction is severe, however, it would be a good idea to do a skin sensitivity patch test to test skin tolerance first. Record the results of the skin sensitivity patch test on the client's record card.

There are three ways that potentially harmful chemicals can enter the body and if each of these 'routes of entry' is prevented as far as possible, all hazards are avoided. The 'routes' are:

1 **Inhalation**: that is, *breathing in* vapours or dust.

2 **Ingestion**: that is, *through the mouth*.

3 **Absorption**: that is, chemicals can enter *through the skin*.

Inhalation

Vapours

◆ Many nail products involve *volatile chemicals* and even the tidiest technician cannot totally prevent some of the **vapours** escaping into the air. Vapours are molecules of chemicals in the air and, although most nail products have strong odours, if there is no obvious smell it does not mean the vapour is not there. Adequate ventilation is therefore essential using efficient filtration of the air through several specific filters, usually activated carbon or charcoal.

◆ *Contact lenses*: Never wear contact lenses when working with nail products. It is possible that vapours can be absorbed by soft lenses and seriously affect the eye.

◆ *Safety glasses*: Wearing plain safety glasses is highly recommended to protect eyes from harmful vapours and dust.

Vapours might be present even if there is no obvious odour; adequate ventilation is essential

Keep vapours to a minimum There are a few simple rules that can be followed to keep vapours to a minimum:

◆ keep all bottles and jars closed

◆ keep any dishes covered at all times other than for the few seconds you are using them

◆ do not wipe your liquid and powder brush on a tissue. If you need to wipe your brush have a small wipe dampened with an alcohol-based liquid on the desk for this purpose

◆ clean your brush in **monomer** after every use, wipe it dry with a pad and discard this pad in a metal bin with a lid

◆ store your brushes flat in a closed container in a drawer, not open on the desk

◆ have a metal waste bin with a lid at every nail desk

◆ put all nail wipes/cotton wool straight into the bin after use

◆ change the paper towel under client's hands after each stage and put into the bin

◆ wipe up spills immediately with absorbent paper and put paper in an outside waste bin

◆ when using a solvent to remove artificial nails, keep the bowl covered with a towel and remove directly after use

◆ keep the use of sprays to a minimum

◆ discard all unwanted solvents and nail monomers immediately by soaking in absorbent paper and placing in a covered waste bin; larger quantities should be placed in a safe place in the open and allowed to evaporate – do not pour down sinks or lavatories

◆ maintain adequate ventilation at all times, and make sure the salon is not too hot

◆ follow all these rules if working in a client's home and have several windows open.

Disposable dust mask

Dust

Dust is a major problem in the salon. Although the amount of dust can be minimized by correct working procedures, it is impossible to avoid the production of quantities of dust.

◆ Dust falls into two categories: the dust you can see and the dust you cannot see. All dust is potentially harmful, but the dust you can see is slightly less harmful than the dust you cannot see. Larger dust particles will settle on surfaces and not float around in the air to be breathed in.

◆ Particles that cannot be seen can be so small that they can be inhaled right into the lungs. Inhaled dust is an irritant and excess dust can cause respiratory problems.

Avoiding excess dust There are a number of ways that excess dust can be avoided using appropriate extraction units. Collected dust should be disposed of correctly according to the manufacturer's guidelines. For those technicians who feel particularly susceptible to dust, a disposable mask can be worn. Dust masks are only effective if they are worn correctly.

Ingestion

To avoid ingestion of dust and vapours:

◆ do not drink hot liquids at the work station; it is possible for them to absorb vapours from the air

◆ avoid placing any drinks on the work station, as the container could collect dust

◆ wash your hands before eating anything.

Absorption

Every time a chemical touches the skin or nails, some of it will be absorbed into the skin. Some chemicals are recognized by the skin cells as harmful and a skin reaction will occur as it defends itself.

◆ The most obvious reaction is irritated skin in the area of absorption.

◆ Local irritation is not always the first sign of an allergic reaction. Puffy or itchy eyes could be a reaction to a product on the nails. Headaches, tiredness, mood swings, nosebleeds, dizziness, coughs, or a sore throat can also be signs of a reaction to chemicals via any of the routes of entry.

Ways to avoid **sensitization**:

◆ nail products are designed for the nail, therefore keep them off the skin

◆ do not touch the skin with your brush. If you find this difficult when applying a liquid and powder overlay, use a smaller brush

◆ do not wipe your brush on the towel your hand is resting on

◆ when removing the sticky inhibition layer (which is uncured monomer, one of the most active allergens in nail products) on a **UV light cured** material, start with the smallest nail up to the largest nail to avoid putting the residue on the skin

◆ wipe the nail away from the cuticle area towards the free edge

TOP TIP

Hot drinks

It is safe for a client to drink a hot drink at the work station as they are in the salon so infrequently.

HEALTH & SAFETY

Contact with a skin irritant If the irritating chemical is removed, the symptoms should also disappear. They will, however, reappear if the chemical is reintroduced, as once the body is sensitized it will always be sensitized to that substance. From the point of view of a technician, if this sort of sensitivity is created to a commonly used product it may be difficult to find an alternative. This could mean you can no longer work in the industry without appropriate PPE. If a client develops a sensitivity it could mean they can no longer receive nail enhancements.

◆ make sure all the inhibition layer is removed as this will fall into your hand as you are shaping the overlay

◆ wear protective gloves if you are susceptible to allergic reactions and always wear gloves if you notice any redness or itching of your skin.

Allergic reactions

Although allergies can be caused by just about any product, they are more common when providing nail enhancement treatments because of the products involved. Following simple working procedures will help minimize the possibility for both the technician and their clients:

◆ keep the nail desk clean and free from dust

◆ change the disposable towel between clients and several times during the treatment when dust is created

◆ avoid any skin contact with the liquid monomer:

– avoid the skin surrounding the nail during application

– do not touch the brush with your fingers

– do not have a patch wet with monomer where you have wiped your brush and then lean in it.

◆ if using 'low odour' or UV-cured liquid and powder systems, be aware of the dust on the client's fingers, your fingers and in the palm of your hand that is holding

ACTIVITY

Would you like to see how much dust is generated during an artificial nail treatment?

Start with a clean nail desk and equipment. Provide an artificial nail treatment, such as applying tips and overlays or a maintenance treatment without using any local dust extraction and just a towel on the desk.

When you have finished, get a vacuum cleaner and 1–3 sheets of kitchen roll. Layer the sheets and push the centre down inside the hose, then attach the small flat attachment of the vacuum (the number of sheets will depend on their thickness and the size of the hose and its attachment). Make sure the corners of the sheet are outside the hose and held firmly in place. Vacuum your desk and towel. Then remove the vacuum attachment very carefully and tip out the contents of the sheets!

the client's finger. This usually has some unreacted monomer in it and can cause problems

◆ wipe away the inhibition layer on light-cured gels starting with the smallest finger first, wipe from cuticle to the free edge and avoid smearing uncured monomer onto the skin.

Disinfection

Hygiene must be maintained in a number of ways:

◆ ensure all tools and equipment are cleaned and disinfected before use

◆ disinfect work surfaces after every client

◆ use disposable products and tools wherever possible

◆ always follow hygienic working practices

◆ maintain a high standard of personal hygiene.

The nail technician's hands should be washed before and after every treatment for the safety of themselves and their clients. It not only limits the spread of bacteria but also removes traces of artificial nail products and dust.

Clients should also have clean hands and nails. A huge amount of debris can collect under the free edge and on the surface of the nail. Ask the client to wash their hands with soap and water before treatment. To ensure that under the nails are clean, ask the client to use a nail brush that is provided at the sink. Have a dish with clean nail brushes for this purpose plus a dish for used brushes. Disinfect these brushes at the end of the day.

Store sterilized tools in a clean, covered container before use

As an extra precaution, both the nail technician and the client should use a hand sanitizer at the work station.

Wear gloves and safety goggles while handling disinfectant

Nail technician personal presentation

There is a large aspect of 'nails' that is connected with image and a professional working within that type of industry should promote a good image. It is not always necessary for a nail technician to wear a clinical white uniform, unless the workplace has such a dress code, but a nail technician should be suitably dressed in clean and pressed clothes. A nail technician's nails should be well cared for and immaculate. Jewellery on the hands should be kept to a minimum for the safety of the nail technician (products could get trapped under jewellery and cause a skin reaction) and hair should be worn in a way that does not impede working.

Consultation

Reception

When a new client makes an appointment for nail enhancement treatment, the receptionist should ask the client:

◆ if they have had nail enhancements before

◆ what type of extension do they have (acrylic, gel, etc.)?

◆ do they require application or maintenance?

This will guide you on the time required to complete the treatment.

Client consultation and assessment

A thorough client **consultation** will help you to provide the best possible service for your client. Assessing the client for treatment is a very important part of every client's appointment and the keeping of records is a requirement for insurance purposes. A full client consultation should provide a great deal of important information, including:

◆ Occupation: to give an idea of the type of nails a client could cope with. It could also offer clues to any nail and skin problems.

◆ Medical history: with nail treatments, it is unnecessary to go into any medical history in any depth. There are some that are relevant in a general way and the main questions that should be asked are:

— **Allergies**: if a client is prone to allergies, there is a good chance that they may be allergic to some of the products that will be used. If this is the case, it would be a good idea to carry out a skin test on a test nail.

— **Diabetes**: if a client suffers from this condition great care must be taken with all treatments. Circulation is often poor and consequently diabetics are slow to heal. Obtain approval from their doctor before embarking on any course of treatment.

— **Other**: a general enquiry of the client should be made to ascertain whether there is any other condition that may be relevant to nail treatment.

◆ **Previous nail treatments**: ask if the client has received nail treatments in the past. Results from these treatments would be useful to know, as a sensitivity to

> A consultation is only as good as the questions that are asked of the client. The nail industry has moved on. No longer is it acceptable to just offer 'a set of nails'. Each of the three systems of enhancements are more suited to some nail types and client lifestyle than others. The choice of system used should be a collaboration based on your knowledge and your client's choice.
>
> *Liza Smith*

TOP TIP

Client communication

When dealing with the public, especially in the service industries, you must have good communication skills. Your approach, while professional, should also be friendly and interested. You should make the client feel at ease and comfortable, and genuinely important. Use the time during a treatment usefully and educate your client in understanding what they need to do with their nails, hands and feet.

Examine the client's nails carefully before every nail enhancement treatment

ALWAYS REMEMBER

Minors

If the client is a minor under the age of 16, it is necessary to obtain parent/guardian permission for the service. The parent/guardian will also have to be present when the service is received.

Bacterial nail infection

products may have occurred or the client may be unable to keep on artificial nails owing to lifestyle or habits (like nail biting or picking).

◆ **The condition of the skin and nails**: this should be noted on the client's record card at this early stage. If everything looks healthy and in good condition, it should be noted in case something changes at a later stage. If there is any indication of a skin or nail condition, whether it restricts treatment or not, *it must be noted*.

Skin and nail disorders

It is important to be able to recognize various nail and skin conditions. There are many common conditions that do not prevent the application of nail enhancements, others which restrict and, less commonly, some which prevent treatment.

It is worth pointing out that if a client has an obvious medical condition of the skin or nails and is treated by a nail technician without an agreement from their GP or specialist, the nail technician's insurance can be void and they would be directly responsible for any claim against them should problems arise.

For detailed information on specific nail disorders refer to pages 394–399.

Contra-indications

Contra-indications that prevent treatment include fungal infection, bacterial infection, viral infection, infestations, severe nail separation, severe eczema, severe psoriasis and severe skin conditions.

Contra-indications that restrict treatment include broken bones, recent scar tissue, skin allergies, cuts and abrasions, diabetes, skin disorders, recent fractures and sprains, undiagnosed lumps and swellings, product allergies.

Treatable nail conditions

These are conditions of the hands, feet and nails that do not prevent treatment, but an understanding of each condition is important as suitable care and the appropriate action needs to be taken. These include pterygium, onychopaghy, weak, dry, brittle, split nails, hangnails, longitudinal or horizontal ridges and allergies to products.

Common and avoidable nail conditions

Bacterial infection This is, unfortunately, a common condition seen during nail treatments. It is caused by an overlay lifting from the nail plate and bacteria entering. The warm, moist environment is a perfect condition for the bacteria to grow. It is seen as an area that is discoloured. This starts as a faint yellow and can progress, if left untreated, to a very dark green. This colour is a by-product of the bacteria and not the bacteria itself. It will remain as a stain on the nail plate even after the bacteria has gone. If this is treated early it will not cause any long-lasting problem. But, if left, can, eventually destroy the nail plate!

This is virtually always associated with an area of lifted overlay and can be treated by a nail technician if caught early. To do this, remove all the existing overlay by gently buffing or soaking in **acetone** depending on the type of overlay. Throw away the buffer used and the disposable towel that has caught the dust. Then dehydrate the nail. Now the environment does not support the bacterial life. The stain will remain until it grows out but should not change in colour or size. It is safe to reapply the overlay.

Other common skin conditions

Dermatitis this is a general term that describes a non-specific inflammation of the skin. This is common with nail technicians and often due to overexposure. This type is called allergic contact dermatitis. This is not necessarily localized and can be anywhere on the skin. Another type commonly seen in salons is irritant contact dermatitis. This is caused where the skin has been irritated by contact with some substances.

Contact dermatitis

> ### TOP TIP
>
> **Treating clients with dermatitis**
>
> If a client already has dermatitis then any nail treatments will need some restrictions. The client will probably be aware of what products affect their skin so these should be avoided. If they do not know what causes their condition all skin products should be avoided. If the skin around the nail is unaffected, treatments that treat just the nail can be provided but extra care must be taken to avoid touching the skin.

Treatment plan

The information obtained from the consultation should enable the nail technician to provide clear treatment recommendations to the client. An important piece of information to find out is exactly what the client expects from the treatment. Include discussion of the possible **contra-actions** and the appropriate action to be taken by the client.

Contra-actions A contra-action to nail enhancement is an adverse or unwanted condition. Examples include:

- ◆ allergies
- ◆ infection
- ◆ lifting of the nail enhancement product.

It is best practice to provide the client with written aftercare instructions.

Once this discussion has taken place it is worth reminding the client of all the options available in order that both parties are sure the correct choice is being made. The nail technician should note down on the record card what the treatment is and what the client's expectations are. This can be referred to later to see if the expectations were fulfilled and it is also useful if another nail technician treats the client. The client should then sign this and a note made of which nail technician carried out the treatment.

> ### Knowledge Check
>
> Name five functions of the skin.
>
> Refer to Chapter 2 Anatomy and Physiology pages 35–37 to help you.

> " When looking for a new member of my team, I am obviously looking for personality and skill level. However, there are many components that are in the mix. The two at the top of my list are (a) creativity and enthusiasm, and (b) people skills. If I was interviewing two candidates, I might choose the one who had better people skills and was more easily motivated.
>
> *Liza Smith*

A sample client record card

Date	Nail technician name	
Client name	Date of birth (identifying client age group)	
Home address	Postcode	
Email address	Landline phone number	Mobile phone number
Name of doctor	Doctor's address and phone number	
Related medical history (Conditions that may restrict or prohibit treatment application.)		
Are you taking any medication? (This may affect the sensitivity of the skin to the treatment.)		

CONTRA-INDICATIONS REQUIRING MEDICAL REFERRAL
(Preventing nail enhancement application.)

- ☐ bacterial infections (e.g. paronychia)
- ☐ viral infections (e.g. plane warts)
- ☐ fungal infections (e.g. tinea unguium)
- ☐ parasitic infections, (e.g. scabies)
- ☐ severe nail separation
- ☐ severe eczema and psoriasis
- ☐ severe bruising
- ☐ severe skin conditions

CONTRA-INDICATIONS WHICH RESTRICT TREATMENT
(Treatment may require adaptation.)

- ☐ minor nail separation
- ☐ minor eczema and psoriasis
- ☐ recent scar tissue
- ☐ severely bitten nails
- ☐ severely damaged nails
- ☐ broken bones
- ☐ recent fractures and sprains
- ☐ minor cuts or abrasions
- ☐ minor bruising or swelling
- ☐ undiagnosed lumps or swellings
- ☐ product allergies
- ☐ diabetes

NAIL ENHANCEMENT SYSTEM

- ☐ liquid and powder
- ☐ fibre
- ☐ UV gel

NAIL ENHANCEMENT TREATMENT

- ☐ full set
- ☐ infill
- ☐ re-balance
- ☐ natural nail overlays
- ☐ removal

EQUIPMENT AND MATERIALS

- ☐ nail enhancement application tools
- ☐ nail cleanser
- ☐ cuticle softener
- ☐ nail dehydrator
- ☐ plastic nail tips
- ☐ adhesives
- ☐ liquid monomer and powders
- ☐ primers

NAIL, CUTICLE AND SKIN CONDITION
Nails

- ☐ healthy ☐ brittle ☐ split
- ☐ dry ☐ weak ☐ bitten
- ☐ ridged (horizontal (longitudinal)
  or onychopagy)

Cuticle

- ☐ healthy ☐ split ☐ overgrown
- ☐ dry ☐ hangnails (pterygium)

Skin

- ☐ healthy ☐ dry ☐ hard

CONTRA-ACTIONS FROM PREVIOUS TREATMENT

- ☐ artificial nail fitted incorrectly ☐ structural damage
- ☐ tip fitted incorrectly ☐ chemical damage
- ☐ overexposure ☐ contamination
- ☐ natural nail infected ☐ missing nail(s)
- ☐ accidental damage ☐ chipping
- ☐ mechanical damage ☐ discolouration
- ☐ lifting

NAIL SHAPE

- ☐ oval ☐ claw
- ☐ tapered ☐ fan
- ☐ square ☐ pointed
- ☐ squoval

Nail technician signature (for reference)
Client signature (confirmation of details)

A sample client record card (continued)

TREATMENT ADVICE	TREATMENT PLAN, ACTIONS FOR DURING AND AFTER TREATMENT, RETAIL OPPORTUNITIES AND HEALTH & SAFETY
Full set – *allow 120 minutes* Maintenance (infill or re-balance) – *allow 90 minutes* Removal – *allow 60 minutes* Natural nail overlays – *allow 75 minutes*	See the client record card on page 402 of Chapter 11 Manicure Treatments for more information.

Outcome 2: Be able to provide nail enhancement services

Learn how to provide nail enhancement services

PRACTICAL SKILLS

Communicate and behave in a professional manner

Follow health and safety working practices and industry Code of Practice for Nail Services

Position yourself and client correctly throughout the service

Use products, tools, equipment and techniques to suit client's service needs and nail conditions

Complete the service to the satisfaction of the client

Record the results of the service

Provide suitable aftercare advice

UNDERPINNING KNOWLEDGE

State how to communicate and behave in a professional manner

Describe health and safety working practices and industry Code of Practice for Nail Services

Explain the importance of positioning yourself and the client correctly throughout the service

Explain the importance of using products, tools, equipment and techniques to suit client's service needs, nail and skin conditions

Describe how services can be adapted to suit client service needs and nail conditions

Describe how to maintain and remove nail enhancements

State the contra-actions that may occur during and following service and how to respond

State the importance of completing the service to the satisfaction of the client

State the aftercare advice that should be provided

Describe the chemical process involved in the nail enhancement system

Describe the structure and functions of the nail and skin

Describe the different natural nail shapes

Client preparation

After the client consultation has finished, prepare the client for the chosen nail enhancement treatment. The hands and nails of the nail technician and client should be clean as discussed previously.

> If you are visiting someone's house, hotel or studio, be conscious to protect furniture and soft furnishings. Plastic-backed table towels underneath your towel help against splashes of products like acetone. Keep lids on bottles to protect against smells and do not wipe your brush on a tissue excessively. Place paper roll under where you are filing to keep dust under control, then fold away the paper and place in bin.
>
> *Liza Smith*

Various tip shapes

Applying tips to the nails

The application of plastic tips is relevant to all the different nail systems, as it forms the basis of this method of applying artificial nails.

Plastic tips come in many shapes and sizes, colours and lengths.

Good quality tips are made from 'virgin' ABS plastic; a plastic within the acrylic family. Some tips are made from another type of plastic called acetate, which is often cheaper but these are unsuitable for artificial nail systems as they are difficult to blend into the natural nail and have a higher oil content than ABS tips that may affect the overlay.

Every tip, whatever its shape or size, has a number of features that are relevant to the nail technician.

(a)
- Side walls
- Stop point
- Contact area

(b)
- Upper arch
- Lower arch

(c)
- 'C' curve

Features of tip: (a) the front, (b) the side, (c) the end

1   **Contact area or well.** This is a thinner area and the part that is in contact with the natural nail.

2   **Stop point.** This is the demarcation point of the contact area and the actual tip. When the tip is properly blended, this line will produce a natural-looking smile line.

3   **Side walls.** Tips either have parallel or tapered side walls to suit the natural shape.

4   **Upper arch.** Tips have differently curved upper arches from flat to very curved. Choose the one that fits the natural nail shape or, if the natural upper arch is flat, it will need some correcting and a tip with a curved upper arch will help. If the nail has a high arch, a curved tip will exaggerate this, even more so a flatter tip will help compensate.

5   **Lower arch.** A tip needs to have a lower arch so that it looks as if it has grown from the finger and not been stuck on top.

'C' curve of a nail looking from the nail down the length of the finger

6 **'C' curve.** As with the upper arch, this can vary between types of tip, and the shape of the natural nail should dictate which is most suitable. Unlike the upper arch, it is not advisable to choose a shape that is different from the natural 'C curve. The tip needs to sit on the nail comfortably without distorting the shape of the tip.

Choosing the correct tip

Some guidelines

◆ The first thing to look for when choosing the correct tip is the 'C curve of the natural nail. Match the shape of the natural nail.

◆ The next area to take into account is the natural upper arch. Again, match the natural shape, or choose a tip to correct an over- or under-exaggerated arch.

Size and width Choose the right size or width. Most tips come in 10 or 11 different sizes with 0 being the biggest and 10 the smallest. Sizes 4–6 are the most commonly used.

When choosing the correct size, the width of the contact area must be ignored as it is the width at the stop point that is important. This must be exactly the same width as the nail at the smile line (also referred to as the onychodermal band) without any gaps when the skin is pulled back from the sides.

If one size is too wide and the next is too narrow, choose the wider one and file away a very small amount from either side until it fits perfectly.

Full contact area versus reduced contact area Many tips have a full contact area. These can be applied directly to the nail plate with adhesive or they can be tailored beforehand.

There are two methods of removing the contact area:

1 *Using a file.* By holding the tip and the file at the appropriate angle (see picture), the contact area can be removed very quickly leaving a curved edge. By leaving this shape as opposed to a straight edge, the side walls of the free edge of the natural nail are provided with extra protection and support.

2 *Using scissors or clippers.* Scissors with a curved blade are ideal for snipping around the contact area, following the shape of the stop point. Nail clippers can also be used to cut out a 'V' shape.

Exactly the same process applies when enhancing toenails but remember that the feet are often the perfect environment for infections and toenails are often 'wetter' than fingernails.

Removal of contact area using a file

Removal of contact area using scissors

TOP TIP

Shape to fit

Always pre-tailor or shape a tip to fit before application as it cannot be changed when it is on the finger.

ACTIVITY

Problem nail shapes

Research techniques for customizing tips and methods for applying tips to problem nail shapes, including:

◆ ski-jump or spoon shaped nail
◆ fan shaped nail
◆ hooked or claw nail
◆ bitten nails.

(a)

(b)

Tip and upper arch: (a) tip with complete contact area producing wrong upper arch curve, (b) tip with reduced contact area producing correct upper arch

STEP-BY-STEP: PREPARING THE NATURAL NAIL

Before any artificial product is applied to natural nails, they must be carefully prepared.

1 Sanitize the hands and the nail plate. Clean the nail plate of surface debris and oils using a solvent applied from free edge to cuticle.

2 Shape the nail to fit the 'stop point' of the tip, which is the demarcation point between the contact area and the rest of the tip.

3 Apply cuticle remover to soften the cuticle.

4 Remove all traces of cuticle from the nail plate with a clean cuticle knife. Carefully check the whole nail for cuticle, paying special attention to the sides of the nails.

5 Wash the nail to remove cuticle remover. Dry the nail thoroughly. Careful preparation is essential to avoid potential problems later.

6 Two shiny surfaces do not bond together well as there is not enough 'grip', so the shine on the surface of the natural nail must be carefully removed (but only the shine). Use the end of a 240 grit file (the lowest grit that should be used on the natural nail) with gentle strokes from cuticle to free edge. Make sure the file is angled down towards the side walls. There should not be any scratches on the nail.

7 **Dehydrate** the nail plate with a specialist dehydrator to remove all traces of oil or moisture.

Adhesives

Tips are attached to the nails with an adhesive. The adhesives used in the nail industry are cyanoacrylates, specifically ethyl cyanoacrylate. It is widely used in artificial nails, as it is used for applying tips and is also the basis of the **resin** in the fibre system. Nail adhesive is available in different viscosities (thicknesses) and curing speeds. You should always use a high grade adhesive but the viscosity and speed is up to personal preference. Nail adhesives are broken down by solvents, the most efficient being acetone.

Cutting the tip

Use clippers or scissors to cut each side separately, never straight across. If the clipper is angled under the client's hand it will cut a slightly curved shape at the tip. The more upright the clipper is held, the straighter the edge.

Blending the tip

Once all the tips have been applied to the nails with adhesive and cut to the required length the tips must be blended to the natural nails. The result should be perfectly natural in appearance and look as if the nail grew there. More importantly, there must be no damage to the nail plate.

There are two methods of blending the tip: manually with a file (shown in step-by-step that follows), or chemically with acetone or a branded tip blender which melts the plastic when applied to the contact area. The chemical method is not the most effective but it is useful when blending a tip to a very small nail plate, e.g. a nail biter or for a client who has very sensitive nail beds and buffing is uncomfortable. A fine file is then used to file away the melted plastic when it appears shiny.

Cutting tips with clippers

In addition to the resources listed on page 465, you will require the following products, tools and equipment for applying tips to the nails.

Products, tools and equipment
Additional equipment for applying tips

◆ **Tissues or disposable towels** To cover the work area and protect the client's clothing

◆ **Nail tips** A selection of tips in assorted sizes, styles and colours

◆ **Adhesive** To attach the tip to the natural nail

◆ **Tip cutters** To cut the tip to the desired length

◆ **Files (240 and 180 grit)** To file the tip to the desired length and shape and blend the tip with the natural nail

STEP-BY-STEP: APPLYING TIPS TO THE NAILS

1 Choose the correct tip for the nail and pre-tailor by removing the contact area. Shape the sides if necessary.

2 Place a small amount of adhesive in the contact area of the tip. Fit the free edge into the stop point at a 45 degree angle, as shown (this will avoid air bubbles under the tip).

3 Lift the end of the tip so the contact area closes down onto the nail plate pushing out any bubbles that may be under the tip. Make sure the angle of the tip on the nail is correct by looking at the side view. Hold in place for a few seconds pushing the finger up from underneath by the hand that is holding it.

4 Cut the tip to the chosen length and roughly shape the free edge.

5 Using a thin file and holding the file parallel to the side walls, blend the side walls first so that the tip is the same width as the nail plate.

6 Using two-thirds of a 240 grit file blend the tip contact area taking great care to avoid the nail plate. Gently blend until there is no sign or shadow of the tip contact area. Refine the shape. Check that the upper arch and lower arch is correct and even. Refine the 'smile line' to produce a neat, natural looking effect. The dust created from filing must be removed from the nails.

7 The finished nail. The tip should look like it 'grew there'! Perfect fit. Note the side walls are perfectly in line.

TOP TIP

Nail wraps

An overlay can be applied to a natural nail (without an artificial tip) to strengthen and protect the nail. Some clients like to wear a natural nail overlay just to keep their nail varnish in perfect condition as it does not chip. **Fibre mesh** may sometimes be used under the free edge to seal the nail and strengthen it. This treatment is often called a **nail wrap** and the process is exactly the same as applying an overlay to a nail with a blended tip.

HEALTH & SAFETY

Nail files Only a fine grit file of 240 or more should be used on the natural nail. Great care must be taken to avoid buffing the nail plate. This is the stage that causes many problems for beginners and removing the contact area of the tip may help.

Applying overlays

The perfect foundation has been created with the application of tips. Now is the time to create the perfect artificial nail that looks good and is very durable and strong. The tip has provided the required length, now the overlay on that tip will provide the required strength.

All products in artificial nails belong to the acrylic family of chemicals. Acrylics are a vast family of various types of plastic. The word 'system', when it is related to artificial nails, describes the specific method and type of acrylic that produces the overlay.

We will look at the following three systems:

◆ **liquid and powder**

◆ **UV gel**

◆ **fibre.**

The structure of the overlay

When applying an overlay, it will help to think of the nail with its tip in terms of three different **zones**:

1 **Zone 1** is the free edge where the overlay needs to be thin on the edge so that the finished nail does not look artificial.

2 **Zone 2** is the area beside the smile line and onto the **nail bed** where maximum strength is needed. This is the area of the nail that receives the most stress. It is often called the 'stress area' and should have a highest point that is called the 'apex'. The strongest natural structure is a curve (pressure is dispersed along the curve and is not concentrated over one point). The apex should be where two curves, the upper arch and the 'C' curve, come together at their highest and thickest part. This will create maximum strength for the whole nail without putting any stress on the natural nail, the nail bed, or the matrix.

3 **Zone 3** is the area near the base of the nail. Like Zone 1, this should be thin so that any ridges on the nail bed are avoided and, by being thin, it will be more flexible and able to move with the softer natural nail in this part of the nail plate.

Zones of the nail

Curves of the nail

There are two types of nail treatment environment:

◆ The spa arena demands a highly professional interaction between nail technician and client. You should keep your voice low and engage your client in conversation that also enables the client to benefit from the relaxing environment provided.

◆ A nail salon is similar to a hair salon in atmosphere. Even though conversation and background music is more upbeat, subject matter should be varied and geared around each client's interests. It MUST be all about them.

Liza Smith

If these zones are always kept in mind when applying an overlay, the correct shape and strength will be easier to achieve.

Liquid and powder

Liquid and powder products with coloured powders

This system (usually referred to as L&P) uses a liquid monomer and powder **polymer** that cure to form a solid polymer.

The liquid monomer is quite volatile and has a strong odour. Working cleanly, correctly and hygienically can minimize this problem.

A version of this system is the UV light-cured liquid and powder system. These are applied in a very similar way to traditional acrylics; the main difference is that they do not polymerize until UV light is applied as the **catalyst**.

Most brands of L&P have powders in several colours. This gives the nail technician the ability to create very natural looking artificial nails that suit the client's preferences.

Application to the nails

The liquid and powder systems are applied with a brush made of natural hair, by dipping the tip of the brush first into the liquid monomer and then into the powder polymer where it forms a 'bead' of the material. This bead is then applied to the nail and pressed into place. **Polymerization (curing)** either occurs within a few minutes or when placed under a UV light if it contains a **photoinitiator**.

Knowledge Check

At what angle should the nail tip be applied to the nail?

Refer to page 476 to help you.

Picking up the product with a brush in such a way that it can be applied to a nail takes practice. The bead must be the correct consistency and size for the nail and zone of application. Some liquid and powder brands need a specific ratio of liquid to powder, others are less sensitive. The 'bead' that needs to form on the tip of the brush should look smooth and glassy.

There are different methods of picking up powder: little circles can be drawn in the surface of the powder or the brush can be drawn through in a line. It helps to tap the dish of powder on the desk to create a smooth surface.

Dipping a brush in powder

When working, the brush should be cleaned periodically by dipping it into the liquid and taking it straight out without touching the sides of the dish and then wiping it on a disposable towel. This will remove the build-up of powder that accumulates in the hairs and then goes into the liquid. When using **white-tip powder**, the brush should be cleaned in this way after each nail.

In addition to the resources listed on page 465, you will require the following products, tools and equipment for liquid and powder treatments.

Products, tools and equipment
Additional equipment for liquid and powder overlays

◆ **Tissues or disposable towels** To cover the work area and protect the client's clothing

◆ **Liquid monomer in a clean, covered dappen dish** The volatile liquid acrylic component used in the L&P system

◆ **Powder polymer in a clean, covered dappen dish** The dry powder acrylic component used in the L&P system; available in a variety of colours

◆ **Clean sable brush** To apply beads of the liquid and powder to the nail

◆ **Files (240 grit)** To refine and smooth the nail overlay

◆ **Nail oil** To condition the nail and surrounding skin

◆ **Primer (if required)** Prepares the nail for the application of the L&P system

◆ **Glosser or three-way buffer** To add shine to the finished nail overlay

STEP-BY-STEP: APPLYING LIQUID AND POWDER USING WHITE-TIP POWDER

If the **overlay** is being applied without white tip, it should still be applied in zones, but it would not be necessary to create a smile line (step 6), otherwise the process is the same.

1 Nails should have the tips perfectly blended (if tips are applied), the dust removed and be clean and oil-free. Using a pipette, place a small amount of monomer liquid in a dappen dish that has a lid. Do not put too much in the dish. It is easy to top up.

2 If necessary, apply primer (check manufacturer's instructions) sparingly around the base of the nail. Make sure the primer is dry before applying the overlay.

3 Clean the brush first by dipping it into the liquid monomer, taking it straight out and wiping it on disposable tissue.

4 Dip the brush in the liquid monomer and then the powder to form a bead.

5 Place a small bead of white powder in the centre of Zone 1, closer to the smile line than the edge. Holding the brush at the same angle as the upper arch and using the tip of the brush, press the bead.

6 Using small pressing movements, take some of the bead out to one side and create a sharp smile line with a pointed 'dog ear'. Repeat the process on the other side. Make sure the 'C' curve is even and the extreme edge is thin. Tidy up the smile line if necessary.

7 Pick up a medium bead of clear or pink powder and place in the centre of Zone 2 close to the smile line. Using small pressing movements take some of the bead to either side of the nail, angling the brush to create a thin and even overlay at the side walls. Blend the overlay into Zone 1 for a smooth finish. Check the 'C' curve and side view for the correct structure.

8 Pick up a small bead of clear or pink powder and place centrally in Zone 3. Angle the tip of the brush and, using gentle pressure, move the bead across Zone 3, taking care not to touch the skin. Flatten the brush against the nail, press and blend the overlay up the nail into Zone 2. Check the shape and smoothness of the overlay.

9 Repeat the process for each finger. Make sure the overlay has cured sufficiently by tapping with the handle of the brush. It should 'click' and not be a dull sound. Ideally, the nail should need minimal refining at this stage.

10 Using a thin file, refine the side walls. Then, with a 240 grit file, gently buff to refine and smooth the overlay. Check from all angles to make sure the structure is correct. Make sure there are no dull or flat spots.

11 When the overlay is a perfect shape, use a glosser or three-way buffer to shine the surface.

12 Massage nail oil into the nail and surrounding skin.

UV gel

The UV gel system could be considered to be a 'pre-mixed' system, as there is only one material that is applied. The only other necessity is a UV light source. The gels are available in many different versions, all with different features and benefits. The main difference that will be immediately noticed by a nail technician is the viscosity (thickness) and how it flows. Some gels are very runny, others are very thick. Some thick gels will eventually flow, others will stay where they are put. Gels are available coloured or clear.

Another benefit of this system is that it is virtually odour-free and therefore may be more suitable for use in areas where stronger odours are a problem. In addition, the gels can be very flexible and therefore move more with the natural nail.

The disadvantages of the UV gel system are that some gels and their application methods cannot produce an overlay that is as strong as the liquid and powder systems and are therefore suitable only for those clients who are not too hard on their nails. Many of the gels on the market can be removed only by buffing and not by soaking off with a remover. Some consider this to be a benefit, others consider it to be a disadvantage.

UV gel system products

Knowledge Check

What are the different overlay systems available?

Refer to page 481 to help you.

Application to the nails

The gel 'system' can comprise a single component – that is, one type of gel – or it can comprise several gel components, all of which are needed to create an artificial nail.

UV gels are applied to the nail and moved around with a brush before being polymerized (cured) under a UV light source. Following cure, most gels have a sticky layer (inhibition layer) on the surface. This is uncured monomer and needs to be removed. Most brands have a specific product to do this but an alcohol-based solvent or nail polish remover can be used.

With a one-component gel system, the gel is applied to the nail in one or more layers to build up strength. In a system with two or more components, there is usually a gel that acts as a bonding layer; it is compatible with the nail plate and also with the next layer of gel; next there is a thick gel that can build an overlay with the required structure, that is curves, and then a sealer gel that provides a high-gloss shine and protection. The manufacturer's instructions should always be followed.

Products, tools and equipment
Additional equipment for UV gel overlays

- ◆ **Tissues or disposable towels** To cover the work area and protect the client's clothing
- ◆ **Gels** UV activated gels; available in a variety of colours
- ◆ **UV lamp** To activate the polymerization process
- ◆ **Primer (if required)** Prepares the nail for the application of the UV gel
- ◆ **Clean brush (either nylon or natural hair)** To apply the gel(s) to the nail
- ◆ **Files (240 grit)** To refine and smooth the nail overlay
- ◆ **Nail oil** To condition the nail and surrounding skin
- ◆ **Finishing wipe (if required)** To remove the inhibition layer
- ◆ **Glosser or three-way buffer** To add shine to the finished nail overlay

STEP-BY-STEP: APPLYING UV GEL

1 Most UV gel systems have a bonder layer or primer. On a nail that has had a tip applied and has been prepared, apply a very thin layer of bonder gel to each nail on the first hand making sure the whole nail is covered and the gel does not touch the skin.

2 Cure for the manufacturer's recommended time. While the hand is in the UV lamp repeat Step 1 for the second hand. It may be necessary to cure the thumbs separately if a 'whole-hand' lamp is not being used.

3 Apply a second layer of the builder gel. Notice how the brush is used to build an apex in the centre of the nail. At the free edge pull the brush down to seal the edge. Cure in the UV lamp for the recommended time. Depending on the viscosity of the gel, it may be necessary to 'fix' the layer on two nails at a time to prevent the gel from moving while you apply a layer to the next two nails. A third layer may be necessary if the nails are very long. Alternate the hands so one hand is always under the lamp.

4 Using an alcohol-based product, remove the inhibition layer (the sticky surface of uncured monomer) from each nail, wiping from the cuticle to the free edge.

5 If necessary, use a 240 grit file to refine the shape of each nail looking at it from all angles to make sure it is even and has a good structure and a thin free edge. A three-way buffer may be used to create a shine or a further layer of gel may be applied. Remove all traces of dust with a cotton pad dampened with an alcohol-based product.

6 A thin layer of gloss top coat may be applied, making sure the whole nail is covered, the edge is sealed and the surface is smooth. Cure for the recommended time in the UV lamp.

7 Remove the inhibition layer. The nails are now finished and ready for massaging in some nail oil.

STEP-BY-STEP: UV GEL NAILS WITH A WHITE TIP

Follow steps 1—5 for a straightforward gel overlay. The white tip product should be applied after the nail has been refined and before the gloss top coat.

1 When all the dust has been removed from the nails, apply the white-tip product just as if painting a French manicure. The smile line can be sharpened by using a clean gel brush. Cure in the UV lamp for the recommended time. Then apply the gloss top coat.

2 Finished nail.

In addition to the resources listed on page 465, you will require the following products, tools and equipment for liquid and powder treatments.

Products, tools and equipment
Additional equipment for fibre overlays

◆ **Tissues or disposable towels** To cover the work area and protect the client's clothing

◆ **Fibre mesh, silk or fibreglass** To wrap around the nail as the basis of the overlay

◆ **Fibre scissors with very fine and sharp blades** To cut and trim the fibre mesh to fit the nail

◆ **Resin with long nozzle** To soak the fibre mesh to create the overlay

◆ **Activator, spray or brush-on** To initiate the polymerization process

◆ **Files (240 grit)** To refine and smooth the nail overlay

◆ **Nail oil** To condition the nail and surrounding skin

◆ **Glosser or three-way buffer** To add shine to the finished nail overlay

Fibre

The third main system involves the application of a fibre mesh (wrap fabrics are usually silk or fibreglass) with a cyanoacrylate resin. This is polymerized or activated with a spray or paint-on chemical. This system is quite gentle on the natural nail and odours are kept to a minimum, especially if a paint on resin activator is used instead of a spray.

A fibre system

Fibre overlays are very popular as a natural nail wrap, as they are quick and fairly easy to apply and easy to remove.

Fibre overlays are not as strong as the structured nails of other systems and some nail technicians find the application techniques 'fiddly'.

Application to the nails

The fibre system uses a fibre mesh with a cyanoacrylate resin which is then activated. Either silk or fibreglass can be used as the mesh. The mesh is placed on the nail and then soaked with the resin. The resin is sometimes called a no-light gel (not to be confused with a UV gel). There are two different ways of activating the resin: a spray or a brush-on activator.

Fibre overlays are not solvent resistant at all. If nail varnish is worn then a very gentle remover should be used otherwise the surface of the overlay will be destroyed.

STEP-BY-STEP: APPLYING THE FIBRE SYSTEM

1 Using scissors and avoiding handling the fibre too much, cut a piece of fibre which is approximately the width of the nail. Remove the backing paper and place the fibre onto the nail, close to but not touching the nail fold.

2 Trim the sides if necessary by sliding the blade of the scissors down the side wall and cutting away the excess. Trim the excess length by angling the scissors backwards on the nail tip so the fibre is slightly shorter than the tip.

3 Apply a very small amount of resin down the centre of the nail and, with the side of the nozzle, use small circular movements to spread the resin over the nail and work it into the mesh. The mesh should be wet but visible.

4 Apply further resin down the centre of the nail and spread using the nozzle if a brush-on activator is not being used. If using spray activator, hold it at least 30 cm away from the nails and spray once.

5 If using brush-on activator, have brush cleaner ready. Spread the activator over the resin with the brush to cover the nail while keeping the product off the skin and leaving a tiny margin around the edge.

6 Clean the activator brush before replacing it in the bottle.

7 Apply a further layer of resin and smooth over either with the nozzle or, if using a brush-on activator, the brush.

8 Activate the same way as before.

9 Refine the surface with a white block. The overlay should be relatively smooth and should need minimal buffing to refine and smooth the surface.

10 Bring the nails to a high shine with a three-way buffer.

11 Remove all dust and apply oil.

There are two things that have progressed my career: education gives you the knowledge and competition allows you to perfect your craft to a higher level than doing clients alone can.

Liza Smith

TOP TIP

Fibre mesh with UV gel

Due to the nature of the resin, it is not possible to create any additional curves in the overlay, as can be done with a L&P or UV gel overlay. However, it is possible to use fibre with a UV gel to give added strength or for free-form sculpting.

Aftercare advice

The following **aftercare advice** should be given to clients after every artificial nail treatment:

◆ return for recommended maintenance treatments

◆ keep the nails clean

Aftercare Advice

Aftercare leaflet

◆ if there appears to be discoloration under the artificial nail, return immediately

◆ do not pick off the overlay or try to remove the artificial nail product

◆ do not use nails as tools

◆ massage nail oil into the cuticle area every day

◆ do not file the surface of the nail

◆ it is not advisable to shorten the nail as the thin layer at the free edge will be filed away to a thicker area

◆ use acetone-free varnish remover if necessary

◆ contact the salon if there is any sign of a contra-action including infection indicated by swelling, inflammation or discoloration. This could indication a bacterial or fungal infection.

Potential retail product recommendations

◆ Nail oil.

◆ Polish remover.

◆ Nail polish.

◆ Hand cream.

◆ Top coat.

Knowledge Check

Briefly explain the overlay application for each of the following systems:

a) liquid and powder

b) UV gel

c) fibre.

Refer to pages 482–488 to help you.

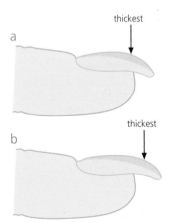

Nail growth: (a) Position of overlay at application stage, (b) Position of overlay at two weeks' growth

Maintaining artificial nails

Skilful maintenance is as important as skilful application and will keep clients returning on a regular basis.

The appearance of an outgrown artificial nail is one consideration, but there are two more important reasons for regular maintenance treatments:

1 The nail technician will have explained to the client that they must watch out for any changes to the nail, and return immediately if anything is noticed. However, some slight changes may not be noticed by the client. There may be some lifting of the overlay, a slight reaction to the products or some minor nail separation. It is important that the nail technician monitors the health of the nail and skin.

2 After a period of natural nail growth, the structure that was created during application with the two curves (upper arch and 'C' curve) meeting at the apex or stress point of the nail to create the strongest nail possible, will have moved.

The apex will have moved further away from the nail bed and could be on the free edge, making it susceptible to breakages. The smile line that was created either by the tip application or by a white tip overlay will also have moved and there will be a band of natural nail growth that will be a different colour to the tip.

new nail growth

growth at free edge

1. Infill procedure: (a) Buff overlay near cuticle, (b) Replace overlay in shaded area

2. Rebalance procedure: (a) Remove most of overlay, (b) Replace with complete overlay

3. Smile line at 2 weeks' growth

ALWAYS REMEMBER

Only maintain nails that you have applied

If you have not applied a set of nails you cannot be sure of the procedures followed or the preparation, and there may be a problem that the nail is hiding. The products used previously may also not be compatible with the ones you use. Either suggest the client returns to their original nail technician for maintenance or, preferably, explain why you cannot provide a maintenance treatment and suggest that the nails are removed and a new set applied by you.

Maintenance treatments

Infill or rebalance?

There are two types of maintenance treatments. One, called an **infill**, is a short treatment that allows the nail technician to check for any problems and fill in the small area of growth to make the artificial nail look smooth without a ridge at the base (1). The other is called a **rebalance**, as it removes the apex that has moved to the wrong place and replaces it in the right place, it fills the regrowth area at the base (2) and, if required, will put the smile line back to where it should be and cover the band of natural nail growth (3).

The decision as to which treatment is needed should depend on the rate of nail growth. If growth is slow to average, it is likely that an infill will be required 2 weeks after the first application and a rebalance 2 weeks after that. These treatments can then be alternated. If nail growth is average to fast, then a full rebalance may be needed every 2 to 3 weeks.

Assessment of client's nails

Before the maintenance treatment assess the client's nails, especially on the first maintenance visit after application of a first full set.

What did the client want to achieve? When providing a maintenance treatment, always remember what the client wanted to achieve at the beginning.

Is the client happy? There should be discussion with the client as to how they are getting on and if they are happy with their nails. It may be that the original plan needs changing to achieve another goal.

ACTIVITY

Maintenance – observation

When performing a first maintenance, write a log of your observations including a description of each section of each nail, including:

a. shape on looking down onto nail

b. shape from sides

c. shape of barrel

d. smile line

e. clarity of overlay

f. Zone 3

g. general.

Contra-actions

Contra-action	Reason	Solution
Broken nails (if some product is left on the remaining nail plate)	1 Too long. 2 Weak.	Shorten all nails. Rebuild stress area
Missing nails (nothing is left on the nail plate)	1 Oil or moisture on nail plate (if no damage to the nail plate). 2 Client picking nails (if damage to the nail plate is obvious).	Careful preparation. Discussion
Lifting in Zone 3	1 Cuticle on nail. 2 Oil on nail. 3 Overlay too thin. 4 Overlay too thick. 5 Overlay touching skin.	Careful preparation. Careful preparation, dehydrate twice or second coat of primer (if applicable). Add slightly more. Refine overlay in Zone 3. Take more care in application
Chipping at cuticle	1 Overlay too thick. 2 Overlay too brittle. 3 Client picking.	Apply smaller beads. Use wetter ratio in L&P system or less activator in fibre system. Discussion
Chipping at free edge	1 Overlay too brittle. 2 Overlay too thin.	Use wetter ratio or less activator. Apply more, but taper at free edge

Contra-action	Reason	Solution
Discoloration of overlay	1 Contamination. 2 Affected by UV light. 3 Coloured varnish.	Use fresh product and clean tools. Cover with UV-resistant sealer. Use base coat under varnish
Discoloration of nail plate under overlay: yellow-green	1 Bacterial infection.	If very superficial (that is very pale colour and small area) remove overlay, dehydrate, prime and reapply; see client 1 week later. If more serious, remove overlay and refer to GP/pharmacist
Discoloration under nail plate	1 Possible infection.	Remove artificial nail and refer to GP

Step-by-step approach to maintenance

At the start of each maintenance treatment, four steps should be followed, then nothing of importance will be missed out.

1 *Observation*: Look carefully at all the nails. The only difference from when they were first applied should be the natural nail growth at the cuticle, leaving a gap, and at the free edge an obvious growth of natural nail. If there is anything more than this, there is a problem that needs solving and correcting and what is noticed should be noted on the client's record card.

2 *Questioning*: The client must be asked how they have managed with the nails.

3 *Diagnosing*: If the nails are less than perfect, the nail technician needs to decide what the possible causes of the problem may be and discuss this with the client.

4 *Treatment*: Having followed the above steps, the most appropriate treatment can be decided upon and suggested to the client.

ACTIVITY

Maintenance – questioning

When performing a first maintenance, record your client's responses to the following questions:

a. How did the nails break? (If appropriate!)

b. How have you managed with them?

c. Have you followed all home care advice?

d. If not, what has been missed?

e. Do you like the length and shape?

f. Have they caused any problem?

Knowledge Check

What are the main points of aftercare advice to be discussed with the client?

Refer to pages 489–490 to help you.

Further contra-actions

ACTIVITY

How would you deal with the following problems that may occur at a maintenance treatment:

a. shape

b. breakages

c. clarity of product

d. lifting

e. chipping

f. allergic reaction or infections.

Discoloration under nail plate at free edge: white This indicates nail separation and may be due to a number of different reasons. The correct treatment would be to remove all products and, if the condition were very minor, wait and see if it improves. A pharmacist should be able to suggest what will keep the area under the nail clean.

Skin reaction If there is any irritation of the skin, such as itching, swelling, redness or a rash anywhere on the body – but especially on the hands, fingers or face – the products must be removed immediately.

A skin sensitivity patch test or a test nail should be performed to see which product or products must be avoided.

The maintenance treatment

The equipment and preparation of the work area, yourself, the client and the nails is exactly the same as for the first application. Any artificial nails that are missing will need to have a tip replaced in the same way as previously described. The step-by-steps that follow describe the general processes for infill and re-balance treatments across the three overlay systems (liquid and powder, UV gel and fibre); you will also need to refer back to the specific step-by-steps for each system to remind yourself of the application process.

Second maintenance As with the record of first maintenance, look at and ask all the same points. Compare results and determine if problems have been solved and results improved. If this is not the case, make a note of what is not right as before and complete a full self-assessment.

STEP-BY-STEP: INFILL TREATMENT

1 Assess the nails. Sanitize the hands and nails. Soften and remove any cuticle that is on the newly grown nail.

2 Using a 240 grit file, gently blend the edge of the overlay in Zone 3. This will also remove the shine. If there is any lifting in this area it will need to be buffed away carefully without over-buffing the nail plate.

3 Remove the shine from the whole nail surface.

4 Remove the dust and apply dehydrator, taking care to clean around the side walls and nail fold. Apply primer if required.

5 Apply a thin layer of product (liquid and powder, UV gel or resin) in Zone 3 as in the original application and blend with the rest of the nail. (Image shows L&P application.)

6 Refine the shape of the overlay as in the first application with a 240 grit file, checking from all angles that the structure of the curves is correct. Further refine the surface with a white block.

7 Finish the nail with a three-way buffer or high gloss sealant (after removing all traces of dust).

8 Apply oil to the finished nail.

STEP-BY-STEP: RE-BALANCE TREATMENT

1 Assess the nails. Sanitize the hands and nails.

2 Shorten the length of the nail. Using a 240 grit file, thin out the whole overlay, removing the apex so that the remaining overlay is thin and even. Ensure the tip of the free edge is thinned as after shortening the nail it will be thicker than the original tip.

3 Remove the dust and apply dehydrator. Apply primer if required.

4 Apply a new overlay in exactly the same way as the original overlay. If it is a fibre system and the original fibre has not been disturbed it is not necessary to apply the fibre mesh to the whole nail as it will get too thick as time goes on. A small piece of fibre placed in Zone 3 will be sufficient. (Images show L&P application.)

5 Refine the shape of the overlay as in the first application, checking from all angles that the structure of the curves is correct.

6 Finish the nail with a three-way buffer or high gloss sealant (after removing all traces of dust).

7 Apply oil to the finished nail.

> " Beware using social media in your private life that may clash with your professional image. I always check people out online to see what it says about them as a person. The Internet, however, is an amazing tool now for people wanting to showcase their work. If you want to work in the session industry and you have great enhancement skills, you have a string to your bow that not everyone has.
>
> *Liza Smith*

The removal of artificial nails

There are many occasions when it is appropriate to remove artificial nails, for example:

◆ the client wanted long nails for a short time only

◆ the natural nail has grown to a length the client is happy with

◆ the regular maintenance required is not possible for the client

◆ the client has had a set of nails applied by someone else

◆ there is a problem with the nails, e.g. allergic reaction, infection, etc.

Liquid and powder and fabric nails are removed in the same way:

◆ remove any coloured varnish

◆ pour enough acetone into a small metal bowl (or one suitable for solvents) to just cover the nails

◆ place bowl in a larger bowl of warm (not hot) water

◆ make sure the client is seated comfortably, preferably at a desk (holding bowls of acetone on laps can result in accidents!)

◆ ask the client to place their fingers in the acetone and cover the bowl and the client's hands with a towel to prevent vapours escaping

◆ liquid and powder nails will take approximately 30 minutes to come off. This time may be longer due to the thickness of the overlay and temperature. Artificial nails that have MMA (Methyl Methacrylate) as the monomer will take a lot longer

◆ the resin used in the fabric system will take only 10–15 minutes

◆ do not remove the nails before the process is complete, as the product will harden immediately and then take longer

◆ when all the product has gone from the nail, remove the fingers and dry them

◆ apply nail oil to the nails and fingers as they will look very white and dry

◆ buff the nails to give them a shine

◆ if artificial nails have been worn for a long time, the natural nail may feel a little weak. Two or three layers of a strengthening top coat (not hardener) will help protect them until they become stronger, which will take a couple of days.

TOP TIP

Oil and barrier cream

Applying oil or a barrier cream to the skin around the nails will help prevent the extreme drying effect of the acetone. This effect is very temporary and moisture will be replaced immediately but the skin does look unpleasant following the removal.

HEALTH & SAFETY

Acetone Always dispose of the used acetone safely and always have the room well ventilated.

HEALTH & SAFETY

Important reminder Always follow the manufacturer's instructions.

UV gel nails are removed as follows:

◆ many UV gels are resistant to acetone, so the only way to remove them is by buffing the nails off

◆ great care must be taken when doing this, as it is very easy to buff the nail plate without realizing

◆ remove any colour first

◆ using a course grit file, but taking great care when near the skin or new nail growth, remove some of the overlay

◆ before the overlay gets thin, use a fine grit file

◆ when the overlay is thin, keep wiping the nail with varnish remover. This will show up the overlay as shinier than natural nail and thus prevent buffing the nail

◆ when the overlay and tip have gone, buff the nail for a shine and apply oil

◆ the natural nail may need some protection from a nail strengthener

If the gel used is a type that can be removed with acetone, the procedure for liquid and powder can be followed after breaking up the surface of the gel with a coarse grit file.

ASSESSMENT OF KNOWLEDGE AND UNDERSTANDING

You have now learnt about providing and maintaining nail enhancements in the beauty therapy workplace. To test your level of knowledge, answer the following short questions. These will prepare you for your summative (final) assessment.

1. Nail _____ removes surface moisture and tiny amounts of oil left on the natural nail.

    a. primer
    b. dehydrator
    c. adhesive
    d. abrasive

2. A disease that is communicable or easily spread by contact is a _____ disease.

    a. contaminant
    b. contagious
    c. infection
    d. allergy

3. The portion of the skin that supports the nail plate as it grows towards the free edge is the nail:

    a. groove
    b. fold

    c. plate
    d. bed

4. Visible ridges running across the width of the natural nail plate are:

    a. ridges
    b. leukonychia
    c. melanonychia
    d. Beau's lines

5. Nail _____ is used for securing nail tips to the natural nails.

    a. primer
    b. dehydrator
    c. adhesive
    d. abrasive

6. How often should a client receive nail maintenance treatments?

    a. when the client feels it is necessary
    b. once a week
    c. every 2 weeks
    d. once a month

7. What is applied at the end of every nail enhancement treatment?

   a. cuticle oil
   b. cuticle remover
   c. cuticle cream
   d. hand cream

8. The maintenance procedure that removes the apex, restores and corrects it is a:

   a. re-balance
   b. infill

9. To remove liquid and powder or fibre artificial nails you can use:

   a. acetate
   b. acetone
   c. dehydrator
   d. acrylic

10. When applying overlay, the area behind the smile line where maximum strength is needed is which zone?

Zones of the nail

14 Nail Art

LEARNING OBJECTIVES

There are two learning outcomes for this unit which you must achieve:

1 Be able to prepare for nail art service.

2 Be able to provide nail art service.

From the range statement, you must show that you can:

◆ Use **consultation** techniques to identify the **treatment objectives**.

◆ Use all listed products, tools and equipment and techniques as appropriate

◆ Identify **nail conditions**.

◆ Ensure that the environmental conditions are suitable.

◆ Complete a consultation and skin inspection to identify any contra-indications.

◆ Communicate and behave in an appropriate and professional manner.

◆ Follow all **health and safety** working practices.

◆ Provide relevant aftercare and **contra-action advice**.

KEY TERMS

aftercare advice	glitters	polish secures
blending	health and safety	polishing
client record cards	jewellery tool	treatment objectives
consultation	marbling	treatment plan
contra-action advice	nail art	transfers
contra-actions	nail art techniques	skin colour
dotting	nail conditions	skin condition
dotting tool	nail polish	striping
foiling	nail shapes	
gel polish	painting techniques	

Unit Topic

Provide nail art

This VRQ unit is linked to the Beauty Therapy NOS Unit N4.

INTRODUCTION

This unit is about how to provide nail art. Nail art is an exciting and elaborate form of nail decoration, which may be applied to the hands and feet. There are a variety of nail art techniques which are limited only by imagination and creativity. It can be as simple as a single stripe across the nail or as intricate as a tiny repeated pattern.

The introduction of gel polish into the nail technicians' repertoire has opened a whole new series of nail art techniques and, if anything, has made it easier and more achievable. Before attempting nail art using gel polish, it is important that the subject is learned and practised, as a good application is the basis for every design in that section.

Dealing with people in a polite, efficient manner and using good communication and questioning skills to find out exactly what they require from the nail art treatment forms an important part of this technical service.

You must be able to show you have the necessary practical skills and underpinning knowledge to provide nail art.

INDUSTRY ROLE MODEL

NATALIYA is qualified Master of Science in Finance

" My passion and interest in the nail and beauty industry led me to pursue my dream and change direction in life. I attended Mary Reid International School of Beauty and graduated in 2006 with ITEC qualifications in beauty and body therapy. I then worked as a senior therapist in PURE Spa in Edinburgh. As the only nail professional in the team, I realized that nail design is what I wanted to do for life. Shortly after leaving the spa and opening my first beauty salon, I attended various nail courses in the brand Creative Nail Design (CND). I became a CND Shellac education Ambassador in 2011 and have taken nail art to a new level. In May 2013 I attended CND's Education Boot Camp in San Diego and qualified as a full systems CND Education Ambassador, bringing home two awards. I regularly contribute to the industry with my Nail Trail article in *Scratch* Magazine. I work full time in my own salon N-Style in Edinburgh, with responsibility for hygiene, marketing and business development.

ANATOMY & PHYSIOLOGY
Essential anatomy and physiology knowledge requirements for this chapter are identified on the checklist chart on page 31.

Nail art

Nail art is a skill which takes practice and requires a very good eye for detail.

The nail art skill starts when a 'French manicure' is applied, demonstrated in Chapter 11 Manicure Treatments, as this is actually two colours which need to be painted very accurately. The skill becomes even more advanced when other colours and actual designs are incorporated. You do not need to be a great artist in order to create quite stunning and very commercially acceptable designs. There are many easy nail art techniques and products that allow even the most 'artistically challenged' to produce some stunning designs!

There is an extensive range of nail art products or mediums available on the market today that, with a few guidelines and hints, can create stunning 'masterpieces' at minimal cost and effort. The real effort is practising! Nail art is visual and there are a relatively small number of basic painting techniques that, using readily available products, can be demonstrated in a few step-by-step pictures. Every newcomer to nail art will find that, with the right direction and range of products, a few initial ideas will lead on to many, many more.

" **How to convince clients to try nail art?**
Wear it yourself, usually clients will ask for what you are wearing on your nails. Encourage your clients with a complementary simple design on their ring finger to introduce them to artistic designs. Take into consideration clients' profession, lifestyle and fashion preferences. Ask clients about preferred shape and length, colours they love and dislike, and keep a note of them for future appointments.

Nataliya

Decorated false nails

Although some more unusual designs are included, the aim of this chapter is to provide the underpinning knowledge and practical skills of the various techniques of nail art which may be performed commercially in a beauty salon or freelance situation.

Preparing for nail art

Outcome 1: Be able to prepare for nail art service

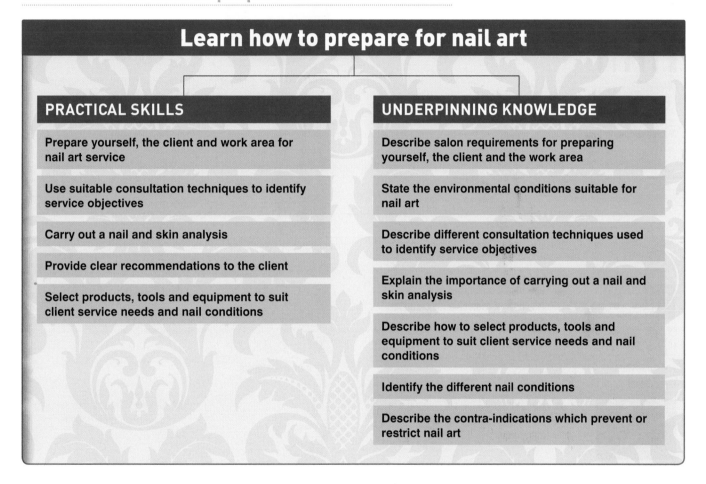

Learn how to prepare for nail art

PRACTICAL SKILLS

Prepare yourself, the client and work area for nail art service

Use suitable consultation techniques to identify service objectives

Carry out a nail and skin analysis

Provide clear recommendations to the client

Select products, tools and equipment to suit client service needs and nail conditions

UNDERPINNING KNOWLEDGE

Describe salon requirements for preparing yourself, the client and the work area

State the environmental conditions suitable for nail art

Describe different consultation techniques used to identify service objectives

Explain the importance of carrying out a nail and skin analysis

Describe how to select products, tools and equipment to suit client service needs and nail conditions

Identify the different nail conditions

Describe the contra-indications which prevent or restrict nail art

Preparing the work area

Prepare the work area to meet the requirments for all related health and safety legislation. The work surface must be stable to avoid products being knocked over or spilt. The area must be free of any other previously used materials and debris, such as dust created from the application of artificial nails. Dust can spoil the effect of a client's newly painted nails. Lighting must be good to enable you to avoid eyestrain, especially when performing intricate artwork. It is a good idea to use a magnifying lamp.

All the health and safety rules and legislation that you learnt in Chapter 3 Health and Safety, Chapter 11 Manicure Treatments and Chapter 12 Pedicure Treatments must be followed.

Ensure all tools and equipment are clean and disinfected as appropriate and are neatly organized on the nail work station. Before beginning nail art service check you have all the necessary products, tools and equipment to hand and that they meet all legal hygiene and industry requirements for nail services.

Products, tools and equipment

Brushes

◆ **Brushes** A variety of shapes and sizes of brushes for freehand painting including detail brush, striping brush, flat brush and fan brush

Polish secures

◆ **Polish secures** Small stones or shapes for attaching to the nail as part of the design

Marbling/dotting tool

◆ **Marbling/dotting tool** For creating 'marbling' or 'dotting' designs with the paint

Specialized nail art sealer/top coat

◆ **Specialized nail art sealer/ top coat** For sealing the design once the paint is dry

Foils/transfers/ tapes/stencils

◆ **Foils/transfers/tapes/stencils** A variety of materials for creating designs

Glitter polishes/dusts

◆ **Glitter polishes/dusts** Can be used to create or enhance nail art designs

Nail piercing tool

◆ **Nail piercing tool** For making small holes in the nail for jewellery attachments

Dappen dishes

◆ **Dappen dishes** For keeping polish secures or glitter in

Nail art paints

◆ **Nail art paints** Specialized water-based acrylic paints for nail art

YOU WILL ALSO NEED:

◆ **Palette** For placing nail art paints on for use or mixing

◆ **Disinfectant solution** To store small stainless steel sterilized tools

◆ **Nail work station** On which to place everything. You will require manicure tools and equipment to prepare the nails

for nail art. A light is useful when carrying out detailed techniques.

◆ **Nail polish remover** to remove nail polish/products as required

◆ **Nail polishes** including base coat and a range of coloured polishes

◆ **Medium sized towels (3)** To dry the skin, nails, etc. and protect the client's clothing

◆ **Water spray** For re-wetting the nail art paints when they start to dry out

◆ **Skin disinfectant** To cleanse and disinfect the client's skin and nails

◆ **Waste container** This should be a lined metal bin with a lid to contain vapours from solvents

◆ **Tissues or disposal towels** To cover the work area when using paints and protect the client's clothing

◆ **Cotton buds** A damp cotton bud can be used to remove mistakes made with nail art paint

◆ **Client record card** To record the client's personal details, products used and details of the service

Disinfection

Hygiene must be maintained in a number of ways to prevent secondary and cross-infection:

◆ ensure that tools and equipment are clean and, where applicable, disinfected before use

◆ disinfect work surfaces after each client

◆ always follow hygienic practices

◆ clear discarded waste after each client

◆ maintain a high standard of personal hygiene.

Reception

Nail art should be priced as a stand alone service, not just included in the cost of a manicure, pedicure or nail extension service. When a client makes an appointment for nail art, discuss the cost of the service; prices will vary depending on the products and materials used, or the time involved to create the design.

Some designs are very quick and use little product, for example a flick of paint with a nail art brush or a simple **marbling** technique using a **dotting tool**. Other designs are very quick but use more costly products, for example, polish secures that are fast to apply, but cost much more than a flick of nail art paint or a couple of 'blobs' of **nail polish**.

Nail art can be time consuming but must be cost effective. If it costs too much this may be a barrier as it will only last a short time. You must always be realistic in your pricing ensuring that the most popular designs are quick to apply but will equally look stunning. The simplest designs are often the most effective and may appeal to a wider client base.

> Don't forget to display your creations at your nail station, so that your clients will see them. If clients don't know what you can do, they will never ask for it. Display artistic designs on colour wheels or colour pops. It is advisable to change your designs according to the seasonal colour schemes and latest colour arrivals by your brand.
>
> Remember, that nail art is an artistic skill and requires a little extra time to the appointment, hence it should be charged accordingly. It is normal practice to add at least 20 per cent extra to the total cost of the appointment.

Nataliya

TOP TIP
Spoilt polish
It is a good idea for the client to pay before the service to prevent spoiling the nail art.

ALWAYS REMEMBER
Be realistic
Although designs look effective displayed on quite large plastic tips, remember that the design will look very different on a much smaller nail on a finger and some designs are much easier to apply on a tip than a real nail as the surrounding skin can get in the way!

ALWAYS REMEMBER
Minors
If the client is a minor under the age of 16, it is necessary to obtain parent/guardian permission for the service. The parent/guardian will also have to be present when the service is received.

If the client's natural nails are in poor condition it will be necessary to allow extra time to perform a simple nail treatment, to improve the nails' appearance, and facilitate application. The client must be aware that it may take time for the nail products to harden.

Commercial timing

Allow 30 minutes for nail art application.

Consultation

If a client shows an interest in nail art, the next step is careful questioning. Find out at the consultation the client's likes and dislikes and how adventurous they are; do they have a specific idea for a design or are they prepared to give you free rein? Make sure you understand what your client is saying and that you are clear about the degree of 'statement' they are interested in making with their nails. For example, a client usually known for their conservative taste in clothes and natural nails with sheer or delicate colours, who is interested in nail art for a special occasion, is only likely to be interested in a very subtle design. Alternatively, a client who likes to try out new ideas, such as the latest fashion trends, may be open to a more interesting suggestion such as rhinestones or an unusual nail polish application technique.

It is a good idea to prepare a number of nail art designs to show the client. These may be applied to artificial nails, or they may be images of nail art designs that you have created and photographed. On your display have designs in two or three colour ways to demonstrate that a design can be customized to suit the client and show how different colour combinations can change the design dramatically. Start the display with the simpler and less expensive designs and progress to the more elaborate and more involved designs.

Assess the condition of the client's nails and cuticles before the service. If the client's expectations are unsuitable because of the client's natural nail shape or size or condition of the nail, offer a suitable alternative. For example, if the client's nails are too short, if qualified, you could apply tips to the natural nail, blend and paint these. Decide upon the nail shape and length. It is important that the nail shape and length selected suits the client's hands and fingers. Refer to page 421 for further guidance on preparing the natural nail.

Contra-indications   Whilst assessing the client's hands/feet you should be looking for any contra-indications to nail art. Contra-indications are the same as for any other nail service (see pages 394–399). If the client has a disease or disorder of the hand or nail it is in the interest of the client and beauty therapist not to proceed with the nail art service. Treating a client with a contra-indication may lead to cross-infection or a worsening of the client's condition. It is important to advise the client to seek medical advice to ensure a correct diagnosis and treatment for their condition. Some conditions will require restriction and adaption of the nail art service.

Contra-actions   Certain cosmetic ingredients are known to cause allergic reactions in some people. These substances are known as allergens and may cause irritation, excessive erythema, inflammation and swelling. This is known as a contra-action and may occur during or following service.

The client may at any time develop an allergy to a nail art product that has been successfully used previously. This could be for a number of reasons, such as new medication being taken or illness. If an allergic reaction occurs, remove the product immediately and a soothing substance may be applied. This product should not be used again. See pages 399–400 for more information on contra-actions.

As with all treatments, accurate client record cards must be kept for clients receiving nail art services. If the client has received nail art services before, consult the record card and review the success and satisfaction of this with the client. Details of the products used should be recorded on the client record card. This is useful if the client returns for this service, also it is important in the event of a contra-action such as an allergic reaction.

Preparation of the nail technician

Sitting properly is important. Ideally sit on a properly designed manicure stool or chair which offers adequate back support. When completing nail art it is important to sit upright with both feet flat on the floor.

Preparation of the client

Ensure that the client is warm and comfortable when preparing them for nail art.

◆ Confirm the client's choice of nail art.

◆ File the nails to achieve the desired shape and length.

◆ Ensure the free edge is clean.

◆ The cuticles should be removed from the nail plate and the eponychium neat.

◆ Ensure the surface of the nail plate is clean and grease-free.

◆ Wipe with polish remover or an alcohol such as isopropyl alcohol to prepare the nail. Use a lint-free pad as cotton wool may leave fibres, which may spoil the application of the nail polish/paint.

◆ Apply the required nail art base (usually a good quality base coat and the chosen base colour).

Basic nail art techniques

The basic techniques are easy! All that is required are ideas, a bit of imagination and the right products, tools and equipment.

The paints used are different from nail polishes. They are usually water-based acrylic artist's paint, as this gives a very dense colour, can be mixed and is easier to use for fine detail. There are lots of effects that can be achieved with paints, a selection of nail art brushes and a 'marbling/dotting tool'.

Nails need to be painted with a base colour that will be part of or enhance the finished design. This is usually a nail polish.

◆ Very simple but effective designs can be achieved by placing dots of colour. Use either a very small round brush or a 'marbling or dotting tool' to apply the dots (1). Care needs to be taken on the size and regularity of the dots as this can spoil a good design.

◆ A very long, thin brush referred to as a '**striping**' brush dipped in paint can achieve fine stripes and create quite sophisticated designs (2).

HEALTH & SAFETY

Dealing with a contra-indication Remember, never advise the client as to what the contra-indication may be; you are not qualified to do so. Always refer the client to their GP if you are at all unsure. Do not treat the client.

TOP TIP

Costing

When allowing for time in costing a design, use an average time that the design would take. Initially, when inexperienced, it will take you longer to achieve the finished nail art but you shouldn't be charging the client extra for that time.

ACTIVITY

Questioning for client satisfaction

Practice some designs on a nail tip and then a real nail plate. You will notice the appearance and application are different.

HEALTH & SAFETY

Avoiding a contra-action Always check at the consultation for any known allergies to substances or ingredients. Formaldehyde is used in some base coats to strengthen the nail plate and it can cause an allergic reaction in some people. Always follow the manufacturer's instructions to ensure that products are used correctly and safely.

Knowledge Check

Name three contra-indications observed at consultation that would prevent treatment being carried out. This can apply to the nails of the hands or feet.

Refer to pages 394–399 to help you.

TOP TIP

Nail polish storage

Store nail polish stock in a cool, dark place to avoid separation and fading. Use good stock control, FIFO – First In, First Out, to ensure optimum quality of resources.

(1) Steps: Base colour, flower centres, flower petals, finished design with stems added

(2) Steps: Base colour and stripes

Outcome 2: Be able to provide nail art service

Learn how to provide nail art

PRACTICAL SKILLS

Communicate and behave in a professional manner

Follow health and safety working practices

Position yourself and client correctly throughout the service

Use products, tools, equipment and techniques to suit client's service needs and nail conditions

Complete the service to the satisfaction of the client

Record the results of the service

Provide suitable aftercare advice

UNDERPINNING KNOWLEDGE

State how to communicate and behave in a professional manner

Describe health and safety working practices

State the importance of positioning yourself and the client correctly throughout the treatment

State the importance of using products, tools, equipment and techniques to suit client's treatment needs and nail conditions

Describe how treatments can be adapted to suit client treatment needs and nail conditions

State the contra-actions that may occur during and following services and how to respond

State the importance of completing the treatment to the satisfaction of the client

State the importance of completing treatment records

State the aftercare advice that should be provided

Describe diseases and disorders of the nail

Describe the structure and functions of the nail

Designs using dotting and marbling techniques

A design achieved with striping brushes

Designs using free hand brush techniques

HEALTH & SAFETY

Legislation It is important that you comply with all relevant health and safety legislation while performing nail art.

Examples include:

◆ Control of Substances Hazardous to Health Regulations (COSHH) (2002)

◆ Personal Protective Equipment (PPE) at Work Regulations (1992)

Remember to use the underpinning knowledge and practical skills you have learnt in Chapter 3 Health and Safety; Chapter 11 Manicure Treatments and Chapter 12 Pedicure Treatments.

Steps: Base colour, add two or more different coloured dots, swirl together

> " Nail Art is all about colour. It is very important to learn and understand colour theory prior to offering nail art to your clients. Understanding colour will help you to identify the client's skin tone correctly and choose a method that would complement, neutralize or accessorize the client's skin tone. Learning colour theory is so much fun, in fact this is my favourite subject to teach. Nail artists must have a colour wheel in their kit; this will be your ultimate partner in choosing the colour schemes for your designs.
>
> *Nataliya*

Abstract patterns or marbling can look stunning with a good choice of colour combinations. Flicking the colour from side to side with a fine brush or placing spots of colour on the nail and mixing them together with the 'marbling tool' achieves this effect.

◆ Those who are not so good at hand painting designs can use stencils. The types that are readily available have a sticky back to keep them in place. These are applied to a dry nail and painted over. When the nail paint is completely dry they are removed, leaving the chosen design behind.

◆ Pictures of all sorts can be painted on a nail with a steady hand, a good imagination or an easy picture to copy. (Most nail artists keep large numbers of pictures to copy onto a nail or just to give them inspiration to create an original design.)

Hand painted designs

Hand painting with a theme

" Arm yourself with plenty of ideas for artistic designs. Where to get ideas? Simply look around, you can see colour everywhere. We are surrounded by colour. I love getting my ideas from the shops – fruit and vegetable arrangements at the supermarket, fashion departments, fabric shops, fashion programmes on TV and the Internet are full of ideas, you just need to learn to see them. Choose colours that are enjoyable to wear and look at, so your designs are very well thought through and are pleasurable to look at.

Nataliya

Knowledge Check

How would you decide upon the recommended nail art for a client?

Refer to page 506 to help you.

TOP TIP

Brush techniques

If you have a very long striping brush, try placing three or four dots of different coloured paint next to each other on a plastic palette (or similar). Lay the brush in the dots and turn it so all the hairs are coated. Then lay the brush on the nail and lift off. An attractive multi-coloured stripe will be left behind. Try different colours and techniques of applying to the nail and see what happens.

◆ Buy or find a palette. This can be any plastic surface that can be easily cleaned with water. This can be used to place nail art paints on for use or mixing. Have a small water spray to hand then, if your paints start drying out, give a small spray of distilled water to keep them workable.

Nail art paint is water-based and any mistakes can be easily removed with a wet nail wipe, or a cotton bud will remove a small part.

In all nail art, sealing the design is very important and, when the paint is dry, a sealer or top coat must be applied to fix the paint and also bring out the colour. The manufacturer's recommended sealer should be used, as some top coats may react to the paints. Clients should be advised to reseal the nails every couple of days to keep them fresh-looking and avoid any chips.

Nail art brushes

There are many brushes specifically sold for nail art purposes but also remember that art shops sell many shapes and sizes too. A small collection of brushes is necessary for the nail technician in order to create a wide range of styles and these can be purchased relatively cheaply from suppliers and, with care, will last a long time.

◆ *Detail brush*. This is the smallest brush and is used for hand painting details or placing dots.

◆ *Striping brushes*. These are available in different sizes. Their length and the number of hairs are relevant. A shorter brush with several hairs will produce lines

TOP TIP

Experimental techniques

Put dots of two different colours on your palette. Dip one corner of a flat brush in one colour and the other corner of the brush in the other colour. Then apply to the nail turning the brush in a circular motion. See what happens!

Designs using striping

> Nail Art requires tools, invest in good quality tools that will last a long time and become your partner in success. Research what is available. It is great to ask for advice from experienced nail artists. Join Salon Geek nail and beauty forum, where you can find vast amounts of helpful advice and connect with industry experts. Take good care of your tools, clean them after every use and store them properly when not in use.
>
> *Nataliya*

that are thick. The longer and thinner the brush, the finer and longer the line they produce. It is worth having at least two of these: a medium one for lines and flicks and a very long one for fine stripes.

◆ *Flat brush*. This is a brush with a small flat head that can create several effects and is used to fill in colours. It can shade and smudge and create swirls.

◆ *Fan brush*. This brush can create texture and blend colours together. It is probably not as versatile as the others but worth having.

Foiling

Foiling is another very easy technique that uses various designs of a foil supplied on a roll. This is almost instant nail art, as some foils have designs on them and just need applying to a painted nail.

◆ Nails should be painted before using foils. They can be painted with a base coat, but it is worth spending the extra time to paint a colour, as this will enhance the effect.

◆ Foils are supplied with a special adhesive that should be painted onto the nail in a very thin coat. The adhesive is usually white and needs to turn clear before the foil is applied; this takes a very short time. The foil is then applied to the tacky adhesive, pattern side uppermost, gently pressed onto the nail with either a finger or a cotton bud and the backing pulled off leaving the foil behind. It is not necessary to cut any foil from the roll, as it will only stick to where the adhesive is.

◆ This is an amazingly quick process that can have spectacular results. As the foil only sticks to where the adhesive has been applied, patterns or pictures can be drawn with the adhesive. The foil needs a special sealer, as most top coats will destroy the delicate layer. Several layers of sealer are also needed, as with all nail art, to keep it intact.

Foiled nail

Polish secures

As the name suggests, this technique requires polish to secure the design. Many different products are available for this easy technique. **Polish secures** is the term for small stones or shapes with a flat back that are placed into the wet nail varnish and held secure when it dries. The products that fall into this category sometimes have different brand names. Most of them are available in different sizes and, although it depends on the design, the smaller versions are usually the most effective.

Knowledge Check

What different brushes are available for nail art? When are each used?

Refer to pages 510–511 to help you.

ACTIVITY

Nail conditions

Identify the cause of the nail conditions below and what salon service and home care/action you would recommend for a client who wished to receive nail art and to improve the appearance/condition of the nail.

◆ Pterygium.
◆ Onychopagy.
◆ Weak, dry, brittle and split nails.
◆ Hangnails.
◆ Longitudinal or horizontal ridges.
◆ Allergies to products.

Polish secures – square rhinestones

Polish secures – flower beads

Polish secures – pearls

◆ *Rhinestones* (or *diamantes* or *crystals*). These are clear or coloured stones that look like precious or semi-precious stones. They are usually made of glass or crystal and cut with facets to reflect light. They can be used to encrust a design or a judiciously placed single stone can bring a simple design to life. In relative terms they are not cheap and the designs using them should reflect this cost. Good quality rhinestones will not dull or lose their sparkle if sealed with a top coat and this will ensure they stay on the nail for the maximum time, especially if the client re-applies a top coat. Although stunning, even the smallest rhinestone stands quite proud from the nail.

◆ *Flat backed beads*. These, like rhinestones are usually coloured glass but they are rounded rather than cut with facets. Applied in the same way to wet polish, they look like beads on the nails.

◆ *Flatstones*. These are a less expensive version of rhinestones. As the name suggests, they are quite flat and usually very small, but they sparkle well. They can, however, lose their sparkle under a top coat. If this is the case, then apply a thicker layer of top coat than usual and push the stones into the wet polish. This should hold them in place without the need to seal them.

◆ *Pearls*. These are flat backed plastic shapes coloured to look like pearls. Although white is the obvious colour, they can be obtained in pastel colours, such as pink or lilac. They can look very pretty, especially in a design for a bride. Again, take account of their size.

◆ *Stone shapes*. There are some interesting shapes available now, such as a flower made of coloured glass.

◆ *Foil shapes*. These are tiny pieces of shiny or holographic plastic cut into different shapes that can look very effective incorporated into a design. The shapes may be circular, stars, moons, hexagons, even tiny hands and dolphins! These are applied in the same way, but care must be taken with the top coat. They need to be sealed, as edges that are not covered by top coat can catch and be pulled off, although some top coats have a solvent that is too strong. This will cause the colour to be affected and it will often streak.

◆ *Metal studs*. A very effective and less 'glitzy' polish secure are metal studs. These are available in gold or silver colours and different sizes.

◆ *Fimo canes*. These can be bought in ready cut or in long 'canes'. There is a vast variety of designs that can be laid on the nail once a very thin 'slice' has been cut. Some of these can be partially transparent.

◆ *Crushed shells*. These are available in many colours and can be applied as a base for other decorations to go on top or can be used alone or with colour variations. They have an opalescence that can look spectacular.

◆ *Dried flowers*. Various tiny dried real flowers and leaves are available and applied in the same way.

After the base colour has been applied (or other design) a top coat or sealer must be painted onto the nail. While this is still wet, the 'secures' can be placed on it. The easiest way to pick up 'secures' is with a wet orange stick or with a small piece of Blu-Tack® on the end of an orange stick. The Blu-Tack® can be shaped into a point to make picking up of the tiny shapes easier.

When all the shapes have been placed, the whole nail needs to be sealed with a thick coat of sealer or top coat. Make sure your top coat does not affect the colour of the foil shapes.

Recommend to your client that they re-apply a top coat every 2 to 3 days to keep the design fresh and avoid damage to or loss of stones.

Alternative application methods:

1 Use a spot of nail adhesive to place the decoration on the nail.

2 Embed in a UV gel top coat before curing.

3 Place on the nail and apply a layer of clear L&P (liquid and powder) or UV gel over the whole design.

Steps: base colour, apply secures

Designs using mixed techniques

Designs using glitter dusts

Designs using transfers

Knowledge Check

What is the purpose of a marbling tool?

Refer to page 507 to help you.

Fimo canes

Flowers and shells

Designs using studs

TOP TIP

Wetting your brush

Never put an orange stick in your mouth to wet it! If Blu-Tack® is not available, dip the stick into varnish remover or a small dish of water to wet it.

Knowledge Check

How does the condition of the client's nails influence timing and choice of nail art?

Refer to page 506 to help you.

Glitter dusts

Glitter polishes and glitter dusts are a very versatile range of products to create or enhance nail art. Obviously, glitter can be applied to the whole nail, but it can also be used to make patterns or designs; a well-placed highlight on a painted or airbrushed design can make a simple piece of nail art spectacular. Make sure your loose glitter is of a cosmetic quality and the colour will not run with the top coat. Cosmetic glitter is plastic rather than metal.

◆ Glitter polishes can be painted straight from the bottle with either the brush supplied or a fine nail art brush. Glitter dusts can be used to create more specific designs by picking up the dust with a brush dipped in sealer, as this will give an effect that is denser than glitter polish. The dust will also stick to wet sealer, so the tip of a nail dipped into the pot will collect the dust on the tip only or where the sealer is wet.

◆ Like all nail art, glitter dusts need sealing. The sealer must be painted on thickly and gently to avoid moving the dust.

Knowledge Check

Name four nail art techniques.

Transfers and tapes

There are many **transfers** available to apply to nails. These are ready-made nail art and can be very effective. Some need to be soaked off their backing with water (place a few drops onto the backing paper to soak through and then the transfer slides off) or they peel off their backing and stick straight on to the nail.

Tapes are also available in many plain colours and patterns. They have a sticky back and must be placed on the nail and then trimmed with a small pair of very sharp scissors.

Nail jewellery

Many different types of nail jewellery are available.

◆ Some of the designs are applied to the nail as a 'polish secure', that is stuck to wet varnish or nail adhesive. These can only be very light and small. Larger designs can be applied to the nail with nail adhesive . Both of these are reusable, as they can be removed with nail varnish remover.

◆ Other types of nail jewellery involve making a small hole in the free edge of the nail. This can be done with ease using a specially made tool that has a very sharp but tiny drill. There is no problem at all when piercing an artificial nail, but care must be taken when piercing a natural nail:

◆ a natural nail should be strengthened with a coating of resin as used in a fibre system.

◆ the free edge must be long enough to provide a space for the hole without being too close to the hyponychium. If the hole is made on a nail that is too short the seal at the hyponychium could be damaged.

◆ There are two types of jewellery that require a pierced nail. One has a post that is put through the hole and secured with a tiny nut on the underside. The piercing tool has both the drill and the socket to tighten the nut. The other type has a clasp or ring that is attached to the nail through the hole. The first type usually sits on top of the nail plate and the second hangs from the edge.

Nail piercing tool and nail pendant attached

To pierce the nail:

1 Make sure there is sufficient free edge to safely pierce.

2 Turn the finger over so that the underside of the nail is visible and the nail and finger are resting on a soft surface, for example, a piece of cork or several layers of tissues.

3 Place the tip of the drill on the nail, not too near the edge but also in the right place for the jewellery to fit on the nail (not too far away from the free edge for a pendant or ring).

4 Gently turn the drill until a neat hole is made; withdraw the drill by turning in the opposite direction.

5 Turn the finger over and smooth the surface of the nail with a white block.

> Photograph finished designs and use those to promote your business on your website or Facebook. The best advertisement is word of mouth, make your clients' nails stand out with beauty and fashion. Always give your clients a couple of extra business cards so they can recommend your services to their friends.
>
> *Nataliya*

6   Apply the nail jewellery.

7   If a pendant has been applied, advise the client to remove it while dressing, doing housework, washing hair, etc., as it is possible to catch it and split the nail.

These are some basic instructions for starting off in the realms of nail art. All the various techniques can be mixed and matched. Foil can be mixed with polish secures, paint mixed with glitter. The possibilities are endless and the only limit is imagination.

Water Marbling (Technique and images courtesy of Natash Lee, Divine by Design)

The marbling technique is a quick and fun way to create very impressive designs that will impress clients. It produces an effect that would be very time-consuming if painted by hand and would not be as sharp. It can be a messy process but this method is quick and clean.

There is very little special equipment required:

Products, tools and equipment

◆ A variety of contrasting colours (avoid mixing creams, metallics and shimmers) including a very pale cream colour, e.g. white
◆ A dotting tool (or other sharp object, e.g. an orange stick)
◆ Cotton buds
◆ Cotton pads (plastic backed pads are more effective)
◆ Polish remover
◆ A small dish with a wide surface (e.g. a ramekin dish)
◆ Top coat
◆ A small stiff brush with square shape (optional)

STEP-BY-STEP: WATER MARBLING

1 Prepare all your equipment. Fill the dish with room temperature water.

Paint the nails with a very pale colour (e.g. the white). Have the caps of all the bottles unscrewed.

2 Drop the white from the brush into the water. Follow with each of the colours, dropping each one into the middle until you are happy with the number of colours.

With a fine dotting tool, place it into the middle and draw it out so the polish touches the side of the dish. Repeat a few times around the circle.

Place your dotting tool between each line drawn into the colour next to the white (not the whole as that will break the pattern) and draw into the middle. This will give you a flower-like pattern.

3 Choose an area of the pattern you like and place the finger, nail side down, into the pattern, tip first and hold the finger there.

With a cotton bud, sweep around the water to pick up all the remaining pattern. When all the polish is cleared away lift out the finger.

4 The nail (and some of the skin) will have the pattern on it.

With your dotting tool, run the tip around the base of the nail to break the polish seal, leaving the polish on the nail separate from that on the skin.

5 Soak your plastic backed cotton pad with polish remover.

With the plastic side against the nail, carefully remove the polish by the nail and the skin.

With your brush dipped in remover, carefully run it around the edges of the nail to tidy up the design. Repeat with the other fingers.

6 The finished design. Apply a top coat to give it shine.

Gel Polish Nail Art

If anything, gel polish makes nail art even easier! The coloured polish does not dry like traditional polish does until it is cured under a UV lamp so there is much more time to create the designs and, once cured, is immediately dry so no chance of smudging!

Before starting, the nails must be prepared and painted with the appropriate base coat following the application techniques recommended by the brand manufacturer.

Cut outs (peekaboo)

The nature of gel polish and its instant drying when cured allows for this fabulous technique to be achieved quickly during a service. A colour or effect (e.g. glitter, pigments, etc.) is applied to the nails, then covered by a contrasting colour. The top coat can be 'carved' away in a pattern to show the base effect through. So effective and so versatile.

Products, tools and equipment

◆ **Nails prepared and with the chosen base colour or effect** This can be a polish colour, a glitter or pigments. They need to have a cured top coat applied but it is not necessary to remove the sticky layer

◆ **The chosen top colour** (this can be any colour but darker and bolder colours usually work best)

◆ **Dotting tools of various sizes**

◆ **A clean gel brush**

◆ **Gel polish top coat**

◆ **UV lamp**

◆ **Cotton wool pads**

◆ **Gel cleanser**

STEP-BY-STEP: CUT OUTS (PEEKABOO)

1 Apply one good layer of the chosen colour to the cured top coat on each nail of one hand but DO NOT cure. If you are only doing one nail, let the polish sit for 30 seconds before 'carving'.

2 Take your dotting tool and 'carve out' a pattern until you are happy with it (mistakes can be rectified by applying more colour). Keep wiping the dotting tool on the pad soaked with gel cleanser. Cure as usual. Apply the gel polish top coat and cure. Remove sticky layer.

3 The finished cut out nail.

Removal of any gel polish nail art is the same as removal of gel polish on page 409.

Knowledge Check

What is a contra-action? What could be a contra-action to a nail art service?

Refer to page 518 to help you.

Knowledge Check

What aftercare advice should be given to a client following a nail art service?

Refer to page 518 to help you and remember also to look at Chapter 11 Manicure Treatments and Chapter 12 Pedicure Treatments.

Aftercare advice

Confirm with the client that the finished result is to their satisfaction. Complete details of the nail art service on the client record card. Clear instructions should be provided on how to care for their nails and also what action to take in the event of a contra-action.

Aftercare advice will differ for each client according to their individual needs, but generally it will be as manicure aftercare advice: see pages 426–427.

When giving aftercare advice, it is a good opportunity to recommend retail products, such as nail polish or hand cream, thereby enhancing retail sales and the salon profits. It is a good idea to have the nail polish colours that you have used available for sale. The client can then touch up any accidental chips. Recommend the use of a top coat applied every 3 to 4 days to protect the nail art, increase its durability and impart shine if traditional nail polish has been used.

Nail art will last approximately 5 to 10 days with traditional polish and 2 to 3 weeks with gel polish, so recommend the client books their next appointment after this. Ideally, the client should return to the salon to have their nail art removed. However, nail art with traditional polish can usually be removed with nail polish remover. Care should be taken to remove attachments such as polish secures and nail jewellery. ALWAYS recommend that gel polish is removed in the salon.

Contra-actions A contra-action is an unwanted reaction to the service. An unwanted reaction to the nail art service might include an allergic reaction. This occurs when a person becomes sensitized to a product ingredient. It is possible to become allergic to a product after having been in contact with it for years. The reaction would be recognized if the skin becomes red, itchy and inflamed.

Advise the client that if an allergic reaction occurs, all nail products should be removed and a cool compress and soothing agent applied to the skin to reduce redness and irritation.

ACTIVITY

Create a design plan for each of the following. Include the created design on a nail tip or a photograph(s) of your nail art.

1 A design plan for a photographic shot using a fantasy image. The image is to appear on the CD cover of a girl group called 'Heavenly'.
2 A design to be used on all the female models of a bridal fashion show.
3 A design for a client who is going to a Christmas party. She has asked you to create a design that includes snow!
4 A design for a mature client who will be celebrating her golden wedding with a big family party.

ASSESSMENT OF KNOWLEDGE AND UNDERSTANDING

You have now learnt about the underpinning knowledge and practical skills for providing nail art in the beauty therapy workplace. To test your level of knowledge, answer the following short questions. These will prepare you for your summative (final) assessment.

1. Pterygium is a nail condition recognized by:

   a. overgrown thickened cuticles
   b. pitting of the nail plate
   c. grooves in the nail plate
   d. swelling, redness and pus appearing in the cuticle area of the skin of the nail wall

2. When storing nail products, which legislation acronym applies?

   a. PPE
   b. PUWER
   c. COSHH
   d. RIDDOR

3. A marbling tool can be used:

   a. for creating thick, straight lines
   b. where detail is required
   c. to sweep products across the nail
   d. to apply dots

4. A contra-action allergy will normally affect:

   a. the nail plate
   b. the nail bed
   c. the free edge
   d. the cuticle

5. A *squoval* nail shape is a:

   a. combination of square and oval shape free edge
   b. rounded free edge
   c. square shape free edge
   d. nail plate that becomes broader at the free edge

6. Foil is applied to the nail:

   a. pattern side uppermost
   b. pattern side facing down

7. Polish secures 'cut with facets to reflect light' are referred to as:

   a. flatstones
   b. rhinestones
   c. stone shapes
   d. flat backed beads

8. The crescent shaped part of the nail which can be defined when painting the nails is called the:

   a. lunula
   b. mantle
   c. leuconychia
   d. free edge

9. To maintain the appearance of the nail art, what should the client apply at home?

   a. base coat
   b. top coat

10. Which of the following conditions would prevent nail art from proceeding?

    a. diabetes
    b. product allergies
    c. scar tissue
    d. severe onycholysis

15 Waxing Treatments

LEARNING OBJECTIVES

There are two learning outcomes for this optional unit which you must achieve:

1 Be able to prepare for waxing treatments.

2 Be able to provide waxing treatments.

From the range statement you must show you can:

◆ Use consultation techniques to identify the treatment objectives.

◆ Carry out the necessary tests before treatment.

◆ Use all the listed products, tools and equipment as appropriate.

◆ Ensure the environmental conditions are suitable.

◆ Use hot, warm and roller wax hair removal methods.

◆ Describe alternative methods of hair removal and their effects on the skin.

◆ Complete a consultation and skin inspection to identify any contra-indications that may affect if and how the treatment can proceed.

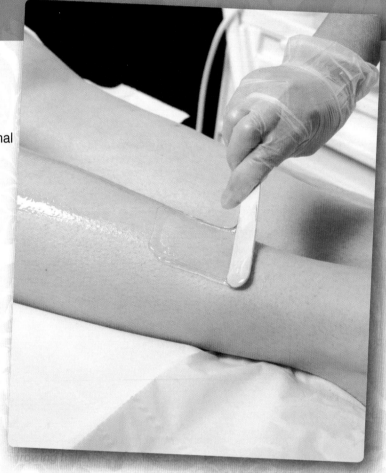

◆ Communicate and behave in an appropriate and professional manner.

◆ Follow all health and safety working practices.

◆ Adapted treatments to suit all skin types and conditions.

◆ Provide relevant aftercare and contra-action advice.

KEY TERMS

after-wax lotions
aftercare advice
anagen
burns
catagen
cold wax
consultation
contra-action advice
contra-actions
contra-indications
depilatory creams
disposable applicator
electrolysis
environmental conditions
erythema
folliculitis
hair growth cycle

hairy moles
health and safety
heat rash
heat sensitivity skin test
histamine
hot wax
ingrowing hair
IPL (intense pulse light)
laser hair removal
photothermolysis
pre-wax lotion
razoring
roller wax
skin conditions
skin removal
skin sensitivity patch test
skin tags

skin types
strip sugar
sugar paste
sugaring
superfluous hair
tactile skin sensation test
telogen
terminal hair
threading
treatment objectives
treatment plan
varicose veins
vellus hair
warm wax
wax depilation
waxing products

Unit Topic

Remove hair using waxing techniques
This VRQ unit is linked to the Beauty Therapy NOS Unit B6.

INTRODUCTION

This unit is all about how to remove facial and body hair temporarily using appropriate wax removal products and techniques for the skin type, hair type, growth and area including hot wax, warm wax and roller methods. Areas for hair removal include the eyebrows, face, forearms, under arms, legs and for female clients the bikini line area. Aftercare advice is an important part of this treatment which the client should follow to ensure skin healing and to prevent possible infection.

Dealing with people in a polite, efficient manner and using good communication and questioning skills to find out exactly what they require from the waxing treatment forms an important part of this technical service.

You must be able to show you have the necessary practical skills and underpinning knowledge to remove hair using waxing techniques.

INDUSTRY ROLE MODEL

JANICE BROWN Director Hof Beauty Ltd.

"As director of Hof Beauty Ltd, one of the leading suppliers to the Beauty industry, I am privileged to meet some amazing beauty therapists who build fantastic businesses. The common factors to success are passion, learning and determination.

My career journey included: therapist, managing single and groups of salons, sales, teaching and training. I am author of the *Encyclopedia of Hair Removal* and *Practical Electrolysis*. I can honestly say that I have loved every single role.

My greatest passion remains hair removal; it is both emotionally and financially rewarding – people will not in the foreseeable future want to have excess hair!"

ANATOMY & PHYSIOLOGY
Essential anatomy and physiology knowledge requirements for this chapter are identified on the checklist chart on page 33.

Hair removal methods

Hair removal is a popular treatment in the beauty salon, where both temporary and permanent methods of removal are usually available. Temporary removal must be repeated regularly, as the removed hair will regrow. With permanent methods, the client needs to visit the salon regularly, initially to have the hair removed; thereafter, the part of the hair responsible for its growth has been destroyed and the hair will not grow again (see the hair growth diagram on page 68).

Knowledge Check

What are the three stages of the hair cycle? Briefly explain what happens to the hair at each stage.

Temporary methods of hair removal

Depilatory waxing to the bikini area using warm wax, spatula method

Depilatory waxing Wax depilation, using a warm wax, hot wax or cold wax, involves applying wax to the treatment area and embedding the hairs in it. When the wax is removed from the area, the hairs are removed at their roots so the regrowth is of completely new hairs with soft, fine-tapered tips. They grow again in approximately 4 weeks.

Plucking Plucking or tweezing uses a pair of tweezers to remove the hair. These grasp the hair near the surface of the skin, and the hair is then plucked in the direction of growth, again removing it at its root. The hair grows again in approximately 4 weeks.

Due to the sensitive nature of the eye tissue, tweezing is often considered the most suitable choice for temporary hair removal from eyebrows.

Depilatory waxing using roller wax method

Plucking may be used after waxing to remove the hairs too short for the wax to remove or to remove specific hairs, i.e. to define the final brow shape following eyebrow wax hair removal.

Plucking or tweezing hair following eyebrow wax hair removal

Some clients may use an electrical depilatory device, which performs the function of mass plucking. As the device is moved over the skin's surface, hairs are grasped and removed. This does not consider the way the hair grows and therefore can be problematic when the hair regrows as it can lead to distortion of the hair follicle affecting the way the hairs lie when they regrow; hair breakage and ingrowing hairs may also occur.

Threading Threading involves the use of a thread of twisted cotton, which is rolled over the area from which the hair is to be removed: the hairs catch in the cotton, and are pulled out. This skill is frequently practised by people of Asian or Mediterranean origin. See Chapter 9, for more information on this technique.

Waxing, plucking and threading removes the entire hair, including the visible hair above the skin's surface (the hair shaft) and the part that cannot be seen in the hair follicle.

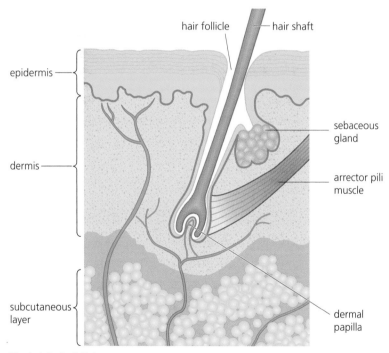

The hair in its follicle

ACTIVITY

Hair removal

Make short notes on the advantages and disadvantages of the different methods of hair removal available.

Threading eyebrow hair

Other methods of hair removal

There are other methods of hair removal that the client may have used at home. At the client **consultation** it is important to find out which method of hair removal the client has used previously and discuss suitability. If a client chooses waxing as their preferred hair

Electrolysis

Laser hair removal

removal method, temporary methods such as those discussed later should stop being used unless recommended by the beauty therapist.

◆ *Cutting the hairs with scissors* Scissors are used to trim the hair close to the skin's surface. This does not affect hair growth as only the dead hair above the skin's surface, the hair shaft, is removed. The hair, however, is left with a blunt end and feels stubbly. This leaves the skin hair-free for a very short time, usually only 1 to 2 days, dependent upon the client's hair growth.

◆ *Shaving* A razor blade is stroked over the skin, against the natural hair growth after the skin has been prepared with a suitable skin lubricant such as shaving foam or oil. This removes the hair at the skin's surface. This leaves the skin hair free for a very short time, usually only 1 to 2 days, dependent upon the client's hair growth. The hair feels sharp as it grows because the hair is left with a blunt end. Shaving is unsuitable for sensitive, thinner areas of skin such as the eyebrow area. Accidental damage to the skin can result in skin scarring.

◆ *Depilatory cream* A strong alkaline chemical cream containing ammonium thioglycolate is applied to the hair, and removed after 5 to 10 minutes: the hair will have been dissolved at the skin's surface. As the chemical is strong enough to dissolve the hair protein keratin, it can sometimes cause skin irritation as the skin contains keratin too.

◆ *Abrasive mitt* An abrasive glove is rubbed against the skin and the hair is broken off at the skin's surface. The result and its effectiveness are similar to shaving and is unsuitable for a sensitive skin as the skin can become reddened quickly and become more sensitive.

Permanent methods of hair removal

Electrical current methods Galvanic electrolysis, electrical epilation and the blend epilation technique are all techniques that use an electrical current. The current is passed to the hair root via a fine needle inserted into the hair follicle. The current destroys the hair root, preventing hair regrowth.

HEALTH & SAFETY

Laser hair removal Registration with the Care Quality Commission (CQC – www.cqc.org.uk) is a requirement to practise laser hair removal.

Part of their remit is to drive up quality of health care and they have a wide range of enforcement powers.

Laser hair removal Laser energy works by producing light at various wavelengths, energy output and pulse widths. It is passed through the epidermis of the skin, which stops the activity of the hair follicle creating hair growth through a process called photothermolysis. The melanin pigment that provides hair colour absorbs the laser energy that is converted to heat, which at a sufficient temperature destroys the part of the hair follicle where the cells divide to create the hair.

The more melanin, the more destruction occurs. Therefore, generally laser hair removal works best for light-skinned people with dark hair.

> For waxing treatments, it is important to keep your client warm. If your client becomes cold, the hair follicle will tighten around the hair, making the treatment more uncomfortable and the hair difficult to remove.
>
> If it's a very cold day, at the skin preparation stage briskly rub or massage your client's skin with the preparatory products as this will increase blood supply thereby increasing skin temperature.
>
> *Janice Brown*

HEALTH & SAFETY

Sensitive skin Products are increasingly being formulated which contain only natural ingredients which can reduce skin irritation. Ingredients include sugar and plant extracts such as chamomile and lavender to soothe the skin.

Organic sugar-based hair remover

A course of laser treatments is required. Treatment length will depend on the coarseness of the hair type and the size of the hair follicle. The treatment is most effective when the hair is in the **anagen** (growth) stage of the **hair growth cycle**. Subsequent treatments therefore target different hairs in their anagen stage of growth until all hairs cease to grow.

The client needs to understand that the hair will never grow back if effectively treated with any of the above permanent methods. This is an important consideration when treating the brow hair, as the desired shape and thickness of the brows change frequently under the influence of fashion.

Intense pulsed light Intense pulsed light (IPL) systems work on the same principle as laser; that of absorption of light energy into melanin in the skin and hair. The light energy is converted to heat energy, which causes damage to the specific target area. There are two beams of light, one yellow and one red, which together affect both the existing hair and the follicles where the hair grows. The high-energy light pulses remove the hair.

IPL systems differ to laser in that they can deliver hundreds of wavelengths of light in each burst of light instead of just one wavelength, increasing the area of skin that can be treated. Certain filters are used that target these flashes of light so that they can work in a similar way to lasers.

Hair re-growth

Because of the cyclical nature of hair growth and the fact that follicles will be at different stages of their growth cycle when the hair is removed, the hair will not all grow back at the same time. Waxing, along with threading and plucking, can therefore appear to reduce the *quantity* of hair growth. This is not so, however, and the hair will all grow back eventually; waxing is therefore classed as a temporary form of hair removal.

Nevertheless, certain bodily changes (such as ageing), when *combined* with waxing, can result in permanent hair removal. This effect is so erratic and unpredictable, though, that waxing cannot reliably be sold as a permanent method of hair removal. Occasionally hair re-growth will increase, which is not a normal reaction and may be related to medication being taken or the medical health of the client. That is why it is important to carry out a thorough consultation before waxing treatment is provided. Waxing is unsuitable as a hair removal method in this instance.

ACTIVITY

Methods of hair removal

As well at the professional use of depilatory waxing, threading and plucking, other methods of temporary hair removal include the home use of plucking, cold wax using ready-waxed strips, sugaring, electrical devices, chemical depilatory creams, shaving and pumice powder. Find out how each method works to remove the hair shaft and assess its effectiveness. Are any of them potentially hazardous?

Preparing for waxing

Outcome 1: Be able to prepare for waxing treatments

Learn how to prepare for waxing treatments

PRACTICAL SKILLS

Prepare yourself, client and work area for a waxing treatment

Use suitable consultation techniques to identify treatment objectives

Carry out necessary tests prior to the treatment

Provide clear recommendations to the client

Select products, tools and equipment to suit client treatment needs

UNDERPINNING KNOWLEDGE

Describe salon requirements for preparing yourself, the client and work area

State the environmental conditions suitable for waxing treatments

Describe different consultation techniques used to identify treatment objectives

Describe the types of tests that are carried out prior to waxing treatment

Describe how to select products, tools and equipment to suit client treatment needs

Identify the different types of waxing methods and products available

State the advantages and disadvantages of alternative methods of hair removal

Describe the effects alternative methods of hair removal may have on the skin and waxing treatments

Describe the contra-indications which prevent or restrict waxing treatments

Preparing the work area

Check the suitability of the **environmental conditions** in the work area.

To enable the hairs to be removed effectively, the treatment area should be well lit; a magnifying lamp may be available to assist observation of the area. It must also be warm, as the client must be made as comfortable as possible when performing the treatment. If the client is cold, the hair follicles will restrict, making hair removal more difficult. Ensure ventilation is adequate to remove odours and remove humid air, providing sufficient air movement to keep the air fresh.

Before the client is shown through to the work area its contents should be checked to ensure that they are clean and tidy. The bins should have been emptied following the previous client.

Check the trolley to ensure that you have all that you need for carrying out the treatment and that it is suitably positioned to prevent unnecessary stretching or walking which will affect commercial timing and could cause RSI. The wax should be of a suitable consistency, i.e. ready for application.

The plastic-covered couch should be clean, having previously been washed with hot soapy water and wiped thoroughly with a disinfectant which is bactericidal, fungicidal and virucidal. The use of an additional heavy-duty plastic sheet is recommended: this is easier to wipe than the couch, and can be replaced if damaged.

All disinfectable surfaces must be disinfected after thorough cleaning between treatments.

The couch should then be covered and protected with a long strip of paper-tissue bedroll. Place a towel(s) neatly on the couch, ready to protect the client's clothing and to cover them, protecting modesty, when they have undressed. These tend to be of a medium size as large towels can make the client too warm. The tissue should be disposed of after use, and the towel freshly laundered for each client.

The couch should be in the sit-up position, unless the client is only having their bikini line or underarm areas waxed, in which case it should be flat.

Before beginning the waxing treatment, check that you have the necessary products, tools and equipment to hand and that they meet legal hygiene and industry requirements. Metal tools such as scissors and tweezers should be sterilized in an autoclave prior to use.

> " Waxing is one of, if not the most popular treatments on offer in most salons. Clients therefore have a vast choice of salons. By creating the right atmosphere, giving excellent service and paying attention to details you will encourage the client to return to YOUR salon.
>
> *Janice Brown*

Types of wax product

Warm wax This first became available in 1975 and remains the market leader for hair removal, its advantage being it is clean and easy to use.

Warm wax is used at a low temperature, around 43°C, so there is little risk of skin burning, and in less sensitive areas the wax can be re-applied once or even twice if necessary.

Warm wax does not set but remains soft at body temperature. It adheres efficiently to hairs and is quick to use; treatment is relatively pain-free. It can remove even very short hairs (2.5 mm) from legs, arms, underarms, the bikini line, the torso, the face and the neck.

Warm wax

Warm waxes are frequently made of mixtures of glucose syrup, resin to help the wax stick, oil to help removal (e.g. almond oil), water and fragrances. Honey (fructose syrup) can be used instead of glucose syrup and this formulation is often called honey wax. Zinc oxide is added to cream wax to provide an opaque colour. This type of warm wax is capable of providing a thin, liquid consistency at lower temperatures making it less sensitizing to the skin.

Hot wax This takes longer to heat than warm wax, and is relatively slow to use, taking approximately double the time of a warm waxing. This time reduces when skill is attained.

As hot wax is used at quite a high temperature, 50°C, extra care must be taken to avoid accidental **burns**. Because of this risk, hot wax cannot be re-applied to already treated areas.

Hot wax cools on contact with the skin. It contracts around the hair shaft, gripping it firmly. This makes it ideal for use on stronger, short hairs.

Hot wax (discs)

Strip sugar wax

Hot waxes for hair removal need to be a blend of waxes and resins so that they stay reasonably flexible when cool. Beeswax is a desirable ingredient, and often comprises 25–60 per cent of the finished product.

Cetiol, azulene and vitamin E are often added to wax preparations to soothe the skin and minimize possible skin reactions.

Cold wax

This is already applied to a strip. The pre-coated strip is applied firmly to the area of skin for hair removal and then removed quickly against hair growth. The hair sticks to the wax and is removed as the wax strip is removed, against hair growth.

Sugar wax

There are two methods of sugar wax hair removal – **sugar paste** and **strip sugar**.

Sugar paste is applied to the skin, using the hands, in the direction of hair growth. The hairs embed in the wax, which is then removed swiftly against hair growth, removing the hairs. This method is ideal for a sensitive skin as the wax does not stick tightly to the skin. On removal it will remove surface loose skin cells with the hair, improving overall skin appearance.

Strip sugar is similar in application and removal to warm wax and requires a wax removal strip to remove the wax, against hair growth. Sugar wax has pure sugar as the main ingredient, plus other natural ingredients such as lemon. Resins may be added to help skin adherence.

When choosing a wax, select one with the following qualities:

- it should be easy to remove from equipment
- it should be able to remove short, strong hairs (2.5 mm)
- it should have a pleasant fragrance or no smell
- it should not stick to the skin, but only to the hair
- wherever possible, it should be suitable for all **skin types** including sensitive skin type and all facial and body areas. Although it is common to have different waxing products to suit the removal of different hair strengths.

Trolley prepared

TOP TIP

Accommodating clients with disabilities

Hydraulic couches are effective as they enable clients with mobility problems easier access onto the couch. Always tactfully confirm, prior to the treatment where possible, if there are any special mobility considerations and these can be prepared for.

Products, tools and equipment

◆ **Couch** With sit-up and lie-down positions and an easy-to-clean surface

◆ **Trolley** To hold all the necessary products, tools and equipment

◆ **Disposable wooden spatulas (a selection of differing sizes)** For use on different body areas

◆ **Wax-removal strips** Thick enough that the wax does not soak through, but flexible enough for ease of work. These strips should be cut to size and placed ready in a container. These may be paper or muslin

◆ **Cotton wool** For cleaning equipment and applying various skin soothing/cleansing preparations

◆ **Tissues (white)** For blotting skin dry and protecting the client's clothing in the area

◆ **Anti-bacterial skin cleanser** (Also known as pre-wax lotion) or professional antiseptic wipes

◆ **Wax heater** With a thermostatic control, a lid and a central bar for spatula methods

◆ **Tweezers** For removing stray hairs following wax depilation or defining the brow shape following a brow waxing treatment

◆ **Single-use disposable synthetic powder-free gloves** To comply with Personal Protective Equipment (PPE) at Work Regulations and ensure a high standard of hygiene and to reduce the possibility of contamination

◆ **Waste container** This should be a lined metal bin with a lid. Specific disposable bags may be required for contaminated waste

◆ **Hand disinfectant** To clean hands before each waxing treatment

YOU WILL ALSO NEED:

◆ **Magnifying lamp** To provide additional assistance when observing the area of hair removal

◆ **Disposable tissue couch roll** Disposable consumable placed over the couch cover prior to each treatment to prevent the client sticking to the couch cover and for reasons of hygiene

◆ **Protective plastic couch cover** A durable covering which can be cleaned with a disinfectant agent before each client treatment. It is then covered with disposable tissue roll

◆ **Professional talcum powder** Or alternative talc free powder formulation to avoid allergic responses in some clients. To absorb body perspiration and to facilitate hair removal

◆ **Disposable panties** These may be provided when carrying out bikini waxing

◆ **Surgical spirit** Or a commercial cleaner designed for cleaning waxing equipment

◆ **Towels (medium-sized)** For draping around the client

◆ **Small scissors** For trimming over-long hairs

◆ **Disinfecting solution** In which to immerse small metal tools following sterilization in the autoclave. This must be changed regularly as stated in manufacturer's instructions

◆ **Wax** A choice to suit skin types and conditions and hair types

◆ **After-wax lotion** With soothing, healing and antiseptic qualities

◆ **Mirror (clean)** For facial waxing treatments

◆ **Apron** To comply with Personal Protective Equipment (PPE) at Work Regulations and protect work wear from spillages

◆ **Client record card** Confidential card recording details of each client registered at the salon, to include personal details, products used and details of the treatment

◆ **Aftercare leaflets** Recommended advice for the client to refer to following treatment

> Selling is a vital part of the role of a beauty therapist. It is important that the client gets the right treatment and products in order to get the results they are after. Clients do not buy our treatments or products, they buy the benefits and results. It is your job to help them imagine how using the products and treatments will make them look and feel. Remember that we all hate to be sold to but love to buy; so practise and perfect your selling skills.
>
> *Janice Brown*

ACTIVITY

Wax heaters

Research using current beauty trade magazines, online manufacturers/suppliers, visits to wholesale suppliers or tradeshows for at least five different types of wax heater and applicators. Where possible, try to see demonstrations of them working. Discuss their suitability in terms of size (important if to be transported), design features, cleaning practicalities, safety features, hygiene and any other points that you think are important. Which heater would you choose and why?

TOP TIP

After-wax lotions

After-wax lotions reduce redness and promote skin healing. They contain ingredients such as tea tree, aloe vera, azulene and witch hazel. These are an ideal retail product to recommend to your client to ensure effective skin healing.

ACTIVITY

Safe storage of related products

How should flammable products used in the waxing treatment be stored? Consider the environmental conditions also.

Disposable applicator warm wax system

HEALTH & SAFETY

Avoiding cross-infection Never filter hot wax after use: it cannot be used again as it will be contaminated with skin cells, tissue fluid, and perhaps even blood.

ACTIVITY

Electrical testing

How can you ensure that your wax heater is safe to use?

What checks should you make before use?

How can you ensure you comply with the Electricity at Work Regulations (1989)?

Sterilization and disinfection

Disposable waste from waxing may have body fluids on it: potentially it is a health risk. It must be handled, collected and disposed of according to the local Environmental Health Regulations. It is a requirement to wear disposable gloves while carrying out bikini and underarm wax treatments, to protect yourself from body fluids and the client from contamination. Care should be taken when removing the gloves to prevent contamination. These too should be disposed of after each waxing treatment. Wash your hands regularly with anti-bacterial soap, before and after preparing the work area and before application of the disposable gloves. This shows the client that you have a high standard of hygiene.

An apron should be worn for reasons of hygiene and to protect work wear from wax spillage.

HEALTH & SAFETY

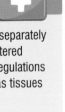

Contaminated waste Any wax waste that contains bodily fluids should be bagged separately from other regular waste and special arrangements made for its disposal by a registered waste carrier in an approved incinerator in accordance with the Controlled Waste Regulations (1992). This may include spatulas, wax strips and wax waste, consumables such as tissues and cotton wool, disposable underwear, aprons and tissue couch roll.

All metal tools should be sterilized in the autoclave before use. This includes tweezers and scissors.

After the waxing treatment they must be replaced and re-sterilized.

Increasingly systems which minimize the risk of cross-infection are being adopted. These include single use tubes and cartridges using disposable applicator heads.

TOP TIP

Habia guidance

See the Habia *Hygiene in Beauty Therapy* booklet for further guidance to hygiene best practice. Also check the Habia website www.habia.org for specifications and updates.

ACTIVITY

Maintaining hygiene

Spreading wax on the client and dipping the used spatula back into the tub with the spatula method creates the possibility of cross-infection between clients. How can cross-infection be avoided, with this method and the use of roll-on wax applicators?

Reception

When the client is booking their treatment they should be asked whether they have had a wax treatment before in the salon. If they have not, a small area of waxing should be carried out as a skin sensitivity patch test, to ensure that the client is not sensitive to the technique or allergic to any of the ingredients contained in the product. If the sensitivity test, commonly referred to as a patch test, causes an unwanted reaction within 48 hours, then the treatment must not be carried out. Unwanted reactions include excessive redness, irritation and swelling, referred to as **contra-actions**.

> " When carrying out a consultation for waxing treatments always consider the client's social, work and holiday commitments; this will enable you to get the best result at the right time for the client.
>
> *Janice Brown*

Wear disposable gloves when carrying out waxing treatments

Treatment	Warm waxing (minutes)	Hot waxing (minutes)
Half leg	20–30	30
Half leg and bikini	30	45
Full leg	50	60
Full leg and bikini	60	60–70
Bikini	15	15–20
Underarm	10–15	15–20
Half arm	10–15	15–20
Full arm	20–30	20–30
Top lip	5	5–10
Chin and throat	10	15–20
Top lip and chin	15	15–20
Eyebrows	10–15	15

HEALTH & SAFETY

Couch covers If the salon chooses to use stretch-towelling couch covers or additional towels to provide extra comfort, these must be provided clean for each client and laundered in hot soapy water at a temperature of 60°C after use.

Wear disposable gloves when carrying out waxing treatments

Advise the client not to apply any lotions or oils to the area on the day of the treatment– these could prevent the adhesion of the wax to the hairs being removed. Ask them also to allow at least 1 week, and preferably 2, between any home shaving or other depilatory treatment and a salon waxing treatment. This is to let the hairs grow to a length sufficient to be waxed.

When a client makes an appointment for a wax depilation treatment, the receptionist should advise the client how long the treatment will take.

It is important to complete the treatment in the time allowed in order to be efficient in treatment application and to ensure the appointment schedule runs smoothly and clients are not kept waiting.

Knowledge Check

Following waxing treatment how should the waste be disposed of?

Refer to page 530 to help you.

ALWAYS REMEMBER

Treatment of minors

Check the salon's insurance guidelines relating to age restrictions for waxing treatment. Check age restrictions in your area (note that in England a minor is under 18, whereas in Scotland it is 16) – refer to current guidance.

ALWAYS REMEMBER

Client record card

Accurately record your client's answers to necessary questions to be asked at consultation on the record card. This is necessary for future reference.

Inform them briefly what the waxing treatment will involve so that they have an understanding of what will be required from them. This will help clients who have not received the more intimate wax removal treatments, i.e. to the underarms and bikini area, to relax.

> Waxing removes the dead skin cells from the surface of the skin and as a consequence will lighten natural tans and may completely remove some self tans. You must advise your clients of this effect as they may then choose to delay treatment.
>
> *Janice Brown*

Allow a 4- to 6-week interval between successive wax depilation appointments. Following set intervals between waxing treatments will improve the effectiveness of the treatment as this will follow the hair growth cycle. The times to be allowed for wax treatments are as shown in the table previously mentioned. However, repeat bookings vary according to the natural hair re-growth and client requirements.

All staff, especially the staff communicating with clients at reception, should be familiar with the different pricing structures for the range of waxing treatments and products available for retail.

Minors (clients under 18 years of age in England; 16 in Scotland) must be accompanied by a parent/guardian who will be required to sign a consent form for treatment to proceed.

Consultation

A consultation must be performed for all clients who have not received the treatment before or are new clients to you. Discuss what methods of hair removal have been used before and when they were last used. Discuss the known sensitivity of the client's skin. If the client is taking any medication that causes skin thinning, such as tetracycline, or has received facial chemical peels or retin-A, skin lifting may occur because the wax is designed to stick to the skin before removal. This will result in skin damage so waxing must not be performed. If necessary a skin sensitivity patch test should be provided to assess tolerance. A positive reaction where there is redness, irritation or swelling means that the treatment cannot proceed. A negative reaction means that it can. Maintain client privacy at all times during the consultation. Explain what is involved with the method of hair removal technique to be used, the expected costs, sensations, treatment reactions and aftercare requirements.

It is a good idea to discuss the hair growth cycle with the client using a visual aid. This will help the client to understand that hairs that grow through following hair removal were at a different stage of the hair growth cycle and were below the skin's surface at the time of the treatment. It also is beneficial to support the need for regular intervals between waxing appointments as hairs will be at a similar hair growth pattern.

Immediately following hair removal, the skin becomes slightly red around the follicle where the hair has been removed. There may also be slight swelling of the skin in the area. This will soon disappear following treatment, but will vary according to skin sensitivity and hair strength and the quantity of hair that has been removed. Occasionally spot bleeding may occur where a particularly strong hair has been removed, usually when in the anagen stage where it is receiving blood from the dermal papilla resulting in capillary damage. This too may be explained at consultation.

> " Consultation is the key to a successful treatment. You may be asking yourself why you need to consult your client, you may feel you already know what they want, or see it as a card filling exercise, so you should just get them on the couch and get started. However, you'd be wrong. Consultation is your opportunity to gain the information you need to enable you to give a safe effective treatment. Learn exactly what your client wants and needs, in order to sell them the suitable products and treatments. It is also your opportunity to impress potential clients with your knowledge and professionalism to ensure they build a trust in you and become a regular customer.
>
> *Janice Brown*

Invite the client to ask questions. It is important that they understand fully what the treatment includes.

Advise the client following the consultation and completion of the record card of the most appropriate method of waxing temporary hair removal having considered the type of hair (vellus/terminal) and amount, and the sensitivity of the skin.

Contra-indications

When a client attends for a wax depilation treatment, the beauty therapist should always check that there are no **contra-indications** that might prevent treatment.

Certain medical conditions or medications and hormonal changes in the body such as those that occur at pregnancy, puberty and menopause can affect hair growth, causing an increase, so it is important to discuss the hair growth observed in the area to be removed with the client. This will confirm client suitability for treatment. Types of hair growth and factors affecting hair growth are discussed on page 69.

If the client has any of the following, wax depilation must not be carried out:

◆ *skin conditions* such as thin and fragile skin

◆ *skin disorders* such as severe eczema or psoriasis

◆ *eye disorders* such as conjunctivitis when treating the face

◆ *swellings* – the cause may be medical

◆ *diabetes* – a client with this condition is vulnerable to infection as they have slow skin healing

◆ *defective circulation* – poor skin healing, burning and infection may occur. This may be a symptom of conditions such as diabetes, heart disease and multiple sclerosis

◆ *recent scar tissue (under under 6-months old)* – the skin lacks elasticity

◆ *broken bones*

◆ *fractures or sprains* – discomfort may occur

◆ *phlebitis* – an inflammatory condition of the vein

◆ *retin-A, tetracycline medication* – the skin is more sensitive, delicate and prone to skin irritation and tearing

◆ *recent exfoliation treatments* – including micro-dermabrasion

TOP TIP

Describing the sensation

Here are some useful explanatory phrases: 'It's a bit like quickly ripping a plaster off and taking the hairs with it.' 'It isn't so bad, or so many people wouldn't have it done time and time again!' 'The skin looks and feels great after hair removal, making any possible discomfort experienced worthwhile!'

TOP TIP

Examples of waxing treatment modification

◆ Hair removal around contra-indications that restrict treatment (such as hairy moles and skin tags).

◆ Altering the choice of wax to suit skin sensitivity and hair type.

◆ *loss of skin sensation* – the client would be unable to identify if the wax was too hot

◆ *scar tissue* – under 6-months old

◆ *allergies to products* – such as the ingredient resin, an ingredient found in wax.

Name	Description
Bruising	Injury to an area causes blood to leak from damaged blood vessels. Bruises may swell, appearing dark purple or blue at first and then turn, brown, green or yellow as they fade
Folliculitis	A bacterial infection where pustules develop in the skin tissue around the hair follicle
Severe varicose veins	Veins are vessels that carry blood away from the body tissues and back to the heart. Veins have valves to prevent backflow as they carry blood under low blood pressure back towards the heart. If valves become weak and their elasticity is lost, it becomes a *varicose vein*. The area appears knotted, swollen and bluish-purple in colour

Certain contra-indications restrict treatment application. This may mean that the treatment has to be adapted for the client. For example, in the case of a small, localized bruise the area could be avoided.

Other contra-indications that restrict treatment include:

◆ *Cuts* – secondary infection could occur.

◆ *Mild skin disorders* – such as psoriasis or eczema and skin tags.

◆ *Abrasions* – secondary infection could occur.

◆ *Self tan* – waxing will remove the surface skin cells and the chemically tanned skin.

◆ *Bruises* – client discomfort may be caused and the condition made worse.

◆ *Sunburn* – the skin is damaged and there is excessive heat in the area due to acute over-exposure to the sun.

◆ *Varicose veins* (non-severe) – avoid the area.

◆ *Moles* – avoid wax application to the area.

◆ *Ingrowing hairs* – the area should be avoided as the hair will not be removed; additionally, infection commonly occurs at the site of an ingrowing hair, leading to folliculitis.

Further contra-indications that prevent waxing treatment

Name	Description
Heat rash	A reaction to heat exposure where the sweat ducts become blocked and sweat escapes into the epidermis. Red pimples occur and the skin becomes itchy
Warts and verrucas	Small epidermal skin growths. Warts may be raised or flat, depending upon their position. Usually they have a rough surface and are raised
Hairy moles	Moles exhibiting coarse hairs from their surface. Hair growing from a mole may be cut, not plucked: if plucked, the hairs will become coarser and the growth of the hairs further stimulated
Skin tags	Skin-coloured threads of skin 3–6 mm long, projecting from the skin's surface. Skin tags often occur under the arms

HEALTH & SAFETY

Precaution if there is a restrictive contra-indication present If there is a hairy mole, skin tag or small abrasion you may apply petroleum jelly to avoid wax adherence.

Petroleum application to a skin tag in the bikini line area. Contact with the skin tag must be avoided

TOP TIP

Tanned clients

Waxing a client with a recent well-established suntan may cause the loose sun-damaged epidermis to peel and be lost, along with the hair. Inform the client of this at consultation. This information is also applicable to a client who has recently had a self-tanning treatment.

Knowledge Check

What are the necessary environmental conditions required for waxing? Consider lighting, heating and ventilation in your answer.

Refer to pages 526–527 to help you.

TOP TIP

Bruising

If there is any bruising on the client's legs, tactfully draw their attention to these bruises, or they might later think that the treatment has caused them.

Knowledge Check

How often should a client have waxing treatments?

Refer to page 532 to help you.

Refer to page 532 to help you.

HEALTH & SAFETY

Contra-actions If a contra-action, an unwanted reaction during treatment occurs, discontinue the treatment and provide appropriate advice.

TOP TIP

Sensitive skin

Waxing products designed for sensitive skin are available. It is a good idea to have such products available to accommodate all skin types.

Wax for sensitive skin

Coiled ingrowing hair

TOP TIP

Habia skin safety awareness

Remember your role in helping your client stay safe by informing them of any mole that appears to have changed in size, shape or colour. See www.habia.org

Contra-actions

Inform the client at consultation of any contra-actions that may occur and the action to take.

A contra-action is an unwanted reaction to a waxing treatment which may occur during or following the treatment.

Contra-actions which are quite common with waxing include:

- *Ingrowing hairs.*
- *Removal of skin.*
- *Burns* – caused by both excessive wax temperature and friction burns.
- *Excessive erythema* – increased blood flow to the skin, causing an extreme redness.

Ingrowing hairs Ingrowing hairs can arise in three ways:

- *Over-reaction to damage* An excessive reaction by the skin and the follicle to the 'damage' produced by depilation may cause extra cornified cells to be made. These may block the surface of the follicle, causing the newly growing hair to turn around and grow inwards.

- *Overtight clothing* If after the treatment the client wears clothing that is too tight, this too can block the follicle.

- *Dry skin* Likewise dry skin can cause blockage of the follicle.

Ingrowing hairs can usually be recognized to be one or other of three types:

- *A hair growing along beneath the surface of the skin* Identify the tip (the pointed end); then pierce the tissues over the root end with a sterile needle. Free the tip and leave it in place so that the follicle can heal around it.

- *A coiled ingrowing hair* This looks like a small black spot or dome on the skin. If this is gently squeezed and rolled between the fingertips, using a tissue, it will release the coiled ingrowing hair and some hardened sebum. If the hair does not fall out, it should be left in place (as above).

- *An infected ingrowth* If the trapped sebum or hair starts to decay, either of the two preceding forms can become infected or begin to display an immune response. The area first becomes red (irritation); then an infected white dome-shaped pustule develops. Release the trapped tissue (as above), and cover the affected area – which may bleed, or leak tissue fluid – with a sterile non-allergenic dressing.

Skin removal If the upper, dead, protective cornified layer of the skin is accidentally removed during a treatment – leaving the granular layer of the living, germinative layer exposed – the skin should be treated as if it has been burnt. This is often a result of poor removal techniques such as not holding the skin sufficiently taut or lifting the wax too high rather than parallel to the skin. This can also occur as a result of the client having used exfoliating skin medications, cortisone steroid medications and recent exfoliating beauty treatments such as micro-dermabrasion. Cool the area immediately by applying cold-water compresses for 10 minutes. Dry it carefully; then apply a dry, non-fluffy dressing to protect the area from infection. The dressing should be worn for 3 to 4 days, and the area then left open to the air. (Antiseptic cream by itself should be used only when the injury is very minor.) Medical attention should be sought if necessary.

Burns A burn should be treated the same as for 'skin removal'. If blisters form, they should not be broken – they help prevent the entry of infection into the wound. Medical attention should be sought. Always remember the importance of testing the wax temperature on yourself and the client before treatment commences and make ongoing checks throughout the treatment.

Erythema Erythema is a visible redness which is a normal reaction to skin waxing treatment. If excessive, it will be accompanied by an increase in warmth on the surface of the skin. This is created by an increased blood flow through the capillaries near the surface of the skin, caused by the histamine reaction after waxing. Ask the client to follow the recommended aftercare advice.

Certain waxing ingredients such as rosin, a resin, may cause an allergic reaction in some people.

The symptoms of an allergic reaction could be:

◆ redness of the skin (erythema) ◆ itching

◆ swelling ◆ blisters.

Poor hygiene practice such as inadequate skin cleansing, application of aftercare lotion infecting the area of treatment and non-compliance by the client with aftercare instructions may result in bacterial infection seen as erythema and pustules in the area.

If an allergic reaction occurs during waxing application, stop treatment and remove any remaining product. Apply a cool compress and soothing agent to the area to reduce redness and irritation. Identify the possible cause of the allergic reaction. If symptoms persist, seek medical advice.

Always record any allergies on the client's record card, so that the offending product may be avoided in the future. Try an alternative waxing product to assess skin tolerance. In some cases the skin is too sensitive and intolerant to waxing treatment.

Always date and record any contra-actions on the client record card, with actions taken/recommendations provided and outcome.

After the record card has been completed, the client should be asked to read the list of contra-indications and sign to state that they are not suffering from any of the problems stated.

The beauty therapist must not carry out a wax treatment immediately after a heat treatment, such as a sauna, or steam or UV treatments, as the heat-sensitized tissues may be irritated by the wax treatment.

If you are unsure if treatment may commence, tactfully refer the client to their general practitioner for permission to treat. A copy of the GP's letter on receipt should be kept with the client's record card. If the treatment cannot be carried out for any reason, always explain why, without naming a contra-indication, as you are not qualified to do so. Clients will respect your professional advice.

ALWAYS REMEMBER

Reactions to treatment

Damage to the skin that occurs during a waxing treatment causes cells called *mast cells* to burst in the skin releasing a chemical substance called histamine. Histamine is released into the tissues causing the blood capillaries to dilate, giving the redness called erythema. The increased blood flow limits damage and begins repair. There can also be an increase in keratinized cells in the area seen as flaky patches of skin as the skin heals.

Normal erythema skin reaction following leg wax hair removal

TOP TIP

Contra-indications

While assessing the client's skin for waxing treatment, you should also be looking for contra-indications to treatment.

ACTIVITY

Ensuring client comfort

Imagine that you are a client who has never had a waxing treatment before. You are shown through to a cubicle and left to 'Get yourself ready, please'. How would you feel? What would you do? What clothing would you think it necessary to remove for each area of waxing?

If the client had mobility issues identified at consultation how could you prepare the work area to accommodate this need?

Following the consultation an appropriate **treatment plan** will be confirmed with the client. Their understanding of the treatment is important to ensure that their needs are met and that they will not be disappointed.

Record all client details accurately on the client record card. A sample record card follows.

Sample client record card

Date	Beauty therapist name
Client name	Date of birth (identifying client age group)
Home address	Postcode
Email address	Landline phone number · Mobile phone number
Name of doctor	Doctor's address and phone number
Related medical history (Conditions that may restrict or prohibit treatment application)	
Are you taking any medication? (This may affect the sensitivity and skin reaction following treatment.)	

CONTRA-INDICATIONS REQUIRING MEDICAL REFERRAL
(Preventing hair removal treatment.)

- ☐ bacterial infection (e.g. impetigo, conjunctivitis)
- ☐ viral infection (e.g. herpes simplex/warts)
- ☐ fungal infection (e.g. tinea corporis)
- ☐ severe skin conditions
- ☐ diabetes
- ☐ severe varicose veins
- ☐ phlebitis
- ☐ deep vein thrombosis
- ☐ client is undergoing chemotherapy or radiotherapy treatment

TEST CONDUCTED

- ☐ self ☐ client

WAX PRODUCTS

- ☐ hot wax
- ☐ warm wax – spatula method
- ☐ warm wax disposable applicator/tube/cartridge system
- ☐ strip sugar
- ☐ sugar paste

WORK TECHNIQUES

- ☐ keep the skin taut during application and removal
- ☐ speed of product removal
- ☐ direction and angle of removal
- ☐ ongoing wax product temperature checks

CONTRA-INDICATIONS WHICH RESTRICT TREATMENT
(Treatment may require adaptation.)

- ☐ cuts and abrasions
- ☐ bruising and swelling
- ☐ self tan
- ☐ skin disorders
- ☐ heat rash
- ☐ sunburn
- ☐ hairy moles
- ☐ mild eczema/psoriasis
- ☐ broken bones
- ☐ recent fractures
- ☐ recent scar tissue
- ☐ hyperkeratosis
- ☐ skin and product allergies
- ☐ circulatory conditions

AREAS TREATED FOR HAIR REMOVAL
(Treatment may require adaptation.)

- ☐ eyebrows
- ☐ face
- ☐ upper lip
- ☐ chin
- ☐ legs
- ☐ full leg
- ☐ half leg
- ☐ underarm
- ☐ bikini line

SKIN TYPE

- ☐ normal ☐ oily
- ☐ dry ☐ combination

SKIN CONDITION

- ☐ sensitive ☐ mature ☐ dehydrated

Beauty therapist signature (for reference)
Client signature (confirmation of details)

Sample client record card (continued)

TREATMENT TIMINGS*

Half leg wax – *allow 30 minutes*   Eyebrow wax – *allow 15 minutes*

Full leg wax – *allow 50 minutes*   Facial wax   top lip or chin – *allow 10 minutes*

Bikini wax – *allow 15 minutes*   top lip and chin – *allow 15 minutes*

Underarm wax – *allow 15 minutes*

*Waxing timings may differ according to the system used. Always allow slightly longer when using hot wax.

TREATMENT PLAN

Record relevant details of your treatment and advice provided for future reference.

Ensure the client's records are up-to-date, accurate and fully completed following treatment. Non-compliance may invalidate insurance.

DURING

Monitor:

◆ client's reaction to treatment to confirm suitability.

Note:

◆ any adverse reaction, if any occur.

AFTER

Record:

◆ results of treatment

◆ any modification to treatment application that has occurred

◆ what products have been used in the wax removal treatment

◆ the effectiveness of treatment

◆ any samples provided (review their success at the next appointment).

Advise on:

◆ use of aftercare products following wax removal treatment

◆ maintenance procedures

◆ the recommended time intervals between treatments.

RETAIL OPPORTUNITIES

Advise on:

◆ products that would be suitable for the client to use at home to care for and maintain the treatment area (these include body exfoliation and moisturizing skincare products)

◆ recommendations for further treatments

◆ further products or treatments that the client may or may not have received before.

Note:

◆ any purchase made by the client.

EVALUATION

Record:

◆ comments on the client's satisfaction with the treatment

◆ if poor results are achieved, the reasons why

◆ how you may alter the treatment plan to achieve the required treatment results in the future, if applicable.

HEALTH AND SAFETY

Advise on:

◆ how to care for the area following treatment to avoid an unwanted reaction

◆ avoidance of any activities or product application that may cause a contra-action

◆ appropriate **necessary action** to be taken in the event of an unwanted skin or eye irritation.

CourseMate video: Bikini Waxing

Preparing the client

The client should be shown through to the treatment cubicle, and asked to remove specific items of clothing or accessories in the area as necessary, so that the treatment may be carried out. Disposable briefs may be provided if a bikini wax treatment is to be received.

If it is the first time the client has had the treatment, explain to them that the treatment can be uncomfortable, but it is quick and any discomfort experienced is tolerable.

Be efficient and quick, so that the client does not have to wait. Try to get the client talking about something pleasant, such as a holiday, to take their mind off the treatment. Throughout the treatment, reassure them, praising them in order to motivate them to continue with the treatments. Do try to be sympathetic to your client's feelings, and provide support and encouragement when necessary. Waxing, although a necessity for many people, is not a particularly pleasant or relaxing treatment.

How to prepare the client for treatment

1   Use a towel to protect the client's remaining clothing. Even if performing an eyebrow wax, protect the chest area in case of wax spillage.

2   Wipe the area to be waxed with a professional antiseptic pre-wax cleansing lotion on cotton wool. This should be dispensed from a pump or spray bottle or removed with a spatula if in a container. Blot the area dry with tissues before applying the wax. While wiping the skin, look for contra-indications that restrict the treatment, e.g. varicose veins.

3   Record any bruising or contra-indications that restrict treatment on the record card to avoid potential problems later.

4   If the client's skin is very greasy (they may for example have applied oil before coming to the salon), cleanse it using an astringent lotion such as witch hazel. Talcum powder may be applied lightly to the area to facilitate hair removal.

5   Immediately before starting the treatment, wash your hands. Apply PPE as required according to the body part being treated.

6   Perform a **thermal skin sensitivity test**: before applying the wax, check its temperature. Test the wax on yourself first, to ensure that it's not too warm; then try a little on the client on the area to be treated (to check tolerance to the heat) before spreading it on other areas.

Cleansing the skin to be waxed

Testing wax temperature on inner wrist

ALWAYS REMEMBER

Angled follicles

An angled follicle may cause the hair to be broken off at the angle during waxing, instead of being completely pulled out with its root. If this happens, broken hairs will appear at the skin's surface within a few days.

By causing damage to the follicle and changing its shape, waxing can cause the re-growth of hairs to be frizzy or curled where previously they were straight.

Knowledge Check

If the client has a sensitive or allergic skin type, what must be performed in advance of the waxing treatment?

Refer to page 531 to help you.

Waxing treatments

Outcome 2: Be able to provide waxing treatments

Learn how to provide waxing treatments

PRACTICAL SKILLS

Communicate and behave in a professional manner

Follow health and safety working practices and industry Code of Practice for Waxing Services

Position yourself and client correctly throughout the treatment

Use products, tools, equipment and techniques to suit client treatment needs, skin type and condition

Complete the treatment to the satisfaction of the client

Record the results of the treatment

Provide suitable aftercare advice

UNDERPINNING KNOWLEDGE

State how to communicate and behave in a professional manner

Describe health and safety working practices and industry Code of Practice for Waxing Services

State the importance of positioning yourself and the client correctly throughout the treatment

State the importance of using products, tools, equipment and techniques to suit client's treatment needs

Describe how treatments can be adapted to suit client treatment needs, skin types and conditions

State the contra-actions that may occur during and following treatments and how to respond

State the importance of completing the treatment to the satisfaction of the client

State the importance of completing treatment records

State the aftercare advice that should be provided

Describe the structure and functions of the skin

Describe the structure and growth cycle of the hair

Describe diseases and disorders of the skin

TOP TIP

Thin wax application

The thinner the wax, the easier the treatment is to carry out when using a strip removal technique and the better the result. Also, less wax and fewer strips are used.

CourseMate video: Underarm Waxing

HEALTH & SAFETY

Avoid cross-contamination
It is unhygienic to return a spatula to the wax after it has been in contact with the body part. It is therefore required that a new spatula be used for each entry to the wax. This applies to warm, hot and sugar-strip wax.

Warm wax application to the bikini area

Warm waxing

Warm waxing has a few basic rules which must be followed to ensure a good result.

Observe the direction of hair growth. Warm wax must always be **applied with** the direction of hair growth, and **removed against** the direction of growth. This ensures both maximum adhesion between the hair, the strip and the wax, and that the hair will be pulled back on itself in the follicle and thus removed complete with its bulb.

> " Keep your client warm. If your client becomes cold, the hair follicle will tighten around the hair, making the treatment more uncomfortable and the hair difficult to remove.
>
> *Janice Brown*

Spatula application technique

1   Dip the spatula into the wax. Remove the excess on the sides and tip by wiping the spatula against the metal bar or the sides of the tub. Place the strip under the spatula while transferring it to the client: this will control dripping and improve your technique.

2   Place the spatula onto the skin at a 90° angle, and push the wax along in the direction of the hair growth. Do not allow the spatula to fall forward past 45°. The objective is to coat the area with a very thin film of wax. Quite a large area can be spread with each sweep of the spatula, as warm wax does not set. Do not attempt to smooth out or go over areas on which wax has already been spread, however, as the wax will have become cooler and will not move again, but will drag painfully on the client's skin.

3   Fold back 20 mm at the end of a strip and grip the flap with the thumb widthways across the strip. The flap should provide a wax-free handle throughout the treatment.

4   Place the strip at the bottom end of the wax-covered area, and make a firm bond between the wax and the strip by pressing firmly along the strip's length and width, following the direction of hair growth. If the strip is placed anywhere but at the bottom of a waxed area, the hairs at the **bottom** of the strip will become tangled together and held in the wax on the area below the strip: the removal of the strip will then be far more painful for the client.

5   Using the non-working hand, stretch the skin to minimize discomfort. Gripping the flap tightly, use the working hand to remove the strip against the direction of hair growth. Use a firm, steady pull. Make sure that the strip is pulled back on itself, close to the skin. (To obtain the correct angle of pull, stand at the side of the client, facing them.) Maintain this same horizontal angle of pull until the last bit of the strip has left the skin: **do not pull the strip upwards at the end of the pull** as this would break the hairs at the end of the strip and be very painful.

6   The strip may be used many times; in fact it works best when some wax builds up on its surface. When there is too much wax on the surface it will stop picking up more: throw it away and start with a new one.

7 Do not repeatedly spread and remove wax over one area. In particular, wax should not be spread and removed more than twice on sensitive areas such as the bikini line, the face and the underarms. Any remaining stray hairs must instead be removed using sterilized tweezers.

Alternatively, warm wax may be applied using a disposable cartridge/tube applicator system. This system is discussed on page 555.

Different temperatures Summer heat and winter cold can each give rise to application and removal problems during the wax treatment. In summer, the wax can stay too warm on the body, becoming sticky and difficult to work with, and tending to leave a sticky residue on the treated areas. In winter, the client's legs may be cold, causing the wax to set too quickly as you spread it, so that it becomes too thick. This prevents the efficient removal of both the wax and the hair growth.

To some extent these problems can be overcome by using thicker waxes with higher melting points in the summer, and thinner waxes with lower melting points in the winter.

Warm wax spatula application to the lower leg

 Removing the entire hair including the bulb is the aim of waxing (though many beauty therapists do not always achieve this goal). To ensure you always remove all the hair and so provide a lasting treatment, get two things right:

◆ when removing the wax, hold the skin taught this will 'open the follicles', which means you are more likely to remove the entire hair

◆ master an effective 'flicking' action when removing the wax strip; flick backwards, keeping it parallel to the skin, always against the direction of hair growth. Do not pull upwards as this is more likely to 'snap' off the hairs at the surface of the skin.

Janice Brown

TOP TIP

Take the sting out

To take the sting out of the removal, immediately place a hand or finger over the depilated area.

Wax removal from the forearm

How to provide a half-leg wax treatment

The areas of the body where warm-wax hair removal is most frequently used are the lower legs. This is often referred to simply as a half-leg treatment. A 'pair of half legs' should take 20–30 minutes to treat, and use no more than three or four wax removal strips.

1 Prior to the treatment, the area to be waxed should be cleansed as previously described.

2 Sit the client on the upraised couch, with both legs straight out in front of them.

3 Spread the wax on the *front* of the leg further away from you. Use three sweeps of the spatula: each sweep should go from just below the knee to the end of hair growth at the ankle.

Repeat this pattern of spreading on the leg nearer to you. (By spreading the further leg first, you will not have to lean over an already waxed area.)

4 Starting with the nearer leg, remove the wax using the strip. Start at the ankle and work upwards towards the knees.

Repeat for the other leg.

Warm wax removal, a wax strip is used to remove the layer of wax and hair from the skin.

HEALTH & SAFETY

Contra-action as a result of waxing treatment If any contra-action (unwanted skin reaction following treatment) appears to be more than minor, advise the client to see their GP straight away after treatment.

TOP TIP

Winter and summer problems

Thick lumps of wax stuck to the legs (the winter problem) after wax strip removal. These can be removed by pulling more slowly than normal, or by reversing the direction of pull on the strip. A sticky residue on the legs (the summer problem) must be removed using after-wax lotion.

Removal of warm wax from the back of the client's lower leg

Tweezer hair removal

5 Ask the client to bend their legs to one side. Beginning again with the further leg, spread wax on one *side* of the leg, from the knee to the ankle, using two sweeps of the spatula.

Repeat for the nearer leg.

6 Starting with the nearer leg, remove the wax from the bottom upwards.

Repeat for the other leg.

7 Repeat steps **5** and **6** for the other side of the legs.

8 Bend one knee. Spread the wax from just above the knee, downwards.

9 Remove this wax from the bottom upwards, remembering that strips cannot pull around corners effectively. To keep the angle of the pull horizontal, remove wax below the knee first, then that above the knee.

10 Repeat steps **8** and **9** for the other knee.

11 Lower the backrest and ask the client to turn over.

12 On the *back* of the legs, the direction of hair growth is not from the top to the bottom but sweeping at an angle, from the outside to the inside of the calf muscle.

Starting with the further leg, spread wax following the direction of the natural hair growth.

Repeat for the nearer leg.

13 Starting with the nearer leg, remove the wax against the direction of the natural hair growth.

Repeat for the other leg.

14 Finally, apply after-wax lotion to clean cotton wool and apply this to the back of the client's legs. As you apply the lotion, check for hairs left behind; if there are any, remove them using tweezers.

Ask the client to turn over, and repeat application on the front of the legs. Remove any excess using a tissue.

TOP TIP

Troubleshooting

The faults most commonly seen in warm-wax depilation are these:

◆ spreading the wax too thickly
◆ placing the strip in the middle of a wax-spread area, instead of starting at the bottom and working up
◆ pulling the strip upwards instead of backwards, away from the leg, causing breakage of the hair
◆ wax left on the skin after strip removal – this may be because of poor skin preparation; the skin was damp before wax application; the skin was not held sufficiently taut on removal; insufficient pressure applied when rubbing the wax strip before removal.

> Different brands of wax have a range of melting point temperatures so it is important to follow manufacturer's instructions regarding melting times and advised heats.
>
> *Janice Brown*

Disposable warm wax application to leg Wax is heated in its container applied through the disposable applicator head directly to the skin area. A wax strip is used to remove the hairs from the area removing the wax strip against hair growth.

Toes Clients frequently request that their toes be waxed in conjunction with a half-leg or full-leg treatment. When doing this, follow the normal guidelines for waxing, but be aware that hair may grow in many directions. Cut strips into small pieces to effectively remove hair.

Full-leg wax treatment

A full-leg wax should take 40–50 minutes and four to six strips should be sufficient.

When doing a full-leg wax, follow the same sequence of working as with the half-leg. On the thighs, observe the direction of hair growth carefully, as the hair grows in different directions. It is best not to spread wax on too large an area at once, or you may forget the direction of growth. Each direction of hair growth should be treated as a separate area. It is of prime importance that you support the skin on the thighs as you remove the strip – the tissues in this area can bruise very easily. The two essential factors in preventing bruising, pain and hair breakage are:

◆ the correct angle of pull
◆ adequate support for the tissues.

How to provide a bikini-line wax treatment

A bikini-line treatment takes 10–15 minutes, and requires a new strip for each section to ensure effective hair removal from this delicate area.

1 Treat one side at a time. It is best if the client lies flat, as the skin's tissues are then pulled tighter, but the treatment can be carried out in a semi-reclining position if the client prefers. Bend the client's knee out to the side, and put their foot flat against the knee of the other leg. This is sometimes referred to as the figure-four position.

2 Tuck a protective tissue along and under the lower edge of the client's briefs. Raise this edge and agree with the client where they want the final line to be. Hold the briefs slightly beyond this line, and ask the client to place their hand on top of the protective tissue to hold everything in place. This leaves you with both hands free, one to pull the strip and one to support the skin.

3 Cleanse and dry the areas to be waxed.

4 Using sterilized scissors, trim both the hair to be waxed and the adjacent hairs down to about 5–12 mm in length. This is essential to avoid tangling, pulling and pain, and to prevent wax going onto hair that you do not want to remove.

5 Spread and remove the wax in two or three separate and distinct areas, the number of application areas will depend on the directions of hair growth.

Applying warm wax to the bikini line

Removing the wax strip holding the skin taut

Disposable warm wax application technique to bikini area

CourseMate video: Facial Waxing

CourseMate video: Male Eyebrow Waxing

6 Use half of the strip length to remove the wax. Do not cover the whole area and tear it off at once! Treat the top plane of the thigh (Plane 1) and then the plane underneath this (Plane 2).

As soon as an area is completed, apply after-wax lotion. If necessary, use a clean tissue to remove excess lotion.

7 With both legs straight out in front on the couch, place a protective tissue along the top edge of the client's briefs, against the abdomen. Lower the briefs as necessary to expose just the hair to be removed – check this with your client. Usually the direction of hair growth here sweeps in from the sides and then up to the navel.

8 Trim the hair as before.

9 Apply and remove the wax in small sections, carefully observing hair growth. On completion, apply after-wax lotion.

Disposable warm wax application to bikini area Wax is applied in small sections through the applicator head to the skin area. A wax strip is used to remove the hairs from the area removing the wax strip against hair growth.

How to provide an underarm wax treatment using setting wax

An underarm treatment should take 5–15 minutes and two strips, one for each underarm.

1 With their bra still on, ask your client to lie flat on their back with their hands behind their head, elbows flat on the couch.

2 Cleanse both underarms with pre-wax lotion on clean cotton wool; blot with a tissue.

3 Place a protective tissue under the edge of the bra cup on the side away from you. Ask the client to bring their opposite arm down and over, and to pull the breast away from the underarm being waxed and across towards the middle of their chest. This pulls the tissues tight, making the treatment a lot more comfortable for them; it also leaves you with both hands free, one to pull and one to support.

4 Underarm hair usually grows in two main directions. Observe the directions of hair growth, then apply and remove the wax separately for each small area.

5 Apply after-wax lotion to the treated area. Check for stray hairs; remove these with sterile tweezers.

6 Blot any excess cream with a clean tissue.

STEP-BY-STEP: UNDERARM WAX TREATMENT

4a Applying hot setting wax to the underarm   **4b** Removing the wax   **4c** The completed area

Knowledge Check

What could be three undesirable post treatment skin reactions? How would these be avoided?

CourseMate video: Forearm Waxing

Warm wax spatula application technique to underarm Wax is applied in small sections using a spatula to the skin and hair in the area. A wax strip is used to remove the hair from the area, removing the wax strip against hair growth.

How to provide an arm waxing treatment

Depilation in this area should take 10–15 minutes for a half-arm treatment and 20–30 minutes for a full-arm treatment. Half the length of the strip should be used.

Arms are usually waxed with the client in the sitting position, with their general clothing protected with a towel. Sleeve edges can be protected with tucked-in tissues; ideally, though, upper outer clothing should be removed.

The roundness of the arm means that in order to effect a horizontal pull the work must be done in short lengths. Other than this, follow the general rules for waxing.

Warm wax spatula application to underarm

STEP-BY-STEP: ARM WAX TREATMENT

1 Wax applied in the direction of hair growth using disposable applicator warm-wax technique.

2 Wax is removed against hair growth commencing at the wrist area, ensuring that the skin is held taut to minimize discomfort and ensure effective hair removal. Hair removal continues until the area is hair-free.

3 Mild erythema of the skin following hair removal. Check the area from all angles to ensure all hairs have been removed. A soothing antiseptic lotion is applied to reduce erythema and any discomfort and to prevent secondary infection.

How to provide a face wax treatment

The face treatment must always be approached with extra care as facial skin is more sensitive than skin elsewhere on the body. Faulty technique can result in the top layer of skin being removed. (If this happens, a scab will form after about a day and the mark will take days to heal and fade completely.)

STEP-BY-STEP: FACE WAX TREATMENT

1 The client should be in a semi-reclining position, with their head supported and a clean towel draped across their shoulders to protect their clothing. A clean headband can be used to keep the hair away from the face.

2 Cleanse and wipe over the area thoroughly until the cotton wool or pre-wax cleansing wipe shows clean using an antiseptic cleansing lotion. Blot the area dry with a tissue.

3 Application of warm wax to the upper lip using a disposable applicator, paying close attention to the direction of natural hair growth. Hair removal is only required to the outer upper lip area for this client. You might need to spread one-half of the top lip with wax; remove this in three or four narrow strips; repeat the process on the other side of the face; and finally treat the central section immediately under the nose.

4 Removal of wax against hair growth. The area is held taut to minimize discomfort and ensure effective hair removal.

5 Pressure is applied to the area to minimize discomfort.

6 Application of wax to the upper lip area immediately below the nose. The client is requested to pull the skin taut using their facial muscle, moving the skin over the upper teeth. This position will assist hair removal.

7 Application of antiseptic soothing lotion follows to the hair-free area to promote skin healing, reduce redness and prevent secondary infection.

ALWAYS REMEMBER

Bleached hair

Previously bleached hair when waxed tends to break off at skin level. Clients should be told not to bleach facial hair if it is to be waxed.

TOP TIP

Dark superfluous facial hair

Avoid obvious lines when removing facial hair. Ensure the outer border of the area treated blends into the adjacent area of skin.

ALWAYS REMEMBER

The lips

The lips are extremely sensitive. To avoid possible irritation, do not allow the wax to come into contact with them.

A top-lip wax should take approximately 5 minutes, a chin and neck wax approximately 10 minutes, and a lip and chin wax approximately 15 minutes. A removal strip of no more than one-eighth normal size should be used on the face. Do not allow wax to build up on the facial wax strips – such a build-up could lead to skin removal. Use a new wax removal strip for each area.

If the chin is to be treated this area is less sensitive than the upper lip so if treating both areas complete the chin area last. Apply the wax according to the type of wax used. You may find that when treating a female client there may be small groupings of hairs and the wax may be applied to these areas only. If the client has dark superfluous facial hair it may be necessary to treat the sides of the face also.

A disposable warm wax application to facial area Wax is applied in small sections through the applicator head to the skin area. A wax strip is used to remove the hair from the area removing the wax strip against growth.

Facial wax application using disposal applicator warm wax technique

How to provide an eyebrow wax treatment

Eyebrows, as a part of the face, are treated accordingly (see above). An eyebrow wax should take approximately 10–15 minutes.

1 Study the eyebrows and decide upon their final shape and proportions.

2 Brush the eyebrows and separate the unwanted hair (**superfluous hair**) from the line of the other hairs.

3 Commence waxing between the brows, the skin is firmer in this area and allows the client, especially if this treatment is new to them, to become accustomed to the sensation.

4 Using a small spatula, apply a thin film of wax to the unwanted hairs in a small area. Remove the wax and hair using a clean strip. Repeat application to, and removal from, the different areas, using a clean strip each time, until all the unwanted hairs have been removed.

5 Apply a soothing antiseptic cream and use sterile tweezers to remove any stray hairs.

TOP TIP

Protect against spillage

When performing an eyebrow wax, eyebrow hair that does not need to be removed may be protected with petroleum jelly. This is a useful tip when first performing eyebrow waxing to prevent mistakes!

Cotton wool pads may be placed over the eyes to protect the eye and eyelashes from accidental wax spillage.

STEP-BY-STEP: EYEBROW TREATMENT

3a Applying wax between the eyebrows

3b Removal of wax using a wax strip

Application of wax under the brow

5 Apply a soothing antiseptic cream and use sterile tweezers to remove any stray hairs

Finished look

A disposable warm wax application to the eyebrow area Wax is applied in small sections through the applicator head to the skin area. A wax strip is used to remove the hair from the area removing the wax strip against growth.

Aftercare and advice

The following aftercare and advice should be provided after each waxing treatment is completed to reconfirm the client's understanding of these important procedures.

An after-wax antiseptic, soothing lotion should be applied, using clean cotton wool, at the end of the treatment. This breaks down any wax residue, helps to guard against secondary infection and irritation, and takes away any feelings of discomfort. Encourage your client to continue with the use of such a lotion at home for up to 3 days: it will protect against dryness, discomfort, infection and ingrowing hairs.

> Always let your client know that if there are hairs just under the skin at time of treatment they are likely to be visible above the skin in just a few days following, this is not re-growth but the growth of hairs which are not long enough for removal at that time.
>
> *Janice Brown*

Products have been formulated to apply to the skin following wax depilation to slow hair re-growth. When entering the empty hair follicle the product aims to weaken the cell's matrix, slowing cell division in this area which is responsible for creating the new hair. These are available for your client to purchase as a retail product.

Advise the client against wearing any tight clothing (such as tights or hosiery) over the waxed areas for the 24 hours following a treatment. Such clothing could lead to irritation and ingrowing hairs.

If the client suffers from ingrowing hairs, they should exfoliate their skin every 4 to 7 days, starting 2 or 3 days after the treatment. Exfoliation prevents the build-up of dead skin cells on the surface of the skin; these would otherwise block the exit from the follicle and cause a growing hair to turn back on itself and grow inwards. Ingrowing hairs should be freed and, if possible, left in place so that the follicle exit will reform around the hair's shaft. Demonstrate to the client the correct use and benefits of the exfoliant product.

Advise the client that for the 24 hours following their treatment they should not apply any talcum powders, deodorants, antiperspirants, perfumes, self-tanning products or make-up over the treated areas. Any of these products could block the pores or cause irritation or allergy reactions on the temporarily sensitized area. During this time they must use only plain, unperfumed soap and water on the treated area.

For the same 24-hour period they should preferably avoid exercise, especially swimming, and not apply heat or UV treatments – hot baths, for example, or the use of a sun bed or sauna – as these would add to the heat generated in the skin following the treatment and would probably cause discomfort or irritation. They must also refrain from touching or scratching the area, so as to avoid infecting the open follicles.

Aftercare leaflets should contain this information: as best practice these can be given to the client at the end of the treatment to remind them what to do at home.

If there is a contra-action following treatment such as excessive redness and irritation, advise the client to apply a cool compress with soothing antiseptic lotion. If the redness does not disappear they must contact the salon. Advise the client to receive the treatment as follows: facial waxing 3–4 weeks; body waxing 4–6 weeks. Repeat bookings vary according to the natural hair re-growth and client requirements.

Ensure that the client's records are up-to-date, accurate and complete following the waxing treatment and provide written instructions in an aftercare leaflet.

Hot waxing

In hot waxing, the wax is applied at a higher temperature than warm wax. The hairs embed in the wax and are gripped tightly as the wax cools and contracts. When the wax is pulled away, it removes the hair from the base of the follicle.

Equipment and materials

The equipment and materials required for hot waxing are the same as for warm waxing (page 529), except that:

◆ *a wax heater* suitable for hot wax should be selected

◆ *wax-removal* strips are not necessary

◆ *pre-wax oil* may be applied to the skin before wax application to make wax removal easier.

Some people prefer to apply the hot wax with disposable brushes rather than spatulas, but either can be used.

How to carry out the treatment

1 Ensure that the area to be waxed is clean and grease-free.

2 Apply a small amount of talc against the direction of hair growth. This will make the hairs stand on end and stick more firmly into the wax. Alternatively oil may be applied. Preparation will depend upon manufacturer's instructions.

3 Keep the same order of work as for warm waxing.

4 Carefully observe the direction of hair growth and the size of the area to be waxed.

5 Test the heat of the wax on the inside of the wrist.

6 Using a disposable spatula, apply a layer of wax about 5 cm × 10 cm *against* the direction of hair growth. Apply a second layer *with* the direction of growth; and a third layer against the direction of growth. (If two or three strips are applied at the same time, you can work faster.) Keep the edges of the wax thicker than the middle, to make it easier to remove. Overlap the lower edge by about 2 cm onto a hair-free area: this makes it less painful later, when you lift the edge to make a lip to pull.

Curl up the lower end of the wax to make a lip, and press and mould the wax firmly onto the skin.

ACTIVITY

Aftercare leaflets

Discuss why aftercare leaflets should be given to clients, as well as giving them the advice verbally.

What could happen if aftercare advice is not given?

Design a suitable aftercare leaflet you could provide for your clients following waxing treatment.

Knowledge Check

If your client suffers from ingrowing hairs, what advice would you give them that could possibly prevent them recurring?

Refer to page 536 to help you.

TOP TIP

Choosing a hot wax

When selecting a hot wax, choose one that does not go brittle when cool. Wax sold as small blocks or pellets is often preferable as this melts quickly.

Applying hot wax to plane 1 of the bikini line area

Hot wax removed when set but still pliable

Removing hot wax from plane 1, wax has been applied to plane 2

7 Leave the wax for a minute or so to cool. The wax has to cool sufficiently to grip the hairs, but not so much that the wax becomes brittle and breaks on removal. As it sets, it starts to lose its gloss: it should be removed when this happens and while it is still pliable.

8 Support the area below the wax, grasp the lip, and tear the wax off the skin *against* the direction of hair growth in one movement (as with warm-wax removal). Immediately press or firmly stroke the area with your hand: this takes away some of the discomfort.

9 Check the area for any remaining wax and any stray hairs. Remove using tweezers. (Second applications are not advisable when using hot wax, because of the risk of burning.)

If this general application technique is followed, any area of the body can be depilated – use the same order of work as for warm waxing: observe the direction of hair growth and take into account the body area; use smaller strips in smaller areas; support the skin; and use the correct angle of pull for removal.

Apply a soothing antiseptic cream and use sterile tweezers to remove any stray hairs. Follow with appropriate aftercare advice.

Sugaring and strip sugar

Sugaring is an ancient and popular method for hair removal. The superfluous hairs become embedded in a pliable organic paste of sugar, lemon and water. The sugar paste is then removed from the skin's surface, against the hair's growth, leaving the skin hair-free.

Sugaring may be applied using a paste formulation removed with the hands, referred to as sugar paste, or in a formulation similar to warm wax, removed with material strips, referred to as strip sugar. Sugaring is effective on fine hair growth, and as it contains fewer ingredients or additives this method is less likely to cause an allergic reaction.

Reception

Re-book the client for sugaring hair removal every 4 to 6 weeks, dependent upon the hair growth rate and area. For effective hair removal, the hairs must be at least 2 mm long.

Equipment and materials

The equipment and materials required for sugaring are the same as for warm waxing (page 529), except for the following differences.

Sugar paste

◆ *Wax heater (with a thermostatic control) or microwave* – to heat the paste.

◆ *Sugaring paste* – either soft or hard, depending on your personal preference and the temperature of the working environment: hard paste is a better choice in warmer temperatures and when working on coarser hair.

◆ *Talc (purified)* to reduce stickiness and absorb perspiration – to prevent the sugar sticking to the skin.

◆ *Bowl of clean water* – to remove the sugar paste from the hands, reducing stickiness.

Strip sugar

◆ *Wax heater (with a thermostatic control)* – to heat the strip sugar.

◆ *Strip sugar*.

◆ *Talc (purified)* to reduce stickiness and absorb perspiration – to prevent the sugar sticking to the skin.

◆ *Disposable wooden spatulas* – a selection of differing sizes, for use on different body areas.

◆ *Wax-removal strips (bonded-fibre)* – thick enough that the wax does not soak through, but flexible enough for easy working.

◆ *Disposable gloves*.

ALWAYS REMEMBER

Talcum powder

Talc aids the sugaring treatment technique, by reducing stickiness when working with the paste, and by absorbing perspiration (particularly in areas such as the underarms).

Sterilization and disinfection

As sugar paste is water-soluble, it is easily cleaned from any surface. However, the wax heater containing the sugar wax must be regularly disinfected.

STEP-BY-STEP: PREPARING THE CLIENT

1 Cleanse the area to be treated, using an antiseptic cleansing tissue. Blot the skin dry.

2 Apply talc to cover the area: this prevents the sugar from sticking to the skin.

3 Rubbing in the talc.

How to provide a sugar paste treatment

The sugar paste adheres to the hair and not to the skin, which allows the sugar to be reapplied to a treatment area. Technique is important and it takes practice and experience to become skilled.

1 Heat the sugar gently, to soften it.

2 Apply talc to the area.

3 Apply the sugar paste to the skin by hand. Select the amount used according to the treatment area. Draw the paste over the area *in the direction* of the hair

4   To complete the treatment, a cooling spray may be applied to the area, followed by a soothing cream.

5   Record details of the treatment on the client's record card.

Disposable applicator roller waxing systems

Using a **roller wax** system is a hygienic method, using disposable applicators that are new for each client. A disposable applicator head screws onto the wax applicator tube in place of a cap. This reduces the possible risk of contamination through cross-infection. The method is less messy, as the wax is contained in the tube or cartridge and is not exposed until application.

Each tube/cartridge of wax as needed is heated to working temperature, which minimizes the risk of burning.

CourseMate video: Leg Waxing

Disposable applicator starter kit

STEP-BY-STEP: WAXING THE LEGS USING DISPOSABLE APPLICATOR

1 Remove the disposable applicator from the right-hand heating and storage compartment.

2 Remove the cap from the tube of wax. Attach the applicator head to the tube.

3 Release the applicator by lifting the lever upwards. Squeeze until a small amount of wax appears on the front of the applicator, then apply the wax. Hold the applicator at a 45° angle to the leg, and glide it smoothly down the leg.

4 Apply a thin film of wax to the front of both legs, then press down the closing device on the applicator to stop wax flow.

5 Wipe any wax residue from the front of the applicator and return the tube to heat.

6 Remove wax from the leg, starting at the ankle and working towards the knee. Support the skin with one hand, and firmly stretch it against the removal of the wax. Continue application and removal to the sides and back of the legs.

7 When treatment is complete, apply antiseptic soothing lotion (shown). Record details of the treatment on the client's record card.

8 Remove the applicator from the tube, replacing the cap and returning the tube to the heater. Dispose of the applicator head.

ASSESSMENT OF KNOWLEDGE AND UNDERSTANDING

You have now learnt about removing hair using waxing techniques treatment in the beauty therapy workplace. To test your level of knowledge, answer the following short questions. These will prepare you for your summative (final) assessment.

1. Hair removal using waxing techniques is:

   a. temporary hair removal
   b. permanent hair removal

2. The act of accurately sharing information between two people or groups of people is called:

   a. clarification   c. client consultation
   b. communication   d. reflective listening

3. The hair shown below is in which growth cycle stage?

   a. **catagen**
   b. **telogen**
   c. anagen

4. Diabetes is a medical condition which if present will:

   a. prevent treatment   b. restrict treatment

5. The part of the hair shown in the cross section below which is not always present in **vellus hair** type is:

   a. cuticle   b. cortex   c. medulla

6. Warm wax and roller wax is applied:

   a. with the natural hair growth pattern
   b. against the natural hair growth pattern

7. When performing waxing, surface skin cells are also removed from the following layer:

   a. stratum germinativum
   b. stratum corneum
   c. subcutaneous
   d. stratum granulosum

8. Following a skin sensitivity patch test, an allergic reaction resulting in swelling and excessive erythema is referred to as:

   a. a positive skin reaction
   b. a negative skin reaction

9. The skin condition folliculitis is a:

   a. bacterial infection
   b. viral disorder
   c. fungal disorder

10. Lemon can be an ingredient in formulations of:

    a. hot wax
    b. cold wax
    c. honey wax
    d. sugar wax

16 Ear Piercing

LEARNING OBJECTIVES

There are two learning outcomes for this optional unit which you must achieve:

1   Be able to prepare for ear piercing.

2   Be able to provide ear piercing.

From the range statement, you must show you can:

◆ Use consultation techniques to identify the treatment objectives.

◆ Use the listed products, tools and equipment as appropriate.

◆ Ensure the environmental conditions are suitable.

◆ Complete a consultation and skin inspection to identify contra-indications. that may affect if and how the treatment can proceed

◆ Follow all health and safety working practices.

◆ Provide relevant aftercare and contra-action advice.

KEY TERMS

aftercare advice

certificate of registration

clinical waste

consent form

consultation

contra-action advice

contra-actions

Dangerous Substances and
Preparations (Nickel) (Safety)
Regulations (2005)

ear piercing

Ear piercing gun

external ear structure

Greater London Council
(General Powers) Act 1981

health and safety

keloid

Local Government Act (2003)
(section 120 and schedule 6)

London Local Authorities Act
(1991 and 2007)

treatment objectives

treatment plan

Unit Topic

Provide ear piercing

This VRQ unit is linked to the Beauty Therapy NOS Unit B7.

INTRODUCTION

Ear piercing creates a hole in the skin and underlying tissues where jewellery is inserted. This unit is all about carrying out the skin piercing of the earlobe safely to ensure the correct placement and healing of the skin tissue avoiding any contra-action complications.

Dealing with people in a polite, efficient manner to reassure them and using good communication and questioning skills to find out exactly what they require from the ear piercing service forms an important part of this technical service. You must be able to show you have the necessary practical skills and underpinning knowledge to provide ear piercing.

INDUSTRY ROLE MODEL

KATHRYN DARWIN Sales and Training Manager, Studex UK Ltd

"Having worked for Studex now for over 10 years, I truly love the variety of work that my job brings. With a background in sales, my work with Studex has allowed me to develop new skills and explore areas, such as teaching and working on industry policies and procedures. On a day-to-day basis I could be working on marketing material for national customers, reviewing new products, teaching in colleges or presenting our Ear Piercing Systems to local councils. Life is certainly never dull and I love that I have the opportunity to travel the country and sometimes internationally.

> **ANATOMY & PHYSIOLOGY**
> Essential anatomy and physiology knowledge requirements for this chapter are identified on the checklist chart on page 33.

Earlobe piercing

Ear piercing is a quick, profitable and popular service, which also has the potential to generate further custom. This may be the client's first visit to a beauty salon, and the service they receive may encourage them to return for further treatments.

Outcome1: Be able to prepare for ear piercing

Learn how to prepare for ear piercing

PRACTICAL SKILLS

Prepare yourself, client and work area for ear piercing

Use suitable consultation techniques to identify treatment objectives

Provide clear recommendations to the client

Select products, tools and equipment to suit client treatment needs

UNDERPINNING KNOWLEDGE

Describe the environmental conditions **suitable for ear piercing**

Describe different consultation techniques used to identify treatment objectives

Describe how to select products, tools and equipment to suit client treatment needs

Describe the contra-indications to ear piercing

Knowledge Check

What is the helix part of the ear composed of that makes it unsuitable for piercing?

Refer to page 63 to help you.

Preparing the work area

Ear piercing can be carried out either in a private cubicle or at reception. Use your discretion to decide which would be more appropriate.

Check the suitability of the environmental conditions. Good ventilation and lighting is important – some clients may feel faint following the treatment, usually caused by feelings of tension and anxiety beforehand. As clients may be anxious before having their ears pierced, a calm environment should be provided, and restful, background music will help to create a relaxing environment. The client should be seated on a seat with a stable surface, without wheels.

All furniture and fittings in the treatment area should be kept clean and in good repair so that they can be cleaned effectively.

The surface that the ear piercing equipment is to be placed on should be cleaned immediately prior to service with detergent and disinfectant. It should then be covered with disposable tissue roll, which is disposed of immediately following treatment. All work surfaces must be kept clean at all times and covered with a smooth, impervious surface.

Check that the client is positioned at a suitable height when performing the treatment. The earlobe should be easily accessible without risk of injury to the client. Remember, awkward positioning for the beauty therapist may result in uneven piercing and can also lead to RSI and must be avoided.

Piercing ear stud display board

> ### Training
>
> Education is key to providing a first class service. A recognized qualification or certification is necessary for insurance and licensing as well as providing an opportunity to learn everything, including tips and techniques from an industry expert. The opportunity to perform a piercing under the watchful eye of an ear piercing trainer is so important for competence and confidence. Many manufacturers offer training with some starter kits, so make sure you do your research.
>
> *Kathryn Darwin*

TOP TIP

Cosmetic piercing

Skin piercing of the earlobe and cosmetic body piercing are classified in the single term *cosmetic piercing*.

Before carrying out the ear piercing, check that you have the necessary equipment and materials to hand and that they meet legal hygiene and industry requirements for ear piercing.

Products, tools and equipment

- **Couch or chair** For client to sit on, with easy-to-clean surface
- **Trolley** On which to place products, tools and related equipment
- **Ear piercing gun (also referred to as ear piercing instrument)** Ear piercing gun that complies with current health and safety legislation
- **Pre-packed alcohol-based sterile cleaning tissues (2) or manufacturer's cleansing solution** Used to cleanse the ear area

YOU WILL ALSO NEED:

- **Studs** A variety of styles and designs to accommodate differing client preferences. These must be manufactured from hypo-allergenic metal to minimize allergic reactions in people with metal allergies, e.g. nickel
- **Non-toxic surgical skin-marker pen** To mark where the piercing will be. This is usually in gentian violet ink
- **Disinfectant (70 per cent alcohol)** For example surgical spirit for cleaning the gun after use
- **Clean cotton wool** To apply lotions/cleaning products

◆ **Single use disposable synthetic powder-free gloves such as nitrile or PVC formulation** To ensure a high standard of hygiene and to reduce the possibility of contamination

◆ **Disposable tissue couch roll** To protect the clean, disinfected work surfaces; client clothing at the neck area

◆ **Waste container (with yellow coloured waste liner to collect contaminated waste)** This should be a lined metal bin with a lid to collect waste

◆ **Sharps box** To dispose of studs when necessary

◆ **Headband (clean) or clip** To hold the hair away from the ear during ear piercing

◆ **Hand mirror (clean)** To show the client the proposed placement of the earrings after marking and after the completed ear piercing

◆ **Client record card** For recording confidential details of each client registered at the salon, including personal details, products used and details of the treatment

◆ **Aftercare solution** Either to offer for sale or to include as part of the cost of the service to promote skin healing and avoid secondary infection

◆ **Aftercare instruction leaflet** Instructions for the client to keep to minimize healing times and reduce the risk of secondary infection

◆ **Hand disinfectant** Usually containing chlorhexidine to cleanse and disinfect hands

Examples of ear piercing guns

Disposable cassette

Ear piercing gun

HEALTH & SAFETY

Hygiene practice information from Habia See the Habia *Hygiene in Beauty Therapy* booklet for more information about the types of infection that occur in a salon, the requirements of the law and inspection, and practical advice on how to avoid the spread of infection. It is available as a download from the Habia website www.habia.org.uk

HEALTH & SAFETY

Manufacturer's systems Be aware the manufacturer's systems may vary depending on the type of ear piercing gun you are using.

Sterilization and disinfection

The premises should be kept clean and hygienic. The floor covering should be such that the surface can be cleaned with a disinfectant and hot soapy water; work surfaces likewise should be washed regularly with detergent and water and wiped with a disinfectant. Hypochlorite solutions (bleach) are recommended for disinfecting work surfaces. Potential hazards include skin infection and cross-infection including the transmission of blood borne viruses such as hepatitis or HIV due to poor hygiene practice to both client and beauty therapist.

HEALTH & SAFETY

Ear piercing marker pens Keep the non-toxic marker pen in a safe hygienic place – if left out, somebody might mistake it for an ordinary felt-tip pen!

HEALTH & SAFETY

Avoidance of cross-infection If you have any cuts on your hands or fingers, these should be covered with a clean dressing before you treat the client. It is a requirement to wear disposable gloves.

Also, if you have an acute cold, e.g., a respiratory infection, do not perform ear piercing service. This will prevent airborne transfer of infection. A protective face mask may be worn for reasons of hygiene when working in close proximity to the client.

Knowledge Check

How should the client be positioned for ear piercing treatment and why is this important?

Refer to page 561 to help you.

Some salons that offer ear piercing treatment also retail earrings. Those designed for pierced ears should never be tried on by a client, in the interest of health and hygiene. Such earrings may instead be attached to a special clear acrylic slide that can be held against the ear to assist in selection.

HEALTH & SAFETY

The Control of Substances Hazardous to Health (COSHH) Regulations (2002) – including biological agents The Control of Substances Hazardous to Health (COSHH) Regulations (2002) require employers and the self-employed to prevent or control the exposure of employees and clients to hazardous substances. This includes exposure to biological agents such as bacteria, fungi and viruses and chemical cleaning/sterilizing agents. Records of the COSHH assessment must be available for inspection.

A COSHH essential information document is available for cosmetic piercers at www.coshh-essentials.org.uk

The gun approved for ear piercing is designed so that it does not come into contact with the client's skin, and is used with pre-sterilized ear studs and ear clasps.

The **ear piercing gun** may be placed in the UV cabinet before use, although this is not a mandatory requirement due to the hygienic operational design of the gun. The studs are provided in sterile packs. Many give a date after which their sterility can no longer be assumed; others have a seal that changes colour when the expiry date has been reached. Only use studs that come from a sealed package, check before use that the packaging is not damaged in any way.

Ensure that all recommended skin cleansing solutions are in date and that packaging has not been damaged in any way.

The Local Government (Miscellaneous Provisions) Act (1982) requires that salons offering any form of skin piercing be registered with the local health authority. This registration includes both the operators who will be carrying out the treatment and the salon premises where the treatment will be carried out. There is a requirement by some local health authorities to display a certificate that training has taken place. In some cases this may be a manufacturer's product training certificate.

The **Local Government Act (2003) (section 120 and schedule 6)** has amended the 1982 Act to enable each local authority to regulate businesses providing differing types of cosmetic piercing and skin colouring. Each local authority can introduce its own bye-laws to set the standards as required. For information and guidance on skin piercing visit your local council website.

Premises are inspected by a local authority enforcement officer, who checks that relevant local bye-laws are being followed. (The bye-laws are to ensure that treatment is carried out in a healthy, safe and hygienic manner.)

If the inspector is satisfied, the salon will be issued with a **certificate of registration**; this should be displayed in the reception area at all times. Any breach of the Act or the bye-laws could result in a fine, and permission to carry out the treatment could be withdrawn.

The London local authorities mainly use the **Greater London Council (General Powers) Act 1981** and **London Local Authorities Act (1991 and 2007)** which covers the London local authorities and enables them to regulate special treatment businesses including cosmetic piercing and micro pigmentation.

The HSE have a guidance publication for those involved in work where exposure to blood or other body fluids may occur titled *Blood-borne viruses in the workplace: Guidance for employers and employees.*

Reception

When making an appointment for this service, allow 15 minutes. Although ear piercing is completed quickly, time must be allowed to complete the client's record card, determine the client's service plan and give clear concise aftercare instructions. Good communication is important. Speak clearly, establish what the client's requirements are and listen to ensure communication is effective and that a professional relationship is developed with the client, gaining client confidence.

A record card should be prepared for the client, recording just the information that is relevant to the ear piercing service. Record-keeping protects both the beauty therapist and client. While completing the record card you will be able to ascertain whether the client is suited to this treatment – if the client is under 16 years of age (a minor), for example, it is necessary for a parent or guardian to accompany them and sign a **consent form** containing a disclaimer in the event of contra-indications. It is recommended to prevent parental complaints. These should be kept for a period of 3 years for inspection, enabling checks to be made on clients' ages.

Contra-indications to ear piercing should be checked for. If the area for piercing is unsuitable, politely explain to the client why this is so.

> ❝
> **Paperwork**
>
> Completing a client consultation form for every piercing not only allows a technician to record all important information, but also ensures that clients have been informed about the process and expectations. Technicians can identify any contra-indications, record where the piercing was positioned as well as the jewellery selected. Most consultation forms supplied by manufacturers will also provide clients with a copy of the aftercare advice to take away with them.
>
> *Kathryn Darwin*

Contra-indications

In certain circumstances you should not carry out the ear piercing treatment. Medical conditions which make the skin prone to the possibility of poor skin healing or infection will prevent ear piercing being carried. Advise the client to consult their GP and always obtain confirmation that ear piercing treatment can be carried out.

Use your professional judgement to assess the suitability of each client. The **consultation** will draw any contra-indications to your attention.

◆ *If a client is particularly nervous* it would be inadvisable to pierce their ears – they might faint or jump while the service was being carried out, causing incorrect placement of the earring.

◆ *Do not pierce the ears of a client who may have allergies* to the metal used for the jewellery stud.

If any of the following are present, do not proceed with ear piercing:

◆ *Diabetes* – the skin is very slow to heal, taking longer to heal following the piercing so infection of the area would be a strong possibility.

◆ *Epilepsy* – the stress before the service and the possible shock incurred during it might induce a fit. If GP permission to treat is received, it is a good idea to recommend that a client with this condition is accompanied.

◆ *Skin disease or disorder*.

◆ *Hepatitis B or HIV (Human Immunodeficiency Virus)* – though the client may not know that they are a carrier, or may choose not to disclose the fact if they do (hygienic practice is vital, for this reason).

Knowledge Check

Which branch of the external carotid artery supplies blood to the ear?

Refer to page 94 to help you.

ACTIVITY

Costs

Research ear piercing service in three local salons. These may include hairdressing salons as it is a popular service to perform in the hair salon.

What is the cost of this service?

TOP TIP

Treatment modification

Examples of ear piercing service modification include:

◆ if a second piercing is requested, ensure the first stud is placed to accommodate, leaving a 9 mm distance for the second piercing

◆ if the client has fat lobes, adjust the tightness following piercing to allow for swelling following the skin piercing which could cause discomfort and lead to infection

◆ if 6 mm or more thickness, the lobe requires a 'long post' stud.

Knowledge Check

Provide five examples of how you can prevent infection when performing ear piercing treatment.

Refer to pages 563–564 to help you.

Inflammation of the ear

Keloid scarring of the ear

◆ *Open wounds, cuts or abrasions* in the area.

◆ *Moles or warts* in the area.

◆ *Circulatory disorders* such as high or low blood pressure.

◆ *Following an operation* – piercing must not be carried out at the site of a recent operation.

◆ *Anti-coagulant drugs* – these drugs affect blood clotting so individuals are likely to bleed persistently.

◆ *Inflammation of the ear* – the skin in the area appears red, swollen, and pus, a sign of infection, may be present.

◆ *Keloid scarring* – **keloids** occur following skin injury and are overgrown abnormal scar tissue which spreads, characterized by excess deposits of collagen. The skin tends to be red, raised and ridged at the site of the wound.

Where there is any contra-indication or a suspected contra-indication to ear piercing, the client must seek written permission from their GP before service can be carried out.

Feel the area to be pierced to check for cysts or keloids at consultation wearing disposable gloves for protection. Do not pierce through cysts or keloids or infection could occur.

Inform the client of possible **contra-actions** that could happen, especially if the correct aftercare procedures are not followed.

Contra-actions

◆ *Infection* – redness, swelling, inflammation and the exudation (oozing/weeping) of serum all signify that the ear is infected. If this occurs, the client should contact the salon. Depending on what they describe, it may be possible to give them adequate instructions over the telephone, or it may be necessary to make an appointment for the beauty therapist to look at the ear. If, following action by the beauty therapist, the infection persists, the client should be advised to contact their GP. Infection usually results from incorrect aftercare, Closed holes are caused by removing the studs too early, or by not continuing to wear earrings after the removal of the original studs.

Infections of the ear can be painful, and if ignored lead to scarring and at worst the skin tissue can die leading to disfigurement of the area.

◆ *Jewellery embedding* – this occurs when the ear jewellery descends beneath the skin's surface. This is usually a sign of infection, rejection or allergy to the metal of the ring. The client should contact the salon for advice. If, following action by the beauty therapist, the jewellery remains embedded, the client should be advised to visit their GP.

◆ *Keloids* – overgrowths of scar tissue – sometimes occur at the site of ear piercing. If a client suffers from keloids, advise them not to have their ears pierced more than once – further **keloid** tissue could develop, giving an unsightly appearance.

◆ *Dizziness and fainting* – may occur if the client was particularly nervous beforehand. The shock of the ear piercing service may cause a short period

HEALTH & SAFETY

Secondary infection If the client's ears become slightly red, indicating a possible infection, they should cleanse the area more frequently.

of unconsciousness due to insufficient blood flow to the brain. If a client faints, loosen any restrictive clothing. Reassure the client, and position them lying flat with their feet raised higher than their head, or sat with their head bent forwards between their knees. Instruct them to breathe deeply and slowly. Increase ventilation in the area.

◆ **Allergy to the aftercare lotion** – the client may be allergic to the aftercare lotion. Check for known allergies to products at the client consultation.

Knowledge Check

If you suspected a client had a contagious contra-indication what actions would you take for the welfare of the client, yourself and others?

Refer to page 566 to help you.

❝❝ **Pricing**

Ear piercing can be a very profitable addition to your business where a simple pricing structure and competitive package are put into place. Always research competition and consider your client base. There are a huge variety of earrings available, however bear in mind that whether you showcase five or 50 styles a client will nearly always be able to choose one pair of earrings. You can always add to your range as your business grows.

Kathryn Darwin

All details recorded on the client record card are confidential and should be stored in a secure area following service. Access to this information will require written consent from the client. This is enforced through the Data Protection Act (1998) – legislation designed to protect the client's privacy and confidentiality. These records should be kept for at least 3 years, and be available for inspection as required. This may be by an authorized officer from the local health authority.

Explain the simple service procedure. Tell them that the ears will be cleansed and marked to show where the ear stud will be placed following piercing. This mark must be agreed with the client. The gun will be loaded with sterile ear studs which will enter the ear, performing the piercing. The back clasps will be fitted at the same time. A tight pinch will be experienced and some initial discomfort, with redness and slight swelling in the area which varies between clients. Most clients will be interested to know what to expect – usually the client's first question is 'Will it hurt?'. You may also demonstrate the noise and action of the gun, this familiarity will provide reassurance when the ear piercing is completed, reducing the possibility of the client moving.

Discuss aftercare: the client should be provided with this in written format and sign to confirm that these instructions are understood and will be followed. It is important to check that the client does not have any known allergies that may be contained in products to be used in the service, e.g. the aftercare lotion. Also, clients are more likely to pay attention at this stage.

Prepare the equipment required for ear piercing, and show the client the range of studs available. The stud's post has a larger diameter than regular earring posts to allow for shrinkage during the healing process; explain this to the client.

Some salon receptionists are trained to carry out this service. This is practical: many clients will be acting on impulse in deciding to have their ears pierced, and will not have made an appointment.

ALWAYS REMEMBER

Client record card

Accurately record your client's answers to necessary questions asked at consultation on the record card.

A sample client record card

Date	Beauty therapist name

Client name	Date of birth (identifying client age group)

Home address	Postcode

Email address	Landline phone number	Mobile phone number

Name of doctor	Doctor's address and phone number

Related medical history (conditions that may restrict or prohibit service application)

Are you taking any medication? (e.g. anti-coagulant drugs may affect the sensitivity of the skin and reaction to the service)

CONTRA-INDICATIONS REQUIRING MEDICAL REFERRAL (Preventing ear piercing service.)	*CONTRA-INDICATIONS WHICH RESTRICT SERVICE* (Service may require adaptation.)
☐ bacterial infection ☐ cardio-vascular problems ☐ viral infection ☐ dysfunction of the ☐ fungal infection ☐ nervous system ☐ severe skin conditions ☐ allergies to metals ☐ diabetes ☐ epilepsy ☐ ear infections ☐ anti-coagulant drugs	☐ cuts and abrasions ☐ bruising and swelling ☐ recent scar tissue ☐ skin disorders ☐ moles ☐ skin inflammation ☐ keloid scar tissue (piercing around the keloid permitted)
EQUIPMENT, MATERIALS AND PRODUCTS	*AREA TREATED*
☐ ear piercing gun ☐ surgical skin marker pen ☐ sterile pre-packed alcohol skin-cleansing wipes ☐ personal protective equipment ☐ sterile pre-packed ear studs (metal type identified) ☐ consumables ☐ aftercare products ☐ mirror ☐ sharps disposal box (for use in the event of disposing of a contaminated ear stud) ☐ waste bin (with disposable liner)	☐ earlobe

Beauty therapist signature (for reference)

Client signature (confirmation of details)

A sample client record card (continued)

SERVICE ADVICE
Ear piercing – *allow 15 minutes*

SERVICE PLAN
Record relevant details of your service and advice provided for future reference.
Ensure the client's records are up-to-date, accurate and fully completed following service. Non-compliance may invalidate insurance.

DURING
Discuss:

◆ details that may influence the client's ear piercing service (e.g., thickness of earlobes).

Note:

◆ any adverse reaction, if any occur.

AFTER
Record:

◆ results of service

◆ any modification to service application that has occurred

◆ what type of ear studs have been used in the ear piercing service

◆ the effectiveness of service.

Advise on:

◆ use of specialized aftercare products following ear piercing service for homecare use to promote skin healing and prevent contra-actions from occurring

◆ aftercare product application in order to gain maximum benefit from their use

◆ general ear piercing and maintenance advice

◆ the recommended time interval before removal of the stud

◆ the recommended time interval between ear piercing services.

Provide:

◆ an aftercare ear piercing leaflet.

RETAIL OPPORTUNITIES
Note:

◆ any purchases made by the client.

EVALUATION
Record:

◆ comments on the client's satisfaction with the service

◆ if poor results are achieved, the reasons why

◆ how you may alter the service plan to achieve the required service results in the future, if applicable.

HEALTH AND SAFETY
Advise on:

◆ how and when to turn the ear stud

◆ how and when to remove the ear stud

◆ recommended replacement of the ear stud used for piercing

◆ appropriate action to be taken in the event of an unwanted reaction to the service.

HEALTH & SAFETY

Recommended metals for ear piercing Certain metals may cause an allergy. These include non-compliant nickel, poor quality gold-plated metals and 9ct gold. The use of nickel-containing jewellery is subject to the Dangerous Substances and Preparations (Nickel) (Safety) Regulations (2005). Manufacturers should ensure that their earrings are regularly tested and comply with the Nickel Directive.

Recommended metals are surgical stainless steel grade 316, silver plate, titanium (6AL4V) and 9ct, 14ct and 18ct gold.

Check what metal is used for your ear jewellery with your supplier, and that it complies with the Regulations.

Knowledge Check

How would you describe the procedure of ear piercing to ensure a client was confident in the procedure?

Refer to page 567 to help you.

Professional

Remain professional at all times. It sounds simple, however this will have an incredibly calming effect on any clients who may be a little nervous or unsure. Be confident in how you address your client and be sensitive to any questions and queries, ensuring that they are comfortable throughout. Word of mouth is a vital marketing tool where ear piercing is concerned so always ensure that your client leaves 100 per cent satisfied with their piercing.

Kathryn Darwin

Preparation of the beauty therapist and client

1 Wash your hands using a hand disinfectant that contains chlorhexidine as an active ingredient and apply a fresh pair of disposable gloves.

2 Secure the client's hair away from the treatment area. Place paper tissue roll over client's shoulder. If the client already has ear piercings, ask them to remove the existing earrings.

3 Thoroughly cleanse the back and the front of the client's earlobes using the recommended cleaning lotion. Check the ears for contra-indications. Each ear should be cleaned separately, using new, sterile cleansing lotion or alcohol-based tissues. Allow the skin to dry. (If moisture is present, the mark will blur.)

4 Holding a mirror in front of the client, discuss with them where the stud should be placed. Mark the position using the sterile pen. Ensure client satisfaction with the placement of the stud, gain their confirmation and satisfaction to proceed. If the client prefers a different position, wipe off the marking with an antiseptic wipe, allow to dry and remark the position.

Remember that the ears are not at the same level on each side of the head, and may protrude at different angles. Take time when marking the position of the studs, to ensure that the final appearance is balanced and that the client is in agreement with the proposed placing of the ear stud.

STEP-BY-STEP: PREPARING THE CLIENT

2 Hygienically preparing the ear for piercing

3 Ear cleansing

4 Marking the agreed position for piercing

HEALTH & SAFETY

Secondary infection As you cleanse the client's earlobes, you may notice that their skin, ear or hair is dirty. You may proceed, but reinforce the aftercare instructions politely, tactfully stating the importance of cleanliness in preventing secondary infection.

Ear studs Studs are preferable to hooped earrings or sleepers, as dirt is less likely to cling to the stud and infect the ear.

ALWAYS REMEMBER

Fat lobes

If the client has fat lobes explain that the studs may feel a little tight.

Adjust tightness of stud in each ear using a clean tissue to hold the stud. Fresh disposable gloves must be worn if adjustment is necessary. Lobes more than 6 mm thick need special care and may require a long post stud.

Piercing the ears

Outcome 2: Be able to provide ear piercing

Learn how to prepare for ear piercing

PRACTICAL SKILLS

Communicate and behave in a professional manner

Follow health and safety working practices

Position yourself and the client correctly throughout the treatment

Use products, tools and equipment and techniques to suit client's treatment needs

Complete the treatment to the satisfaction of the client

Record the results of the treatment

Provide suitable aftercare advice

UNDERPINNING KNOWLEDGE

State how to communicate and behave in a professional manner

Describe health and safety working practices

State the importance of positioning yourself and the client correctly throughout the treatment

State the importance of using products, tools and equipment and techniques to suit client's treatment needs

State the contra-actions that may occur during and following treatments and how to respond

State the importance of completing the treatment to the satisfaction of the client

State the importance of completing treatment records

State the aftercare advice that should be provided

Describe the blood and lymph supply to the ear

Describe the external structure of the ear

HEALTH & SAFETY

Piercing ears Never perform multiple piercing in each ear. The ears will swell, causing discomfort and possible infection.

When more than one hole is required in the same ear the piercing must be at least 9 mm apart from the existing hole.

ALWAYS REMEMBER

Piercing placement

Try to aim for a central position on the earlobe – this will achieve the best result.

HEALTH & SAFETY

Hazards caused by poor practice Medical complications can occur where conditions that are contra-indicated are not diagnosed or treated. Poor technique due to poor anatomy and physiology knowledge and understanding can cause damage to blood vessels, nerves and skin tissue, e.g. keloid scarring.

Accuracy

The most common concern is the marking of the dots. When training I always remind students that we are not symmetrical and therefore our ears are definitely not the same. Clients should be sitting straight and you need room around you to manoeuvre. Check alignment by holding the ears out to see both dots at the same time. Insist that clients have a really good look before piercing and check where there is any hesitation.

Kathryn Darwin

STEP-BY-STEP: PIERCING THE EARS

The following procedure illustrates the general technique, with the beauty therapist wearing synthetic, powder-free vinyl gloves such as nitrile or PVC formulation. The details differ according to the ear piercing gun you are using. Always follow the manufacturer's instructions.

Ensure the service is cost-effective and completed in a commercial time, 15 minutes.

1 Holding the stud pack firmly, remove the backing paper. Complete this over your prepared work surface. Take care not to drop the cartridge on the floor! (If you do drop it you will have to throw it away.)

2 Pull back the plunger knob on the back of the gun, until it is fully extended – you will hear it click.

3 Remove the plastic cartridge from the package, holding it by the plastic mount. To avoid contamination, make sure that you do not touch the stud or backing clasp.

4 There are two parts, which must be separated. One part holds the back clasps: this is positioned in the slot. Push the cartridge down until it will go no further. The second holds the studs: position this against the stud barrel of the gun, which places a protective plastic ring around the barrel of the gun and stud.

5 Gently pull the holder upwards, away from the barrel: this will deposit the stud in the barrel.

6 Holding the gun horizontally, position the stem of the stud at right angles to the ear so that it is accurately placed over the mark on the earlobe.

Gently squeeze the trigger until it stops. Check that the point of the stud is still in the correct position. If it is, squeeze the trigger again. The ear will be pierced, with the back clasp placed onto the back of the stud.

Check that the earring and back clasp are securely connected.

7 Gently move the gun down from the lobe. Hold the gun upside down and discard the plastic ring into the waste bin. Pull back the plunger knob and insert the next stud and protective ring.

8 Holding the gun in one hand, grip the back-clasp holder (using the mount in the other hand) and remove the holder from the gun. Invert the holder and place it back into the gun, with the remaining clasp in the top position.

HEALTH & SAFETY

Never handle studs with your bare hands Follow the manufacturer's instructions for correct loading. There should never be a need to touch the studs or stud-holding devices as contamination can occur leading to infection.

9 Now pierce the second ear, repeating stage **6**. If only one piercing is required where double packs of studs are used, the other stud should be discarded.

10 Using the hand mirror, show the client their pierced ears and check that the result is to the client's satisfaction.

ALWAYS REMEMBER

Technique

Always hold the gun either horizontally or upwards. Never point the gun downwards once it has been loaded – if you do, the studs will fall out.

ALWAYS REMEMBER

Gun malfunction

If the piercing is successful but the clasp fails to attach to the post, firmly attach this manually without causing the client unnecessary distress.

If the ear stud needs adjustment following piercing, re-wash your hands and apply a fresh pair of gloves before touching the pierced ear.

TOP TIP

Technique

To avoid anxiety to the client, pierce the second ear without hesitation, yet safely.

How to complete the service

1 Discuss the aftercare instructions with the client (see later). Record details of the ear piercing treatment on the client's record card.

2 When the service has been completed, invert the gun, eject the protective ring, and remove the empty back-clasp holder. Dispose of the plastic cartridges into the waste bin.

3 Clean the gun using clean cotton wool and surgical spirit, and place it in the UV sterilizing cabinet. Always refer to manufacturer's instructions for guidance on hygiene maintenance of the gun.

4 Dispose of all used products in the covered lined waste bin.

5 Any item that is not disposable and that has been used on a client must be sterilized (or cleaned to ensure hygiene compliance for equipment such as towels) before use on another client to prevent *secondary infection*, or *cross-infection*.

Any item that has penetrated the skin (e.g. ear studs that required replacement during the procedure), must be disposed of hygienically immediately in a sharps box and should be disposed of safely in compliance with **clinical waste** procedures.

Knowledge Check

Why should only one pair of studs be fitted at once?

Refer to page 572 to help you.

TOP TIP

Client comfort

Allow the client to sit still for a few minutes following the service. Offer them tea or coffee. Some clients may be very anxious and need time to relax.

HEALTH & SAFETY

Disposal of waste Waste from skin-piercing procedures is classed as clinical waste.

All consumable materials used during the ear piercing service should be placed in a covered, lined waste bin, and disposed of in a sealed bag.

Waste materials that have come into contact with body fluids must be collected and disposed of by special arrangement.

The disposal of clinical waste is controlled by the Environment Agency. *The Environment Protection Act (1990): Waste Management: The Duty of Care, A Code of Practice* (ISBN 011 752577 X) provides further information on this subject.

Detailed information on safe disposal of health care waste is available from the Department of Health.

ACTIVITY

Differing procedures

The procedure for loading the different ear piercing guns varies. The procedure given above is one example. Referring to the literature you have collected on the different guns, note ways in which the various service procedures differ.

TOP TIP

Technique

The gun should not point down or up when piercing. If the angle of piercing is incorrect, the earring will hang forward, sideways or backwards. Hold at a right angle to the ear.

Aftercare advice

After the ear piercing, complete details of the service on the client's record card. It is normal to experience minor pain and redness on the area following the service, explain this to the client. The client should be given clear instructions on how to care for their ears to prevent secondary infection and promote skin healing. The studs must not be removed for 5 to 6 weeks to enable effective skin healing and prevent infection. The earrings should not be removed if there are any signs of inflammation or infection. If this occurs the client should contact their GP. Invite the client to return to the salon after this period for you to remove the studs.

Remind the client always to wash their hands before cleaning the ear area. (If someone else is going to clean the ears, they also must wash their hands with soap and warm water before touching the client's ears.) The ears should be cleaned twice daily, using an aftercare lotion. The lotion must be applied as directed by the manufacturer. It should be applied to clean cotton wool, and the cotton wool squeezed to allow the lotion to run around the stud, at the front of the ear and then at the back. While the ears are being bathed with the cleansing solution, the stud should be rotated by holding it firmly at the front.

Even if the client cleanses their ears effectively, infection could still occur in other ways. These include the following:

◆ long nails harbour germs. Infection of the ear can occur while the client is turning the stud

◆ the client may touch the stud and ear at times other than when cleaning the ear

◆ shampoo and dirty water may collect around the ear while shampooing the hair. Remind the client to rinse the ear thoroughly with clean water after shampooing

Sharps box

HEALTH & SAFETY

First Aid There must be a first aid kit available that complies with the Health and Safety (First Aid) Regulations (1981). It is recommended that there is a person trained in first aid holding a recognized certificate such as the HSE approved Basic First Aid Qualification.

Knowledge Check

Following ear piercing, consider the waste which will require disposal and how this waste should be disposed of.

Refer to page 575 to help you.

HEALTH & SAFETY

Antiseptic lotions Remind the client that if an antiseptic lotion is applied to the ear area, it must be diluted as directed or skin burning may occur.

TOP TIP

Legal requirements

Always check with your insurance company which areas of the body you are able to pierce.

- the area can get wet, e.g. after showering. Dry the area with a clean tissue if so
- the client should protect their ears when applying hair lacquer or perfume, to avoid sensitizing the ear
- following the removal of the studs, the client should only wear gold, hypoallergenic or nickel-compliant earrings. Cheap fashion earrings should be worn only for short periods of time, or allergic reactions and ear infections may occur. Avoid heavy earrings as these may stretch the holes and cause a slit effect. Post-style earrings should be worn continuously for at least 6 months to ensure the pierced hole doesn't heal following removal of the stud posts

After oral instructions have been given, the client should be provided with an aftercare leaflet containing these instructions.

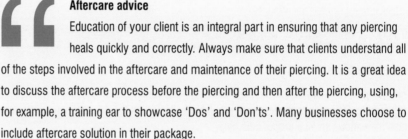

Aftercare advice
Education of your client is an integral part in ensuring that any piercing heals quickly and correctly. Always make sure that clients understand all of the steps involved in the aftercare and maintenance of their piercing. It is a great idea to discuss the aftercare process before the piercing and then after the piercing, using, for example, a training ear to showcase 'Dos' and 'Don'ts'. Many businesses choose to include aftercare solution in their package.

Kathryn Darwin

Body piercing

You may advance your piercing skills further to perform body piercing. Body piercing is currently very fashionable. Common areas for piercing include the nipples, the eyebrows, the nose and the navel. Note that body piercing is inappropriate for clients under 17 years of age, as the body is still growing.

Beauty therapy salons that offer ear piercing are often also asked for body piercing. Body piercing should be undertaken only if you have had thorough training, however, and only if you have the necessary specialized equipment and appropriate insurance cover.

Equipment

The equipment for piercing is either a body piercing gun, which inserts a hollow reed, or the needle and clamp method. With the latter, the clamp reduces circulation in the area, thereby anaesthetizing it, and the needle is inserted into the skin. The opening made by the needle is then filled with a ring or stud of high-quality non-reactive surgical steel or gold (above 16 carat).

Aftercare and advice

Special care should be taken of the area for 1 month following piercing. Ideally the jewellery must not be changed for 4 to 6 months to avoid tissue damage and possible infection. If infection occurs, causing excessive redness, swelling or a discharge, the client should return to the salon.

HEALTH & SAFETY

Body piercing Before performing body piercing, approval is required from your local Environmental Health Authority and registration is required.

Age and consent issues can be confirmed with your local authority who may use licensing powers to impose licensing conditions relating to the age of the client.

Knowledge Check

What aftercare instructions should be given to a client following ear piercing?

Refer to pages 575–576 to help you.

ASSESSMENT OF KNOWLEDGE AND UNDERSTANDING

You have now learnt about ear piercing in the beauty therapy workplace. To test your level of knowledge, answer the following short questions. These will prepare you for your summative (final) assessment.

1. The part of the ear that is recommended for ear piercing is the:

   a. helix
   b. lobule
   c. pinna

2. Which part of the ear is considered unsuitable and can result in keloid scarring?

   a. lobule
   b. helix
   c. pinna

3. What is the healing period before the removal of the initial jewellery used to pierce the ears?

   a. 6 weeks
   b. 5–6 weeks
   c. 6–8 weeks
   d. 3–4 weeks

4. The legislation that enables each local authority to regulate businesses providing cosmetic piercing is the:

   a. Control of Substances Hazardous to Health (COSHH) Regulations (2002)
   b. Management of Health and Safety at Work Regulations (1999)
   c. Local Government Act (2003)

5. How often is it recommended the ear studs be rotated during the healing period?

   a. once a day
   b. twice a day
   c. three to four times a day
   d. once per week

6. The group of lymph nodes that drain the ear area are the:

   a. parotid nodes
   b. occipital nodes
   c. buccal nodes
   d. sub-mental nodes

7. Which of the following contra-indications would require to be verbally checked for?

   a. anti-coagulant drugs
   b. epilepsy
   c. diabetes
   d. all of the above

8. Disposable gloves must be worn when performing ear piercing service. Which legislation does this comply with?

9. The image below shows skin healing contra-action in the ear tissue, known as what?

10. Poor aftercare may result in secondary infection – how would this be recognized?

17 Head Massage

LEARNING OBJECTIVES

There are two learning outcomes to achieve for this optional unit:

1 Be able to prepare for head massage.

2 Be able to provide head massage.

The assessment range applied requires you to:

◆ Use consultation techniques to identify the treatment objectives.

◆ Meet all treatment preparation requirements.

◆ Carry out checks before treatment takes place to consider any factors which may affect the treatment plan.

◆ Ensure the environmental conditions are suitable.

◆ Follow and take into consideration all health and safety working practices.

◆ Use all listed products, tools and equipment as appropriate.

◆ Complete a consultation and skin inspection to identify any contra-indications that may affect if and how the treatment can proceed

◆ Communicate and behave in an appropriate and professional manner.

◆ Identify contra-actions.

◆ Provide relevant aftercare and contra-action advice.

◆ Use different methods of evaluation to assess the success of the treatment, including observation, written, verbal and self-evaluation.

KEY TERMS

aftercare advice

aseptic

consultation

contra-action advice

contra-actions

effleurage

frictions

hair condition

hair density

hair length

health and safety

massage techniques

Oils

petrissage

skin sensitivity patch test

treatment objectives

treatment plan

vibrations

Unit Topic

Head massage

This VRQ unit is linked to the Beauty Therapy NOS Unit B23.

INTRODUCTION

This unit is all about how to provide head massage treatment. The massage is applied to the head, neck and scalp providing both a physiological and psychological effect. Application is modified to achieve the client's treatment objectives identified at consultation. This includes for the purpose of relaxation, well-being and stimulation. Oils may be used, selected to enhance the treatment results, improving the condition of both the skin and hair.

Dealing with people in a polite, efficient manner to reassure them and using good communication and questioning skills to find out exactly what they require from the head massage treatment forms an important part of this technical service.

You must be able to show that you have the necessary practical skills and underpinning knowledge to provide head massage.

INDUSTRY ROLE MODEL

ELEANOR WRIGHT Training Manager, Sanctuary Spa, Covent Garden

"After spending many years as a beauty therapist in salons and spas I went on to be involved in a Boutique Hotel and Spa start-up. Here I was responsible for everything from concept to opening. After establishing myself as an accomplished manager, I went on to train as a lecturer and assessor. I continued to work in my management role whilst teaching and assessing at college. I gained experience as a session nail technician and trainer for the Leighton Denny brand, working on magazine shoots and London Fashion Week. My experience led me to the role of Training Manager at the prestigious Sanctuary Spa, Covent Garden where I am responsible for the training and ongoing development of all team members within the business, which employs a team of approximately 110.

I am also lucky enough to develop new treatments, which are delivered by our expert beauty therapists to the 64 000 women who visit the spa every year.

ANATOMY & PHYSIOLOGY
Essential anatomy and physiology knowledge requirements for this chapter are identified in the checklist chart on page 33.

Purpose of head massage treatment

Head massage is a treatment applied to the neck and head using the hands. It helps to relieve stress and tension, and can create a feeling of well-being. Head massage combines modern Swedish body **massage techniques** with the traditional techniques of Indian head massage. This unit will cover the application of massage technique movements **effleurage**, **petrissage**, tapotement, **frictions** and **vibrations**. These techniques can be developed further at Level 3 to provide Indian head massage treatment.

As the therapeutic effects of massage become increasingly popular, head massage is an ideal treatment to offer and has many advantages that can meet the needs of a range of different clients. It can also be used to enhance other treatments such as facials, e.g. you may perform a scalp and neck massage after the face mask has been applied. There is no need for the client to undress, it is relatively quick to perform, can be performed almost anywhere and does not require related expensive equipment.

Benefits of head massage

There are many general benefits of head massage that address the symptoms of everyday working, including:

◆ headaches caused by stress and tension

◆ aches and pains caused by poor posture in the neck and shoulder area, i.e. long periods working on a computer

◆ poor sleeping problems are improved.

Oils may be incorporated into the massage to condition the skin of the scalp and hair. Their application within massage can also help to induce relaxation.

Massage is adapted to both the client's physiological and psychological needs. These are identified and agreed during the client **consultation** and are termed the objectives of the treatment.

These objectives may include:

◆ relaxation

◆ creating and maintaining a feeling of well-being

◆ an uplifting or stimulating effect

◆ improving the condition of the skin of the scalp and hair.

Physiological effects of head massage

Head massage application

◆ The muscles receive an improved supply of oxygenated blood, essential for cell growth. The tone and strength of muscles are improved. Areas of muscular tension will become relaxed.

◆ Increased joint mobility in the neck area occurs through massage movement to the area.

◆ The increased blood circulation in the area warms the tissues. This induces a feeling of relaxation, which is particularly beneficial when treating tense muscles.

◆ As the blood capillaries dilate and bring blood to the skin's surface, the skin colour improves.

◆ The lymphatic circulation and the venous blood circulation increase. These changes speed up the removal of waste products and toxins. The removal of excess lymph improves the appearance of a puffy oedematous skin, it also improves production of white blood cells which help fight infections.

◆ Sensory nerve endings can be soothed or stimulated, depending on the massage movements selected.

◆ Massage stimulates the sebaceous and sudoriferous glands increasing the production of sweat and sebum. This helps to increase the skin's natural oil and moisture balance.

◆ Applying oil to the scalp and hair (optional) adds moisture and improves the condition of hair or scalp according to the oil used.

◆ Massage to the scalp may stimulate hair growth by increasing blood supply to the hair follicle, e.g. in cases of alopecia, hair loss.

❝ Think about your environment! Massage treatments are relaxing treatments for your client to enjoy. It is amazing how much people will notice, so always ensure your work area is clear from clutter, has the right lighting, use music and candles to create ambience. The right environment will enhance your client's enjoyment of their treatment.

Eleanor Wright

Effleurage – stroking technique to the forehead frontal bone. This technique can be used all over the whole scalp area

The psychological effects of massage are broad, and when performed on a regular basis can benefit the client. The client may feel less stressed, fresher, more invigorated and healthier.

Psychological effects of head massage

◆ Helps to improve concentration – increased oxygen to the brain

◆ Relieves tension

◆ Induces relaxation

◆ Relieves stress and anxiety

◆ Confidence-raising following the removal of tension.

Massage techniques

Head massage is based on a series of classic Westernized and Indian massage movements, applied to create different effects. There are five basic massage techniques:

◆ effleurage

◆ petrissage

◆ tapotement (percussion)

◆ frictions

◆ vibrations.

The beauty therapist can adapt the way each massage movement is applied, according to the **treatment objectives**. Either the *speed* of application or the *depth of pressure* can be altered.

Effleurage Effleurage is a stroking movement, used to begin the massage, as a link movement, and to complete the massage sequence. This movement can be applied lightly or briskly, has an even pressure and is applied in a rhythmical, continuous manner to induce relaxation. The speed of application depends upon the effect to be achieved and according to the underlying structures and tissue type, but it must *never* be unduly heavy. Movements also include stroking. Effleurage has the following effects:

- desquamation (skin removal) is increased

- arterial blood circulation is increased, bringing oxygen and fresh nutrients to the area, energizing the client and warming the tissues

- venous circulation is improved, aiding the removal of congestion from the veins

- lymphatic circulation is increased, improving the absorption of waste products and elimination of toxins from the tissues

- the underlying muscle fibres are relaxed

- relaxes and soothes sensory nerve endings.

Uses in treatment: to relax tight and contracted muscles.

Petrissage

Petrissage involves a series of movements in which the tissues are lifted away from the underlying structures and compressed, including kneading and squeezing and releasing the muscles along their length. The whole hands or just the fingers and thumbs may be used. Pressure is intermittent, and should be light yet firm. Petrissage has the following effects:

- improvement of muscle tone, through the compression and relaxation of muscle fibres

- improvement in blood and lymph circulation, as the application of pressure causes the vessels to empty and fill

- increased activity of the sebaceous glands, due to the stimulation effect on the skin tissues.

Movements include picking up, kneading, pinching and rolling.

Uses in treatment: to stimulate a sluggish circulation; to increase sebaceous gland and sudoriferous gland activity when treating a dry skin condition.

Percussion

Percussion, also known as tapotement, is performed in a brisk, stimulating manner. Rhythm is important as the fingers are continually breaking contact with the skin; irritation or damage can occur if this movement is performed incorrectly. Percussion has the following effects:

- stimulation of the nerves

- a fast vascular (skin reddening) reaction because of the skin's nervous response to the stimulus – this reaction, erythema, is a sign of skin stimulation

- increased blood supply, which nourishes the tissues

- improvement in skin and muscle tone in the area.

Movements include hacking and tapping. When performed on the scalp, only light pressure should be used. In facial massage only light tapping should be used.

Uses in treatment: to tone areas of loose skin and improve blood and lymphatic circulation in the area.

Frictions

Frictions cause the skin and superficial structure to move together over the underlying structures. These movements are performed with either the fingers or the thumbs and concentrated in a particular area, applied with regulated pressure. Frictions have the following effects:

TOP TIP

Relief from tension and stress

Massaging the scalp and neck can relieve symptoms of stress such as stiffness in the neck and headaches.

HEALTH & SAFETY

Skin elasticity As the skin ages it becomes thinner and less elastic. Take care when using petrissage movements to avoid skin tissue damage.

Also, any areas of scar tissue will not be as supple as normal skin, care in handling is required.

Petrissage – picking up the muscle and skin at the back of the neck

Percussion – hands positioned for hacking movement. This movement is applied lightly to the scalp

Frictions to the scalp

Vibrations to the scalp

- ◆ desquamation (skin removal) is increased

- ◆ gentle stimulation of the skin and superficial tissues improving functioning

- ◆ improves scar tissue by breaking down the tissue adhesions

- ◆ improved lymphatic and blood circulation

- ◆ breaks down tight nodules (tension in the muscle fibres), improving mobility.

Uses in treatment: to help break down fatty deposits, fibrous thickening and the removal of non-medical oedema (fluid retention). To stimulate and improve a dry skin condition.

Vibrations   Vibrations are applied on the nerve centre. They are produced by a rapid contraction and relaxation of the beauty therapist's arm, resulting in a fine trembling movement. Vibration has the following effects:

- ◆ stimulation of the nerves, inducing a feeling of well-being

- ◆ gentle stimulation of the skin.

Movements include *static* vibrations, in which the pads of the fingers are placed on the nerve and the vibratory effect created by the beauty therapist's arms and hands is applied in one position; and running vibrations, in which the vibratory effect is applied along a nerve path. Static vibrations are shown where the fingers grasp the hair, carrying the vibratory effect to the scalp.

Uses in treatment: to stimulate a sensitive skin in order to improve the skin's functioning without irritating the surface blood capillaries. Stimulation of the scalp; increasing blood and lymphatic circulation in the area and nerve endings relieving tension.

> "Don't over-complicate your treatment when you explain it to your client. It is so easy as a beauty therapist to get carried away with the physiological effects when speaking to our clients that sometimes we end up confusing them with the language we use. Keep it simple by giving them a key benefit and effect of the treatment that links to any concerns they discussed in their consultation.
>
> *Eleanor Wright*

Preparing the working area

Prepare the work area to meet all **health and safety** legislation requirements.

The treatment area should be clean and at a warm, comfortable working temperature for both the client and the beauty therapist, between 18 and 21°C. Adequate ventilation should be provided to create a hygienic environment, preventing cross-infection through viral airborne spores, drowsiness through carbon dioxide-saturated air and the removal of stale smells and odours. The treatment area should make the client feel comfortable and relaxed. Lighting should be soft, the colour of the decor should be subtle and non-gender biased. Sound levels should be low and selected for relaxation. If performing the treatment over a couch there should be adequate support in the form of a bolster (a pillow) cushion to support the head and neck and ensure client comfort. Place all the products, tools and equipment required on the trolley prior to the treatment, to ensure that an efficient treatment is provided without unnecessary disruptions.

Outcome 1: Be able to prepare for head massage

Learn how to prepare for head massage

PRACTICAL SKILLS

Prepare yourself, the client and work area for head massage

Use suitable consultation techniques to identify treatment objectives

Advise the client on how to prepare for the treatment

Identify influencing factors

Provide clear recommendations to the client based on factors

UNDERPINNING KNOWLEDGE

Describe salon's requirement for client preparation, preparing yourself and the work area

Identify different consultation techniques used to identify treatment objectives

Describe the factors that need to be considered when selecting techniques, products and equipment

Describe the environmental conditions suitable for head massage treatment

Describe the safety considerations that must be taken into account when providing head massage treatment

Identify the range of equipment used for head massage treatment

Identify products used and their key ingredients

Describe contra-indications that prevent or restrict head massage treatment

Sterilization and disinfection

Prior to the head massage treatment, make sure that the work area is hygienic. The surface of the massage chair/couch and the trolley surface should be wiped over with disinfectant.

Plastic spatulas, if used, should be cleaned and placed in an UV cabinet prior to use to ensure they are free from bacteria. Disposables are ideal for this purpose.

An **aseptic** condition should be maintained, a situation where you are trying to eliminate bacteria. The treatment area should remain in a safe and hygienic state throughout the day, ready for each treatment. Waste at the end of each treatment should be disposed of in a sealed polythene bag and used towels removed ready to be laundered.

Clean towels should be provided for each client to prevent cross-infection. Disposable paper roll may be used to cover work surfaces.

Remember to use the underpinning knowledge you learnt about in Chapter 3 Health and Safety.

ALWAYS REMEMBER

Treatment timing

It is important to complete treatment in the given time. This will ensure that:

- each client receives a treatment meeting their treatment requirements
- clients are not disadvantaged by receiving a hurried treatment
- a relaxing treatment environment in which clients are not made to feel anxious or stressed due to treatment delay is maintained.

Products, tools and equipment

- ◆ **Massage chair or couch**
- ◆ **Chair** With adjustable height, low back support without an arm rest

Specialist head and neck massage treatment chair shown. Alternatively a treatment couch may be used

On-site massage chair

- ◆ **Organic massage oil** For example almond, olive, mustard, sesame, coconut or pre-blended oil. The oil is warmed before application to aid absorption and induce relaxation
- ◆ **Trolley** Or other surface on which to place everything
- ◆ **Combs** To allow the client to comb their hair following treatment
- ◆ **Plastic bowls (2)** To dispense products into as necessary and hold consumables
- ◆ **Clean towels** Freshly laundered for each client

Combs

A towel may be placed over the client's shoulders if using oils

- ◆ **Hair clips** Used to secure long hair away from the neck area
- ◆ **Client record card** To record confidential details of each client registered at the salon including personal details, products used and details of the treatment

Hair clips

YOU WILL ALSO NEED:

- ◆ **Paper tissue disposable bedroll** To cover the treatment couch cover if used
- ◆ **Dry and damp cotton wool and tissues** To apply skin-cleansing agents and dry the skin
- ◆ **Skin cleansing agent** Such as witch hazel or eau de cologne
- ◆ **Cosmetic cleansing preparations** To remove facial make-up (as necessary)
- ◆ **Waste container** Metal lined bin with a disposable liner
- ◆ **Aftercare advice** Recommended advice for the client to refer to following the treatment

HEALTH & SAFETY

Legislation It is important that you comply with all relevant health and safety legislation while performing head massage.

Examples include:

Workplace (Health, Safety and Welfare) Regulations (1992)

Control of Substances Hazardous to Health Regulations (COSHH) (2002)

Electricity at Work Regulations (1989)

HEALTH & SAFETY

Allergies Refer to the client record card to check for any known allergies to products, which could cause a contra-action, e.g., sesame oil can cause skin irritation. Where possible select an alternative such as olive oil.

Reception

Head massage can be carried out as required, but is usually recommended once or twice a week, and preferably as a course for maximum effect. Regularity of treatments will depend upon the client's personal circumstances including their financial position and time constraints. When a client is booking for this treatment, allow 10–15 minutes (excluding consultation and preparation time), which includes practical treatment and **aftercare advice**. Warn the client that they may have a reaction after treatment. Symptoms can include tiredness, muscular aches and possibly headaches. This reaction will normally subside after 24 hours. If the client is wearing a false hair piece warn them that this will have to be removed.

If using oils a **skin sensitivity patch test** should be carried out in advance, usually 24 hours before treatment, to assess the client's tolerance to the recommended products to be used in the treatment.

Before beginning the head massage treatment, check that you have the necessary products, equipment and materials to hand and that they meet the legal, hygiene and industry requirements for head massage treatment.

Preparation of the beauty therapist

The beauty therapist should wear a professional work uniform which does not restrict movement. Full, enclosed shoes should be worn with low or medium-height heels. Optionally shoes may be removed when performing the massage to assist energy flow through the body. (Always follow your workplace policy.) Jewellery must be removed from the hands and wrists.

Before preparing the client for the treatment, wash your hands. The hands need to be flexible in order to fit the contour of the client's upper body. Shake the hands to remove any tension from the wrists and hands. Practise deep slow breathing technique before applying massage. This will help you to relax and focus your concentration on the massage treatment.

Collect the client's record card from reception prior to their arrival. A full client consultation should be carried out before the treatment commences, including a postural check of the neck area. This will help you to identify any areas of tension.

Is the neck straight or is there an exaggerated curve? Is the neck drawn towards the left or right shoulder? Does the chin poke forwards causing the neck to curve forwards? Make the client aware of this so that they can consciously correct the problem. Treatment can only proceed if the reason for the curvature is non-medical and it is related to tension or poor posture.

Beauty therapist's hands The beauty therapist should always disinfect their hands prior to the treatment. Nails should be short, to avoid scratching the client and to facilitate massage application. The hands also need to be flexible in order to fit the contours of the client's body. Mobilizing the joints of the hands and fingers will loosen the hands and facilitate good movements. Hand exercises should be practised on a regular basis.

> " Consultation is key! Find out as much as you can about your client and their expectations of the treatment. You will not only check their medical information, but find out how they have come to book this treatment with you. You will always be able to provide a fabulous treatment and please your client following a thorough consultation.
>
> *Eleanor Wright*

Hair analysis

Hair length If the client's hair is long it may be necessary to clip the hair away to perform certain massage movements. Ensure the hair is tangle-free before you begin.

Hair texture The thickness or diameter of the individual hair strand. Hair texture can be classified as coarse, medium or fine. It is not uncommon for hair from different areas

TOP TIP

The number of hairs on the head generally varies with the colour of the hair.

Hair colour	Average number of hairs on head
Blonde	140 000
Brown	110 000
Black	108 000
Red	80 000

ALWAYS REMEMBER

Postural check of the neck

If the head pokes forward this can lead to neck and shoulder pain, headaches, tiredness and backache caused by unnecessary strain on the ligaments and muscles of the neck.

ALWAYS REMEMBER

Local Authority Licensing Regulations (2003)

Massage treatments must apply for a licence to practise from their local authority's environmental health department. Your local authority will advise you on the requirements for a licence and how to obtain a licence.

TOP TIP

Breathing technique

Advise the client that breathing should be deep and slow, not shallow and rapid.

Before treatment encourage the client to breathe in slowly through the nose – the stomach should move out slightly – and out through the mouth.

TOP TIP

Long hair

If the client has long hair secure it with a clip while performing massage to the neck.

of the head to have different textures. Coarse hair texture has the thickest diameter and is the strongest. Care must be taken with fine hair to prevent breakage when performing movements which pull at the base of the hair. If the hair is thick in diameter it will be more difficult to access the scalp.

Hair density Relates to the amount of hair the client has on their scalp. Hair density can be classified as low, medium or high. The average hair density is about 2200 hairs per square inch. Hair with high density (thick or dense hair) has more hairs per square inch, and hair with low density (thin hair) has fewer hairs per square inch. Density of hair will affect the quantity of oil required, if used, thick density requiring more oil. The average head of hair contains about 100 000 individual hair strands. If the hair density suddenly changes this may be related to the client's health, refer the client to their GP before treatment.

Degree of curl This is determined by the wave pattern of the hair which refers to the shape of the hair shaft, and is described as straight, wavy, curly, or extremely curly. Natural wave patterns are genetic. Although there are many exceptions, as a general rule Asian hair tends to be extremely straight hair, European hair tends to be straight to wavy and African hair tends to be extremely curly. But anyone of any race, or mixed race, can have hair with varying degrees of curliness from straight to extremely curly. Care must be taken when performing head massage on extremely curly hair as it often has low elasticity, breaks easily, and has a tendency to knot, especially on the ends. It will benefit from the oil application to condition, strengthen and reduce tangling.

Hair porosity Hair porosity is the ability of the hair to absorb moisture. The degree of porosity is directly related to the condition of the cuticle layer. Healthy hair has a compact cuticle layer and is naturally resistant to penetration. Porous hair has a raised cuticle layer that easily absorbs moisture. Chemically treated hair is more porous and will benefit from the moisturizing effect of the chosen oil. Overly porous hair is often dry, fragile and brittle. It can also often feel rough to the touch. Care must be taken with very porous hair to avoid breakage.

Hair and scalp conditions

Dry hair and scalp Dry hair and scalp can be caused by underactive sebaceous glands, and can be made worse by excessive shampooing or exposure to dry, warm air, such as during winter. The lack of natural oils (sebum) leads to hair that appears dull, dry and lifeless. Dry hair and scalp should be treated with oils that stimulate the sebaceous glands and have an emollient effect.

Oily hair and scalp Oily hair and scalp can be caused by improper shampooing or overactive sebaceous glands, and is characterized by a greasy build up on the scalp and an oily coating on the hair. Oily hair and scalp can be improved by properly washing and rinsing the hair and using an oil regulating shampoo. A well-balanced diet, exercise, regular shampooing and good personal hygiene are essential to controlling oily hair and scalp.

Hair loss Under normal circumstances, some hair is lost every day. Normal daily hair loss is the natural result of the three phases of the hair's growth cycle. Abnormal hair loss is called alopecia. Head massage must not be provided in the case of abnormal hair loss. Massage is beneficial to perform when healthy hair begins to grow back following abnormal hair loss, with GP consent. Care must be taken to avoid irritating the scalp when massaging a client with low hair density as the scalp will have less protection and may easily become sensitized.

Dandruff (Pityriasis) A scalp condition is characterized by the excessive production and accumulation of skin cells and is thought to be caused by a fungus. Instead of the normal shedding of tiny individual skin cells, one at a time, dandruff results from the removal of an accumulation of large visible clumps of cells. Some individuals are more susceptible to the irritating effects of dandruff and factors such as stress, age, hormones and poor hygiene can cause dandruff symptoms to worsen. Dandruff is not contagious and may be treated when controlled by a specialist shampoo. Sometimes when not treated, scales may build up and the scalp may be itchy and irritated which should not be treated and referred to a GP.

Psoriasis A non-contagious skin condition involving abnormal cell growth (see page 59). Psoriasis can appear on the scalp. Do not treat severe psoriasis where the skin is broken, as bacterial infection could occur. If there are scales present avoid these areas as bleeding can occur if these are removed whilst massaging. Only ever treat mild psoriasis where there is no risk of harm to the client or contact with tissue fluid.

Seborrheic warts Raised, pigmented rough patches of skin (see page 59). These are non-contagious and may occur on the scalp of elderly clients. Avoid massaging over the area but if unsure refer the client to their GP before treatment.

Selecting massage oils

Suitable massage oils If using oils, organic oils are the most suitable oils when massaging the scalp. High in polyunsaturated fats, these oils are very soft and liquid at room temperature. They have healing benefits from their fatty acid, vitamin and nutrient content. They absorb easily through the skin, and have both an internal and external effect. Approximately 2–5ml is required for the scalp massage, this will, of course, vary according to the length of the client's hair and condition of the scalp. The oil is applied at body temperature or 1 to 2 degrees above. The choice of oil depends on its texture, smell and specific properties to meet the treatment objectives agreed at consultation. Popular oils are sesame, mustard, almond, olive and coconut. Pre-blended oils can also be used which are essential oils, aromatic substances which can be hazardous if applied to the skin. They are added to a vegetable oil called a carrier oil, which enables the oils to penetrate into the skin in order to achieve different therapeutic effects dependent upon the oils chosen.

> " If you are applying a product to work with during your massage sequence then remember to consider when and how you do this. For a client trying to relax there is nothing worse that hearing the flip of a capped bottle, the squirt of oil and the beauty therapist rubbing their hands together. Remember to decant this discretely so that they are not disturbed. It is considerations like this that will set your treatment apart from others!
>
> *Eleanor Wright*

ALWAYS REMEMBER

Pre-blended oils

The smell of the essential oil, when inhaled, is picked up by the olfactory nerve, a nerve found high up inside the nose and responsible for the sense of smell. The odour molecules, simple chemical units from the essential oils, dissolve in the nasal mucus. The receptor cells cause a nerve impulse to the olfactory nerves. The smell can influence the behaviour of the person causing stimulation or relaxation. Choose an oil that your client will enjoy the smell of when inhaled as well as the physiological benefit.

Massage oils

Name	Plant	Use
Sesame oil		This oil is high in minerals which nourish the skin and hair. Sesame oil has a high lecithin content (a fat-like substance) thought to relieve swelling and muscular pains. Sesame oil may irritate sensitive skin and scalps
Mustard oil		A strong-smelling oil which creates an intense heating, invigorating action. Popular for use in winter due to its warming action. The increase in body heat relieves pain, swellings and relaxes stiff muscles. The skin's pores open and a cleansing action is created. Not suitable on sensitive skin and scalps as it may cause irritation
Almond oil		A light-textured oil, it is warm pressed and good to moisturize dry skin and hair as it is high in unsaturated fatty acids (essential fats derived from food), protein and vitamins A, B, D and E
Olive oil		Cold pressed from olives and has an emollient, healing and nourishing effect. It has a thick consistency high in unsaturated fatty acids, suitable for excessively dry hair and skin. It also creates a heating action which helps to relieve pain, swellings and relax stiff muscles
Coconut oil		A medium-to-light oil with skin and **hair conditioning** and emollient properties; particularly suitable for dry, brittle, chemically-treated hair. Popular for use in summer as it induces a cooling action on the scalp

Head massage treatment should be adapted in application to meet the client's physiological and psychological needs obtained at the consultation.

Once the consultation is complete, the beauty therapist should ensure that all details are recorded accurately and that the client has signed their record card. This enables continuity of service and up-to-date tracking of the treatments received. An example of a typical record card is provided in this chapter on page 54.

Preparation of the client

Take the client through to the treatment area. Preparation will depend upon how the client is being positioned for the treatment. The client will need to remove any outdoor clothing such as a coat or jacket. Footwear may be removed and the feet placed flat on the floor. Clients can generally receive head massage through their outdoor clothing, but bulky clothing which may restrict treatment application should be removed. Shirt or blouse collars should be loosened to allow access to the neck region. If oil is to be used for the massage, upper clothing should be removed and the client provided with a towel. Any jewellery in the area of massage application should be removed – this includes earrings, necklaces, bracelets and watches. Other accessories such as glasses should also be removed. False hairpieces will also need to be removed before treatment. If you are using screens, ensure that these are fully closed to maintain the client's privacy. This will enable the client to feel more comfortable and relaxed – essential if they are to gain treatment benefit. Seat the client on a low-backed massage chair or alternatively they can be positioned lying on a treatment couch. If the client is in a wheelchair it may be possible to treat them while sitting in their chair, which means minimum disturbance to the client. Ensure the client is seated comfortably; correct positioning will optimize the massage treatment effects. If the client is lying down for the head massage prepare the client as if receiving a facial.

While performing Indian head massage and all treatments it is very important to remember the medical contra-indications and the health and safety aspects at all times.

Make sure you are aware of your spa or salon's operating procedures and follow them with every treatment to continually provide safe treatments to a high standard.

Consultation

Discuss with the client their treatment requirements. Explain clearly to the client what the head massage treatment involves and the effects that can be gained. Treatment objectives must be realistic and achievable. Discuss the way the treatment application can be modified or adapted to meet their specific needs including the use of oil. Agree the treatment objectives with the client to meet their needs, both physically and psychologically. Allow time and invite the client to ask questions – the client should fully understand what the treatment involves including costs, duration, frequency recommendations including post-treatment reactions.

The beauty therapist needs to obtain relevant details from the client before starting the head massage treatment. The beauty therapist must ensure that their communication skills make the client feel welcome and comfortable. The client should be at ease throughout the treatment and a good, professional rapport should be built between client and beauty therapist. Personal details taken from the client are recorded on a record card. These should include medical history, doctor's details, and contra-indications that may be present.

Lifestyle

It is important to find out about the lifestyle habits of the client at the consultation. These include:

◆ *Occupation* – the client's occupation may be stressful or contribute to poor posture and muscle fatigue.

◆ *Family situation* – the client's domestic situation may affect their stress levels and limit their opportunities to take exercise or relax.

◆ *Dietary and fluid intake* – a nutritionally balanced diet is vital to the health of the body and the appearance of the skin. Lack of energy, skin allergies and disorders are, in part, the result of a poorly balanced diet. A healthy diet contains all the nutrients we need for health and growth. *Caffeine*, which is a stimulant, is found in

Sample record card for head massage

Date	Beauty therapist name	
Client name	Date of birth (identifying client age group)	
Home address	Postcode	
Email address	Landline phone number	Mobile phone number
Name of doctor	Doctor's address and phone number	
Related medical history (conditions that may restrict or prohibit treatment application)		
Are you taking any medication? (i.e. if taking medication to control blood pressure, head massage will alter blood pressure temporarily)		

CONTRA-INDICATIONS REQUIRING MEDICAL REFERRAL
(Preventing Indian head massage treatment application.)

☐ bacterial infection, e.g. impetigo
☐ viral infection, e.g. herpes simplex
☐ fungal infection, e.g. tinea unguium
☐ skin disorders, i.e. sebaceous cyst, eczema, acne vulgaris
☐ skin disease
☐ hair and scalp disorders
☐ high or low blood pressure
☐ recent head and neck injury
☐ severe bruising
☐ severe cuts and abrasions
☐ hair disorders
☐ medical conditions
☐ diabetes
☐ recent scar tissue
☐ dysfunction of the nervous system
☐ epilepsy
☐ during chemotherapy and radio therapy

TREATMENT AREAS

☐ scalp
☐ head
☐ neck

MASSAGE TECHNIQUE

☐ effleurage   ☐ petrissage
☐ tapotement   ☐ frictions
☐ vibrations

MASSAGE MEDIUM (IF USED)

☐ organic oil – type _____

CONTRA-INDICATIONS THAT RESTRICT TREATMENT
(treatment may require adaptation)

☐ cuts and abrasions   ☐ bruising and swelling
☐ recent injuries to the treatment area
☐ medication   ☐ mild eczema/psoriasis
☐ recent scar tissue (avoid area)
☐ undiagnosed lumps, bumps, swellings
☐ migraine   ☐ product allergies

LIFESTYLE

☐ occupation   _____
☐ family situation   _____
☐ dietary and fluid intake (including allergies) _____
☐ hobbies, interests, means of relaxation   _____
☐ exercise habits   _____
☐ smoking habits   _____
☐ sleep patterns   _____

PHYSICAL CHARACTERISTICS

☐ posture   ☐ hair condition
☐ health   ☐ scalp condition
☐ muscle tone   ☐ age
☐ skin condition

OBJECTIVES OF TREATMENT

☐ relaxation   ☐ stimulating and uplifting
☐ health and well-being
☐ improvement of hair and scalp condition

PRODUCTS, TOOLS AND EQUIPMENT

☐ towels   ☐ comb
☐ spatulas   ☐ protective covering
☐ consumables   ☐ hair clip
☐ massage chair/couch

Beauty therapist signature (for reference)
Client signature (confirmation of details)

Sample record card for head massage (continued)

TREATMENT ADVICE

Head massage treatment – *this treatment will take approximately 10–15 minutes*

TREATMENT PLAN

Record relevant details of your treatment and advice provided for future reference. Ensure the client's records are up-to-date, accurate and fully completed following treatment. Non-compliance may invalidate insurance.

DURING

- ◆ explain choice of massage medium and its benefits
- ◆ explain the treatment procedure at each stage of the massage to meet the treatment needs
- ◆ explain how the massage products should be applied and removed for home use
- ◆ note any adverse reaction, if any occur, and action taken.

AFTER

- ◆ record the areas treated
- ◆ record any modification to treatment application that has occurred
- ◆ record what products have been used in the treatment as appropriate
- ◆ provide postural advice
- ◆ provide hair and scalp advice
- ◆ provide advice to follow immediately following treatment, to include suitable rest period following treatment, general advice regarding food and drink intake, avoidance of stimulants
- ◆ recommended time intervals between treatments
- ◆ discuss the benefits of continuous treatments
- ◆ record the effectiveness of treatment
- ◆ record any samples provided (review their success at the next appointment).

RETAIL OPPORTUNITIES

- ◆ provide guidance on progression of the treatment plan for future appointments
- ◆ advice regarding products that would be suitable for home use and how to gain maximum benefit from their use to care for the skin and continue the treatment benefits
- ◆ recommendations for further treatments including heat treatment and body massage treatments
- ◆ advice of further products or treatments that you have recommended that the client may or may not have received before
- ◆ note any purchase made by the client.

EVALUATION

- ◆ record comments on the client's satisfaction with the treatment
- ◆ record if the treatment objectives were achieved, e.g. relaxation, if not, explore the reasons why not
- ◆ record how you will progress the treatment to maintain and advance the treatment results in the future.

HEALTH AND SAFETY

- ◆ advise on avoidance of activities that may cause a contra-action, including strenuous exercises and stimulants such as caffeine and alcohol
- ◆ advise on appropriate necessary action to be taken in the event of an unwanted reaction (an allergy to the oil used, headaches, and aching muscles.

TREATMENT MODIFICATION

Examples of massage treatment modification includes:

- ◆ altering the pressure or choice of movement during massage to suit the client's skin and muscle tone
- ◆ adapting the massage to achieve an effect of relaxation, stimulation
- ◆ altering the choice of massage medium to treat the skin/hair condition.

tea, coffee and some fizzy drinks. Excessive amounts can interfere with digestion and block the absorption of vitamins and minerals. *Water* is important to avoid dehydration of the body and *at least* one litre of natural water should be drunk per day.

◆ *Alcohol* – alcohol is a toxin (poison) and deprives the body of vitamin reserves, especially vitamins B and C. It also causes dehydration.

◆ *Hobbies and interests* – these leisure activities can be a form of relaxation and method to alleviate stress.

◆ *Exercise taken and regularity* – a lack of exercise leads to poor lymph and blood circulation and poor muscle tone, resulting in slack contours and weight gain due to inactivity. Lack of exercise also results in lethargy.

◆ *Smoking habits* – smoking interferes with cell respiration and slows down the circulation. This makes it more difficult for nutrients to reach the skin cells and for waste products to be eliminated. The skin looks dull with a tendency towards open pores. Nicotine is a toxic substance.

◆ *Sleeping patterns* – disturbed sleeping patterns are often a result of raised stress levels. Disturbed sleep can result in exhaustion, fatigue, irritability and poor concentration.

Questioning the client on expectations and outcomes ensures that the client gains satisfaction from the treatment. Listen carefully to make sure you fully understand the client's treatment requirements. You will need to assess the client's skin type, hair and scalp condition in order to check client suitability for treatment, plan the treatment and select suitable massage medium oils.

TOP TIP

Healthy diet

Although a healthy diet does not always guarantee healthy hair and scalp, you are what you eat. Your body cannot produce healthy hair without the proper nutrients. The body can produce 11 of the 20 amino acids that make up hair, but the remaining nine must come from your daily diet. This is why crash dieting and anorexia can cause hair loss, lacklustre hair and unhealthy scalp conditions. Proteins in meat, fish, eggs, and dairy products are good sources of these amino acids, as are food combinations such as peanut butter and bread, rice and beans, and beans and corn.

Contra-indications

Certain contra-indications prevent or restrict head massage. These can be divided into three categories: general, local and temporary. General contra-indications affect the whole body or part of the body; local contra-indications are concentrated in a particular area; the symptoms of temporary contra-indications have only a short time span and clear up quite quickly. If the beauty therapist has any concern over the client's health or well-being, medical advice should be sought prior to the treatment. GP approval should be obtained before treatment is carried out.

Those requiring GP referral should be tactfully and clearly discussed to ensure client understanding.

Contra-indications

General	Local	Temporary
Heart conditions	Recent operations*	Medication
High or low blood pressure	Recent scar tissue (up to 6 months)*	Severe bruising*
Medication	Psoriasis or eczema*	Skin cuts and abrasions*
Diabetes	Skin disease	Pregnancy
Cancer	Skin disorder	Medical oedema
Rheumatism and arthritis (especially of the neck)	Recent injury*	Skin disease
Undiagnosed, lumps, bumps and swelling		Skin disorder
Loss of skin sensation		Intoxication
High temperature		Flu, cold symptoms
Migraine or severe headaches		Scalp disorders
Disorders of the nervous system		Infestations such as head lice
		Headaches
*Only apply if located in the area		

Always check for contra-indications at the consultation, and if present do not proceed with the treatment. The following contra-indications may be present in the scalp area and cannot be treated:

Fungal infections (tinea capitis) A fungal disease, for more information see page 52. It is characterized by itching, scales and sometimes painful circular lesions. Several such patches may be present at one time. The hair can also become brittle, often breaks off, leaving only a stump, or may be shed. All forms of tinea are contagious and can be easily transmitted from one person to another. Infected skin scales or hairs that contain the fungi are known to spread the disease. A client with this condition should be referred to their GP for medical treatment.

Parasitic infestations

◆ Scabies or itch mites (sarcoptes scabiei) are highly infectious (see page 51). A client with this condition should be referred to their GP for medical treatment.

◆ Pediculosis capitis A highly infectious condition in which small lice parasites infest scalp hair (see page 51). A client with this condition should be referred to their GP for medical treatment.

Staphylococci infections Staphylococci are harmful bacteria that can infect the skin of the scalp, for further information see pages 48–49. The two most common types of staphylococci infections are furuncles and carbuncles (see page 49). A client with either condition must be referred to their GP for medical treatment.

HEALTH & SAFETY

Avoid excessive use of oil which would hinder effective treatment application and possibly could enter the eyes.

Knowledge Check

Name three benefits to the skin that occur as a result of a head massage treatment.

Refer to page 580 to help you.

Walk standing

Contra-actions

A contra-action is an unwanted reaction to Indian head massage treatment which may occur during or following the treatment. **Contra-actions** to the treatment should be discussed at the consultation so the client would recognize symptoms if experienced.

Contra-actions occur mainly as a result of the increased circulation of waste products following the massage. Monitor the contra-actions to confirm client suitability for further treatment.

These might include:

◆ nausea or headache caused by increased circulation of waste products transported in the lymphatic system

◆ fainting caused by dilation of the blood capillaries, altering blood pressure levels

◆ tiredness

◆ skin reactions, such as an allergy to the massage oil

◆ aching muscles.

If the client suffers any contra-action, you must assist the client before letting them leave the salon:

◆ ensure the client can breathe properly and that the room is well ventilated

◆ offer the client a glass of water

◆ remove product and apply a cold compress if a skin reaction occurs

◆ advise the client to seek medical advice if the symptoms persist.

Allow time and invite the client to ask any questions before treatment commences. Be honest and concise in your answers. Confirm the objectives of the treatment.

Before the head massage is applied, the face may be cleansed to remove facial make-up. Use suitable facial products for their skin type with your regular cleansing routine. If the head massage follows a facial the skin will already have been cleansed.

After preparing the client, and before touching the skin, wash your hands again.

If your client is having a treatment using oils you will need to select and warm a suitable oil to use.

Place a towel over their shoulders if applying a massage oil medium.

Massage position or stance

When performing the head massage it is important to position yourself correctly. Massage may be performed with the client seated or lying on the couch. This will prevent pain and fatigue while working. Working positions are *walk standing* and *stride standing*. If performing the head massage with the client seated it is important to consider your working position or stance.

Walk standing The beauty therapist stands with one foot in front of the other, two foot lengths between the heels and the weight evenly distributed. This enables the beauty therapist to work longitudinally (along the length) of the body.

Outcome 2: Be able to provide head massage

Learn how to provide head massage

PRACTICAL SKILLS

Communicate and behave in a professional manner

Position yourself and the client correctly throughout the treatment

Select and use products, equipment and techniques taking into account identified factors

Follow safe and hygienic working practices

Identify contra-actions and take appropriate action during treatment

Provide suitable aftercare advice

Complete the treatment to the satisfaction of the client

Evaluate the results of the treatment with the client

UNDERPINNING KNOWLEDGE

Describe how to communicate and behave in a professional manner

State the importance of positioning yourself and the client correctly throughout the treatment

Describe safe and hygienic working practices

Describe contra-actions which might occur during and following the treatment and how to respond

Describe the aftercare advice that should be provided

State the importance of completing the treatment to the satisfaction of the client

State the methods of evaluating the effectiveness of the treatment

Describe the basic structure and function of the skin

Describe the basic structure and functions of the bones of the neck and skull

Describe the functions of the muscles of the scalp and neck

Describe the massage movements used in head massage treatments

TOP TIP

Relaxation practices

Music is available for the purpose of relaxation and this makes an excellent accompaniment to create a calm environment in the treatment room.

Aromatherapy burners can be used to create a specific atmosphere in the treatment room. Essential oils which create different therapeutic effects when inhaled can be burnt.

Crystals may be placed in the work area.

Selected for their therapeutic properties, crystals mined for thousands of years have their own energy and are used to help balance the body's energy channels.

Knowledge Check

Why is the positioning of the client an important consideration when performing head massage treatment?

Refer to page 591 to help you.

Stride standing

Knowledge Check

To perform an effective consultation you need the client to feel confident about providing you with positive, honest answers to your questions.

You should have good:

a. communication skills
b. questioning techniques
c. listening skills
d. answering techniques.

Give examples of what you understand by good skills and techniques for each of the above. Refer to pages 154–156 to help you.

Client position - lying down

HEALTH & SAFETY

Stance and health Failure to adopt the correct stance will result in the beauty therapist not being able to work without strain and pain, muscle fatigue will occur and eventually serious neck or back injury could develop.

Stride standing The beauty therapist stands with feet side-by-side, positioned two foot lengths apart and the weight distributed between them. This allows the beauty therapist to work transversely (across) the body. This is the most common position when performing head massage treatment.

If performing the massage whilst the client is positioned on the treatment couch ensure good sitting posture. The chest up and shoulders back; body weight evenly distributed along the thighs; feet together and flat on the floor; avoid sitting on the edge of your seat.

Examples of a head massage routine are provided with clients in both lying and sitting positions.

STEP-BY-STEP: HEAD MASSAGE WITH CLIENT SITTING

1 With both feet placed firmly on the floor, place the hands on the client's shoulders. Ask the client to close their eyes and relax.

2 Place your hands on the client's scalp on the crown area.

3 Then place the hands, one on the forehead and one on the occiput (anatomical term for the back part of the head), hold this position for 2 minutes.

4 Rest your forearms on the client's shoulders – ask the client to slowly breathe in and then slowly breathe out. This will cause the client to relax and feel calmer. As the client breathes out apply gentle pressure with your forearms onto the client's shoulders. If oil is to be used when performing the scalp massage this is applied now, selected according to the treatment effect required.

The hair is gently parted and oil is applied to the partings. Massage the oil in using the fingers with a rotary movement. Ideally apply the oil to a position between the hairline and the crown of the head.

HEALTH & SAFETY

Client posture If the client is uncomfortable, they will be unable to relax and will not gain maximum benefit from the treatment. Check on client comfort before and during treatment application.

CourseMate video: Head Massage

5 Pick up the muscle and skin at the back of the neck. Gently lift the tissue with each hand alternately.

6 Apply frictions under the occiput. Using both thumbs apply gentle pressure in a circular movement.

7 Apply petrissage under the occiput. Using the heel of one hand, apply a gentle circular pressure.

8 Apply frictions with both thumbs in a triangular movement under the occiput.

9 Apply effleurage strokes to the scalp. Place each hand alternately on the hairline and stroke hand upwards, covering the whole scalp.

10 Apply frictions to the scalp using the pads of the fingers to apply small circular movements.

11 Apply finger stroking, place the fingertips on the hairline and draw them in a combing action through the hair.

12 Apply vibrations: gently grasp the hair and pull in a vibrating manner.

13 Apply light hacking using both hands to cover both sides of the head.

14 Using flat hands, place one hand on the forehead and the other over the occipital bone and gently lift the head. Move the hands, place one hand over the corner of the forehead, the other over the corner of the back of the skull, and lift. Repeat on remaining corners of the head.

15 Stroke over the forehead using alternate hands.

16 Apply circular pressure to the temples simultaneously using the fingertips.

17 Finally, apply effleurage to the scalp as in step 9. Wash your hands. Remove excess oil if used, using damp warm towelling mitts or sponges and warm water.

STEP-BY-STEP: HEAD MASSAGE WITH CLIENT LYING DOWN

1 Apply effleurage strokes to the scalp. Place each hand alternately on the hairline and stroke hand downwards, covering the whole scalp.

2 Interlock fingers and place joined hands above the forehead. Using the heel of the hands simultaneously perform circular, petrissage movements, moving the hands to cover the scalp.

3 Place the thumbs on the scalp at the hairline and gently apply frictions. This helps to relieve stress and tension as the pressure points are on the meridians of energy pathways that connect the body. This in turn stimulates the nerve pathways, frees blockages on the meridian lines of the body and helps to balance the body.

4 Place one thumb above the other. Each thumb alternately applies pressure in a 'C' shape moving from the hairline towards the crown area.

5 Position both thumbs at the crown area. Rotate both thumbs simultaneously in a clockwise direction, increasing pressure with each rotation: check pressure with client for comfort. Follow by rotating thumbs anticlockwise, reducing pressure with each rotation.

6 Apply petrissage movement over the scalp as if shampooing the scalp, using the fingertip pads to move the scalp gently.

7 Place the knuckles of each hand against the scalp and apply gentle pressure, rotating the knuckles of each finger to cover the scalp.

8 Grasp sections of hair between the fingers of each hand and gently pull the hair at the roots.

9 Alternating the fingers of each hand, use the fingers to slowly comb through the hair from the scalp to the end of the hair. Cover the scalp.

10 To complete the massage apply effleurage strokes to the scalp. Place each hand alternately on the hairline and stroke hand upwards, covering the whole scalp. Wash your hands following scalp massage.

11 Apply gentle pressure at the temples to indicate to the client that the massage routine is completed.

TOP TIP

Checking body language for effectiveness

The client posture should become more relaxed during application of the treatment. The shoulders should drop and breathing should become deeper.

Encourage the client to relax if their shoulders appear stiff.

Knowledge Check

How should the massage medium be stored and why?

Refer to page 589 to help you.

Knowledge Check

How should the client be advised to breathe to induce relaxation?

> "Think about your touch and pressure. As an experienced beauty therapist you will learn to gauge your client almost immediately and be able to create pressure that suits their needs straight after consultation. Experience like this comes with time, so until then make sure you ask your client after your first few movements and then again if you move onto their area of concern.
>
> *Eleanor Wright*

Adapting the massage

Relaxing massage Avoid stimulating movements and incorporate more effleurage, light petrissage movements. Pressure should be firm and rhythm slower. Concentrate massage application on areas of tension. Remember these areas may feel uncomfortable initially until the muscle tissue warms due to stimulation and increased blood flow in the area and relaxation is induced.

Tight or contracted muscles Avoid excessive use of percussion movements. Slow, rhythmical movements should be used to stretch the muscles. Again, concentrate massage application on these areas and recommend the client has a regular massage treatment to gain cumulative benefits.

Slack muscles Stimulating percussion massage movements should be used to help to tone and firm the area being treated.

Massage for excess weight Incorporate stimulating movements such as hacking over fatty areas, to help soften adipose (fatty) tissue.

Massage for males Muscle bulk tends to be larger and firmer, the epidermal skin is thicker. The massage usually needs to be firmer.

> "Make sure you always have a clear start and finish. Opening and closing movements are often overlooked, but these are the key communicator to our client of when it is time to relax and then when their treatment is coming to an end. A definite finishing pressure will let your client know their treatment is finishing before you need to say a word!
>
> *Eleanor Wright*

Aftercare advice

Before the client gets up, encourage them to rest for a few minutes to allow the blood circulation to return to normal. Provide water for hydration and to refresh the client. A relaxation massage can leave the client feeling light-headed. Sudden movement may result in a light-headed feeling as the brain is temporarily starved of blood; they may even faint. You may have a relaxation room where the client could go following treatment. You can also assist the client as they stand.

As the client's circulation returns to normal, the blood vessels will constrict.

While resting, use the time to discuss with the client suitable aftercare and home care to complement the massage. The client will probably feel extremely relaxed at this point. It is important they do not leave the salon until they feel fully awakened.

If the massage was for relaxation, you might give advice on relaxing bath products and massage techniques that could be used at home. Recommend the client increases their water intake to help detoxification and encourage good eating habits.

Remind the client about the benefits of deep breathing. Encourage them to practise breathing exercises at home, and at any time of anxiety.

Provide hair and scalp care advice, including the avoidance of excessive chemical hair treatments, the importance of hair protection when exposed to UV, and the application of specialized hair/scalp treatment products. If the treatment was for alopecia to stimulate new hair growth, clients should massage their scalp gently at home between treatments.

For the following 24 hours avoid:

◆ stimulants such as caffeine or alcohol

◆ heavy or highly spiced meals

◆ strenuous exercise.

For several hours:

◆ avoid shampooing the hair, especially if oils have been used to maximize treatment effects. To remove the oil advise the client to apply shampoo directly to the oil before wetting the hair, massage the shampoo into the hair and rinse, this will break down the oil.

Warn the client of post-treatment reactions including:

◆ emotional anxiety

◆ headaches

◆ aching muscles.

These reactions will normally subside within 24 hours. Remind the client what action to take in the event of a contra-action previously discussed at the consultation.

Ask the client how they feel to establish if the treatment has achieved the outcome agreed at consultation. Explain the benefits of regular treatment to achieve maximum benefit.

You should complete the client's record card fully so that continuation of the treatment can be tracked and any adverse reactions noted for future reference.

TOP TIP

The client may fall asleep during the massage, a benefit of relaxation technique. Awaken them into consciousness by gently speaking to them to say that their treatment has completed.

TOP TIP

Drink and rest

Offer the client a glass of water following the treatment to rehydrate and allow a suitable rest period to avoid feelings of dizziness caused by changes to blood pressure.

Knowledge Check

How can the massage be adapted to achieve different effects?

Refer to page 582 to help you.

ACTIVITY

As part of the client's home-care programme, simple massage techniques could be taught.

Think of three simple self-massage techniques that the client could use at home.

These may also be applied to relax the face during the day if working in an office, looking at the computer screen for long periods.

Knowledge Check

After the massage treatment the client should be given advice to follow to ensure that they gain maximum benefit from the treatment. Discuss the advice to be given.

Refer to page 602 to help you.

ASSESSMENT OF KNOWLEDGE AND UNDERSTANDING

You have now learnt about the knowledge and skills for applying head massage treatment in the beauty therapy workplace. To test your level of knowledge, answer the following short questions. These will prepare you for your summative (final) assessment.

1. Which of the following massage oils is unsuitable for sensitive skin and scalps?

   a. olive oil
   b. almond oil
   c. mustard oil
   d. coconut oil

2. Which of the following is a temporary contra-indication to head massage?

   a. heart condition
   b. scalp disorder
   c. diabetes
   d. dysfunction of the nervous system

3. Which massage oil is particularly suitable for chemically treated hair?

   a. coconut oil
   b. sesame oil
   c. almond oil
   d. olive oil

4. Does all hair on a person's head have the same texture?

5. Which of the following is not a cause of dry hair and scalp?

   a. winter weather
   b. hot, dry climate
   c. underactive sebaceous glands
   d. overactive sebaceous glands

6. Match the following scalp disorders with its definition:

   1. pityriasis
   2. tinea

   a) medical term for ringworm
   b) bacterial infection of numerous hair follicles

   3. scabies
   4. pediculosis capitis

   c) medical term for dandruff
   d) bacterial infection, with red, painful pustular lumps around the hair follicle

   5. furnucle
   6. carbuncle

   e) the infestation of the hair and scalp with head lice
   f) caused by a parasite called a 'mite'

7. Which muscle of the neck flexes, lowers and rotates the head?

8. Match the following bones of the cranium with its correct description:

   1. parietal
   2. occipital
   3. frontal
   4. temporal

   a) forms the forehead
   b) lower back of the cranium
   c) form the sides of the cranium
   d) form the sides and crown of the cranium

9. What is the term for light, continuous stroking massage movement applied with the fingers or the palms in a slow rhythmic manner?

   a. petrissage
   b. effleurage
   c. friction
   d. tapotement

10. Which layer of the skin contains numerous blood vessels, lymph vessels, nerves, sweat and oil glands and hair follicles?

   a. subcutaneous
   b. dermis
   c. adipose
   d. epidermis

18 Skin Tanning

LEARNING OBJECTIVES

There are two learning outcomes to achieve for this optional unit:

1 Be able to prepare for self-tanning techniques.

2 Be able to provide self-tanning techniques.

The assessment range applied requires you to:

◆ Use consultation techniques to identify the treatment objectives.

◆ Carry out client preparation and adapt treatment to suit different factors, including client's skin type and condition.

◆ Use all listed products, tools and equipment as appropriate.

◆ Ensure the environmental conditions are suitable.

◆ Demonstrate knowledge of the benefits and effects of tanning techniques and the product key ingredients.

◆ Complete a consultation and skin inspection to identify any contra-indications that may affect if and how the treatment can proceed.

◆ Follow all health and safety working practices including skin sensitivity testing.

◆ Communicate and behave in an appropriate and professional manner.

◆ Identify contra-actions and provide relevant contra-action and aftercare advice.

◆ Use different methods of evaluating the results of the treatment including observation, written and verbal.

◆ Describe the structure and function of the skin.

KEY TERMS

aftercare advice

consultation

compressor

contra-action advice

contra-actions

DHA – dihydroxyacetone

erythema

exfoliation products

faux tan

health and safety

Management of Health and
    Safety at Work Regulations
    (1999)

melanocytes

moisturizers

PSI (pounds per square inch)

self-tan products

skin pigmentation

Skin sensitivity test

Sun Protection Factor (SPF)

spray-gun

skin condition

treatment plan

treatment objectives

watery eyes

Unit Topic

Apply skin tanning techniques

This VRQ unit is linked to the beauty therapy NOS Unit B25.

INTRODUCTION

This unit is all about how to provide skin tanning treatments and self-tanning products both manually, by hand, and with tanning equipment which will create the appearance of tanned skin. The ingredients in these products react with the skin to darken the skin coloring temporarily. Application can be modified to achieve the client's treatment objectives which is agreed at consultation. Related health, safety and hygiene practice must be effectively implemented throughout the treatment.

The communication of pre- and post-tanning information and advice is essential to ensure the effectiveness of the treatment and client satisfaction with the result.

Dealing with people in a polite, efficient manner to reassure them and using good communication and questioning skills to find out exactly what they require from the self tanning treatment forms an important part of this technical service.

You must be able to show you have the necessary practical skills and underpinning knowledge to apply skin tanning techniques.

INDUSTRY ROLE MODEL

NICHOLA JOSS Celebrity beauty therapist/facialist and St Tropez Global Brand Ambassador

" I work with the film, television, beauty and fashion industries to create a natural looking, golden glow that is essential for a healthy, youthful appearance. I also work closely with the world's most prominent women's magazines such as *Vogue, Glamour, Elle* and *Marie Claire*.

I became fascinated with skin as a child through watching the women in my family fuss over cleansing, creams and skincare. Not content with a beauty diploma, I went on to earn a degree in biology and physiology, to more fully understand the holistic entirety of beauty therapy.

Upon completing my studies, I did a one-on-one apprenticeship in Malaysia with a local lymphatic drainage therapist. When I returned to the UK, my freelance career skyrocketed. As the St Tropez Skin Finishing Expert, I head up the backstage skin teams at London Fashion Week and as a global ambassador for the brand, I represent St Tropez at the Oscars. I work closely with make-up artists and stylists to ensure the A-list gleam on the red carpet.

Alongside the product development team, I am able to actively participate in the creation of new products offering my skin expertise every step of the way.

ANATOMY & PHYSIOLOGY
Essential anatomy and physiology knowledge requirements for this chapter are identified on the checklist chart on page 31.

ALWAYS REMEMBER

Faux tan is an alternative word for fake tan.

Self-tan applied in an automated booth

Skin tanning

UV light exposure may be outdoor (natural sunlight) or indoor (artificially created by UV tanning equipment). Sensible UV exposure minimizes the associated risks and enables the associated benefits of tanning. An artificial tanned appearance can be created by the application of self-tanning product ingredients to the skin.

A tan created by UV exposure is the skin's method of protection. When the skin darkens this is in order to protect itself from further sun exposure. The **melanocytes**, cells in the stratum germinativum of the epidermis which create **skin pigmentation**, are stimulated to produce the skin's pigment, melanin, which provides skin with its natural colour.

Melanosomes are small organs called organelles found in the melanocyte cell which make and store the skin's pigment melanin. When the melanocytes increase melanin production to absorb harmful rays of UV light, pigmentation changes can occur in the skin due to the changes in activity and numbers of melanocytes. This can result in areas of irregular pigmentation and increased ephelides (freckles) and solar lentigines or chloasma (liver spots).

Pigmentation changes are not uncommon in Asian skin and often result in large hyper-pigmentation marks. The skin also thickens as the cells in the epidermis multiply to absorb UV and reduce its penetration.

The quantity and distribution of melanocytes differs according to race. In a white skin the melanin tends to be destroyed when it reaches the stratum granulosum layer of the epidermis. With stimulation from UV exposure, however, melanin will also be present in the upper layers of the epidermis. In a black skin, melanin is present in larger quantities throughout all the layers, a level of protection that has genetically evolved to deal with bright UV light exposure. The increased protection allows less UV to penetrate the dermis below. The less melanin there is in the skin the less natural protection the skin has from the harmful UV rays.

On exposure to UV the melanin that is already available will produce a tanned effect, which will quickly disappear. It can take between 3 and 7 days before new melanin is released following UV exposure, so the tanned appearance gradually develops. The development of a gradual tan without burning should be aimed for.

Overexposure to the sun results in an **erythema** of the skin as the blood capillaries dilate. The skin will also feel sore as the nerve endings become stimulated. The skin may blister and then form a crust as the skin begins to heal. This can lead to skin hyperpigmentation and hypopigmentation. In hypopigmentation the skin loses colour caused by decreased melanin production and therefore has less protection.

HEALTH & SAFETY

DHA Dihydroxyacetone (DHA) is only recommended for external use to the body, so care must be taken to avoid inhaling the product, ingesting the product or contact with the eyes.

The purpose of self-tanning treatment

The application of self-tanning products creates a healthy, artificially tanned appearance to the skin without any of the harmful effects of UV light.

The effect of tanned skin created as a result of self-tanning treatment is temporary: as dead skin cells are shed, so too is the colour. This process of losing the tan usually takes 5–6 days. However, the life of the tan can be extended through good skin preparation and maintenance procedures following the treatment.

There are many different self-tan applications to choose from for professional or retail use, including self-tan tissues, mousses, **spray-gun**, airbrush, automated spray booth, aerosols, creams and gels.

Formulations differ as they are often created for different parts of the face or body, for various skin tones – light, medium and dark – and also to achieve a subtle hint of colour to give a healthy look. Maximum tanning result takes between 8 to 24 hours depending upon the tanning product and the client's natural skin type/colour.

Self-tanning is ideal for clients who want an immediate colour, have light skin with a tendency to burn in UV light or who are concerned with the associated risks of UV exposure.

HEALTH & SAFETY

Manufacturer's guidance The product manufacturer will guide you if Sun Protection Factor (SPF) is required – inform the client of this requirement as necessary.

> " Identify any contra-indications to the treatment that your client may have so that they can be safe in the context of the treatment they are about to receive. This involves ensuring that the client information sheet is fully filled in and you have read it properly, clarifying anything that is unclear with your client!
>
> *Nichola Joss*

Self-tanning ingredients

The active ingredient in **self-tan products** is **dihydroxyacetone (DHA)**, a colourless sugar which reacts with the amino acids – proteins found in the stratum corneum, the skin's epidermal skin cells – creating the pigmented, tanned look, referred to as Maillard's reaction. DHA reacts differently to everyone's amino acids, producing different tanning colourations. DHA concentrations range from 1–15 per cent affecting the depth of colouration. A fast acting solution will be 10–12 per cent DHA.

TOP TIP

Light-skinned clients

If the client has a light skin, choose a self-tanning product with a low content percentage DHA.

Erythrulose may also be used, a natural based sugar similar in composition to DHA, which produces a lighter and slower developing tan taking between 24–48 hours to develop. This can be combined with DHA to enhance the overall result to create a more natural skin tone.

Some contain UV protection and have a SPF, however, the skin still requires protection.

It is essential that exfoliation is performed before the self-tanning treatment is carried out to remove dry, flaky skin cells which would create a patchy uneven colouration.

Plan and prepare for the treatment

Outcome 1: Be able to prepare for self-tanning techniques

Learn how to provide self-tanning techniques

PRACTICAL SKILLS

Prepare yourself, the client and work area for a self-tanning treatment

Use suitable consultation techniques to identify treatment objectives

Advise the client on how to prepare for the treatment

Identify influencing factors

Provide clear recommendations to the client based on factors

UNDERPINNING KNOWLEDGE

Describe your salon's requirement for client preparation, preparing yourself and the work area

Identify different consultation techniques used to identify treatment objectives

Describe the factors that need to be considered when selecting techniques, products and equipment

Describe the environmental conditions suitable for self-tanning treatment

Describe the safety considerations that must be taken into account when providing self-tanning treatment

Identify the range of equipment used for self-tanning treatments

Identify products used and their key ingredients

Compare the benefits and effects of self-tanning treatments with UV tanning treatments

Explain the importance of regular disinfecting and sterilizing of equipment between self-tanning sessions

Explain the effect self-tanning products have on the skin and the reasons the effect has limited duration

Describe contra-indications that prevent or restrict self-tanning treatment

Before beginning the self-tanning treatment, check that you have the necessary products, tools and equipment to hand and that they meet legal, hygiene and industry requirements for self-tanning.

Products, tools and equipment

- **Couch** Required when performing a manual skin tanning treatment
- **Record card** Confidential card recording details of each client registered at the salon including personal details/ products used and details of the treatment
- **Disposable gloves** To comply with Personal Protective Equipment (PPE) at Work Regulations. Thin enough to enable even application and protect the beauty therapist's hands from staining and skin irritation
- **Unperfumed soap** To cleanse the skin if taking a shower before self-tanning treatment.
- **Self-tan products** These may include exfoliation products, barrier creams and self-tanning gels, spray, cream and lotions
- **Bin** This should be a lined metal bin with a lid and should be emptied after each client.
- **Mirror** Full length to allow the client to prepare skin before treatment and to view afterwards
- **Shower** To cleanse the skin, if applicable, prior to the self-tan system
- **Beauty therapist face mask** With carbon filter to filter out any excess airborne particles during spray-tan application
- **Exfoliating mitt** Used to remove dead skin before self-tanning application

Beauty Therapist face mask

Exfoliating mitt

YOU WILL ALSO NEED:

- **Cosmetic cleansers** To remove make-up if worn
- **Cleansing wipes/tissues** Used following tanning application to remove product from the eyebrows, fingers, toenails, palms of the hand and soles of the feet

- **Buffing mitt** To remove excess tanning product during manual self-tan application
- **Self-tanning guidance instructions – visual and audio especially** If using the spray booth system where the client independently operates the self-tanning equipment
- **Barrier cream/oil** For the palms of the hands, soles of the feet, nails/cuticles and any area of dry skin, e.g. ankle area
- **Self-tan equipment** As appropriate, e.g. spray-gun and compressor, spray-tan cubicle (usually constructed of fibreglass, acrylic or aluminum), extractor fan
- **Disposable briefs/bra** (if required)
- **Protective nose filters** For client and beauty therapist to use to avoid inhalation of airborne particles during spray-tanning techniques
- **Protective apron** To protect workwear from spillages
- **Protective hair covering** To prevent hair staining
- **Protective eyewear** To avoid eye irritation during spray-tanning application techniques
- **Lip balm/barrier cream** Should be provided to protect the lips
- **Protective disposable, self-adhesive foot pads** Secured to the sole of the feet during tanning preventing contact with the solution which could lead to skin staining.
- **Tissues** To protect against staining and for removing cleansing preparations and self-tan product
- **Protective tissue disposable coverings** Paper tissue for covering trolley surfaces and flooring and for cleaning the area
- **Cleaning agents** To clean equipment and work area
- **Lighting** Extra lighting (daylight lamp), a low voltage lamp which does not cause burning if accidently touched
- **Aftercare advice** Recommended advice for the client to refer to following the treatment to ensure the optimum result is obtained and the result is maintained

Sterilization and disinfection

The beauty therapist's hands should be protected with disposable gloves. Regular exposure of the skin to self-tanning preparations without protection may lead to contact dermatitis. Contact dermatitis is a skin problem caused by intolerance of the skin to a particular

Parts of the spray-gun

St Tropez tan range

Spray booth

substance or a group of substances. On exposure to the substance the skin quickly becomes irritated and an allergic reaction occurs. This may occur when a beauty therapist's skin is exposed to self-tanning chemicals on a regular basis. It is recommended that the beauty therapist wears additional PPE such as a protective apron to protect workwear from staining, especially during manual application technique. A face mask with a nose filter can be worn to filter excess airborne particles that are transient in the tanning mist created. A charcoal filter may be fitted in the face mask to remove the perfume component of the self-tanning product. Long hair should be tied back. The hands should be disinfected before the protective gloves are applied.

The shower if used must be cleaned after each client to avoid cross-infection. The treatment floor where the client stands during a spray-tan application treatment must be cleaned with a disinfectant cleaning agent and protected as appropriate using a disposable non-slip covering to avoid slips. The self-tan liquid used in spray systems is a hazard if not adequately removed through ventilation systems and could cause slippage if not removed with cleaning.

An automatic wash cycle cleans the automated spray-tanning booth after each use. Waste is collected in floor filters which will require regular cleaning.

Spray-tan extraction booths require cleaning and have filters which may be disposable or can be cleaned. Follow your manufacturer's instructions.

Airbrush spray-tanning has less opportunity for cross-infection in application as there is no direct contact apart from with the floor, and sole protectors should be worn.

Waste bins in the area should be emptied after each client.

Waste generated from automated spray-tan systems is classed as trade effluent requiring a trade effluent licence. Check your responsibilities with the local water authority.

As water is held in small holding tanks in automated spray booths it is necessary to carry out a risk assessment of the safety levels of bacteria and possible legionella bacteria which can lead to legionnaire's disease by inhaling small droplets of water suspended in the air which contain the bacteria.

Preparation of the work area

Floors in the work area should be non-slip and easy to clean to eliminate the possibility of cross-infection.

Ensure that tanning equipment is serviced regularly as per the manufacturer's instructions. Electrical equipment should be checked every 12 months in compliance with the Electricity at Work Regulations Act.

HEALTH & SAFETY

Compressors The automated spray booth and spray-gun tanning systems use a **compressor** to apply the tanning product.

The use and system must comply with the Pressure System Safety Regulations (2000).

A pressure system is a piece of equipment containing a fluid under pressure.

Some compressors are noisy, so this should be considered when choosing where the treatment is carried out.

For the spray-tan automated application technique a cold water supply and waste pipe for drainage is required. It is essential that spray-tan booths are sealed adequately to prevent chemical leakage into the atmosphere. Ventilation must also be adequate to avoid excessive chemical fumes and extraction of airborne particles. Filters and extraction systems should be checked for efficiency.

Ensure there is sufficient tanning product to operate the spray-tanning systems.

For automated booth spray systems check pressure gauges and fluid tank levels.

There must be sufficient room in the working area to adequately perform the treatment.

Ensure there is adequate lighting when applying self-tan manually to ensure an even application.

Any equipment that comes into contact with clients should be cleaned immediately after use, to prevent cross-infection, using cleaning materials specified by the manufacturer.

Trolley surfaces should be protected against accidental spillage of self-tan product from manual and spray-tan techniques.

Trailing wires should be taped down to avoid trips.

Disposable sole protectors

Disposable underwear

TOP TIP

Self-tan product ingredients

Some self-tan products contain alpha hydroxy acids (AHA) which continue to gently remove dead skin cells, aiming to produce a more even colour as the product achieves the skin's colour change.

Some products contain ingredients to achieve a sparkly finished effect.

Products can also be selected according to their aroma!

HEALTH & SAFETY

Occupational exposure limit (OEL) Each self-tanning product contains different ingredients. Check with your supplier the ventilation/extraction requirements for the tanning system. Visit www.hse.gov.uk to ensure that you comply with COSHH Regulations 2002.

HEALTH & SAFETY

COSHH assessment The safety of the selected tanning product should be assessed by obtaining a MSDS to learn the safe use and handling of the product. Obtain this from the product manufacturer/supplier.

Remember to use the underpinning knowledge you learnt in **CHAPTER 3 Health and Safety**.

HEALTH & SAFETY

Choice of disposable gloves Gloves should be powder-free nitrile gloves or powder-free vinyl gloves to avoid possible allergic reaction to known allergens such as latex.

TOP TIP

Link selling

It is a good idea for clients to receive an exfoliation treatment professionally applied before their treatment. This must be compatible with the self-tanning product or the final tan colour may be affected and the desired colour not achieved.

Disposable floor coverings and disposable sole protectors for the feet should be provided if carrying out spray self-tanning technique.

Treatment couches required for the application of manual self-tan applications must be adequately protected with disposable coverings to prevent staining and cross-infection.

> Always adhere to best practice, listen to your manager and show care and empathy towards your clients. Be open to advancement and change, there is always something else to learn and any extra information will help build the confidence your client has in you and will improve your relationship with them.
>
> *Nichola Joss*

Reception

Preparation procedures should be given in advance of the treatment where possible so that the client's skin is compatible with effective tanning. A skin preparation information sheet is a good idea to give your client when booking the appointment which can detail all aspects of the treatment including aftercare requirements.

If the client has hypersensitive skin or known allergies, a skin sensitivity patch test should be performed to assess skin suitability. This should test the product(s) to be used in the self-tanning treatment. The self-tanning application can only proceed if the client has a negative skin reaction – no skin reaction. Manufacturer's guidance instructions should be followed with regard to the application of skin sensitivity patch tests before treatment application.

Depending on the system used, time should be allowed when booking the treatment for client preparation, self-tan application and drying off.

Advise the client that it may be necessary to wear disposable underwear which will be provided and costed into the treatment. Some clients, however, will be happy not to wear any underwear (follow your workplace policy). Ideally, loose, dark coloured clothing should be worn to avoid removal of product and staining following the treatment.

Waxing, shaving, electrical epilation or injectable treatments such as Botox® injections should be carried out 24–48 hours prior to treatment to avoid skin irritation and skin staining in the follicles.

Body lotions, especially those containing therapeutic/perfumed ingredients should not be applied to the skin on the day of self-tan application as this may affect the result obtained.

Beauty therapy treatment where therapeutic products are applied to the skin or remove the surface skin cells should not be performed before or after the treatment, such as galvanic therapy, micro-dermabrasion or massage using pre-blended aromatherapy oils.

Where you require the client to shower and exfoliate before the treatment, explain this when they book. An oil-free exfoliating, shower or bath product should be used. Attention should be given to the ankles, heels, elbows and knees to remove dead skin to ensure even tanning. Inform the client not to apply deodorant or body lotions following showering which can cause uneven skin tanning.

Consultation

On arrival, complete the client's personal details on the client record card. Question the client to check for suitability and for possible contra-indications. If contra-indications are present do not proceed with the treatment. Carry out a client consultation to assess the client's treatment objectives and expectations.

HEALTH & SAFETY

Skin sensitivity patch test In order to assess skin tolerance to the self-tan product, a **skin sensitivity patch test** may be performed on a small area of skin. This is usually done in the crook of the elbow or behind the ear. This must be completed a minimum of 12–24 hours before treatment application dependent upon manufacturer's recommendations.

Some products contain 'walnut oil' which creates a dark toned effect. This may be unsuitable for use on a client with nut allergies.

If the client has stretch marks or recently healed skin, the colour result will differ. Inform the client of this.

If the client is a minor under the age of 16 years of age, it is necessary to obtain parent/guardian permission for treatment. The parent/guardian will also have to be present when the treatment is received. Check local bye-laws with regard to spraying children.

Explain what is involved in the different self-tanning treatments, timings, how long the effect will last and costs – a choice will then be able to be agreed on the most suitable technique.

Agree with the client the colour required and what can be achieved with the chosen tanning system. Consider the client's natural skin colouring. Ideally the colour result should be realistic; two to three shades darker. A light-skinned client will not achieve the possible dark tanning of a darker skinned client. The tan may initially appear too dark for a fair skinned client as they do not usually tan. Explain this, but cautiously apply a lighter application of tan if spray-tanning using a spray-gun on a client's first treatment.

> Before the treatment starts make sure all the tools you need are in place and you are presentable. Your client should have all the information they need about the treatment and know what to expect. Their skin should also be ready-exfoliated and moisturized especially the areas like elbow, knees, ankles and heels that tend to have rough skin. If the client has not done this at home, it can be done in the salon before the treatment.
>
> *Nichola Joss*

Knowledge Check

How can a hygienic environment be maintained when providing self-tanning treatment? Give five examples of necessary cleaning regimes.

Refer to page 611 to help you.

TOP TIP

Communication

Always use 'open-ended' questions which encourage conversation. Make the occasion even more special for the client: find out the reason why the client is having the self-tanning treatment.

ST.TROPEZ

TANNING TREATMENT CONSULTATION

	YES	NO
Have you used self-tanning products before?	☐	☐
How were the results? POOR ☐ AVE ☐ GOOD ☐		
Have you had a St.Tropez tan before?	☐	☐
If yes, were you pleased with the results?	☐	☐
Do you require an all over tan?	☐	☐
Is the tan for a special occasion?	☐	☐
Are you going on holiday?	☐	☐
Is your skin free from SPF and salt water?	☐	☐
Have you removed all deodorant/perfume/make-up?	☐	☐
Have you shaved or waxed less than 24 hours ago?	☐	☐
Do you have bleached hair or eyebrows?	☐	☐
Are you on any medication?	☐	☐
Have you recently had a course of antibiotics or chemotherapy?	☐	☐
Have you any known allergies?	☐	☐
Have you any open cuts, wounds, rashes or grazes?	☐	☐
Do you suffer from any skin disorders?	☐	☐
Do you have any pigmentation patches or pigmentary disorders?	☐	☐
Would you describe your skin as hyper-sensitive?	☐	☐
Do you suffer from any respiratory problems?	☐	☐
Are you pregnant or breastfeeding?	☐	☐
Have you recently had any body piercings or tattoos?	☐	☐
Have you received a pre-treatment advice slip?	☐	☐
Have you any queries from this advice or any other questions?	☐	☐
How will you maintain your tan?		

What concerns do you have with home tanning?

PATCH TEST

We recommend that you have a patch test prior to every treatment.	YES	NO
Have you taken the patch test?	☐	☐
If no, are you happy to receive a tan without a patch test?	☐	☐

DETAILS

Name:

Address:

Date of Birth:

Telephone:

E-mail:

INDEMNITY

I have read and understood the recommendations. To the best of my knowledge, there is no reason why I should not tan.

Signed:

St.Tropez and its agents would like to be able to advise you of products, services and special promotions in the future. If you do not wish to receive further communications, please tick the box ☐

ST.TROPEZ

DATE	TREATMENT/COMMENTS	INITIALS

Record card for self-tanning

Explain how the client will be prepared for the treatment and how long the treatment will take.

If the client is receiving an automated spray-tan booth application they will need to be instructed to adopt different poses between each spray application exposure. For some clients with mobility issues these may be difficult to adopt and they should be advised accordingly. For clients who suffer from claustrophobia this method of self-tanning treatment may be an unsuitable choice.

Discuss the expected skin colour, expected skin reactions following treatment and aftercare requirements. If the client has a tattoo it will appear faded when the tan is initially applied.

Once the consultation is complete, the beauty therapist should ensure that all details are recorded accurately and that the client has signed their record card. This enables reference for future treatments and up-to-date tracking of treatments received. A sample of a record card is shown here.

Invite the client to ask questions, the client should fully understand what the treatment involves.

Contra-indications

Certain contra-indications prevent a self-tanning treatment. If there is any concern over the client's suitability, GP approval should be sought before the treatment proceeds.

During the client consultation, if you find any of the following, self-tan treatment must not be recommended or carried out.

◆ Pregnancy – due to the hormonal changes in the body, the colour result may change. There is also an insurance implication as no body treatments should be carried out in the first 3 months of pregnancy (often referred to as the first trimester).

◆ Hormone Replacement Therapy (HRT) medication – can sometimes affect the tanning result.

◆ Hypersensitive, allergenic skins – an allergic reaction can occur caused by the ingredients in the self-tan product.

◆ The client is undergoing chemotherapy or radiotherapy treatment which can affect cell renewal and the production of melanin and may result in uneven tanning.

◆ Infectious **skin conditions** – fungal, viral or bacterial.

◆ Cuts and abrasions in the area – skin irritation and secondary infection could occur.

◆ Recent tattoo, as scar tissue will not tan evenly and there may be a risk of bacterial infection.

◆ Recent piercings must be covered to prevent skin irritation and bacterial infection. It is best not to treat an area where the piercing is less than 6 weeks old.

◆ Immediately after other heat or sensitizing treatments such as waxing hair removal, micro-dermabrasion, laser, electrolysis or sauna. Again, skin irritation and secondary infection can occur if the skin has been damaged.

◆ Contact lenses, unless removed – to avoid eye irritation.

◆ Skin conditions where the skin is thickened and broken such as psoriasis, eczema and dermatitis. Excessive skin plaques will also result in uneven tanning. A barrier cream should be applied to minor areas of eczema and psoriasis.

Knowledge Check

Which part of the skin is affected by the DHA in the self-tanning treatment?

Refer to page 609 to help you.

TOP TIP

Vitiligo

Vitiligo skin cannot be effectively treated with self-tan as the melanin pigment is not present. A skin coloured make-up camouflage application can help disguise the appearance of the skin condition vitiligo (lack of skin pigment), especially when applied specifically to one area, e.g. using spray-tan airbrush technique. Choose a colour close to the client's natural skin tone.

Vitiligo

◆ Respiratory conditions such as asthma – these may be aggravated by the chemical fumes with spray-tan technique.

◆ Positive (allergic) reaction to a skin sensitivity patch test.

◆ Skin erythema – the skin is already sensitized.

Those requiring GP referral should be tactfully and clearly discussed to ensure client understanding. Never attempt to diagnose a condition as you are not qualified to do so and could cause the client unnecessary concern.

Inform the client at consultation of any relevant **contra-actions** that may occur and the action to take.

Contra-actions

◆ Erythema (reddening of the skin) irritation, burning sensation and swelling caused by an allergic reaction to the self-tanning product used. The allergic reaction is rarely to DHA but other ingredients such as perfume and preservatives. If this occurs, advise that the client showers to remove the product, apply a cool compress with cold water and make a record of this skin response on the client's record card. If the redness does not reduce, the client may need to seek medical attention.

A skin sensitivity patch test may take place in the future using a different skin self-tanning product to assess skin tolerance.

◆ Respiratory problems due to inhalation of airborne self-tanning particles or inadequate ventilation leading to shortening of breath and tightening of the chest.

◆ Respiratory problems should be checked for at consultation and appropriate action taken. A mask or nose filters may be provided for client use and used as a precautionary measure.

◆ **Watery eyes** caused by an irritant effect to the self-tanning product. Protective eyewear is available for use as a precautionary measure.

◆ Fainting may occur if standing during spray-gun tan applications. Check client comfort during application. Have water available to ensure client hydration. Ensure the work area is free from obstacles that could harm the client if they fainted. Have an awareness of what action to take if a client fainted.

◆ Nausea ingestion of the self-tanning product can occur when using spray systems which may cause nausea. Discuss the procedure at consultation to avoid unnecessary ingestion.

◆ Undesirable hair colouration caused by inadequate protection and contact with the self-tanning product, this may include facial e.g. eyebrows and scalp hair.

◆ Undesirable skin colouration caused by poor preparation, consultation, suitability of the client for self-tanning treatment, choice of product, application techniques and non-adherence by the client with **aftercare advice**. This is discussed in more detail on page 627.

Have tanning instructions clearly displayed for use with automated spray-tanning systems.

Preparation of the client

Choose the correct shade for the skin colour – light, medium or dark. Some manufacturers provide shade charts to enable the client to select the colour required. If an automated spray-tan booth is used this cannot be accommodated for. The client must be confident of the poses to adopt during spray-tan application and the treatment sensations.

Best results are achieved on clean skin which has been cleansed and exfoliated to remove skin lotions, sebum and dead skin cells, all of which will act as a barrier. This type of cleansing enables an even application, although not all tanning systems require this.

Poor skin preparation can result in streaking, darker uneven patches or a lack of colour development.

> Look and listen carefully to your client. In that way you can personalize your treatment for each client. Work with your client's shape and contours to create the best tan, working organically from around the shoulders. Always start lighter and build the tan up, rather than create a tan that is too dark for your client's colouring.
>
> *Nichola Joss*

For automated booth spray systems check pressure gauges and fluid tank levels.

Exfoliation may be performed in the salon or by the client at home, depending on the self-tan product. Areas requiring exfoliation attention by the client or beauty therapist are the elbows, knees, ankles and heels, where dead skin cells build up.

A lip balm may be applied before spray-tanning technique to avoid skin staining and mucous membrane irritation. Glasses and jewellery should be removed from the treatment area to ensure an even application, and make-up should be removed.

It is recommended to provide paper underwear to prevent staining the client's underwear. It is the client's choice if worn.

In the self-tan spray techniques a barrier cream is applied to the palms of the hands, soles of the feet, ankles and nails of the client to prevent staining. Disposable foot sole protectors may be used. If used, ask the client to step firmly onto the adhesive surface. Some drier areas of skin such as the elbows and knees may require a moisturizer application to ensure even tanning.

A protective cap is worn to cover the hair. This is lifted at the hairline to expose the ears. Ensure this is not too low on the forehead or a demarcation line will occur. The eyebrow hair may also be protected with a barrier cream.

Remind the client of the procedure and sensations. Invite any questions from the client to confirm understanding. It is a good idea if you ask them to signal to you if you need to stop for any reason during spray-tan manual application.

If using an automated tanning booth, ensure the client is confident on the procedure to ensure their safety and efficiency of the tanning application. Have instructions clearly placed for the client to refer to. Often the booths provide audio instructions also.

TOP TIP

Exfoliation

Dry exfoliation can be performed using an exfoliating mitt before the treatment.

Buffing/exfoliating dual purpose mitt

Knowledge Check

Why is it important not to name specific contra-indications when encouraging clients to seek medical advice before treatment?

Refer to page 618 to help you.

Applying barrier cream to the hands

TOP TIP

Avoid stained nails

If the client has long nails, barrier cream may be applied under the free edge to avoid staining. Nail polish will provide further protection.

Provide self-tanning treatments

Outcome 2: Be able to provide self-tanning techniques

Learn how to prepare for self-tanning techniques

PRACTICAL SKILLS

Communicate and behave in a professional manner

Position yourself and the client correctly throughout the treatment

Select and use products and equipment taking into account identified factors

Follow safe and hygienic working practices

Identify contra-actions and take appropriate action during treatment

Provide suitable aftercare advice

Complete the treatment to the satisfaction of the client

Evaluate the results of the treatment with the client

UNDERPINNING KNOWLEDGE

Describe how to communicate and behave in a professional manner

State the importance of positioning yourself and the client correctly throughout the treatment

Describe safe and hygienic working practices

Describe contra-actions which might occur during and following the treatment and how to respond

Describe the aftercare advice that should be provided

State the importance of completing the treatment to the satisfaction of the client

State the methods of evaluating the effectiveness of the treatment

Describe the structure and function of the skin

Self-tanning products – pre-treatment clarifier, tanning fluid, pure pigment, hydrating mist

HEALTH & SAFETY

When performing a self-tanning treatment consider your responsibilities under the following legislation at all times:

◆ Health and Safety at Work Act (1974)
◆ Control of Substances Hazardous to Health Regulations (2002)
◆ Pressure Systems Safety Regulations (2000)
◆ Workplace (Health Safety and Welfare) Regulations (1992)
◆ Management of Health and Safety at Work Regulations (1999)

How to apply self-tanning products

The following tanning systems application techniques are discussed: automated spray booth, spray-tan using an airbrush or gun and manual hand-applied technique. Always follow the manufacturer's instructions to ensure the optimum effect is achieved.

When applying self-tan to the face, the eyes should be closed or protected as per the manufacturer's instructions and system used. Hair should be protected and covered. Nose filters should be provided to prevent inhalation of tanning particles if using spray systems.

How self-tan is applied using spray-tan automated booth application technique

1   The client and their skin are prepared for spray application.

2   A large air compressor sprays liquid product in a mist evenly all over the client's skin from a set of spray nozzles in a large self-contained booth constructed from fibreglass, acrylic or aluminium. The booth contains filters to remove chemical particles from the air. Some systems also have inbuilt heaters so that the environment is temperature regulated. This feels more comfortable to the client when the cool spray hits the skin and assists drying of the self-tan solution.

3   The client stands in the cubicle in front of the nozzles where, after operating a start button, the front, sides and then the back of the body are sprayed with self-tan. Different positions are adopted by the client, usually four simple standing positions to ensure even application. Some equipment has foot placements marked on the floor of the equipment to ensure the correct position is adopted. Excess product should be removed with a paper towel, including the palms of the hands, soles of the feet and nails. The client should use a paper towel to remove the protective hair cap and foot sole protectors to avoid contact with the solution. This system offers additional privacy for the client.

Application and drying time: *5–10 minutes depending on the system*.

4   If required, a second application may be given when the skin has dried. An immediate colour is achieved, the guide colour indicating where the self-tan has been applied and then the tan continues to develop.

5   Ensure the client is satisfied with the finished result and understands how the finished result will appear. The colour change to the skin will usually last 5–7 days.

A disadvantage of the automated systems is that you cannot control where the product is applied by taking into consideration the size, shape and skin condition of the client, which can be achieved with a personal manual application.

Automated spray-tanning has the following benefits:

◆ it is the quickest self-tanning treatment

◆ there is little time required as a resource for the beauty therapist

◆ it offers the client total privacy.

How to apply self-tan using spray-gun application technique
This technique uses a compressor, which generates pulses of air pressure producing a stream of compressed air, to power an airbrush that directs a fine mist of self-tan product onto the skin through a flexible hose and a spray-gun nozzle.

One to two full body applications may be applied but only one application to the hands and feet, at the end of the treatment.

TOP TIP

Spray booths

Spray booths provide privacy during application of the spray-tan. This may be made of material, which has the benefit of being easily transported if working freelance; or of a solid construction, usually fibreglass, which is designed to be permanently positioned. The permanent spray booths may feature inbuilt fans to clean the air following application, additional lighting to assist application and a protective floor cover.

Knowledge Check

How is the choice of self-tan product and colour selected?

TOP TIP

Avoid stained hands

When removing the protective hair covering, advise the client to use a paper towel to avoid contact with the skin of the hand, which could lead to skin staining.

1   The client and their skin are prepared for application. Explain to the client the treatment sensation of a cool mist of moisture. This prepares the client as it can feel uncomfortable initially if the client is warm.

2   The client stands in an overspray booth, collapsible spray-tan cubicle booth or working area protected from spray, while the beauty therapist applies self-tan with an air gun. It is important that the client does not touch the skin during application to avoid uneven coverage.

3   The client should stand upright with legs apart facing the beauty therapist with arms relaxed at their side. It is important to explain throughout the application how you want them to stand and move different parts of their body.

4   Start spraying the body starting at the face and working your way down.

5   When spraying the face the client should be advised to hold their breath and close their eyes.

6   Overlap each stroke as you work down the body, keeping the spray-gun level.

7   Ensure that you spray underneath the breasts, this will be achieved by asking the client to raise their arms to the sides of the body.

8   Hold and rotate the arms spraying down towards the hand (without spraying the hands), spraying the inside and side of each arm.

9   Spray down each leg (without spraying the feet) and release the trigger on the gun as you reach the ankles. A lighter application is required over the knees where the area is drier.

10   Ask the client to turn around and face the back of the booth.

11   The client should tilt their head forward while you spray the neck. Work your way down the body, spraying over the shoulders and back.

12   Ask the client to point their hands towards the back of the booth with palms facing down and arms held slightly away from their trunk while you spray the back of the arms.

13   Continue spraying down the body, the client may bend forward slightly when spraying over the buttocks in order to tan the crease underneath the buttocks or a lighter line will result in this area.

14   Spray the outside to inside of one leg and the inside to outside of the other. Stop at the ankle.

15   Spray the sides of the body asking the client to turn to one side so that they are facing side on to you. This will require the client to position themselves with one leg in front of the other and one arm raised above their head and elbow pointed back. Spray the sides of the breast and trunk.

16   Spray down the inside of the back leg and then the outside. Repeat this application to the other side of the body which will require the client to alter the position and raise the other arm. Repeat the spray application again.

17   Finally increase the distance from the client and lightly spray each foot and hand. The hands will require the client to move their hands into different positions in order to cover the backs and sides of their hands effectively.

18   Apply the tan in a specific sequence to ensure even coverage. Adjust pressure according to the effect required. Follow your manufacturer's application, including

vertical, horizontal and circular spray patterns. Always try to use the lowest pressure as less fumes will be created and a good coverage achieved.

Any area which appears wet should be gently patted dry.

A cleansing wipe can be used following application to remove product from the fingers, toenails and palms of the hand.

19 Ensure the client is satisfied with the finished result and understands how the finished result will appear. Advise the client to allow the product to dry for approximately 5–10 minutes before dressing.

20 Body moisturizer may be applied to areas that typically can crease and stain such as the wrists, knees and ankles.

21 Following application the client stands in the booth to allow the warm air to dry the skin. Alternatively the hose may be released from the gun and used to direct warm air over the body to dry the self-tan.

22 The sole protectors are removed and any sticky residue may be removed with a cleansing tissue. Clean the work area and dispose of waste.

Application and drying time: *20–30 minutes.*

Airbrush spray booth

STEP-BY-STEP: SPRAY-GUN APPLICATION TECHNIQUE

2 Guidance on client positioning for treatment application

5 Spraying the client's face

8 Spraying the inside and side of each arm

11 Spraying over the shoulders and back

14 Spraying the outside to inside of one leg

15 Spraying the sides of the body

Spray-gun tanning application technique To ensure even application a small rotating platform, which the client stands on, can be used to facilitate application.

◆ To create a more natural, lighter result reduce pressure and increase the distance.

◆ Start moving the air gun before you start spraying to avoid darker areas of application.

◆ Ensure no body parts are missed, e.g. under the chin!

◆ Wipe over fair brow hair to avoid staining, following face application.

◆ If application is excessive, blot the area to avoid too dark a colour developing.

◆ Keep the airbrush at 90 degrees and move at all times to ensure even application. A repetitive finger, hand and arm movement is required. Safe working must be considered to prevent RSI.

◆ Hairy areas require the application to be slower in order that the product is in contact with the skin.

◆ Do not over-wet the skin, this will also waste the product.

◆ If the client has any folds of skin e.g. on the back, it will be necessary for them to stretch while these body parts are sprayed.

◆ When spraying the face, ask the client to inhale through the nose and as they exhale through the mouth spray the face from the chin to forehead to avoid inhalation of the spray. The client's eyes are closed at all times.

◆ Blemished areas, and areas of dry skin absorb more colour and lighter application is required over such areas.

CourseMate video: Spray-Tanning

STEP-BY-STEP: AIRBRUSH TANNING APPLICATION TECHNIQUES

A small pen-like spray-gun applicator atomizes the spray-tan liquid into tiny particles. This is operated by a compressor and is useful for performing corrective work, i.e. concealment of vitiligo.

1 Switch on the compressor and adjust the pressure to create the desired result. Leg application – apply tan to the client's legs as these take the longest to dry. Work down the leg at a distance of 13–21 cm to ensure full, even coverage.

2 Ankle application – this area can be dry, creating a darker effect, so a lighter application is required. Lightly spray the tops of the feet. Increase distance and reduce pressure. Advise the client to lean forward to stretch the skin in this area. Continue to apply tan to the upper body front and back by applying tan in a downwards direction until the area is evenly covered. Ask the client to move their body as required to facilitate application.

3 Arm application – apply tan to the client with their arm raised, working from the wrist down the arm and then apply to the rest of the arm, asking the client to move their arms as required to ensure full, even coverage.

4 Facial application – protect the hair (including brow hair) to prevent staining. Ask the client to close their eyes and take a deep breath while you apply tan to the face. Include the ears, around the ears and the neck area.

5 Finished result – ensure the client is satisfied with the finished result and that the application is even. Re-apply to any lighter areas.

Rinse the air gun immediately with warm clean water to prevent clogging with dried product. Tanning product is water-based.

ALWAYS REMEMBER

Care of the spray-gun

Temporarily between use, store the air gun in water to prevent clogging.

When not in use, store the air gun in an air gun holder.

If clogged, the air gun will not apply the product evenly and will spit the product.

Key pieces of the spray-gun include the spray container, needle, air cap, needle spring and density dial. All should be regularly cleaned as sugar in DHA will crystallize causing blockages, preventing the tan from being applied evenly. Warm water and detergent should be used to clean the parts.

The machine is re-assembled and the needle is inserted into the density dial hole and trigger area. Some resistance may be experienced until it is aligned.

The needle spring follows.

The density dial is attached.

The spray pattern adjuster is firmly attached.

TOP TIP

Check your work

Check your application of the product as you are working. The skin should look initially as if it has a fine mist on its surface which dries quickly. If it is too wet it will run resulting in streaking.

Ensure you have informed your client fully about the aftercare of their tan. They should not shower until the following day, after which they should moisturize. This is an opportunity to sell the products that will optimize your client's tan.

Nichola Joss

Knowledge Check

What is the meaning of the term PSI, and which self-tanning system does this relate to?

Refer to page 622 to help you.

Skin buffing as part of manual self-tan application

TOP TIP

Protecting the hands

The hands have more pores than other body areas and will soon tan. To prevent staining wear thin gloves during application.

ALWAYS REMEMBER

Medication

Some forms of medication can affect how the skin responds to self-tanning product.

Knowledge Check

If the client experienced an allergic reaction following the self-tanning treatment, what action would the client have been advised to take at consultation?

Refer to page 619 to help you.

TOP TIP

Uneven self-tan application

If you make a mistake during application, pat the area dry, do not rub the skin as this will lead to uneven patchy colouration.

You can always apply a further application to produce an even result.

How to apply self-tan using manual hand-applied application technique
This is a luxurious treatment which is recommended if the client would like to benefit from a relaxing massage to the skin's surface.

1 The client should be dressed in disposable underwear, hair secured from the face and covered on the couch with towels for modesty and to keep warm. The client and their skin are prepared for self-tan application. This usually requires showering and the application of an exfoliant. Alternatively the skin can be exfoliated as part of the self-tanning treatment skin preparation.

2 Moisturizer may be applied to the elbows, knees, ankles and feet. Adding moisturizer lightens the result but should only be used if recommended by the manufacturer as it can also create a barrier if too much is used.

3 The self-tan product is applied over the body following the manufacturer's guidelines for application using the hands, which are usually protected with gloves to prevent staining.

4 Treatment must be methodical to ensure no body parts are missed and that an even coverage is obtained.

5 Product should be removed immediately during application, using a clean tissue, from the palms of the hands, toes and fingernails to prevent staining.

6 Time should be allowed for the product to dry, *approximately 10 minutes*.

7 The skin is then buffed to remove excess product, avoid rubbing the skin which could result in uneven colouration. Pay particular attention to areas where the skin is drier, i.e. ankles and wrists.

8 Ensure the client is satisfied and understands how the finished result will appear. Application and drying time: *approximately 1 hour 20 minutes* including pre-exfoliation and post skin buffing.

TOP TIP

Spray faults

No spray may indicate a number of problems:

◆ density dial too tight affecting trigger
◆ nozzle clogged with self-tan product
◆ not holding gun at 90 degrees
◆ air hose blocked
◆ insufficient spray-tan in the spray container.

Excessive spray may indicate:

◆ density dial requires to be tightened
◆ gun not moving at the correct speed over the area.

Poor tanning results

These are commonly caused by the beauty therapist and their choice and application of products, or the client not following the necessary skin preparation/aftercare instructions.

- ◆ **Tan too light in colour:** incorrect colour shade selected. Insufficient application of product to area if using spray-gun tanning, the pressure may have been too low or distance too far away. The addition of too much moisturizer to the tanning product during manual hand application technique.

- ◆ **Tan too dark:** incorrect colour shade selected. Incorrect formulation, percentage of DHA too high for skin colouring. If using spray-gun tanning the pressure used was too high or application distance too near the client.

- ◆ **Uneven application:** the client may have products on the skin which have not been effectively removed before tanning. Insufficient exfoliation and moisturizing of the skin before treatment.

- ◆ **Scaly appearance to the skin:** excessive self-tan application.

- ◆ **Incorrect application technique:** this must be methodical to avoid missing areas of skin. Excessively dry skin conditions can result in a patchy uneven result. Not allowing the skin to dry properly before dressing can result in removal of some of the product. There may be a problem with the quality of the product, if it happens again contact the supplier for guidance.

- ◆ **Tan corrector products:** used with leading tanning manufacturer products usually within 5 hours of application to correct streaking. Alternatively, an exfoliant may be used. Self-tan can be re-applied to the area to even the result, the application may be modified to create the necessary result, i.e. darker or lighter.

- ◆ **Orange or ashy cast to the skin:** caused by over-application or incorrect choice of formulation for the client's skin colour. There may be alkaline products on the skin which will create an orange colour to the skin.

- ◆ **Underarms turn green:** this usually occurs if the client is wearing deodorant or if this has not been properly removed.

> "Identify your clients' needs and listen; which areas of their skincare routine are most important to them, what aspects do they enjoy the most, what are their main concerns? Gain a great understanding of the products and what they can and cannot do, as well as your client's skin. Combining all of this knowledge will increase sales, build confidence in you and build customer retention.
>
> *Nichola Joss*

Aftercare advice

- ◆ Details of the treatment should be entered on the record card, to include date, colour, result, any adverse skin reaction. To ensure effective tan development, avoid streaking and to maintain the result:

  - ◆ avoid anything that will make you sweat immediately following treatment as this will dilute the product, disturb application affecting the finished effect. Therefore no strenuous exercise for approximately 6–8 hours

TOP TIP

Lightening the result

Moisturizer may be used to lighten the result for the areas: face, hairline, inner arm. underarm, hands, ankles, knees and feet.

TOP TIP

Removing unwanted product

Any product applied to unwanted areas should be removed with cotton wool during the application. A specialist product can be used for this purpose – tan remover (corrective lotion).

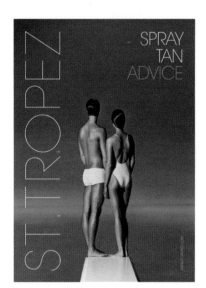

ST.TROPEZ

SPRAY TAN ADVICE

Aftercare leaflet

Knowledge Check

Describe three results that could occur if the client did not follow the pre- and post-treatment self-tanning instructions.

Tan remover
(corrective) lotion

◆ cosmetic products which remove the surface cells such as facial peeling masks should be avoided

◆ avoid tight clothing or friction with any body part immediately following application to avoid product removal

◆ do not bath/shower for at least 8 hours following treatment application. Care should be taken when washing the hands to avoid product removal following treatment

◆ avoid chlorinated pools, excessive bathing and heat treatments such as sauna as they encourage fading. Avoid long baths and showers as they will encourage exfoliation

◆ on showering, excess self-tanning product will be removed making the water appear brown. The skin should be gently patted dry with a soft towel.

◆ Encourage the retail of self-tanning preparations. Tinted products are useful as this assists in even application. They often contain ingredients, such as vitamins and plant extracts, to keep the skin moisturized.

◆ Other relevant products are exfoliators, which can be used between treatments as advised by the beauty therapist and to prepare the skin for future self-tan applications. These must be used cautiously as they will reduce the life of the tan if used incorrectly or too often.

◆ Moisturizer should be applied daily to prevent the skin becoming dry and to keep the skin hydrated. Avoid the use of AHA products, which will encourage skin removal and loss of skin colour.

◆ Encourage the client to use a tan enhancer to maintain and enhance the result.

◆ If a contra-action occurs, follow advice provided and contact the salon for professional advice.

◆ Encourage a repeat appointment booking, usually every 2 weeks as the tan fades. A client, however, requiring a deeper tan could return in 48 hours for a second application if suitable.

◆ Sun protection is necessary on exposure to UV.

> Never worry about asking your colleagues questions if you are not sure. Listen and ask open-ended questions. With your client, empathize; focus on them, using their name; and jot down personal information, such as names and ages of their children so you remember for their next visit.
>
> *Nichola Joss*

TOP TIP

Retail opportunities

Many self-tanning product suppliers have extensive retail ranges to care for and enhance the tanned skin. Explain to your client the unique properties and benefits of each product.

TOP TIP

Oily skin

The result will be better on a client with an oily skin as the product is not absorbed as quickly as on dry skin. However, all skin will require moisturizing to avoid dry, uneven, flaky patches, resulting in uneven desquamation.

TOP TIP

Tan enhancer

The use of tan enhancer will extend the life of the tan as it will keep the skin moisturized and has a small amount of self-tan in its formulation.

ASSESSMENT OF KNOWLEDGE AND UNDERSTANDING

You have now learnt about the knowledge and skills for applying skin-tanning techniques treatment in the beauty therapy workplace. To test your level of knowledge, answer the following short questions. These will prepare you for your summative (final) assessment.

1. The active ingredient in self-tan products is:

    a. amino acetone
    b. hydroxydiacetone
    c. dihydroxyacetone
    d. diacetone–hydroxide

2. The active ingredient in self-tan product is a sugar that reacts with:

    a. amino acids (proteins) in the stratum granulosum
    b. fatty acids in the stratum lucidum
    c. glucose in the stratum spinosum
    d. amino acids (proteins) in the stratum corneum

3. If a client is fair skinned choose a product with:

    a. a higher percentage of DHA
    b. no DHA in it at all
    c. a lower percentage of DHA
    d. the very strongest DHA percentage available

4. The skin condition which is unsuitable for self-tanning as the skin lacks pigment is called:

    a. ephelides
    b. vitiligo
    c. dermatitis
    d. leuconychia

5. A self-tan/treatment can be carried out immediately after:

    a. micro-dermabrasion
    b. waxing
    c. electrical epilation
    d. none of the above

6. To lighten the tanning effect, mix the self-tanning product with a small amount if recommended:

    a. cleanser
    b. moisturizer
    c. massage cream
    d. witch hazel

7. Which health and safety legislation should be considered when applying self-tanning techniques?

    a. Health and Safety at Work Act (1974)
    b. Control of Substances Hazardous to Health Regulations (2002)
    c. Workplace (Health Safety and Welfare) Regulations (1992)
    d. all of the above

8. What time intervals would you advise for a client between each self-tanning treatment?

    a. every 5 days
    b. every 7 days
    c. every 10 days
    d. every month

9. The skin must be exfoliated to remove dead skin cells before the tanning treatment. Which epidermal layer are the cells removed from?

    a. stratum corneum
    b. stratum lucidum
    c. stratum granulosum
    d. subcutaneous layer

10. Melanin is the skin's natural pigment, exposure to UV stimulates the following cells to produce melanin as a protective function:

    a. erythrocytes
    b. leucocytes
    c. melanocytes
    d. pheomelanin

Glossary

Accident book Health and safety legislation requires that a written record is kept of any reportable injury, disease or dangerous occurrence in the workplace. This can be recorded in an accident book. Incidents in the accident book should be reviewed to see where improvements to safe working practice could be made.

Accident form A detailed report form to be completed following any accident in the workplace.

Acetone A solvent commonly used as a tip remover and nail varnish remover.

Acid mantle The combination of sweat and sebum on the skin's surface, creating an acid film. The acid mantle is protective and discourages the growth of bacteria and fungi. The pH scale is used to measure the acidity or alkalinity of a substance using a numbered scale. The skin's pH is acid at 5.5–5.6.

Additional products and services Products and services offered by your workplace which a client may receive or purchase to enhance their service or treatment benefits.

Adhesive A chemical compound used to stick two surfaces together, such as the glue used to attach false eyelashes to the natural lashes or the glue used to attach nail tips to the natural nail.

Aftercare advice Recommendations given to the client following a service to maintain the finished result and enable the benefits to be continued at home.

After-wax lotion A product applied to the skin following hair removal to reduce redness and promote skin healing.

Age groups The different classification of age groups to be covered e.g. 16–30, 31–50 and over 50 years.

Allergic reaction The reaction of the body to a substance or material that could be harmful or that the body has developed a sensitivity to. It produces symptoms including erythema, swelling, itching and bruising.

Anagen The active growth stage of the hair growth cycle.

Antioxidant A molecule found in some foods that maintains the health of the skin by fighting the damaging effects of free radicals (unstable molecules which can cause skin cells to degenerate). Antioxidant ingredients are increasingly being included in skincare preparations to neutralize free radicals or repel them from the skin.

Antiseptic A chemical agent that prevents the multiplication of microorganisms. It has limited action and does not kill all microorganisms.

Apocrine gland Sweat gland found in the armpit, nipple and groin area. Larger than the eccrine sweat gland and attached to the hair follicle. These sweat glands are controlled by hormones and become active at puberty.

Appointment An arrangement made for a client to receive a service on a particular date and time.

Arrector pili muscle A small muscle attached to the hair follicle and base of the epidermis. When the muscle contracts (shortens) it causes the hair to stand upright in the hair follicle.

Aseptic The process of implementing disinfection and sterilization procedures to prevent contamination of tools and equipment which could lead to cross-infection.

Assistance The act of providing help or support.

Autoclave An effective method of sterilization, suitable for small metal objects and beauty therapy tools. Water is boiled under increased pressure and reaches temperatures of 121–134°C.

Ayuveda (Art of life) A sacred Hindu text written around 1800 BC. In Avuyeda life consists of body, mind and spirit – each person is different. By restoring balance and harmony of the body, mind and spirit, the health of the individual improves.

Bacteria Minute, single-celled organisms of various shapes. Large numbers live on the skin's surface and are not harmful (they are non-pathogenic); others, however, are harmful (pathogenic) and can cause disease.

Base coat A nail polish product applied to protect the natural nail and prevent staining from coloured nail polish.

Behaviour This refers to how we conduct ourselves in the workplace. It is important to be polite and friendly at all times, work co-operatively with others and conform with all workplace policies and procedures.

Benefit The gain to be made from using a product or service.

Bevelling A nail filing technique used at the free edge of the nail to ensure it is smooth.

Blending Nail art paints applied and blended together without definite lines creating a 'marbling' or iridescent effect dependent upon products and brushes used.

Blepharitis Inflammation of the eyelid caused by an infection or an allergic reaction.

Blood Nutritive liquid circulating through the blood vessels. It transports essential nutrients and other important substances, such as oxygen and hormones, and removes waste products.

Blood vessel Part of the circulatory system that carries blood around the body. There are three main types of blood vessel: arteries, veins and capillaries, which differ in their structure and role in blood transportation.

Blue nail Nail condition where the nail bed has a blue tinge rather than a healthy pink colour due to poor blood circulation in the area.

Blusher A make-up product applied to add warmth to the face and emphasize the facial contours and draw attention to the cheekbones.

Body language Communication involving the body rather than speech, including facial expressions and hand gestures.

Bone A specialized form of connective, structural tissue that supports, surrounds and connects different parts of the body. Bones support and protect the underlying structures, give shape to the body and provide an attachment point for muscles.

Bones of the chest A group of bones, including the sternum and the ribs, that protect the inner organs and provide a surface for muscle attachment that allows movement.

Bones of the foot and lower leg These include the tarsals, metatarsals and phalanxes in the foot and the tibia and fibula in the lower leg.

Bones of the lower arm and hand These include the carpals, metacarpals and phalanges in the hand and the radius and ulna in the lower arm.

Bones of the neck A group of bones that support the skull and form the neck. The bones in the neck include the cervical vertebrae.

Bronzing products Make-up products applied to create a healthy, natural or subtle tanned look. They are formulated to create a matt or shimmer effect and are also suitable as a highlighting contouring product.

Bruised nail A nail condition where the nail appears blue/black in colour where bleeding has occurred on the nail bed following injury.

Buffer A manicure tool with a pad with a replaceable cover, used on the nail to give a sheen, increase blood supply to the area and, if used with the gritty cream buffing paste, to help smooth out nail surface irregularities.

Bunion A foot condition. The large joint at the base of the big toe protrudes, forcing the big toe inwards towards the other toes.

Burn Injury to the skin caused by excess heat; the skin appears red and may blister.

'C' curve The curve of the nail from side wall to side wall.

Callus A foot condition, displaying thick, yellowish hardened skin, usually found on prominent areas of the foot such as the heel.

Camouflage products Cosmetic make-up products designed to conceal skin imperfections including creams, powders and setting products for the face and body.

Catagen The stage of the hair growth cycle where the hair becomes detached from its source of nourishment, the dermal papilla, and stops growing.

Catalyst A substance that causes or accelerates a chemical reaction.

Cell Basic units of life which specialize in carrying out particular functions in the body. Groups of cells which share function, shape, size or structure are called tissues. The human body consists of trillions of cells.

Certificate of registration Awarded when the premises have been successfully inspected to ensure that the local bye-laws are being followed in relation to cosmetic piercing.

Charge card An alternative form of payment where the complete amount of credit spent must be repaid by the cardholder each month to the card company.

Chemical reaction The process of two or more chemicals combining to create a different substance.

Cheque An alternative form of payment to that of using cash. A cheque must be accompanied by a cheque guarantee card.

Chilblains Poor blood supply where the toes become red, blue or purple in colour and the area may become painful and itchy; aggravated in cold weather.

Chiropodist A person who is trained and qualified to treat minor foot complaints.

Circulatory system The system that controls blood and lymph flow and transports material around the body. It supplies cells with oxygen and nutrients and carries away waste products.

Cleanser A skincare preparation that removes dead skin cells, excess sweat and sebum, make-up and dirt from the skin's surface to maintain a healthy skin complexion. These are formulated to treat the different skin types, skin characteristics and facial areas.

Client care Client service standards on how the client is expected to be treated to ensure their treatment meets their expectations and without harm.

Client record cards Confidential cards recording the personal details of each client registered at the business. This information may be stored electronically on the salon's computer.

Clinical waste Waste from e.g., ear piercing is classed as clinical waste. The disposal of clinical waste is controlled by the Environment Agency. Waste materials that have come into contact with body fluids must be collected and disposed of by special arrangements. The Environment Protection Act (1990): Waste Management: The Duty of Care, A Code of Practice (ISBN 011 752577 X) provides further information on this subject.

Code of conduct Workplace service standards with regard to appearance and behaviour while in the working environment.

Code of practice The expected standards and behaviour for the professional beauty therapist to follow, which will uphold the reputation of the industry and ensure best working practice for the industry and protect members of the public. Beauty therapy professional bodies produce codes of practice for their members. A business may have its own code of practice.

Cold wax A wax already applied to a strip and ready for use. The pre-coated strip is applied firmly to the skin and then removed quickly against hair growth, removing the hair in the area.

Collagen A protein fibre found in the dermis of the skin that provides strength to the skin and other types of connective tissue.

Colour corrector A make-up product applied to target problem areas. It contains pigments which balance skin tone.

Colouring characteristics Identified through consultation with the client and by examining the client's natural hair colouring (e.g. fair, red, dark or white) to determine the correct service plan, e.g. selecting the appropriate tint colour for permanent tinting treatment.

Comedone removal Facial techniques used to extract comedones (blackheads) from the skin. A small tool called a comedone extractor is used for this purpose.

Communication The exchange of information and the establishment of understanding between people.

Complaints procedure A formal, standardized approach adopted by the organization to handle any complaints.

Compressor A piece of equipment used to compress air. The air pressure is then regulated by the attachment of a regulator. It is used in the application of make-up, nail art, airbrushing and self-tan.

Concealer Cosmetic product used to disguise minor skin imperfections such as blemishes, uneven skin colour or shadows.

Confidentiality Keeping information or data private. In order to gain trust between yourself and your client it is important to keep client information confidential. This may also be a legal requirement stipulated by the Data Protection Act.

Conjunctivitis A bacterial infection. Inflammation of the mucous membrane that covers the eye and lines the eyelid. The skin of the inner conjunctiva of the eye becomes inflamed, the eye becomes very red, itchy and sore, and pus may exude from the eye area.

Consent form Written permission obtained from a parent or guardian to perform a service on a minor.

Consultation Assessment of client needs using different assessment techniques including questioning and natural observation.

Consultation techniques Methods used to identify the client's needs using differing assessment techniques, including questioning, manual and natural observation.

Consumer Protection Act (1987) This act follows European Union directives to protect the customer from unsafe, defective services and products that do not reach safety standards.

Consumer Protection (Distance Selling) Regulations (2000) These Regulations as amended by the Consumer Protection (Distance Selling) (Amendment) Regulations (2005), are derived from a European Union directive and cover the supply of goods/services made between suppliers acting in a commercial capacity and consumers. They are concerned with purchases made by telephone, fax, Internet, digital television and mail order.

Consumer Safety Act (1978) This act aims to reduce risks to consumers from potentially dangerous products.

Contact dermatitis A skin disorder caused by intolerance of the skin to a particular substance, or a group of substances. On exposure to the substance the skin quickly becomes irritated and an allergic reaction occurs.

Continuous professional development (CPD) Activities undertaken to develop technical skill and expertise to ensure current, professional experience in the beauty industry is maintained.

Contour cosmetics Make-up products applied to change the shape of the face and the facial features. These cosmetics draw attention either towards or away from the shape of the face or specific facial features, helping to create the optical illusion of balance and perfection.

Contra-action An adverse or unwanted reaction occurring during or after service application.

Contra-action advice Recommended action to be taken to correct an adverse or unwanted reaction.

Contra-indication A problematic symptom that indicates that the service may not proceed or may restrict service application.

Control of risk The means by which risks identified are removed or reduced to acceptable levels.

Control of Substances Hazardous to Health (COSHH) Regulations (2002) (including Biological Agents Regulations) Legislation that requires employers and the self-employed to prevent or control the exposure of employees and clients to hazardous substances.

Controlled Waste (Amendment) Regulations (1993) Categorizes waste types. The local authority provides advice on how to dispose of waste types in compliance with the law.

Corn A small area of thickened skin on the foot. Often white in appearance.

Corrective methods Selection and application of make-up products which aim to change the appearance of the client's skin condition or facial features.

Corrosive A substance capable of causing rapid and sometimes irreversible damage to human tissue or other surfaces.

Cortex The thickest layer of the hair structure.

Cosmetic Products (Safety) Regulations (2004) Part of consumer protection legislation that requires that cosmetics and toiletries are safe in their formulation and are safe for use for their intended purpose as a cosmetic and comply with labelling requirements.

Credit card An alternative form of payment to that of using cash. These cards are held by those who have a credit account, where there is a pre-arranged borrowing limit. These can only be used if your business has an arrangement to deal with the relevant credit card company.

Cross-contamination Transfer of an infection directly from one person to another or indirectly from one person to a second person via an object.

Cross-infection The transfer of contagious microorganisms by direct contact with another person or indirectly by contact with an infected object.

Cure Another word for polymerization; when a liquid turns into a solid structure.

Curing The process of polymerization.

Customer care statement Defined customer service standards that are expected.

Cuticle (hair) The protective outer layer of the hair composed of thin, unpigmented, flat, scale-like cells. These cells contain hard keratin and overlap each other from the base to the tip of the hair.

Cuticle (nail) The overlapping epidermis around and extending onto the base of the nail, developing from the stratum corneum.

Cuticle cream or oil A cosmetic preparation used to condition the skin of the cuticle.

Cuticle knife A metal tool used on the nail to remove excess eponychium and perionychium (the extension of the skin of the cuticle at the base of the nail).

Cuticle nippers A metal tool used to remove excess cuticle and neaten the skin around the cuticle area.

Cuticle remover A cosmetic preparation used to soften and loosen the skin cells and cuticle from the nail.

Cyclical pattern of growth The hair growth cycle, which can be divided into three phases: anagen, catagen and telegen.

Cyst A localized pocket of sebum that forms in the hair follicle or under the sebaceous glands in the skin. Semi-globular in shape, either raised or flat, and hard or soft. Cysts are the same colour as the skin, or red if bacterial infection occurs.

Dangerous Substances and Preparations (Nickel) (Safety) Regulations (2005) The use of nickel has been found to cause allergies. Check what metal is used for your supplier's ear piercing jewellery and that it complies with the regulations.

Data Protection Act (1998) Legislation designed to protect client privacy and confidentiality.

Debit card A method of payment where the card authorizes immediate transfer of the cash amount from the client's account.

Dehydrate To remove water from the surface of the natural nail plate.

Depilatory cream A strong alkaline chemical cream used for temporary hair removal. The disulphide bonds in the hair are broken, the protein keratin dissolved and hair is then removed at the skin's surface.

Dermal papilla An organ that provides the hair follicle with blood, necessary for hair growth.

Dermatitis An inflammatory skin disorder where the skin becomes red, itchy and swollen.

Dermis The inner portion of skin situated underneath the epidermis.

Diabetes A disease that prevents sufferers breaking down glucose in their cells. Insulin, a hormone produced by the pancreas organ, is not produced in sufficient quantities to regulate the sugars and carbohydrates, resulting in excess sugar in the blood.

Dihydroxyacetone (DHA) The active ingredient in self-tan products. A colourless sugar which reacts with amino acids in the skin creating the pigmented look.

Disability Discrimination Act (1996) Implemented to prevent disabled persons being discriminated against. Employers have a responsibility to remove physical barriers and to adjust working conditions to prevent discrimination on the basis of having a disability.

Discrepancy A disagreement over amounts of money etc. This is referred to in instances where a client disagrees with what they are being asked to pay or the amount of change received.

Disinfectant A chemical agent that destroys most microorganisms.

Disposable applicator A piece of equipment used to apply wax hygienically to the area of hair removal without contaminating the wax flowing back into the tube following application. The applicator head is disposed of after each treatment.

Dotting Placement of dots of nail paint or polish using a specialized tool referred to as a dotting/marbling tool. The dots may create a design or blended together creating the 'marbling' nail art technique.

Dotting tool A tool with different sized balls on each end used for applying dots of colour, marbling, water marbling and gel polish cutouts

Ear The external or outer part of the ear collects sound waves and directs these to the inner ear. This part of the ear that stands out at the side of the head is called the pinna, which comprises the helix and lobule.

Ear piercing The perforation of the skin and underlying tissue of the earlobe to create a hole in the skin where jewellery is inserted.

Ear piercing gun Equipment used to perforate the skin and underlying tissue, creating a hole in the skin and the placement of ear stud jewellery.

Eccrine gland Simple sweat producing gland responsive to heat, appearing as tiny tubes which are straight in the epidermis, and coiled in the dermis. Its function is to maintain the body temperature by sweating.

Eczema A skin condition which appears as a reddening of the skin accompanied by itching and sometimes blisters. The blisters can leak tissue fluid which later hardens, forming scabs.

Eczema of the nail A skin condition affecting the nail, resulting in changes to the nail including ridges, pitting, nail separation and nail thickening.

Effleurage A stroking massage manipulation used to begin the massage, as a link manipulation, and to complete the massage sequence. Applied in a rhythmic, continuous manner, it induces relaxation.

Eggshell nail A nail condition where thin, fragile white nails curve under at the free edge.

Elastin A protein fibre found in the dermis of the skin that helps the skin maintain its elastic properties and return to shape.

Electricity at Work Regulations (1989) These regulations state that electrical equipment in the workplace should be tested every 12 months, by a qualified electrician. The employer must keep records of the equipment tested and the date it was checked.

Electrolysis Permanent hair removal method, using an electrical current applied to the base of the hair follicle, via a fine needle. The current or chemicals created destroys the hair root, preventing hair growth.

Emery board A nail file used to shape the free edge of the nail.

Employers' Liability (Compulsory Insurance) Act (1969) This provides financial compensation to an employee should they be injured as a result of an accident in the workplace. A certificate indicating that a policy of insurance has been purchased should be displayed.

Employment rights and responsibilities Employee rights and responsibilities should be provided as part of the content of an employment induction, regardless of previous knowledge and industrial experience. They inform the employee of the essential workplace rights and responsibilities. Employment rights includes details of the contract of employment you have with your employer such as pay and hours of work and health and safety procedures which minimize risk to all in the workplace. Your responsibilities include ensuring health and safety meets legal requirements, where risks to their health and safety are properly controlled.

Enquiries Questions presented by clients or business contacts to find out more information.

Environmental conditions This includes heating, lighting, ventilation and general comfort requirements for the workplace or service.

Epidermis The outer layer of the skin located directly above the dermis. The epidermis is composed of five layers with the surface layer forming the outer skin which has a protective function.

Equal opportunity Non-discrimination on the basis of sex, race, disability, age, etc.

Equipment and tools Used within a service that enable the service to be completed competently.

Erythema Reddening of the skin, caused by increased blood circulation to the area.

Evaluation Method used which measures the value of the instructional activity.

Exfoliant A service used to remove excess dead skin cells from the surface of the skin, which has a skin cleansing, cell rejuvenating action. This process can be achieved using a specialized cosmetic, or mechanically by using facial equipment where a brush is rotated over the skin's surface.

Exfoliation A cosmetic service used to remove dead skin cells from the skin's surface and accelerate the process of natural skin loss – called desquamation.

External client A person who is not an employee of the business i.e. client or other visitor to the business.

External ear structure The visible, outer part of the ear which funnels sound waves into the ear to enable hearing. It comprises the pinna, lobe, cartilage and cartilaginous tissue.

Eye shadow A cosmetic product applied to the eye to complement the natural eye colour, to give definition to the eye area and enhance the natural shape of the eye.

Eyebrow colour A cosmetic product applied to emphasize the eyebrows, alter their shape, and which can make sparse eyebrows look thicker.

Eyebrow shaping The removal of eyebrow hair to create a new shape (reshape) or to remove stray hairs to maintain the existing brow shape (maintenance). Shaping treatments can be performed with tweezers, threading or waxing, or a combination of techniques.

Eyelash adhesive A specialized glue used to apply false strip eyelashes and individual false eyelashes to the natural eyelashes.

Eyelash and eyebrow tinting The permanent colouring of the eyelash or eyebrow hair to enhance and define their appearance by applying specialized dye formulated for use around the delicate eye area.

Eyelash curlers Small flexible rods around which the natural eyelashes are curled during eyelash perming treatment.

Eyelash perming A chemical treatment applied to the eyelashes to permanently curl the lashes, enhancing the appearance of the eyes.

Eyeliner A cosmetic product applied to define and emphasize the eyelid area directly above or below the eyelash hair.

Face shape The size and shape of the facial bone structure. Face shapes include oval, round, square, heart, diamond, oblong and pear.

Facial A service to improve the appearance, condition and functioning of the skin and underlying structures.

Facial bones A type of connective tissue forming a hard structure that forms the face and provides an attachment point for muscles. These include the zygomatic, mandible, maxilla, nasal, vomer, turbinate, lacrimal and palatine.

Facial features The size of a person's nose, eyes, forehead, chin, neck, etc. When applying make-up products, make-up application can emphasize or minimize the appearance of facial features.

Facial products Skincare used with a facial service which have specific benefits to care for and improve the function and appearance of the skin.

False eyelashes Threads of nylon fibre or real hair attached to the natural eyelash hair. There are two main types: individual or strip.

False lashes Threads of nylon fibre which are attached to the natural hair. These are referred to as strip lashes, individual false lashes or single lash extensions.

Faux tan Alternative term for fake tan.

Feature A unique or defining characteristic of a product or service.

Fibre A nail enhancement system that combines a fibre with resin to create an artificial nail overlay.

Fibre mesh Usually silk or fibreglass 'fabric' used in the fibre overlay system to provide strength.

File Used to shape the free edge of the nail.

Fire Precautions Act (1971) Legislation that states that all staff must be familiar with and trained in fire and emergency evacuation procedures for their workplace.

Fitzpatrick Classification System A scale developed to assess the amount of melanin pigment in the skin providing your skin colour and how your skin will react to sun without protection (photo sensitivity). There are six skin type classifications from Caucasian (skin type I) to African-Caribbean (skin type VI).

Foiling A technique used in nail art that uses a foil to decorate the nails.

Folliculitis A bacterial infection where pustules develop in the skin tissue around the hair follicle.

Foot and nail treatments Specialized products and equipment designed to improve the condition and appearance of different nail and skin conditions.

Foot cream lotion/oil A cosmetic mixture of waxes and oils applied to soften the skin of the feet and cuticles.

Foot rasp A pedicure tool used to remove excess dead skin from the foot.

Foot spa A foot bath incorporating massage and water aeration, creating a bubbling effect to cleanse and relax the feet.

Foundation A make-up product applied to produce an even skin tone, to disguise minor skin blemishes and as a contour cosmetic.

Free edge The part of the nail plate that extends past the end of the finger.

Frictions Massage technique using small circular massage movements using the pads of the fingers or thumbs. The skin and muscle below is massaged against the underlying bone. This can be used to loosen any adhesions in the tissues.

Fungus (fungi) A microorganism that can cause fungal diseases of the skin and feed off the waste products of the skin. They are found on the skin's surface or they can attack deeper tissues.

Gel A thickened liquid used as part of the UV gel system to create an artificial nail overlay.

Gel polish A system of base, top coats and colours that are cured under a UV lamp.

Gift voucher A pre-payment method for beauty therapy services or retail sales.

Glitters Sparkly powders or foil material applied to add shimmer to enhance a nail art design.

Greater London Council (General Powers) Act (1981) This act covers the London boroughs and relates to cosmetic piercing. It provides that no person can carry out cosmetic piercing unless they and the business are registered. It also states what records are required to be kept.

Grievance A cause for concern or complaint.

Grit The measure of abrasiveness of nail files and buffers. The higher the number, the finer the abrasive. A level of no less than 240 grit should be used on the natural nail.

Habia The Hairdressing and Beauty Industry Authority; the government appointed standards setting organization for the hair and beauty sector.

Hair A long slender structure that grows out of, and is part of the skin. Each hair is made up of dead skin cells, which contain the protein called keratin.

Hair follicle An appendage (structure) in the skin formed from epidermal tissue. Cells move up the hair follicle from the bottom (the hair bulb), changing in structure, to form the hair.

Hair growth cycle The cyclical pattern of hair growth, which can be divided into three phases: anagen, catagen and telogen.

Hair shaft The part of the hair that can be seen above the skin's surface, extending from the hair follicle.

Hairy moles Moles exhibiting coarse hairs from their surface.

Hand and nail treatments Specialized products and equipment designed to improve the condition and appearance of different nail and skin conditions.

Hand cream/oil A cosmetic mixture of waxes and oils applied to soften the skin of the hands and cuticles.

Hand technique Threading hair removal using thread held and looped between both hands. This technique is also known as cat's cradle, double looped or self technique.

Hangnail Nail condition where small pieces of epidermal skin protrude between the nail plate and nail wall, accompanying a dry cuticle condition.

Hazard A hazard is something with potential to cause harm.

Health and Safety (Display Screen Equipment) Regulations (1992) These regulations cover the use of visual display units (VDUs) and computer screens. They specify acceptable levels of radiation emissions from the screen and identify correct working posture, seating position, permitted working heights and rest periods.

Health and Safety (First Aid) Regulations (1981) Legislation that states that workplaces must have appropriate and adequate first aid provision.

Health and Safety at Work Act (1974) Legislation that lays down the minimum standards of health safety and welfare requirements in all workplaces.

Health and Safety policy Each employer of more than five employees must have a written health and safety policy issued to their employees outlining their health and safety responsibilities.

Heat rash A reaction to heat exposure where the sweat ducts become blocked and sweat escapes into the epidermis. Red pimples occur and the skin becomes itchy.

Highlighter A make-up product that draws attention to and emphasizes features.

Histamine A chemical released when the skin comes into contact with a substance that it is allergic to. Cells called 'mast cells' burst, releasing histamine into the tissues. This causes the blood capillaries to dilate, which increases blood flow to limit skin damage and begin repair.

Hoof stick A nail tool used to gently push back the softened cuticles.

Hospitality This covers welcoming the client, being helpful and offering refreshments and magazines, and ensuring the client is comfortable while at reception.

Hot wax A system of wax depilation used to remove hair from the skin. Hot wax cools and sets on contact with the skin. They are a blend of waxes, such as beeswax and resins, which keep the wax flexible. Soothing ingredients are often included to avoid skin irritation.

Hydrogen peroxide (H_2O_2) An oxidant, a chemical that contains available oxygen atoms and encourages chemical reactions.

Hygiene requirements The expected standards as required by law, industry codes of practice or written procedures specified by the workplace.

Hyperpigmentation Increased pigment production.

Hypopigmentation Loss of pigmentation.

Induction An introductory activity delivered when you start or progress into a new job role. Its aim is to provide you with general and essential information related to the work environment, welfare and your job roles and responsibilities.

Industry Code of Practice A set of guidelines written by the industry to provide a framework for good practice and minimum standards.

Infection The communication of disease from one body to another. An infection is the colonization of a host organism by parasite species. If a client has an infection, do not treat the client.

Infestation A condition where animal parasites live off and invade a host.

Infill A maintenance treatment than compensates for the natural nail growth after the application of artificial nails.

Ingestion One of the main routes of entry into the body; that is via the mouth.

Ingrowing hair A build-up of skin occurs over the hair follicle, causing the hair to grow under the skin.

Ingrowing toenails Nail condition where the side of the nail penetrates the nail wall; redness, inflammation and pus may be present.

Inhalation One of the main routes of entry into the body; that is via the lungs.

Internal client A person who is an employee of the business. In a larger business this will include other departments you may work with.

IPL (intense pulse light) Permanent hair removal method where light energy is absorbed into melanin in the skin and hair. The light energy is converted to heat energy, which causes damage to the specific target area.

Irritant Substances capable of causing inflammation of the skin, eyes, nose, throat or lungs.

Jewellery tool A nail piercing tool which has a sharp, tiny drill used to make a small hole in the free edge of the nail. The hole is used to accommodate jewellery with a post, secured by a tiny nut or ring attached through the hole.

Job description Written details of a person's specific work role, duties and responsibilities.

Joint manipulations Massage technique where the joints of the hand are manipulated through their range of movement dependent upon the type of joint.

Keloids Overgrowths of scar tissue, occurring at the site of the ear piercing.

Keratin A protein produced by cells in the epidermis called keratinocytes. Keratin makes the skin tough and reduces the passage of substances into our bodies. Each hair and nail contains keratin.

Laser hair removal A technique of permanent hair removal. Laser energy is passed through the skin which stops the activity of the hair follicle creating hair growth through a process called photothermolysis.

Legislation Laws affecting the beauty therapy business relating to products and services, the business premises and environmental conditions, working practices and those employed.

Leuconychia Nail condition where white spots or marks appear on the nail plate.

Lifting The separation of an artificial nail from the nail plate.

Limits of own authority The extent of your responsibility as determined by your own job description and workplace policies.

Lip balm A lip moisturiser which may contain pigment.

Lip gloss Cosmetic applied to the lips to provide a moist, shiny look.

Lip liner Cosmetic used to define the lips, creating a perfectly symmetrical outline.

Lip stain Make-up product which adds intense colour to the lips.

Lipstick Cosmetic applied to the lips to add colour and keep the lips soft and supple.

Liquid and powder A nail enhancement system that combines a liquid monomer with a powder polymer to create an artificial nail overlay.

Local Government (Miscellaneous Provisions) Act (1982) Legislation that requires that salons offering any form of skin piercing be registered with the Local Health Authority. This registration includes both the operators who will be carrying out the service and the salon premises where the service will be carried out.

Local Government Act (2003) (section 120 and schedule 6) An amendment to the Local Government (Miscellaneous Provisions) Act (1982) to enable each authority to regulate businesses providing cosmetic body piercing. Each local authority can introduce its own bye-laws to set the standards for cosmetic piercing.

London Local Authorities Act (1991 and 2007) This act states that no person shall carry out cosmetic piercing at an establishment without obtaining a licence from a participating council. Conditions can be attached to the licence, such as hygiene practices, age restrictions, etc.

Longitudinal ridges Nail condition where grooves appear in the nail plate, running along the length of the nail from the cuticle to the free edge.

Lower arch The curve of the lower part of the free edge when viewed from the side.

Lymph A clear, straw-coloured liquid circulating in the lymph vessels and lymphatics of the body, filtered out of the blood plasma.

Lymph vessel Referred to as lymphatics. They transport lymph a watery fluid that flows through the lymphatic system from the tissues to the blood.

Lymphatic system Closely connected to the blood system. Its primary function is defensive: to remove bacteria and foreign materials to prevent infection.

Make-up Cosmetics applied to the skin of the face to enhance and accentuate, or to minimize facial features. Make-up products create balance in the face.

Make-up products Different cosmetics available to suit skin type, colour and condition, i.e. sensitive or mature. Make-up products include concealing and contour cosmetics, foundations, translucent powders, eye shadows, eyeliners, brow liners, mascaras, lipsticks, lip glosses, lip liners, etc.

Management of Health and Safety at Work Regulations (1999) This legislation provides the employer with an approved code of practice for maintaining a safe, secure working environment.

Manicure A service to care for and improve the condition and appearance of the hands and nails.

Manual Handling Operations Regulations (1992) Legislation that requires the employer to carry out a risk assessment of all activities undertaken which involve manual handling (lifting and moving objects).

Marbling A technique used in nail art that mixes two or more colours together to form a design feature.

Mascara Cosmetic that enhances the natural eyelashes, making them appear longer, changed in colour and/or thicker.

Mask A service mask applied to the skin of the feet to treat and improve the condition of the skin; this may include stimulating, rejuvenating or moisturising properties.

Massage Manipulation of the body's soft tissues, using a series of movements or manipulations selected according to their effects which maybe stimulating, relaxing and toning. Their effects produce localized heat and stimulation affecting the circulatory, muscular and nervous systems.

Massage manipulations Movements which are selected and applied according to the desired effect, and which may be stimulating, relaxing or toning. Massage manipulations include effleurage, petrissage, percussion (also known as tapotement) and vibrations.

Massage medium A skincare product which acts as a lubricant to allow sufficient slip over the skin's surface while performing massage.

Melanin A pigment in the skin and hair created by cells called melanocytes. Melanin contributes to the colour of the skin and hair and helps to protect the lower layers of skin from UV damage.

Melanocytes Cells that produce the skin pigment melanin that contributes to skin and hair colour.

Messages Communication of information to another person in written, electronic or verbal form.

Method of payment Different forms of payment that may be accepted to pay for a product or service including cash, cash equivalents, cheque and payment cards.

Milium extraction Skincare technique used to extract milia (whiteheads) from the skin. A small tool called a milia extractor is used for this purpose, which superficially pierces the epidermis, allowing effective removal of the milia.

Mineral make-up Created from finely ground minerals (a process called micronization). It is used in the formulation of different make-up products.

Minor A person classed as a child who is required by law to have a guardian or parent present when undergoing treatment.

Moisturizer A skincare preparation whose formulation of oil and water helps maintain the skin's natural moisture by locking moisture into the skin, offering protection and hydration. The formulation is selected to suit the skin type, facial characteristics and facial area.

Molecule An arrangement of two or more atoms to create specific chemical compound.

Monomer A chemical compound that can be bonded to other molecules to form a polymer.

Mood board A collation or collage of images which have inspired or instigated innovation and creativity used to express your overall ideas. A mood board may include objects such as photographs, fabric swatches, make-up colour samples or anything else that has progressed your ideas.

Mouth technique Threading hair removal where one part of the thread is anchored in the mouth and the other part is looped in the hands.

Muscle Contractile tissue responsible for movement of the body.

Muscle tone The normal degree of tension in healthy muscle.

Muscles of facial expression Muscles which when contracted, pull the facial skin in a particular way and create facial expressions. These include the frontalis, corrugators, temporalis, orbicularis oculi, levator labii, orbicularis oris, buccinators, risorius, mentalis, zygomaticus, masseter, depressor labii.

Muscles of the foot and lower leg The muscles of the foot work together to help move the body. The foot is moved by muscles in the lower leg which pull on tendons that attach the muscle to the bone.

Muscles of the lower arm and hand The hands and fingers are moved by muscles and tendons. The muscles that bend the wrist in towards the forearm are flexors; the extensors straighten the wrist and hand.

Muscles of the upper body These move the arm and include pectoralis and deltoid.

Muscles that move the neck These include sternocleidomastoid, platysma, trapezius.

Nail The structure on the end of each finger and toe formed from hard, horny, epidermal cells that protect the living nail bed of the fingers and toes.

Nail art Nail decoration using a variety of techniques and materials.

Nail art techniques Application styles used to create different effects including dotting, striping, marbling, enamelling, foiling and blending.

Nail bed The area of skin that lies directly under the nail and is protected by the nail plate.

Nail conditions The nail condition is assessed at the nail service consultation. This will identify the nail condition. Nail condition examples include strong, weak, brittle, flaking, discoloured, stained, ridged and bitten.

Nail finish The product finally applied to the natural nail to enhance its appearance, e.g. choice of polish application.

Nail growth Cells divide in the matrix and the nails grow forward over the nail bed until they reach the end of the finger. The nail cells harden as they grow through a process called keratinization.

Nail plate A tough hard covering on top of the nail bed, composed of keratinized skin cells.

Nail polish A clear or coloured nail product that adds colour/protection to the nail. Cream polish has a matt finish and requires a top coat application. Pearlized polish produces a frosted, shimmery appearance and top coat is not required. Nail polish is also referred to as nail varnish and enamel.

Nail polish drier An aerosol or oil preparation applied following nail polish application to increase the speed at which the polish hardens.

Nail polish remover A solvent used to remove nail polish and grease from the nails prior to applying polish.

Nail polish solvent Used to thin nail polish and restore its consistency.

Nail shapes If there is sufficient length at the nail free edge, this can be shaped by filing. There are several popular shapes, selected according to the client's natural nail shape, condition and length, finger length and hand size, fashion and of course client preference. Nail shapes include oval, square, squoval, pointed and round. The shape of the nail free edge can also help disguise the appearance of the natural nail shapes claw, fan and tapered.

Nail strengthener A nail polish product that strengthens the nail plate, which has a tendency to split.

Nail structure Composed for protection the nail is made up of the following parts: nail plate, nail bed, matrix, cuticle, lunula, hyponychium, eponychium, nail wall, free edge, lateral nail fold.

Nail wrap An overlay applied to the natural nail; the fibre system is most commonly used.

National Occupational Standards for Beauty Therapy Standards that set the relevant performance objectives, range statements and knowledge specifications to support performance. These can be obtained from the Hairdressing and Beauty Industry Authority (Habia) website: www.habia .org.uk

Necessary action The action taken or service modification required to deal safely with a contra-action or contra-indication.

Neck technique Threading hair removal where one part of the thread is anchored around the neck and the other part is looped in the hands.

Negative skin sensitivity test A test where result produces no skin reaction. In this case you may proceed with the service.

Nerve A collection of single neurones surrounded by a protective sheath through which impulses are transmitted between the brain or spinal cord and another part of the body.

Nervous system Co-ordinates the activities of the body by responding to stimuli received by sense organs.

Neurones Nerve cells which make up nervous tissue.

Non-verbal communication Communicating using body language, i.e. using your eyes, face and body to transmit your feelings.

Nutrition The nourishment derived from food, required for the body's growth, energy, repair and production.

Oedema Extra fluid in an area, causing swelling.

Oils Oils selected to use with the head massage and applied to the scalp. Usually organic they are high in polyunsaturated fats which have healing benefits from their fatty acid, vitamin and nutrient content. They absorb easily through the skin, and can have an external and internal effect.

Onycholysis Nail condition where the nail plate separates from the nail bed.

Onychophagy Nail condition where a person bites their nails excessively.

Onychorrhexis Nail condition where the person has split, flaking nails.

Orange stick A disposable wooden tool used around the cuticle and free edge of the nail and to apply products to the nail.

Organizational requirements Beauty therapy procedures or work rules provided by the workplace management.

Overlay A coating applied to the natural nail or over a plastic tip that has been blended with the natural nail.

Painting techniques Nail art techniques using specialized paints, tools and brushes to create different effects e.g. freehand, striping, dotting and marbling.

Paraffin wax This is heated and applied to the skin of the feet to provide a heating effect. This improves skin functioning, aids the absorption of service products and is beneficial to ease the discomfort of arthritic and rheumatic conditions.

Paronychia Bacterial infection where swelling, redness and pus appear in the cuticle area of the nail wall.

Payment problems Problems or discrepancies encountered when handling payment transactions ranging from payment disputes to fraudulent use of payment method i.e. forged banknotes or stolen credit cards.

Pedicure A service to care for and improve the condition and appearance of the skin and nails of the feet.

Perm solution Usually contains 6 per cent thioglycolate, which when applied to eyelash hair softens and curls the hair into its new shape.

Personal presentation How you present yourself and how this is judged by others. Your appearance, if face to face, enables the client to make an initial judgment about you but what others see you do and hear you say will also influence their opinion of you. Employees in the beauty industry should always reflect the desired image of the profession they work in and all the personal attributes required. Personal presentation is about presenting yourself positively.

Personal Protective Equipment (PPE) at Work Regulations (1992) This legislation requires employers to identify through risk assessment those activities that require special protective equipment to be worn.

Personal space The space around a person that they see as theirs. Invasion of this can make them feel uncomfortable.

Petrissage Massage movements, including kneading, where the tissues are lifted away from the underlying structures and compressed. Pressure is intermittent, and should be light yet firm.

pH scale A scale from 0–14 used to measure the level of acidity or alkalinity of a substance. In the range of 0–6.9, the lower the pH value, the greater the acidity, 1 being the most acidic. In the range 7+, the greater the pH value, the greater the alkalinity, 14 being the most alkaline. A pH of 7 is neutral, meaning it is neither acid nor alkaline.

Phlebitis Recognized by swelling and pain in the leg caused by inflammation of the vein wall (veins transport blood from the tissues back towards the heart).

Photoinitiator A substance that responds to specific types of light to start a chemical reaction, e.g. UV light.

Photothermolysis An effect created when using a laser for hair removal. The melanin pigment that provides hair colour absorbs the laser energy, which is converted to heat, and at a sufficient temperature destroys the part of the hair follicle where the cells divide to create the hair.

Pigment The colour of skin and hair, called melanin. The amount of pigment varies for each client, resulting in different skin and hair colour.

Pigments A cosmetic grade powdered pigment that adds effects to polishes.

Pilo-sebaceous unit The structure in the skin's epidermis and dermis consisting of the hair follicle and its associated sebaceous gland.

Polish secures Accessories in nail art that stick to the nail using nail polish.

Polishing The application of a nail polish finishing product that adorns the nail to complement the natural nail and effect to be achieved. Polishes can be used to create designs and effects within nail art.

Polymer A long chain of chemically bonded monomers, e.g. the acrylics used in nail enhancement systems.

Polymerization The chemical reaction that creates polymer chains from monomer compounds.

Positive skin sensitivity test An allergic reaction to the skin test. The skin appears red, swollen and feels itchy.

Posture The position of the body, which varies from person to person. Good posture is when the body is in alignment. Correct posture enables you to work longer without becoming tired; it prevents muscle fatigue and stiff joints.

Powder Cosmetic applied to set the foundation, disguise minor skin blemishes and make the skin appear smoother and oil-free.

Pre-wax lotion An antibacterial skin cleanser to clean the skin before wax application.

Prices Act (1974) This act states that the price of products has to be displayed in order to prevent the buyer being misguided.

Primer Provides a base for make-up and acts as a barrier preventing absorption of the make-up products into the skin.

Products The range of different products that may be included with the delivery of a service or available for the client to purchase to meet their needs.

Promotion Ways of communicating products or services to clients to increase sales.

Provision and Use of Work Equipment Regulations (PUWER) (1998) This regulation lays down important health and safety controls on the provision and use of equipment.

PSI Pounds per square inch. Often used in relation to spray-tan guns, meaning the pressure of the air generated by the compressor. This can usually be adjusted to create the required result.

Psoriasis An inflammatory, noncontagious skin disorder where there is an increased production of cells in the upper part of the skin, appearing as patches of itchy, red, flaky skin on the body.

Psoriasis of the nail An inflammatory condition where there is an increased production of cells in the upper part of the skin. Pitting occurs on the surface of the nail plate.

Pterygium Nail condition where the cuticle is thickened and overgrown.

Public liability insurance Protects employers and employees against the consequences of death or injury to a third party while on the premises.

Punctual Arriving at the correct time.

Questioning techniques Enquiries made to gain information, either verbally or non-verbally. Using questioning techniques will assist you in decision making and enable you to provide accurate responses and information when communicating with others.

Razoring Temporary hair removal method, also referred to as shaving. A sharp razor blade is stroked over the skin's surface against the natural hair growth, removing the hair at the skin's surface.

Rebalance A maintenance treatment that corrects the position of the apex when it has moved because of natural nail growth.

Reception The area where clients are received.

Receptionist Person responsible for maintaining the reception area, scheduling appointments and handling payments.

Record cards Confidential cards recording the personal details of each client registered at the business. This information may be stored electronically on the salon's computer.

Regulatory Reform (Fire Safety) Order (2005) This legislation requires that the employer or designated 'responsible person' must carry out a risk assessment for the premises in relation to fire evacuation practice and procedures.

Relevant person The person (or persons) at work to whom you should report any issues which are not within the limits of your own authority e.g. manager, receptionist, senior therapist/nail technician, so they can resolve the problem.

Reporting of Injuries, Diseases and Dangerous Occurrences Regulations (RIDDOR) (1995) These regulations require the employer to notify the local enforcement officer in writing, in cases where employees or trainees suffer personal injury at work.

Resale Prices Acts (1964 and 1976) This act states that the manufacturer can supply a recommended price (MRRP), but the seller is not obliged to sell at the recommended price.

Resin In relation to nail enhancements, a type of cyanoacrylate used in the fibre nail enhancement system.

Resin activator In relation to nail enhancements, a product that speeds up the cure time of cyanoacrylate resin.

Resources The different products, equipment and other things needed to complete an activity.

Responsible persons This term is used in the Health and Safety unit to mean the person or persons at work to whom you should report any issues, problems or hazards. This could be a supervisor, line manager or your employer.

Restriction Something that limits you. Certain contra-indications do not prevent a service completely but they restrict how the service is carried out.

Retail The selling of goods, e.g. products for clients to use at home.

Ridge-filler A nail product used on ridged nails that improves the nail's appearance and provides a more even surface.

Risk The likelihood of a hazard's potential being recognized.

Roller wax A warm wax used to remove hair from the skin. The wax is contained in a cartridge container with a disposable applicator, which rolls the wax onto the skin's surface. The applicator is renewed for each client.

Sale and Supply of Goods Act (1994) Goods must be as described, of merchantable, satisfactory quality and fit for their intended purpose.

Salon policy Covers the documentation prepared by your employer on the procedures to be followed in your workplace. Examples are dealing with payment for products and treatments in line with your salon policy.

Salon requirements Workplace procedures that ensure the smooth running of the business and compliance with any legislation, codes of practices, etc.

Salon services A general term, covering all of the treatments and services offered in a salon or workplace.

Scissors (nail) Tools used to shorten the length of the nail before filing.

Sculptured nails Artificial nails created by building the overlay onto the natural nail and extending it over a form rather than a plastic tip.

Sebaceous gland A minute sac-like organ usually associated with the hair follicle. The cells of the gland decompose and produce the skin's natural oil sebum. Found all over the body, except for the soles of the feet and the palms of the hands.

Sebum The skin's natural oil that keeps the skin supple.

Secondary infection Bacterial penetration into the skin, causing infection.

Self-tan products Cosmetic products containing an ingredient which gives a healthy, tanned appearance to the skin. Different methods can be used to apply self-tan products including spray, manual and airbrush application.

Sensitization The biological process of becoming sensitive to a substance that can then cause an allergic reaction.

Sensory nerve endings These nerves receive information and relay this to the brain. They are found near the skin's surface and respond to touch, pressure, temperature and pain.

Service/treatment plan After the consultation, suitable service objectives are established to treat the client's conditions and needs.

Shader A make-up product that draws attention away from and minimizes certain facial features.

Shoulder girdle bones A type of connective tissue that provides attachment for the muscles which move the arms, and includes the clavicle and scapula.

Skin allergy If the skin is sensitive to a particular substance, an allergic skin reaction will occur. This is recognized by irritation, swelling and inflammation.

Skin analysis Assessment of the client's skin type and condition.

Skin appendages Structures within the skin including sweat glands (that excrete sweat), hair follicles (that produce hair), sebaceous glands (produce the skin's natural oil, sebum) and nails (a horny substance that protects the ends of the fingers/toes).

Skin characteristics While looking at the skin type, additional characteristics may be seen. These include skin that may be sensitive, dehydrated, moist or oedematous (puffy), in addition to dry, oily or combination.

Skin colour The colour of the client's skin tone. This should be considered to select colours which suit the skin colour. Generally lighter skins suit lighter to medium polish colours and darker skins suit medium to dark polish.

Skin condition While looking at the skin type, additional characteristics may be seen that indicate its condition. These include skin that may be sensitive, dehydrated or mature.

Skin removal Accidental removal of the upper, dead, protective cornified layer of the skin, leaving the granular layer exposed.

Skin sensitivity patch test A method used to assess skin tolerance/sensitivity to a particular product or service.

Skin tags Skin-coloured threads of skin 3 mm to 6 mm long, projecting from the skin's surface.

Skin tone The strength and elasticity of the skin.

Skin type The different physiological functioning of each person's skin dictates their skin type. There are four main skin types: normal (balanced), dry (lacking in oil), oily (excessive oil) and combination (a mixture of two skin types, e.g., dry and oily).

Skull bones A type of connective tissue forming a hard structure. It surrounds and protects the brain and forms an attachment point for muscles. These include the occipital, frontal, parietal, temporal, sphenoid and ethmoid.

Smile line Also called the onychodermal band; the curved line on the nail that is created naturally by the hyponychium or artificially with a coloured overlay.

Solvent A product designed to remove and clean false lashes without causing eye irritation.

Specialist skincare treatment products Additional skincare preparations available to target improvement. These products include eye gels, throat creams and ampoule services.

Spray gun Equipment used to apply liquid self-tanning product to the skin.

Steam service A warming effect created by boiling water, which is then vaporized and used on the skin to achieve both cleansing and stimulation.

Sterilization The total destruction of all microorganisms in metal tools and equipment.

Stock-keeping Maintenance of stock levels to anticipate needs. Stock records note how much stock has been used and when a new order is needed. This may be achieved using a manual or computerized system.

Stop point The part of the plastic tip that fits against the free edge of the natural nail.

Striping A nail art technique, creating lines or stripes of different lengths, thickness and definition using a striping brush. These are available in different sizes, lengths and the number of hairs is relevant for the look to be achieved.

Strip sugar A system of wax depilation similar to the warm-wax technique, used to remove hair from the skin. The sugar wax is applied to the skin, and is then removed using a wax removal strip.

Stye Bacterial infection. Infection of the sebaceous glands of the eyelash hair follicles. Small lumps appear on the inner rim of the eyelid and contain pus.

Subcutaneous layer A layer of fatty tissue situated below the epidermis and dermis.

Sugar paste A system of wax depilation. An organic paste made from sugar, lemons and water is used to embed the hair, which is then removed by the paste from the skin.

Sugaring An ancient popular method of hair removal using organic substances, sugar and lemon.

Superfluous hair Hair considered to be in excess of normal hair for the person's age, sex and therefore unwanted.

Sweat gland Or sudoriferous gland is composed of a specialized lining tissue called epithelial tissue. Its function is to control body temperature through the evaporation of sweat from the surface of the skin.

System In relation to nail enhancements, the type of nail enhancement used to overlay the natural nail or plastic tip, e.g. acrylic, UV gel, fibre.

Systemic medical condition A medical condition caused by a defect in one of the body's organs, e.g. the heart.

Tactile skin sensation test A method of assessing skin tolerance/sensitivity to a particular product or treatment.

Tapotement Also known as percussion, massage movements performed in a brisk, stimulating manner to increase blood supply and improve tone of the skin and muscles. Movements include clapping and tapping.

Targets Goals or objectives to achieve, usually set within a timescale.

Teamwork Supportive work by a team.

Telogen The resting stage of the hair growth cycle, when the hair is finally shed.

Terminal hair Deep-rooted, thick, coarse, pigmented hair found on the scalp, underarms, pubic region, eyelash and brow areas.

Thermal booties Electrically heated boots in which the feet are placed following the application of a skin service product, such as a mask. The heat aids the absorption of the product and improves skin functioning.

Thermal mitts Electrically heated gloves in which the hands are placed following the application of a skin service product, such as a mask. The heat aids the absorption of the product and improves skin functioning.

Thermal skin sensitivity test A test performed before wax application to check that the temperature of the wax is not too warm. The wax is tested by the therapist on themselves, usually on the inner wrist, and then on the client on a small visible area such as the inside of the ankle.

Thermometer Equipment used to measure temperature.

Thioglycolate The active ingredient in perm solution.

Threading Hair removal using a length of thread which is moved over the skin's surface, gripping hairs and removing them from the skin against hair growth.

Thrombophlebitis Inflammation of a vein related to a blood clot (see phlebitis).

Tinea corporis or body ringworm Fungal infection of the skin where small scaly red patches, which spread outwards and then heal from the centre, leave a ring.

Tinea pedis or athlete's foot Fungal infection of the foot occurring in the webs of the skin between the toes. Small blisters form, which later burst. The skin in the area can become dry with a scaly appearance.

Tinea unguium Fungal infection of the nails. The nail is yellowish-grey in colour.

Tissues Cells in the body which specialize in carrying out particular functions. These include epithelial, connective, muscular and nervous tissue.

Toluenediamine Small molecules of permanent dye used in tinting service.

Toning lotion A skincare preparation formulated to treat the different skin types and facial characteristics. It is applied to remove all traces of cleanser from the skin. It produces a cooling effect on the skin and has a skin-tightening effect.

Top coat A nail polish product applied over another nail polish to provide additional strength and durability to the finish.

Towel steaming An alternative to facial steaming using an electrical vapour unit. Small, clean facial towels are heated in a bowl of warm water or specialized heater before application to the face to warm, cleanse and stimulate the skin.

Trade Descriptions Acts (1968 and 1972) Legislation that states that information when selling products both in written and verbal form should be accurate.

Transfers Ready-made nail art designs, secured to the nail plate. Transfers are available in water release (decals) and self-adhesive for application.

Transverse furrows Nail condition where grooves appear on the nail, running from side to side.

Traveller's cheques Alternative form of payment used when travelling abroad and must be compared with the client's passport.

Treatment objectives The agreed aims of the treatment which will target or focus on a particular condition or need to be achieved e.g. to improve the strength of weak nails reducing the occurrence of nail breakage.

Treatment plan Following the consultation, appropriate treatment objectives are identified and agreed to treat the conditions and needs of the client.

Tweezers Small metal tools used to remove body hair by pulling it from the bottom of the hair follicle (small opening in the skin where the hair grows from). There are two types: automatic – designed to remove the bulk of the hair, and manual – designed to remove the stray hairs.

Ultra violet (UV) light An invisible part of the spectrum above the colour violet in the visible light bands.

UV gel A nail enhancement system that uses UV light to initiate polymerization in a pre-mixed gel to create an artificial nail overlay.

UV light cured The process of polymerization (curing) using a photoinitiator, in this case UV light, to start the chemical reaction.

Vapour Molecules of a chemical in the air, created by evaporation of the chemical.

Vapour unit An electrical appliance that heats water to produce steam which is applied to the skin of the face and neck, to warm, cleanse and stimulate the skin. Also referred to as a steamer.

Varicose veins Veins whose valves have become weak and lost their elasticity. The area appears knotted, swollen and bluish/purple in colour.

Vellus hair Fine, downy and soft hair – found on the face and body.

Ventilation The transport of fresh air into an area. The spa pool will create heat, humidity and chemical smells. Adequate ventilation is necessary.

Verbal communication Occurs when you talk directly to another person either face to face or over the telephone.

Verruca or plantar wart A viral infection where small epidermal skin growths appear, either raised or flat depending upon their location, and have a rough surface.

Vibrations Massage manipulations applied on the nerve centre. They stimulate the nerves to induce a feeling of well-being and to provide gentle stimulation of the skin.

Viruses The smallest living bodies, too small to see under an ordinary microscope. Viruses invade healthy body cells and multiply within the cell. Eventually the cell walls break down and the virus particles are freed to attack further cells.

Visual aids Another way to communicate information to assist or enhance understanding using an image or illustration – visual communication.

Vitamin D A fatty substance in the skin converted to vitamin D with UV light from the sun. This circulates in the blood and with the mineral salts calcium and phosphorus helps the formation and maintenance of the health of the body's bones.

Warm wax A system of wax depilation. Warm wax remains soft at body temperatures. It is frequently made of mixtures of glucose syrup and zinc oxide. Honey can be used instead of glucose syrup; this is referred to as honey wax.

Warm-oil treatments Involves gently heating a small amount of oil and soaking the nails and cuticles in it to nourish the nails and soften the cuticles and surrounding skin.

Waste Items, substances and materials requiring disposal following a service. Waste must be disposed of safely and in accordance with legal and salon requirements.

Water Marbling A method of mixing coloured polishes on the surface of water and applying to the nail.

Watery eye Over-secretion of tears from the eyes, which would normally drain into the nasal cavity.

Wax depilation The temporary removal of excess hair from a body part using wax.

Waxing products Cosmetic preparations used with a waxing service which have specific benefits to cleanse the skin, assist in hair removal care and improve the appearance and healing properties of the skin following hair removal.

White tip powder A white acrylic powder used to create a white free edge on an artificial nail.

Work techniques The methods you use to carry out waxing services.

Workplace (Health Safety and Welfare) Regulations (1992) These regulations provide the employer with an approved code of practice for maintaining a safe, secure working environment.

Workplace policies This covers the documentation prepared by your employer on the procedures to be followed in your workplace. Examples are your employer's safety policy statement, or general health and safety statements and written safety procedures covering aspects of the workplace that should be drawn to the employees' (and "other persons' ") attention, pricing policies and customer service policies.

Workplace practices Any activities, procedures, use of materials or equipment and working techniques used in carrying out your job. Lifting techniques and maintaining good posture whilst working are also included.

Wrap fabrics Material used in nail enhancements to overlay the natural nail to provide strength, e.g. fibreglass, silk.

Zones In relation to nail enhancements, the three areas of the artificial nail referred to when creating the correct artificial structure.

Index

INDEX

preparation 297–8, 302–3, 306–7, 320–1, 340–1, 403–4, 507, 540, 590–1, 619

record 284–5, 337–8, 401–2, 436–7, 474–5, 532, 538–9, 568–9, 592–3, 631

consultation 136, 215, 216–17, 336, 393, 471, 506, 532, 591, 594, 615–17, 632

Consumer Protection Act (1987) 148, 149, 632

Consumer Protection (Distance Selling) Regulations (2000) 149–50, 632

Consumer Safety Act (1978) 147, 632

contra-actions 139, 260–1, 278–9, 287, 289, 292–3, 320, 339–40, 381, 399–400, 441–2, 475, 506–7, 536–7, 618, 632

contra-indications 116, 217, 220–1, 277–8, 286–7, 289, 291–2, 320, 326, 339, 423, 439–40, 506, 533–5, 594–5, 617, 632

Control of Noise at Work Regulations (2005) 129

Control of Substances Hazardous to Health (COSHH) (2002) 22, 110–12

Controlled Waste (Amendment) Regulations (1993) 125, 447

Cosmetic Products (Safety) Regulations (2004) 149, 632

Crime Prevention Officer 120

Dangerous Substances and Preparations (Nickel) (Safety) Regulations (2005) 633

Data Protection Act (DPA) (1998) 149, 163, 175, 176, 633

Disability Discrimination Act (1996) 633